5 EDITION

The Human Body in Health and Illness

Barbara Herlihy, BSN, MA, PhD (Physiology), RN
Professor of Biology
University of the Incarnate Word
School of Mathematics, Science, and Engineering
San Antonio, Texas

SAUNDERS

3251 Riverport Lane
St. Louis, Missouri 63043

THE HUMAN BODY IN HEALTH AND ILLNESS, FIFTH EDITION   ISBN: 978-1-4557-7234-6

Notices

Knowledge and best practice in this field are constantly changing. As new research and experience broaden our understanding, changes in research methods, professional practices, or medical treatment may become necessary.

Practitioners and researchers must always rely on their own experience and knowledge in evaluating and using any information, methods, compounds, or experiments described herein. In using such information or methods they should be mindful of their own safety and the safety of others, including parties for whom they have a professional responsibility.

With respect to any drug or pharmaceutical products identified, readers are advised to check the most current information provided (i) on procedures featured or (ii) by the manufacturer of each product to be administered, to verify the recommended dose or formula, the method and duration of administration, and contraindications. It is the responsibility of practitioners, relying on their own experience and knowledge of their patients, to make diagnoses, to determine dosages and the best treatment for each individual patient, and to take all appropriate safety precautions.

To the fullest extent of the law, neither the Publisher nor the authors, contributors, or editors, assume any liability for any injury and/or damage to persons or property as a matter of products liability, negligence or otherwise, or from any use or operation of any methods, products, instructions, or ideas contained in the material herein.

Library of Congress Cataloging-in-Publication Data

Herlihy, Barbara L., author.
  The human body in health and illness / Barbara Herlihy.—5th edition.
    p. ; cm.
  Includes bibliographical references and index.
  ISBN 978-1-4557-7234-6 (pbk. : alk. paper)
  I. Title.
  [DNLM: 1. Physiology. 2. Health. 3. Pathology. QT 104]
  QP34.5
  612—dc23
                                        2013030733

Vice President and Content Strategy Director: Linda Duncan
Executive Content Strategist: Kellie White
Content Development Specialist: Joe Gramlich
Content Coordinator: Nathan Wurm-Cutter
Publishing Services Manager: Catherine Albright-Jackson
Project Manager: Rhoda Bontrager
Design Direction: Karen Pauls

Printed in China

Last digit is the print number: 9 8 7 6 5 4 3 2 1

everything but textbook

If you've never considered ebooks before, now may be the time. More than just words on a screen, Pageburst comes with an arsenal of interactive functionality and time-saving study tools that allow you to:

- access your entire course load from one portable device

- instantly swap notes with your instructors and classmates

- quickly search for topics and key terms

- watch videos and animations

- get the same Elsevier content for a lot less money

Discover more at **pageburst.com**

Dedicated to our grandchildren: Grey, Case, Zachary, and Katie Beth

Just when you are convinced that you really haven't survived parenthood, along come the grandchildren and you realize how truly blessed you are.

Grey…11 years…kind, wise, the warmest smile, and fun, fun, fun
…..The one to start
…..Always in Granny's heart

Case…8 years…sensitive…friend to all…artistic beyond belief
…..Called our "bug"
…..For Granny to hug

Zachary…2 years…too cute and just "in there"
…..Zachary's got the beat
…..With those dancin' feet

Katie Beth…2 years…sweet and just "out there"
…..Katie's a honey
…..Ever Granny's bunny

A nod to their parents…well done!

Thank you, Kristan and Joe for Grey and Case

Thank you, Kellie and James for Zach and Katie Beth...and for the "bun in the oven"... Congrats!

Barbara

Mudding with Grey and Case

Acknowledgments

The publishing and republishing of an anatomy and physiology text requires the combined efforts of various persons with diverse talents. I have been blessed to work with many generous and talented individuals at Elsevier and offer my grateful thanks, especially to Karen Pauls, Catherine Jackson, Rhoda Bontrager, Kellie White, and Joe Gramlich.

Many thanks also to my students and friends at the University of the Incarnate Word. They have graciously supported me through all five editions. Thanks to my husband, Jerry, for living with an author and all the associated fallout. He has contributed much to this text by constructing tables, proofreading, and offering many helpful hints; he, too, is a physiologist. Thanks to my daughter Kellie, a NICU nurse, who proofread, rewrote, and photocopied in the midst of being mom to twins. Thanks to my children, grandchildren, and racquetball buddies for their insistence on leisure and play; they are in charge of my mental health. I highly recommend "grannyhood"; it is beyond joy and gets better! My two older playmates and I have graduated from mudding on the ATVs; the boys are rapidly becoming fine young men. Doing it all over again joyfully with our new twins! Beyond cute … and so much fun!

Thanks to my furry friends Annie and Lucy (woof and woof) and Minky (purr) for the hours they hovered around me and my laptop. As usual, a special acknowledgment to my beloved Dachshund, Pretzyl, who labored so hard on the first two editions. Four other furry helpers—Julia, Kenner, Cajun, and Zeke—are missed but certainly not forgotten. With the completion of this edition I will reward myself with a "rescue" Dachshund … or two. To all of you who ask about my pet population, many thanks.

Last but certainly not least, many thanks to those who used previous editions and were kind enough to forward comments and suggestions. Your assistance is so appreciated. Keep the comments coming!

To the Instructor

I would like to present another edition that is older and wiser with the help of your comments and suggestions. Even after minor surgery, a few transplants, and some trimming and plumping, the fifth edition of *The Human Body in Health and Illness* has emerged with the same sense of humor!

The Human Body in Health and Illness tells the story of the human body with all its parts and the way these parts work together. It is a story that we have told many times in our classes. It is also a story that gets better with each telling as the body continues to reveal its mysteries and how marvelously it has been created. I hope that you enjoy telling the story as much as I do.

The Human Body in Health and Illness is a basic anatomy and physiology text addressed to the student preparing for a career in the health professions. It is written for students with minimal preparation in the sciences; no prior knowledge of biology, chemistry, or physics is required. The text provides all the background science information needed for an understanding of anatomy and physiology.

The basic principles of chemistry and biochemistry are presented in Chapters 2 and 4, and they set the stage for an understanding of cellular function, fluid and electrolyte balance, endocrine function, and digestion. Chapter 5, Microbiology Basics, presents clinically relevant microbiological topics. Check out the stories "Rick, Nick, and the Sick Tick" and "Dr. Semmelweis Screams: 'Wash Those Mitts!'" The latter is an amusing presentation of a sad tale in the history of medicine and corresponds to the current emphasis on hand hygiene and healthcare-associated infection.

The anatomy and physiology content is presented in a traditional order, from simple to complex. The text begins with a description of a single cell and progresses through the various organ systems. There are two key themes that run throughout the text: (1) the relationship between structure and function—the student must understand that an organ is anatomically designed to perform a specific physiological function, and (2) homeostasis—the role that each organ system plays in sustaining life and what happens when that delicate balance is disturbed.

The text addresses two concerns about the selection of content. The first has to do with the amount of content. The field of anatomy and physiology is huge; therefore, there must be a selection of content that can be mastered in the short period of time that a semester (or even two) allows. This text focuses on the physiology that is basic and most clinically relevant. Pathophysiology is introduced primarily to clarify physiological function. For instance, the different types of anemias illustrate the various steps in the making of the red blood cell. A second concern has to do with the recognition that we are not preparing physiologists; instead, we want the student to be able to use the physiology to understand clinically relevant content such as pathophysiology, physical assessment, diagnostics, and pharmacology. An understanding of physiology is crucial for advancement in the medically related sciences.

TEXTBOOK STRENGTHS

- Anatomy and physiology are clearly and simply explained. A meticulously prepared set of **illustrations**—complete with amusing cartoons—supports the text. In fact, the story of the body is told as much through the art as through the written word.
- The text **truly integrates pathophysiology;** it is not merely boxed in or tacked on at the end. The integrated pathophysiology is used primarily to amplify the normal anatomy and physiology. The expanded **Medical Terminology and Disorders** tables and frequent references to common medical terminology allow the text to be used for an introductory course in pathophysiology and medical terminology.
- In addition to the pathophysiology, other topics are liberally integrated throughout the text. These include **common diagnostic procedures** such as blood count, lumbar puncture, urinalysis, and electrocardiography. **Pharmacological topics** are also introduced and, like the pathophysiology, are used to amplify the normal anatomy and physiology. For instance, the discussion of the neuromuscular junction is enhanced by a description of the effects of the neuromuscular-blocking agents. Because of the effort of the text to make clinical correlations, it sets the stage for the more advanced health science courses, including pharmacology and medical-surgical nursing.
- **Re-Think** boxes are liberally distributed throughout each chapter and encourage students to master that content before progressing through the chapter. **New Ramp It Up** boxes develop selected clinically

relevant topics that are simply too advanced to be included in the text as critical information. These boxed features contain new or advanced content commonly used in the clinical setting and allow instructors to scale their coverage in a manner appropriate to the course. They offer students the chance to make further connections between the text and their future careers. *(See the To the Student preface on page ix for descriptions and examples of each of the chapter features.)*

- **Medical terminology** is introduced, defined, and used throughout the text. Common clinical terms such as *hyperkalemia, vasodilation, hypertension,* and *diagnosis* are defined and reused so that the student gradually builds up a substantial medical vocabulary. The new and expanded **Medical Terminology and Disorders** tables were deliberately constructed to maximize the use of common medical terms and disorders. To help foster broader understanding of medical terminology, word parts and their meanings are included for nearly every term presented. Repetition of these helps students gain greater ground in understanding the very specific medical language they will be learning to use for a future in the health professions. A description is also provided, which gives the definition or other pertinent information on the topic.
- The **Review Your Knowledge** section has been expanded to include questions that require an analytical response. The **Go Figure** questions are based on the story told by the artwork. The questions can only be answered by analyzing the art and/or the information presented in the tables. This exercise encourages the student to see beyond the "pretty pictures" and realize that a picture is truly worth a thousand words.
- The text is supported by many activities, exercises, puzzles, and games (e.g., Body Bingo) on **Evolve** (http://evolve.elsevier.com/Herlihy). These activities emphasize the focus of this text—clinically relevant anatomy and physiology.
- Last, the text incorporates many **amusing anecdotes** from the history of medicine. Although the human body is perfectly logical and predictable, we humans think, do, and say some strange things. Tales from the medical crypt provide some good laughs and much humility.

CLASSROOM RESOURCES

Materials from the **Study Guide** and **Evolve Instructor Learning Resources** can be used to:
1. Remediate students who are having difficulty in grasping the content
2. Remediate students who have missed class(es)
3. Review students engaged in pathophysiology and pharmacology whose memories need to be refreshed in the physiology

STUDY GUIDE

The Study Guide for *The Human Body in Health and Illness* offers something for students at all levels of learning and is a ready-made resource for instructors looking for homework assignments. Each chapter includes three parts: Part I, Mastering the Basics, with matching, labeling, and coloring exercises; Part II, Putting It All Together, containing multiple-choice practice quizzes, completion exercises, and case studies; and Part III, Challenge Yourself!, which has grouping exercises and word puzzles. Textbook page references are included with the questions, and the answer key is available on the Evolve website, only to instructors.

EVOLVE INSTRUCTOR LEARNING RESOURCES

The Evolve website for *The Human Body in Health and Illness* (http://evolve.elsevier.com/Herlihy) includes all of the Student Resources (see the inside back cover), as well as the following Instructor Resources:
- Answer Key for the Study Guide, Audience Response System questions, Image Collection, Teaching Tips, and ExamView Test Banks that include over 2300 questions—more than 600 questions have been added!
- Instructor's Chapter Exams, Classroom Activities—including Bingo, Line 'Em Up, Sorting, and Word Puzzles—and the TEACH Instructor Resource.

TEACH Instructor Resource on Evolve

Instructors who adopt the textbook will also receive access to the TEACH Instructor Resource, which links all parts of the Herlihy educational package with customizable **Lesson Plans** based on objectives drawn from the text. The TEACH Lesson Plans are based on the chapter-by-chapter organization of *The Human Body in Health and Illness* and can be modified or combined to meet your curriculum's scheduling and teaching needs.

TEACH has been completely updated and revised for this edition. The TEACH Lesson Plans help instructors prepare for class and make full use of the rich array of ancillaries and resources that come with the textbook. The content covered in each textbook chapter is divided across one or more lesson plans, each designed to occupy 50 minutes of class time. Lesson plans are organized into easily understandable sections that are each tied to the chapter learning objectives:
- **Instructor Preparation** This section provides a checklist of all the things you need to do to prepare for class, including a list of all the items you need to bring to class to perform any activity or demonstration included in the lesson plan, and all pertinent key terms covered in that lesson.
- **Student Preparation** Textbook readings, study guide exercises, online activities, and other applicable

homework assignments for each lesson are provided here along with an overall estimated completion time.

- **The 50-Minute Lesson Plan** A lecture outline that reflects the chapter lecture slides that come as part of TEACH is included, as well as classroom activities and online activities, one or more critical thinking questions, and time estimates for the classroom lecture and activities.

- **Assessment Plan** To ensure that your students have mastered all the objectives, the new TEACH includes a separate Assessment Plan section. An easy-to-use table maps each assessment tool to the lesson plans and chapter objectives so you can see all your assessment options—by chapter, by lesson, and by objective—and choose accordingly.

To the Student

This book will take you on an amazing journey through the human body. You will learn many body parts, and more importantly, how they work in an integrated manner to keep you going. You will use this information in your clinical practice when patients become ill with disorders of those structures. The following special features were created to help make learning enjoyable and fun.

TEXTBOOK FEATURES

KEY TERMS

Key terms are listed at the beginning of each chapter along with a page reference. Each is (1) presented in the text in blue print, (2) accompanied by a pronunciation guide, (3) thoroughly explained within the chapter, and (4) defined in the glossary.

OBJECTIVES

Numbered objectives identify the goals for each chapter.

ILLUSTRATIONS

Original illustrations and full-color cartoons help you make sense of anatomy and physiology using humor, clarity, and insight.

DO YOU KNOW...

Most of these boxed vignettes refer to clinical situations; others relate to interesting and amusing historical events related to anatomy and physiology.

RAMP IT UP!

These features challenge you with more advanced anatomy and physiology topics.

RE-THINK

Questions included cover key information found in the chapter and help reinforce important concepts.

AS YOU AGE

These boxed features contain numbered lists describing how human anatomy and physiology is affected by the aging process.

SUM IT UP!

These features appear regularly throughout the chapters and help the student synthesize key concepts.

MEDICAL TERMINOLGY AND DISORDERS TABLES

These tables describe medical terms and specific disorders related to individual body systems, with a focus on developing a strong working vocabulary, which is necessary for a career in the health professions.

END-OF-CHAPTER FEATURES

Summary Outline

A detailed outline at the end of each chapter summarizes key concepts and serves as an excellent review of the chapter content. Use it as a study tool to review your reading and prepare for exams.

Review Your Knowledge

The matching and multiple-choice questions in this section cover the major points of the chapter and allow you to test your comprehension.

Go Figure

This review section asks you to reflect on the figures in the chapter and reinforces the importance of the concepts presented.

ANSWERS TO REVIEW YOUR KNOWLEDGE AND GO FIGURE QUESTIONS

The **Appendix** contains answers to all Review Your Knowledge and Go Figure questions found in the textbook.

GLOSSARY

The glossary includes a pronunciation guide and a brief definition of all key terms and many other words in the text.

STUDY GUIDE

Enhance your learning of the textbook content with the accompanying **Study Guide for *The Human Body in Health and Illness.*** The Study Guide has something to offer students at all levels of learning, from labeling and coloring exercises to multiple-choice practice tests and case studies.

Contents

Introduction to the Human Body

Key Terms

abdominopelvic cavity (p. 10)
anatomical position (p. 6)
anatomy (p. 1)
cranial cavity (p. 9)
dorsal cavity (p. 9)
frontal plane (p. 7)

homeostasis (p. 6)
mediastinum (p. 10)
organs (p. 2)
pericardial cavity (p. 10)
physiology (p. 1)
pleural cavities (p. 10)

sagittal plane (p. 7)
spinal (vertebral) cavity (p. 9)
thoracic cavity (p. 10)
transverse plane (p. 7)
ventral cavity (p. 9)
viscera (p. 9)

Objectives

1. Define the terms *anatomy* and *physiology*.
2. List the levels of organization of the human body.
3. Describe the 12 major organ systems.
4. Define homeostasis.
5. Describe the anatomical position.

6. List common terms used for relative positions of the body.
7. Describe the three major planes of the body.
8. List anatomical terms for quadrants and regions of the body.
9. Describe the major cavities of the body.

The human body is a wonderful creation. Millions of microscopic parts work together in a coordinated fashion to keep you going for about 75 years. Most of us are curious about our bodies—how they work, why they do not work, what makes us tick, and what makes us sick. As you learn more about the body, you will sometimes feel like this cartoon character: "What is this? Why do I need it? How does it work? Why don't I have one?" As you study anatomy and physiology, you will learn the answers to these questions.

ANATOMY AND PHYSIOLOGY: WHAT THEY ARE

WHAT'S IT MEAN?

Anatomy (ah-NAT-o-mee) is the branch of science that studies the structure of the body. For example, anatomy describes what the heart looks like, how big it is, what it is made of, how it is organized, and where it is located. The word *anatomy* comes from the Greek word meaning to dissect. The science of anatomy arose from observations made by scientists centuries ago as they dissected bodies that were usually stolen from the local graveyard.

Physiology (fiz-ee-OL-o-jee) is the branch of science that describes how the body functions. For example, physiology describes how the heart pumps blood and why the pumping of blood is essential for life. Pathophysiology (path-o-fiz-ee-OL-o-jee) is the branch of science that describes the consequences of the improper functioning of the body—that is, how a body part functions when a person has a disease. Pathophysiology describes what happens during a heart attack, when the heart functions poorly, or not at all.

WHY DO I NEED TO KNOW THIS?

Why study anatomy and physiology as part of your professional curriculum? Unless you gain a good understanding of normal anatomy and physiology, you cannot understand the diseases and disorders experienced by your patients, nor can you understand the basis for the various forms of treatment such as drug therapy and surgical procedures. You want to give your patients the best possible care, so you must have a sound understanding of the human body.

Anatomy and physiology are closely related. Structure and function go together. When you examine the anatomy of a body part, ask yourself how its structure relates to its function. For example, the structure of the hand is related to its function: its ability to grasp an object (Figure 1-1). The heart pumps blood, and the long, strong, flexible tail of the monkey allows it to hang from the tree. Structure and function go together.

 Re-Think

Using any household item, explain what is meant by "structure and function are related."

 Do You Know...

Why This Grave Is Being Robbed, and Why the Grave Robber Is in Big, Big Trouble?

Dissection of the human body during medieval times was not allowed. Thus, the only way that the early anatomists had for obtaining human bodies for dissection was to rob graves. Medieval scientists hired people to rob graves. Punishment for robbing graves was swift and severe. This lad will be in big, big trouble if he is caught, and it looks as if he will be. Surprisingly, grave robbing was common early in this century and in this country. Many a medical student who enrolled in the most prestigious medical schools had to "get" his own cadaver.

THE BODY'S LEVELS OF ORGANIZATION

The body is organized from the very simple to the complex, from the microscopic atom to the complex human organism. Note the progression from simple to complex in Figure 1-2. Tiny atoms form molecules. These in turn form larger molecules. The larger molecules are eventually organized into *cells*, the basic unit of life. Specialized groups of cells form *tissues*. Tissues are then arranged into **organs** such as the heart, stomach, and kidney. Groups of organs, in turn, create *organ systems*. Each organ system has a function, such as digestion, excretion, or reproduction. All the organ systems together form the human organism. From simple to complex, the body is built from the tiny atom to the human being.

FIGURE 1-1 Structure and function are closely related.

MAJOR ORGAN SYSTEMS

Twelve major organ systems make up the human body. Each performs specific functions that enable the human body to operate as a coordinated whole. Refer to Figure 1-3 and identify the location and distribution of the organs of each system.

- The integumentary (in-teg-yoo-MEN-tar-ee) system consists of the skin and related structures such as hair and nails. The integumentary system forms a covering for the body, helps regulate body temperature, and contains some of the structures necessary for sensation.
- The skeletal system forms the basic framework of the body. It consists primarily of bones, joints, and cartilage. The skeleton protects and supports body organs and enables us to move around.
- The muscular system has three types of muscles. *Skeletal muscles* attach to the bones and are responsible for movement of the skeleton and the maintenance of body posture. *Smooth* and *cardiac muscles* are found in various organs and tubes; contraction

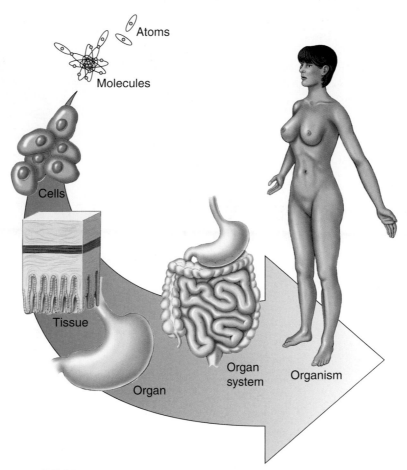

FIGURE 1-2 Levels of organization, from atoms to human organism.

and relaxation of these muscles help the organ systems carry out their functions.

- The nervous system is made up of the brain, spinal cord, nerves, and sense organs. Sensory nerves receive information from the environment and bring it to the spinal cord and brain, where it is interpreted. Decisions made by the brain and spinal cord are transmitted along motor nerves to various body structures.
- The endocrine (EN-doh-krin) system contains numerous glands that secrete hormones and chemical substances that regulate body activities such as growth, reproduction, metabolism, and water balance.
- The circulatory (SER-kyoo-lah-tor-ee) system consists of the blood, heart, and blood vessels. This system pumps (heart) and transports (blood vessels) blood throughout the body. Blood carries nutrients and oxygen to all the body's cells and also carries the waste away from the cells to the organs of excretion.
- The lymphatic (lim-FAT-ik) system is made up of the lymph nodes, lymphatic vessels, lymph, and other lymphoid organs. Lymph and lymphoid structures play an important role in fluid balance

and in the defense of the body against pathogens and other foreign material.

- The immune system is an elaborate defense system that protects the body not only from pathogens, but also from allergens, such as pollens, bee venom, and some of our own cells that have gone awry (cancer cells). The immune system is widely distributed throughout the body (it is not shown in Figure 1-3).
- The respiratory system contains the lungs and other structures that conduct air to and from the lungs. Oxygen-rich air moves into the lungs; the oxygen is picked up by the blood and distributed throughout the body. Carbon dioxide–rich air moves out of the lungs, thereby ridding the body of waste.
- The digestive system is comprised of organs designed to ingest food and break it down into substances that can be absorbed by the body. Food that is not absorbed is eliminated as waste.
- The urinary system contains the kidneys and other structures that help excrete waste products from the body through the urine. More importantly, the urinary system helps control water, electrolyte, and acid–base balance in the body.
- The reproductive system is made up of organs and structures that enable humans to reproduce.

Integumentary system

Skeletal system

Muscular system

Nervous system

Circulatory system

Endocrine system

FIGURE 1-3 Major organ systems of the body.

Lymphatic system

Digestive system

Respiratory system

Urinary system

Reproductive system

FIGURE 1-3, cont'd

HOMEOSTASIS: STAYING THE SAME

Homeostasis (ho-me-o-STAY-sis) literally means staying (*stasis*) the same (*homeo*). The term refers to the body's ability to maintain a stable internal environment in response to a changing environment. For example, in a healthy person, body temperature stays around 98.6° F (37° C), even when room temperature increases to 100° F or decreases to 60° F. The amount of water in your cells stays the same whether you drink 2, 3, or 4 liters (L) of water per day. Your blood sugar remains within normal limits whether you have just eaten a turkey dinner or have fasted for 6 hours.

Mechanisms that help maintain homeostasis are called *homeostatic mechanisms*. The body has hundreds of homeostatic mechanisms, including those for temperature control, blood sugar control, water balance, blood pressure regulation, and regulation of plasma sodium levels. Homeostatic imbalance results in disease or dysfunction.

2+2 Sum It Up!

Anatomy and physiology describes the structure and function of the body. The body is constructed from simple to complex (atoms to molecules to cells to tissues to organs to organ systems to the human organism). The 12 major organ systems are shown in Figure 1-3. Homeostatic mechanisms enable the body to "stay the same" despite changing internal and external environments.

ANATOMICAL TERMS: TALKING ABOUT THE BODY

Special terms describe the location, position, and regions of body parts. Because these terms are used frequently, you should become familiar with them now. People in the medical field are often accused of speaking their own language. Indeed, we do! We always use these terms as if the body were standing in its anatomical position.

ANATOMICAL POSITION

In its **anatomical position**, the body is standing erect, with the face forward, the arms at the sides, and the toes and palms of the hands directed forward (Figure 1-4).

RELATIVE POSITIONS

Specific terms describe the position of one body part in relation to another body part. These are directional terms. They are like the more familiar directions of north, south, east, and west; however, whereas describing Canada as being located north of the United States would be correct, describing the head as "north of the chest" would sound strange. Therefore, in locating body parts, we use other terminology. The terms come

FIGURE 1-4 Anatomical position.

in pairs. Note that the two terms in each pair are generally opposites. Remember, the references are valid only for the body in its anatomical position.

- *Superior* and *inferior. Superior* means that a part is above another part or is closer to the head. For example, the head is superior to the chest. *Inferior* means that a part is located below another part or is closer to the feet. The chest, for example, is inferior to the head.
- *Anterior* and *posterior. Anterior* means toward the front surface (the belly surface). *Posterior* means toward the back surface. For example, the heart is anterior to the spinal cord, but the heart is posterior to the breastbone. Another word for anterior is *ventral,* and another word for posterior is *dorsal.* Consider the dorsal fin of a fish. It is the dorsal part of the shark that can be seen moving effortlessly and very quickly toward your surfboard!
- *Medial* and *lateral.* Imagine a line drawn through the middle of your body, dividing it into right and left halves. This is the midline. *Medial* means toward the midline of the body. The nose, for example is medial to the ears. *Lateral* means away from the midline of the body. For example, the ears are lateral to the nose. In the anatomical position, the hand is closer to the lateral thigh than to the medial thigh.
- *Proximal* and *distal. Proximal* means that the structure is nearer the point of attachment, often the

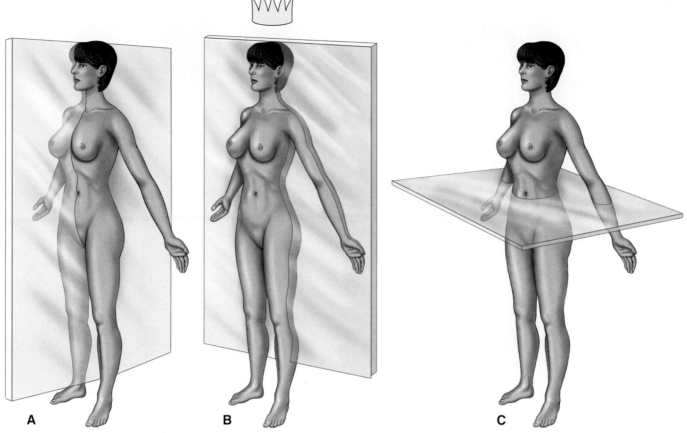

FIGURE 1-5 Planes of the body. **A,** Sagittal. **B,** Frontal (coronal). **C,** Transverse.

trunk of the body. Because the elbow is closer to the point of attachment than is the wrist, the elbow is described as proximal to the wrist. The wrist is proximal to the fingers, meaning that the wrist is closer to the trunk than are the fingers. *Distal* means that a part is farther away from the point of attachment than another part. For example, the wrist is distal to the elbow and the fingers are distal to the wrist.

- *Superficial* and *deep*. *Superficial* means that a part is located on or near the surface of the body. The skin is superficial to the muscles. *Deep* means that the body part is away from the surface of the body. The bones, for example, are deep to the skin.
- *Central* and *peripheral*. *Central* means that the part is located in the center. *Peripheral* means away from the center. The heart, for example, is located centrally, whereas the blood vessels are located peripherally (away from the center and extending toward the limbs). The brain and spinal cord are called the central nervous system and the nerves are called the peripheral nervous system.

? Re-Think

Use the terms *medial* and *lateral* in describing the parts of the thigh. Do the same with the eye.

PLANES OF THE BODY

When we refer to the left side of the body, the top half of the body, or the front of the body, we are referring to the planes of the body. Each plane divides the body with an imaginary line in one direction. Figure 1-5 shows the following three important planes:

1. Sagittal plane (see Figure 1-5, *A*). The **sagittal plane** divides the body lengthwise into right and left portions. If the cut is made exactly down the midline of the body, the right and left halves of the body are equal. This division is a midsagittal section.
2. Frontal plane (see Figure 1-5, *B*). The **frontal plane** divides the body into anterior (ventral) and posterior (dorsal) portions. This plane creates the front part of the body and the back part of the body. The frontal plane is also called the *coronal plane*. Coronal means "crown," so the imaginary line for the coronal plane is made across the part of the head where a crown would sit and then downward through the body.
3. Transverse plane (see Figure 1-5, *C*). The **transverse plane** divides the body horizontally, creating an upper (superior) and a lower (inferior) body. When the body or an organ is cut horizontally or transversely, it is called a cross section.

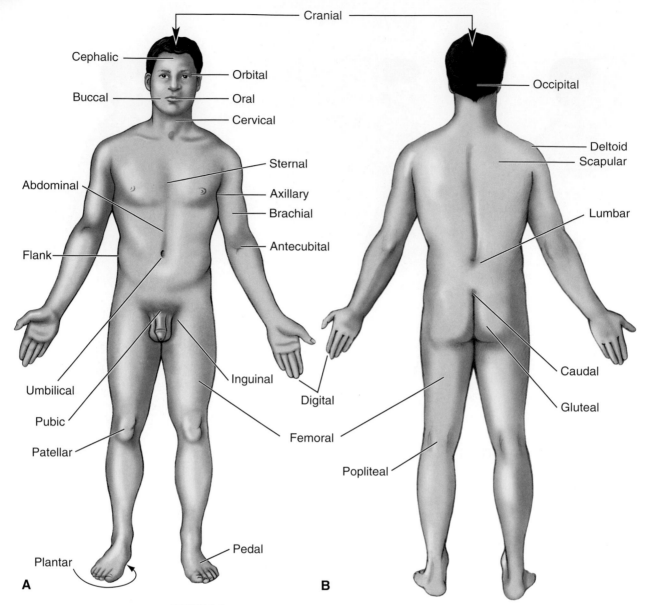

FIGURE 1-6 Regional terms. **A,** Anterior view. **B,** Posterior view.

REGIONAL TERMS

Specific terms describe the different regions or areas of the body. Figure 1-6 illustrates the terms used to identify the regions on the anterior and posterior surfaces of the body.

On the anterior surface, identify the following regions:

Abdominal: anterior trunk just below the ribs
Antecubital: area in front of the elbow
Axillary: armpit
Brachial: arm
Buccal: cheek area; cavity between the gum and cheek
Cephalic: head
Cervical: neck region
Cranial: nearer to the head
Digital: fingers, toes
Femoral: thigh area

Flank: fleshy area along each side between the lower ribs and the top of the hip bones
Inguinal: area where the thigh meets the trunk of the body; often called the groin
Oral: mouth
Orbital: area around the eye
Patellar: front of the knee over the kneecap
Pedal: foot
Plantar: sole of the foot
Pubic: genital area
Sternal: middle of the chest (over the breastbone area)
Umbilical: navel

On the posterior surface, identify the following regions:

Caudal: near to the lower region of the spinal column (near the tailbone)
Deltoid: rounded area of the shoulder closest to the upper arm

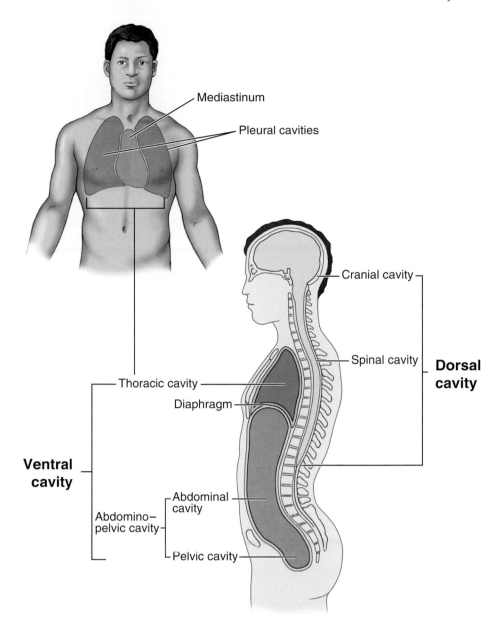

FIGURE 1-7 Major body cavities.

Gluteal: buttocks
Lumbar: area of the back between the ribs and the hips
Occipital: back of the head
Popliteal: behind, or back of, the knee area
Scapular: shoulder blade area

2+2 Sum It Up!

Specific terms describe the relative positions of one body part to the other. The terms are paired as opposites and include superior and inferior, anterior (ventral) and posterior (dorsal), medial and lateral, proximal and distal, superficial and deep, and central and peripheral. The body can be cut into three planes: sagittal (right and left), frontal or coronal (front and back), and transverse (top and bottom) planes. Common terms are used to identify specific areas of the anterior and posterior surface areas.

? Re-Think

Of the following terms, which can be seen only on the posterior view of the body: umbilical, antecubital, gluteal, lumbar, sternal, patellar, and popliteal?

CAVITIES OF THE BODY

DORSAL CAVITY

The organs, called **viscera** (VISS-er-ah), are located within the cavities of the body. Cavities are large internal spaces. The body contains two major cavities: the **dorsal cavity** and the **ventral cavity** (Figure 1-7). The dorsal cavity is located toward the back of the body and has two divisions, the **cranial cavity** and the **spinal (vertebral) cavity**.

Do You Know...

What Your Postsurgical Patient Has Done If He Eviscerated?

His internal organs have protruded through his surgical incision. This word comes from the word *viscera* (organs). The organs must be kept moist and sterile until they can be returned to their home cavity.

The cranial cavity is located within the skull and contains the brain. The spinal, or vertebral, cavity extends downward from the cranial cavity and is surrounded by bony vertebrae; it contains the spinal cord. The cranial and spinal cavities form one continuous space.

VENTRAL CAVITY

The larger ventral cavity is located toward the front of the body and has two divisions, the **thoracic** (thoh-RASS-ik) **cavity** and the **abdominopelvic** (ab-DOM-i-no-PEL-vik) **cavity**.

THORACIC CAVITY

The thoracic cavity is located above the diaphragm and is surrounded by the rib cage. The thoracic cavity is divided into two compartments by the **mediastinum** (MEE-dee-ass-TI-num), a space that contains the heart, esophagus, trachea, thymus gland, and large blood vessels attached to the heart. The **pericardial** (pair-i-KAR-dee-al) **cavity** (not shown) is located within the mediastinum and contains the heart. The right and left lungs are located on either side of the mediastinum in the **pleural cavities**. The lungs occupy most of the space within the thoracic cavity.

ABDOMINOPELVIC CAVITY

The abdominopelvic cavity is located below the diaphragm. The upper portion of this cavity is the abdominal cavity. It contains the stomach, most of the intestine, liver, gallbladder, pancreas, spleen, and kidneys. The lower portion of the abdominopelvic cavity is called the *pelvic cavity*. It extends downward from the level of the hips and includes the remainder of the intestines, the rectum, urinary bladder, and internal parts of the reproductive system.

Because the abdominopelvic cavity is so large, it is subdivided into smaller areas for study. Quadrants and regions divide the abdominopelvic cavity. Note the organs located in each quadrant or region, as shown in Figure 1-8.

Division into Quadrants

The abdominopelvic cavity can be divided into four quadrants (see Figure 1-8, *A*). The quadrants are named for their positions: right upper quadrant (RUQ), left upper quadrant (LUQ), right lower quadrant (RLQ), and left lower quadrant (LLQ).

Quadrant terms are used frequently in the clinical setting. For example, a patient in the emergency room who has acute pain in the RLQ may be diagnosed with appendicitis. Note that the RLQ appears to be on your left. This is similar to looking in a mirror. Keep this in mind when you are studying the diagrams in the text. Here's an easy way to remember this: Lower your right arm. It will be lateral to the RUQ and RLQ.

Division into Regions

A second system divides the abdominopelvic cavity into nine separate regions that resemble the squares for tic-tac-toe (see Figure 1-8, *B*). The three central regions (from top to bottom) include the epigastric, umbilical, and hypogastric regions. The epigastric region is located below the breastbone. Epigastric literally means upon (*epi*) the stomach (*gastric*). The umbilical region is the centermost region and surrounds the umbilicus, or navel (belly button). The hypogastric region is located just below the umbilical region. Hypogastric literally means below (*hypo*) the stomach (*gastric*).

Six regions are located on either side of the central regions. They include the hypochondriac, lumbar, and iliac regions. The right and left hypochondriac regions are located on either side of the epigastric region and overlie the lower ribs. The word *hypochondriac* literally means below (*hypo*) the cartilage (*chondro*) and refers to the composition of the ribs (cartilage). The right and left lumbar regions are located on either side of the umbilical region and are inferior to the hypochondriac regions. The right and left iliac regions, also called the right and left inguinal regions, are located on either side of the hypogastric region. Knowledge of these regions helps you understand terms such as epigastric pain and umbilical hernia. Remember that quadrants and regions refer only to the abdominopelvic cavity and not to the thoracic cavity.

Other Cavities

Four smaller cavities are located in the head. They include the oral cavity, nasal cavities, orbital cavities, and middle ear cavities. (These cavities are described in later chapters.)

 Re-Think

Of the following terms, determine which pertain to the ventral cavity: thoracic cavity, brain, vertebral cavity, abdominopelvic cavity, pleural cavity, dorsal cavity, mediastinum, stomach, heart, and spinal cord.

 Sum It Up!

The organs are located within body cavities. The two major cavities are the dorsal cavity, located toward the back of the body, and the larger ventral cavity, located in the front of the body. The dorsal cavity is subdivided into the cranial cavity and the spinal cavity. The ventral cavity is divided by the diaphragm into the thoracic cavity (including the mediastinum, pericardial cavity, and pleural cavities) and the abdominopelvic cavity. The abdominopelvic cavity is divided into quadrants and regions.

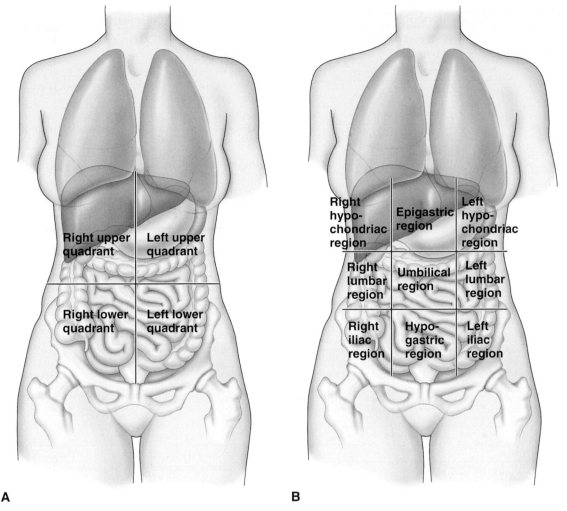

FIGURE 1-8 The abdominopelvic cavity. **A,** Four quadrants. **B,** Nine regions.

👤 MEDICAL TERMINOLOGY AND DISORDERS | Introduction to Medical Terminology

The medical profession has its own language, called **medical terminology**. In general, there are four main types or kinds of word parts. By learning these and how they can be put together, you can often "translate" many long and challenging medical words by breaking them up into their word parts.

A **word root** is *the core of the word* and provides the basic meaning or "subject" of the word. The other word parts, such as suffixes and prefixes, modify the word root so that it takes on a new meaning. For example, in the word **hepatitis,** the word root is **hepat-,** meaning *liver.*

A **suffix** is *a word part attached to the end of the word root;* it modifies the word root. If we add **-itis,** which is a suffix that means *inflammation,* to the word root for liver, **hepat-,** we get **hepatitis,** which means *inflammation of the liver.*

A **prefix** is *a word part attached to the beginning of the word root;* it modifies the word root. For example, the word **nutrition** refers to a normal and healthy food intake. By adding the prefix **mal-** (French for *bad*), as in **malnutrition,** the word root has been modified to mean *poor or bad nutrition.*

Combining vowels are *word parts used to ease the pronunciation,* as in *angioplasty* (angi/o/plasty). **Angi-** means *blood vessel,* and **-plasty** means *repair of.* The -o- joining the word parts eases the pronunciation; it does not modify the meaning of the word. When you see angi/o-, you are seeing the word root and its combining vowel.

On the next page you will see many terms with which you are probably familiar, but what you may not be familiar with is what their individual word parts are and how they are put together to make up many of the words you use every day. For instance, take **-ectomy,** which means *excision* or *removal of.* Think of all the terms that have **-ectomy** at the end—such as lob**ectomy,** vas**ectomy,** hyster**ectomy,** append**ectomy,** tonsill**ectomy**—and you will see how valuable knowing what this one word part is.

Continued

MEDICAL TERMINOLOGY AND DISORDERS Introduction to Medical Terminology—cont'd

Medical Term	Word Parts	Word Part Meaning or Derivation	Description
anatomy	ana-	up or apart	**Anatomy** is *the branch of science that describes the structure of a body, especially as revealed by dissection.* For example, the heart has four chambers.
	-tomy	incision; to cut	
antecubital	ante-	before; in front of	**Antecubital space** is *the area of the arm anterior to the elbow.* A sample of blood is commonly drawn from a vein in the antecubital space.
	-cubital	From the Latin word *cubitum,* meaning "elbow"	
biology	bio-	life	**Biology** is *the study of life and living organisms.*
	-logy	study of	
diagnosis	dia-	apart	**Diagnosis** is *the process of identifying the nature and cause of a disease or injury through an analysis of data such as the patient's symptoms and laboratory and x-ray studies.*
	-gnos/o-	knowing	
	-osis	condition or increase	
pathologist	path/o-	pertaining to disease	A **pathologist** examines tissue for evidence of disease.
	-logist	one who specializes in	
homeostasis	home/o-	sameness	**Homeostasis** refers to *the relative constancy of the internal environment of the body despite many challenges to upset the balance.*
	-stasis	stand still	
transverse	trans-	across	A **transverse** plane cuts across the body; an upper and lower body is created.
	-verse	From the Latin word *vertere,* meaning "to turn"	
midepigastric	mid-	middle	*Related to the middle of the epigastric region of the abdomen.* A person often complains of midepigastric discomfort.
	-epi-	above or upon	
	-gastr/o-	stomach	
	-ic	pertaining to	
prognosis	pro-	before	*Refers to a likely course or outcome of a disease.* For example, the prognosis of a person who seeks early treatment of a basal cell carcinoma (skin cancer) is excellent; the prognosis of a person with metastatic cancer is less favorable.
	-gnos/o-	knowing	
	-osis	process	
quadrant	quadr/i-	four	The abdominopelvic cavity is divided into four equal areas called **quadrants.**
	-ant	performing/promoting	

Get Ready for Exams!

Summary Outline

Anatomy is the study of structure; physiology is the study of function. Structure (anatomy) and function (physiology) are related.

I. The Body's Levels of Organization
  A. From simple to complex: Atoms to molecules to cells to tissues to organs to organ systems to human organism
  B. Major organ systems (12)
   1. Integumentary system
   2. Skeletal system
   3. Muscular system
   4. Nervous system
   5. Endocrine system
   6. Heart and circulatory system
   7. Lymphatic system
   8. Immune system
   9. Respiratory system
   10. Digestive system
   11. Urinary system
   12. Reproductive system

  C. Homeostasis: the body's ability to maintain a stable internal environment in response to various internal and external challenges

II. Anatomical Terms: Talking About the Body
  A. Anatomical position: the body standing erect, arms by the side, with palms and toes facing forward
  B. Relative positions: superior-inferior, anterior-posterior, medial-lateral, proximal-distal, superficial-deep, central-peripheral
  C. Planes (three): sagittal, frontal (coronal), and transverse planes
  D. Regional terms: listed in Figure 1-6
  E. Cavities of the body
   1. Dorsal cavity
    a. Cranial cavity: contains the brain
    b. Spinal (vertebral) cavity: contains the spinal cord
   2. Ventral cavity
    a. Thoracic cavity: superior to the diaphragm; contains the pleural cavities (lungs) and mediastinum (pericardial cavity)

b. Abdominopelvic cavity: located inferior to the diaphragm

c. Abdominal cavity: upper part that contains the stomach, most of the intestines, liver, spleen, and kidneys

d. Pelvic cavity: lower part that contains the reproductive organs, urinary bladder, and lower part of the intestines

e. For reference: the abdominopelvic cavity is divided into four quadrants and nine regions

Review Your Knowledge

Matching: Directions of the Body

Directions: Match the following words with their descriptions below. Some words may be used more than once or not at all.

a. posterior
b. distal
c. medial
d. anterior
e. proximal
f. superior
g. deep

1. ___ Toward the midline of the body; opposite of lateral
2. ___ Structure that is nearer to the trunk than another part; opposite of distal
3. ___ Part of the radius (forearm bone) that is closer to the wrist than to the elbow
4. ___ The lungs are located above the diaphragm; their position relative to the diaphragm is described as being above.
5. ___ Toward the front (the belly surface); another word is ventral

Matching: Regional Terms

Directions: Match the following words with their descriptions below.

a. inguinal
b. oral
c. lumbar
d. axillary
e. buccal
f. patellar
g. flank
h. antecubital
i. sternal
j. scapular

1. ___ Armpit
2. ___ Kneecap area
3. ___ Breastbone area
4. ___ Front part of the elbow area
5. ___ Fleshy area along the side between the ribs and hip bone
6. ___ Pertaining to the mouth
7. ___ Lower back area extending from the chest to the hips
8. ___ Pertains to the space between the cheek and gum
9. ___ Groin region
10. ___ Shoulder blade area

Multiple Choice

1. This part of the humerus (arm bone) is closer to the elbow than to the axillary region.
   a. Anterior
   b. Superior
   c. Distal
   d. Proximal

2. Describe the relationship of the mediastinum to the diaphragm.
   a. Distal
   b. Deep
   c. Anterior
   d. Superior

3. The umbilical area is located
   a. inferior to the inguinal region.
   b. superior to the RUQ.
   c. inferior to the diaphragm.
   d. within the midepigastric region.

4. The sternal area is
   a. superior to the diaphragm.
   b. referred to as the breastbone area.
   c. superficial to the mediastinum.
   d. All of the above are true.

5. Which of the following is not descriptive of the mediastinum?
   a. Thoracic cavity
   b. Dorsal cavity
   c. Ventral cavity
   d. Superior to the diaphragm

6. The frontal plane
   a. splits the body into right- and left-half sections.
   b. is also the coronal plane.
   c. splits the body into a top and a bottom section.
   d. creates a transverse cross section.

7. Which of the following terms best describes when the blood vessels dilate and the person sweats in order to decrease body temperature?
   a. Pathophysiology
   b. Evisceration
   c. Homeostasis
   d. Midsagittal

8. Which of the following is true of these terms: sternal, umbilical, patellar, and antecubital?
   a. All are superior to the inguinal area.
   b. All lie within the ventral cavity.
   c. All can be viewed on the anterior body.
   d. All lie within the dorsal cavity.

Go Figure

1. **According to Figure 1-6**
   a. The brachial, lumbar, and antecubital areas can only be identified on the posterior view of the body.
   b. The inguinal and flank areas are the same.
   c. The gluteal, lumbar, and scapular areas are inferior to the umbilicus.
   d. The popliteal and patellar areas are located in the lower extremities.

2. **Refer to Figures 1-5 and 1-6. A midsagittal section yields half of a body. Which body regions are preserved in this half-body section?**
   a. The patellar (right and left), flank (right and left), and brachial (right and left) are preserved.
   b. Neither the right nor left patellar areas and neither the right nor left antecubital areas are preserved.
   c. All areas displayed in Figure 1-6, *B*, are preserved.
   d. A left or right inguinal, pedal, and axillary area is preserved.

3. **According to Figure 1-7**
   a. The thoracic cavity is a ventral cavity that includes the mediastinum and pleural cavities.
   b. The diaphragm separates the two pleural cavities.
   c. The dorsal cavity includes the pleural cavities and the mediastinum.
   d. All of the above are true.

4. **According to Figure 1-8**
   a. The ventral cavity is divided into quadrants.
   b. The dorsal cavity is divided into regions.
   c. RUQ, LUQ, RLQ, and LLQ describe only the abdominal cavity.
   d. RUQ, LUQ, RLQ, and LLQ are quadrants that define the abdominopelvic cavity.

5. **According to Figure 1-8**
   a. The left iliac region is located within the LUQ.
   b. The hypogastric region is located within the RUQ.
   c. The umbilical region surrounds the navel or belly button.
   d. The right lung is located within the RUQ.

Basic Chemistry

Key Terms

acid (p. 23)

adenosine triphosphate (ATP) (p. 25)

atom (p. 16)

base (p. 23)

catalyst (p. 22)

compound (p. 21)

covalent bond (p. 18)

electrolyte (p. 20)

element (p. 15)

energy (p. 24)

enzyme (p. 22)

hydrogen bond (p. 18)

ionic bond (p. 18)

isotope (p. 17)

molecule (p. 20)

pH (p. 23)

solution (p. 26)

suspension (p. 26)

Objectives

1. Define the terms *matter*, *element*, and *atom*, and do the following:
   - List the four elements that comprise 96% of body weight.
   - Describe the three components of an atom.
   - Describe the role of electrons in the formation of chemical bonds.
2. Differentiate among ionic, covalent, and hydrogen bonds.
3. Explain ions, including the differences among electrolytes, cations, and anions.

4. Explain the difference between a molecule and a compound, and list five reasons why water is essential to life.
5. Explain the role of catalysts and enzymes.
6. Differentiate between an acid and a base, and define pH.
7. List the six forms of energy and describe the role of adenosine triphosphate (ATP) in energy transfer.
8. Differentiate among a mixture, solution, suspension, colloidal suspension, and precipitate.

Why a chapter on chemistry? Because our bodies are made of different chemicals. The food we eat, the water we drink, and the air we breathe are all chemical substances. We digest our food, move our bodies, experience emotions, and think great thoughts because of chemical reactions. To understand the body, we must understand some general chemical principles.

MATTER, ELEMENTS, AND ATOMS

MATTER

Chemistry is the study of matter. Matter is anything that occupies space and has weight. Anything that you see as you look around is matter.

Matter exists in three states: solid, liquid, and gas. Solid matter—such as skin, bones, and teeth—has a definite shape and volume. Liquid matter—such as blood, saliva, and digestive juices—takes the shape of the container that holds it. A gas, or gaseous matter—such as the air we breathe—has neither shape nor volume.

Matter can undergo both physical and chemical changes. The logs in a fireplace illustrate the difference between a physical and a chemical change (Figure 2-1). The logs can undergo a physical change by being chopped into smaller chips of wood with a hatchet. The wood chips are smaller than the log, but they are still wood. The matter (wood) has not essentially changed; only the physical appearance has changed. A chemical change occurs when the wood is burned. When burned, the wood ceases to be wood. The chemical composition of the ashes is essentially different from that of wood.

The body contains many examples of physical and chemical changes. For example, digestion involves physical and chemical changes. Chewing breaks the food into smaller pieces; this is a physical change. Potent chemicals digest or change the food into simpler substances; this is a chemical change.

ELEMENTS

All matter, living or dead, is composed of elements. An element is matter that is composed of atoms that have the same number of positive charges in their nuclei. Even a very small amount of an element such as sodium contains millions and millions of sodium atoms. The same name is used for both the

Physical change   Chemical change

Ashes

FIGURE 2-1 Changes in matter.

element and the atom. Although more than 100 elements exist, only about 25 elements are required by living organisms.

 Do You Know...

Why Children Should Not Be Allowed to Play in Traffic and Chew on Old Paint?

Aside from the obvious safety issues, old paint and emissions from motor vehicles contain high amounts of lead. Exposure to high levels of lead causes lead poisoning, a serious condition that damages the major organs, including the brain, liver, kidney, and bone marrow. The old name for chronic lead poisoning is plumbism, from the Latin word for lead *(plumbum)*. The chemical symbol for lead is Pb. (By the way, a plumber is called a plumber because ancient water pipes were made of *plumbum,* or lead.) Why does plumbism have such a great history? Lead was used to make pipes that carried water and was used to make pottery, particularly drinking vessels. This practice killed many of the rich and famous—those wealthy enough to afford leaded wine goblets. Because of the toxic nature of lead, pipes and pottery in the United States are no longer made of lead, gasoline and paint are now lead-free by law, and the disposal of acid lead batteries is regulated. Is the lead problem a done deal? No! Children are still huffing lead fumes from car emissions, playing with toys laced with lead paint, and wearing clothing impregnated with lead. Go figure!

The most abundant elements found in the body are listed in Table 2-1. Four elements—carbon, hydrogen, oxygen, and nitrogen—make up 96% of the body weight. The trace elements are present in tiny amounts, but despite the small amounts required, the trace elements are essential for life. (Not all the trace elements appear in Table 2-1.)

Each of the elements included in Table 2-1 is represented by a symbol, and the first letter of the symbol is always capitalized. For example, the symbol O is for oxygen, N is for nitrogen, Na is for sodium, K is for potassium, and C is for carbon. These symbols are used frequently, so you should memorize the symbols of the major elements.

ATOMS

ATOMIC STRUCTURE

Elements are composed of atoms, the basic units of matter. An **atom** is the smallest unit of an element with that element's chemical characteristics. An atom is composed of three subatomic particles: protons, neutrons, and electrons. The arrangement of the subatomic particles resembles the sun and planets (Figure 2-2, *A*), with the sun in the center and the planets constantly moving around the sun in orbits, or circular paths. The atom is composed of a nucleus (the sun) and shells, or orbits, that surround the nucleus (see Figure 2-2, *B*).

Where are the subatomic particles located? The protons and the neutrons are located in the nucleus (see Figure 2-2, *C*). Protons carry a positive (+) electrical charge; neutrons carry no electrical charge. The electrons are located in the shells, or orbits, surrounding the nucleus like planets. Electrons carry a negative (−) electrical charge. In each atom, the number of protons (+) is equal to the number of electrons (−). The atom is therefore electrically neutral; it carries no net electrical charge.

All protons are alike, all neutrons are alike, and all electrons are alike. So what makes one atom different from another atom? The difference is primarily in the numbers of protons and electrons in each atom. For example, hydrogen is the simplest and smallest atom.

Table **2-1**	Common Elements in the Human Body	
ELEMENT	**SYMBOL**	**PERCENTAGE OF BODY WEIGHT (%)**
Oxygen	O	65.0
Carbon	C	18.5
Hydrogen	H	9.5
Nitrogen	N	3.2
Calcium	Ca	
Phosphorus	P	
Potassium	K	
Sulfur	S	
Sodium	Na	
Chlorine	Cl	
Magnesium	Mg	
Iron	Fe	
Iodine*	I	
Chromium*	Cr	
Cobalt*	Co	
Copper*	Cu	
Fluorine*	F	
Selenium*	Se	
Zinc*	Zn	

*Trace elements.

A

ATOM

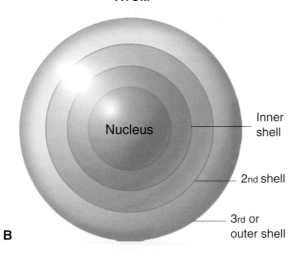

Nucleus

Inner shell

2nd shell

3rd or outer shell

B

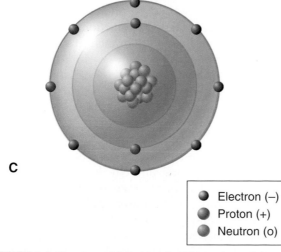

C

● Electron (−)
● Proton (+)
● Neutron (o)

FIGURE 2-2 Structure of the atom. **A,** Subatomic particles arranged like the sun and the planets. **B,** Nucleus and electron shells. **C,** Protons and neutrons located in the nucleus and electrons encircling the nucleus in orbits.

It has one proton and one electron. Helium has two protons and two electrons. Lithium has three protons and three electrons. Hydrogen, helium, and lithium are different atoms because of the different numbers of protons and electrons.

? Re-Think

1. How does the structure of an atom resemble the solar system (sun and planets)?
2. What electrical charge is carried by the proton, electron, and neutron?
3. Identify the locations of the proton, neutron, and electron.

OTHER CHARACTERISTICS OF ATOMS

Two terms describe individual atoms. The atomic number is the number of protons in the nucleus. Thus, hydrogen has an atomic number of 1, helium has an atomic number of 2, and lithium has an atomic number of 3. The atomic mass of an atom is determined by adding the numbers of protons and neutrons in the nucleus. Thus, the atomic mass of hydrogen is also 1 because the hydrogen nucleus contains one proton and no neutrons. The atomic mass of helium is 4 because the nucleus contains two protons and two neutrons. (The atomic mass is roughly equivalent to the atomic weight.)

An **isotope** (EYE-so-tohp) is a different form of the same atom. For example, hydrogen has different forms. Hydrogen has an atomic number of 1 and an atomic mass of 1; it has one proton and no neutrons in the nucleus. A second and less common form of hydrogen is called *heavy hydrogen*. It has one proton and one neutron in its nucleus; thus, its atomic number is 1, but its atomic mass is 2. Because its atomic number is 1, it is still a hydrogen atom. The additional neutron in the nucleus, however, makes it heavy and changes its atomic mass. Heavy hydrogen is an isotope of hydrogen. Remember that an isotope has the same atomic number as an atom but a different atomic mass.

Isotopes are often unstable and their nuclei break down, or decay, giving off energy. In doing so, the unstable nuclei become more stable. Unstable isotopes are called *radioisotopes*. The process of spontaneous breakdown (decay) is called *radioactivity*. Radioisotopes are damaging to tissue and are used clinically to destroy cells. For example, radioactive iodine is used to destroy excess thyroid tissue. Other radioisotopes are used to destroy cancer cells, and radioisotopes can also be used diagnostically. For example, radioactive iodine (^{131}I) is normally taken up by the thyroid gland at a certain rate. Alterations in the rate of ^{131}I uptake can indicate thyroid dysfunction.

? Re-Think

1. What is the difference between the atomic number and atomic mass?
2. What is an isotope? A radioisotope?

ELECTRON SHELLS

Electrons surround the nucleus in orbits called *energy levels* or *electron shells* (see Figure 2-2, C). The number of shells varies from one atom to the next. Some atoms, like hydrogen, have only one shell; other atoms, like sodium, have three shells. Each shell can hold a specific number of electrons. The inner shell closest to the nucleus can hold only two electrons. The second and third shells can each hold eight electrons.

The only electrons that are important for chemical bonding are the electrons in the outermost shell. If it is not filled with its proper number of electrons, the outer shell becomes unstable. It then tries to give up electrons to empty the shell, acquire electrons to fill the shell, or share electrons so that each participating atom acquires the proper number of electrons in its outer shells. The tendency of the outer shell to want to become stable forms the basis of chemical bonding.

CHEMICAL BONDS

Atoms are attracted to each other because they want to achieve a stable outer electron shell. In other words, they want to fill or empty the outer electron shell. The force of attraction between the atoms is similar to the force of two magnets. When you try to separate the magnets, you can feel the pull. The electrical attraction between atoms is a chemical bond. The three types of chemical bonds are ionic bonds, covalent bonds, and hydrogen bonds.

IONIC BONDS

An **ionic** (eye-ON-ik) **bond** is caused by a transfer of electrons between atoms. The interaction of the sodium and chlorine atoms illustrates an ionic bond (Figure 2-3, *A*). The sodium atom has 11 protons in the nucleus and 11 electrons in the shells. Two electrons are in the inner shell, eight in the second shell, and only one in the outer shell. This single electron makes the outer shell unstable. To become more stable, the sodium atom would like to donate the single electron. Donating an electron forms a bond between the two atoms.

Sodium often bonds with chlorine. The chlorine (Cl) atom has 17 protons in the nucleus and 17 electrons orbiting in its shells. The electrons are positioned as follows: two electrons in the inner shell, eight in the second shell, and seven in the outer shell. The seven electrons make the outer shell unstable. The chlorine atom would like to add a single electron. The electrical attraction occurs between the outer shells of the sodium and chlorine atoms. The single electron in the outer shell of the sodium (Na) atom is attracted to the seven electrons in the outer shell of the chlorine atom. Thus, the sodium atom and chlorine atom bond ionically to form sodium chloride (NaCl), or table salt.

COVALENT BONDS

A second type of chemical bond is the **covalent** (ko-VAYL-ent) **bond**. Covalent bonding involves a sharing of electrons by the outer shells of the atoms. Covalent bonding is like joining hands (see Figure 2-3, *B*). The formation of water from hydrogen and oxygen atoms illustrates covalent bonding. Oxygen has eight electrons, two in the inner shell and only six in the outer shell. An oxygen atom needs two electrons to complete the outer shell. Hydrogen has only one electron and requires one electron to complete its inner shell.

Water is formed when two hydrogen atoms, each with one electron, share those electrons with one oxygen atom. By sharing the electrons of the oxygen, each of the two hydrogen atoms has completed the inner shells (capacity is two electrons). By sharing the electrons of two hydrogen atoms, the outer shell of the oxygen is completed, with eight electrons. Water is represented as H_2O (two hydrogen atoms and one oxygen atom).

Carbon atoms always form covalent bonds. A carbon atom has four electrons in the outer shell. Carbon, one of the major elements in the body, most commonly bonds with hydrogen, oxygen, nitrogen, and other carbon atoms. Covalent bonding of carbon with hydrogen, oxygen, and nitrogen forms complex molecules such as proteins and carbohydrates. Covalent bonds are strong and do not break apart in an aqueous (water) solution. The strength of these bonds is important because the protein produced by the body must not fall apart when exposed to water.

Many proteins, such as hormones, are transported around the body by blood, which is mostly water. If the covalent bonds of the protein broke apart in water, the hormones would be unable to accomplish their tasks. So many chemical reactions in the body involve carbon that a separate branch of chemistry—organic chemistry—studies only carbon-containing substances. In contrast, inorganic chemistry studies non–carbon-containing substances.

HYDROGEN BONDS

A third type of bond is a **hydrogen bond** (see Figure 2-3, *C*). It differs from the ionic and covalent bonds in that the hydrogen bond is not caused by the transfer or sharing of electrons of the outer shells of atoms. A hydrogen bond is best illustrated by the weak attraction between water molecules. Water is composed of hydrogen and oxygen. The weak positive charge around the hydrogen of one water molecule is attracted to the weak negative charge of the oxygen in a second water molecule. Because the bond occurs between two molecules it is called an *intermolecular bond*.

POLARITY

Water engages in hydrogen bonding because it is a polar molecule. What makes water a polar molecule?

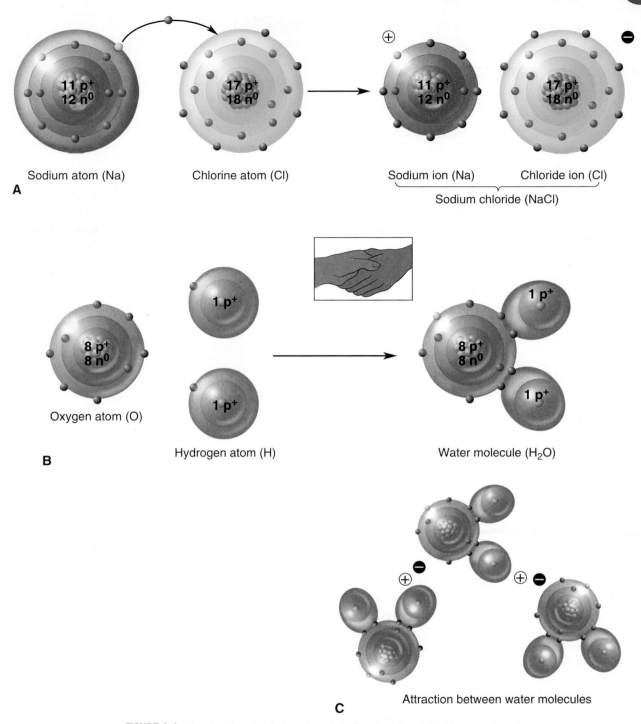

FIGURE 2-3 Chemical bonds. **A,** Ionic bond. **B,** Covalent bond. **C,** Hydrogen bond.

Because of the uneven sharing of electrons within a water molecule, there is a slight positive charge around the hydrogen end of the water and a slight negative charge around the oxygen end. Note how lopsided the water molecule appears in Figure 2-3, *C;* more importantly, the *charges* are lopsided. A polar molecule is defined as a molecule that has a lopsided charge—a positive end and a negative end. The lopsided charge means that the positive end—hydrogen—of one water

molecule is attracted to the negative end—oxygen—of a second water molecule.

? Re-Think

1. Explain the role of the outer electron shell to ionic and covalent bonding.
2. Explain why water is described as a polar molecule.

IONS

CATIONS, ANIONS, AND ELECTROLYTES

Several other terms are related to the activity of the electrons in the outer shells of the atoms. If the negatively charged electrons are lost from or gained by the outer shell of an atom, the electrical charge of the atom changes. In other words, the electrical charge of the atom changes from a neutral charge (i.e., no charge) to a positive (+) charge or negative (−) charge. Atoms that carry an electrical charge are called *ions*. If the ion is positively charged (+), it is a cation. If the ion is negatively charged (−), it is an anion.

An electrolyte is a substance that forms ions when it is dissolved in water. Electrolytes, as the name implies, are capable of conducting an electrical current. For example, the electrocardiogram (ECG) and the electroencephalogram (EEG) record electrical events in the heart and brain.

ION FORMATION

Ions are formed when electrons in the outer shell are lost or gained. For example, the sodium atom has 11 protons (positive charge) and 11 electrons (negative charge). If a single electron is donated, the sodium is left with 11 positive (+) charges and only 10 negative (−) charges. Sodium is said to carry a net charge of +1. The sodium ion, represented as Na^+, is therefore a cation.

The chlorine atom has 17 protons (positive charge) and 17 electrons (negative charge). If an electron is gained, the chlorine then contains 17 (+) charges and 18 (−) charges. Chlorine is said to carry a net charge of −1 and is considered an anion. The chlorine anion is called *chloride* and is represented as Cl^-. Some atoms may give up more than one electron and have a stronger positive charge. Calcium, for example, gives up two electrons. It is represented as Ca^{2+}. Table 2-2 presents other important ions. Note that combinations of atoms, such as bicarbonate (HCO_3^-), carry an electrical charge and are therefore ions.

IONIZATION

When an electrolyte splits, or breaks apart in solution, the electrolyte is said to dissociate (Figure 2-4). For example, NaCl is an electrolyte. In the solid state, it appears as tiny white granules. When dissolved in water, however, the table salt dissociates. What is happening?

$$\underset{\text{salt}}{NaCl} \rightarrow \underset{\substack{\text{sodium ion} \\ \text{(cation)}}}{Na^+} + \underset{\substack{\text{chloride ion} \\ \text{(anion)}}}{Cl^-}$$

When the salt is placed in water, the ionic bonds holding the sodium and chlorine together weaken. The

NAME	SYMBOL	FUNCTION
Cations		
Sodium	Na^+	Fluid balance (chief extracellular cation), nerve and muscle function
Calcium	Ca^{2+}	Component of bones and teeth, blood clotting, muscle contraction
Iron	Fe^{2+}	Component of hemoglobin (oxygen transport)
Hydrogen	H^+	Important in acid–base balance. Its concentration determines the pH of a solution.
Potassium	K^+	Nerve and muscle function, chief intracellular cation
Ammonium	NH_4^+	Important in acid–base regulation
Anions		
Chloride	Cl^-	Chief extracellular anion
Bicarbonate	HCO_3^-	Important in acid–base regulation
Phosphate	PO_4^{3-}	Component of bones and teeth, component of ATP (energy)

Table 2-2   Common Ions

ATP, Adenosine triphosphate.

solid NaCl then splits into Na^+ (sodium ion) and Cl^- (chloride ion). In other words, the NaCl dissociates. Because the products of this dissociation are ions, this dissociation process is referred to as *ionization*. Only electrolytes ionize.

 Do You Know...

What the Patient's "Lytes" Are?

This is medical jargon for electrolytes. One of the most important clinical tools is the assessment of the patient's electrolytes. Actually, the "lytes" are really ions such as Na^+ (sodium), K^+ (potassium), Cl^- (chloride), Mg^{2+} (magnesium), and HCO_3^- (bicarbonate). The terms *electrolytes* and *ions* are used interchangeably in the clinical setting.

? **Re-Think**

Using table salt (NaCl) as an example, explain the difference between an electrolyte, ion, cation, and anion.

MOLECULES AND COMPOUNDS

MOLECULES

When two or more atoms bond, they form a molecule. Two identical atoms may bond. For example, one atom of oxygen may bond with another atom of oxygen to

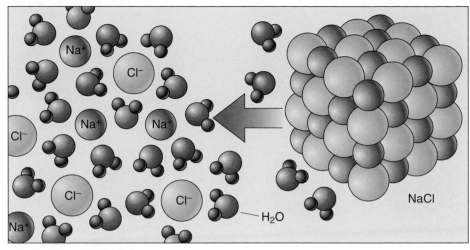

FIGURE 2-4 Ionization—dissociation of NaCl → Na⁺ + Cl⁻ in water.

form a molecule of oxygen, which is designated O_2. The same bonding is true for nitrogen (N_2) and hydrogen (H_2) (Figure 2-5). A molecule can also be formed when atoms of different elements combine. For example, when two atoms of hydrogen combine with one atom of oxygen, a molecule of water (H_2O) is formed.

COMPOUNDS

A substance that contains molecules formed by two or more different atoms is called a **compound**. For example, if two atoms of hydrogen combine with one atom of oxygen, water is formed. Water is considered both a molecule and a compound.

SOME IMPORTANT COMPOUNDS AND MOLECULES

WATER

Water is the most abundant compound in the body. It constitutes approximately two thirds of an adult's body weight and even more of a child's body weight. Water is essential for life. Although we can last for many weeks without food, we can last only a few days without water. What makes water so special?

- *Water as the universal solvent.* Water is called the universal solvent because most substances dissolve in water. Its use as a solvent is one of the most important characteristics of water. The ability to dissolve substances is largely because of the polar structure of water (positive charge on one end, negative charge on the other end). For example, the plasma protein albumin carries a negative (−) charge. It is attracted to the positive (+) end of the water molecule. The attraction of the electrical charges allows albumin to dissolve in water. Many nutrients, waste products, and hormones dissolve in water for transport throughout the body.
- *Water as temperature regulator.* Water has the ability to absorb large amounts of heat without the temperature of the water itself increasing dramatically.

This ability means that heat can be removed from heat-producing tissue, like exercising muscle, while the body maintains a normal temperature. Also, when water evaporates from the skin surface, it carries with it a considerable amount of heat. Water, therefore, plays an important role in the body's temperature regulation.
- *Water as an ideal lubricant.* Water is a major component of mucus and other lubricating fluids. Lubricating fluids decrease friction as two structures slide past each other, thereby minimizing wear and tear.
- *Water in chemical reactions.* Water plays a crucial role in many chemical reactions. For example, water is necessary to break down carbohydrates during digestion.
- *Water as a protective device.* Water may also be used to protect an important structure. For example, the cerebrospinal fluid surrounds and cushions the delicate brain and spinal cord. Similarly, amniotic fluid surrounds and cushions the developing infant in the mother's womb.

❓ Re-Think

1. Physiologically, why is water so important?
2. What characteristic of water allows it to transport solute throughout the body?

OXYGEN

Oxygen (O_2), a molecule composed of two oxygen atoms, exists in nature as a gas. The air we breathe contains 21% oxygen. Oxygen is essential for life; without a continuous supply, we would quickly die. The oxygen we inhale is used by cells to liberate the energy from the food we eat. This energy powers the body; like an engine, if the body has no energy, it stops running. The importance of oxygen accounts for the urgency associated with cardiopulmonary resuscitation (CPR). If the heart stops beating, the delivery of oxygen to the tissue ceases and the brain dies.

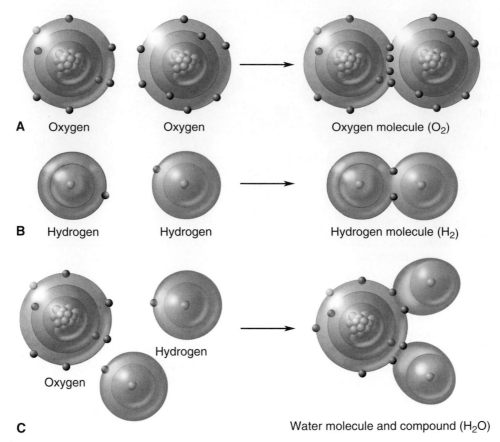

FIGURE 2-5 Molecules and compounds. **A,** Oxygen (O_2). **B,** Hydrogen (H_2). **C,** Water (H_2O).

CARBON DIOXIDE

Carbon dioxide (CO_2) is a compound that consists of one carbon atom and two oxygen atoms—hence the name carbon dioxide (*di-* means "two"). CO_2 is a waste product, so it must be eliminated from the body. It is made when food is chemically broken down for energy.

2+2 Sum It Up!

Chemistry is the study of matter. Matter is composed of elements such as hydrogen, oxygen, carbon, and nitrogen. Each element is composed of millions of the same atoms. Atoms are composed of subatomic particles called protons, neutrons, and electrons. Two characteristics of atoms are the atomic number (number of protons) and the atomic mass (number of protons and neutrons). Chemical bonds are formed through the interaction of one atom with another. The three chemical bonds are ionic, covalent, and hydrogen bonds. The transfer of electrons is responsible for the formation of ions (cations and anions). Cations are positively charged ions, whereas anions are negatively charged ions. Molecules and compounds are formed when atoms interact in a particular fashion. Water (H_2O), oxygen (O_2), and carbon dioxide (CO_2) are examples of important molecules and compounds. Water is the most abundant compound in the body and has numerous characteristics that make it essential to life.

CHEMICAL REACTIONS

A chemical reaction is a process whereby the atoms of molecules or compounds interact to form new chemical combinations. For example, glucose interacts with oxygen to form carbon dioxide, water, and energy. This chemical interaction is characterized by the breaking of the chemical bonds of glucose and oxygen and the making of new bonds as carbon dioxide and water are formed. The reaction is represented as follows:

$$\underset{\text{glucose}}{C_6H_{12}O_6} + \underset{\text{oxygen}}{O_2} \rightarrow \underset{\text{carbon dioxide}}{CO_2} + \underset{\text{water}}{H_2O} + \text{energy}$$

The rates of chemical reactions (how fast they occur) are important. Chemical substances called **catalysts** (KAT-ah-lists) speed up the rate of a chemical reaction. When proteins perform the role of catalysts, they are called **enzymes** (EN-zymes). Most chemical reactions require a catalyst.

ACIDS AND BASES

A normally functioning body requires a balance between substances classified as acids and as bases. Acid–base balance is important because the chemical reactions in the body occur only when these substances are in balance. Imbalances of acids and bases are common and cause life-threatening clinical problems. An understanding of the chemistry of acids and bases is crucial to understanding acid–base balance.

ACIDS

We all recognize the sour taste of an acid. Grapefruit juice, lemon juice, and vinegar are acids. In addition to a sour taste, very strong acids, such as hydrochloric acid (HCl), can cause severe burns. Acid splashed in your eye, for example, can damage the eye tissue to the point of blindness. An **acid** is an electrolyte that dissociates into a hydrogen ion (H$^+$) and an anion. Its dissociation is represented as follows:

$$\underset{\text{hydrochloric acid}}{\text{HCl}} \rightarrow \underset{\text{hydrogen ion}}{\text{H}^+} + \underset{\text{chloride ion}}{\text{Cl}^-}$$

In this reaction, HCl dissociates into H$^+$ and the chloride ion (Cl$^-$). For our purposes, the most important component is the H$^+$. The amount of H$^+$ in a solution determines its acidity.

A strong acid dissociates (breaks apart) completely into H$^+$ and an anion. HCl, found within the stomach, is a strong acid; it yields many hydrogen ions. A weak acid does not dissociate completely. Vinegar, or acetic acid, is a weak acid. Vinegar dissociates slightly into H$^+$. Most of the vinegar remains in its undissociated form, and its dissociation is represented as follows:

$$\text{vinegar} \rightleftharpoons \text{H}^+ + \text{acetate}^-$$

The heavy arrow pointing to the left indicates that the vinegar remains as vinegar, forming very little H$^+$. Because the number of hydrogen ions (H$^+$) determines the acidity of a solution, vinegar is classified as a weak acid. This weakness is the reason that vinegar does not burn your hand. HCl is so strong that it can actually burn a hole through your hand.

BASES

A **base** has a bitter taste and is slippery like soap. Bases are substances that combine with H$^+$. Bases often contain the hydroxyl ion (OH$^-$), such as sodium hydroxide (NaOH). NaOH dissociates into sodium ion (Na$^+$) and the hydroxyl ion (OH$^-$) as follows:

$$\text{NaOH} \rightarrow \text{Na}^+ + \text{OH}^-$$

OH$^-$ is a hydrogen ion eliminator. In other words, the OH$^-$ soaks up a hydrogen ion. The addition of a base makes a solution less acidic.

NEUTRALIZATION OF ACIDS AND BASES

When an acid is mixed with a base, as in the following example, the H$^+$ of the acid combines with the OH$^-$ of the base to form water. In addition, the Na$^+$ and the Cl$^-$ combine to form a salt, NaCl. The reaction is important because the H$^+$ is converted to water. In other words, the acid has been neutralized. This chemical reaction is represented as follows:

$$\underset{\text{acid}}{\text{HCl}} + \underset{\text{base}}{\text{NaOH}} \rightarrow \underset{\text{water}}{\text{H}_2\text{O}} + \underset{\text{salt}}{\text{NaCl}}$$

? Re-Think

1. What makes an acid an acid?
2. What makes a base a base?

MEASUREMENT: THE pH SCALE

One unit of measurement, **pH**, indicates how many H$^+$ ions are in a solution. The pH scale ranges from 0 to 14 (Figure 2-6). At the midpoint of the scale, pH 7, the number of H$^+$ ions in pure water is equal to the number

pH Value	Examples of Solutions
0	Hydrochloric acid
1	
2	Lemon juice
	Stomach contents (1–4)
3	Vinegar, wine
4	
5	Black coffee
6	Urine (5–8)
7	Pure H$_2$O
	Blood (7.35–7.45)
8	
	Intestinal contents (8–10)
9	
10	Soap solutions
11	
12	Household ammonia
13	
14	Sodium hydroxide

Increasingly acidic — Neutral — Increasingly basic

H↑   H↓

FIGURE 2-6 The pH scale. The scale indicates the H$^+$ concentration. Pink indicates the acidic range, and blue indicates the basic, or alkaline, range.

of OH⁻ ions. Therefore, the solution is neutral. A pH that measures less than 7 on the scale indicates that the solution has more H⁺ than OH⁻. The solution is then said to be acidic. Note the pH of lemon juice and vinegar on the scale. They are both less than 7 and are therefore acidic.

A pH measuring more than 7 indicates fewer H⁺ ions than OH⁻ ions. These substances are bases, and the solution is said to be basic, or alkaline (AL-kah-lin). The pH scale measures the degree of acidity or alkalinity. A pH of 0 is most acidic, whereas a pH of 14 is most alkaline. Note that the intestinal contents are alkaline, the pH at which the digestive enzymes are most effective.

READING THE pH SCALE

Each pH unit represents a 10-fold change in H⁺ concentration. For example, a change in 1 pH unit (from 7 to 6) represents a 10-fold increase in H⁺, whereas a change in 2 pH units (from 7 to 5) represents a 100-fold increase in H⁺ concentration. The important point is that very small changes in the pH reading indicate very large changes in the H⁺ concentration.

Do You Know...

Why Antacids Are Used?

Patients with ulcers often have excess stomach acid. The stomach acid (HCl) can be neutralized with a drug that contains a base. Because these drugs oppose acids, they are called *antacids*. One of the most commonly used antacids contains aluminum hydroxide. The hydroxyl ion (OH⁻) of the drug combines with the H⁺ of the stomach acid, thereby neutralizing the acid.

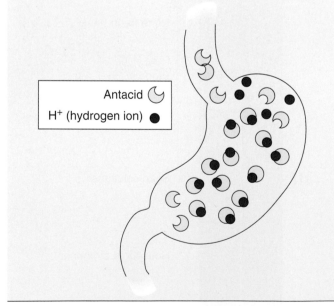

Antacid ☾
H⁺ (hydrogen ion) ●

pH OF BODY FLUIDS

Note the pH of some of the body fluids (see Figure 2-6). The stomach contents are very acidic, with a pH of 1 to 4. The pH of urine is normally acidic, with a pH

range of 5 to 8, although a number of conditions, including diet, can change urinary pH. The intestinal secretions are alkaline, with a pH range of 8 to 10.

Blood pH is maintained within a narrow range of 7.35 to 7.45, a slightly alkaline pH. Because the blood pH is normally slightly alkaline (called the alkaline reserve), a blood pH of less than 7.35 is more acidic than normal, and the patient is said to be acidotic. If the patient's blood pH is higher than 7.45, the patient is said to be alkalotic. Because all of the body's enzymes work best at a normal blood pH, both acidosis and alkalosis cause serious clinical problems and must be corrected. The need to maintain the body's normal alkaline state is the reason for monitoring blood pH closely during the course of a patient's illness.

The blood pH is regulated on a minute-by-minute basis by three means: a buffer system, the lungs, and the kidneys. (These processes of regulation are described in Chapters 24 and 25.)

2+2 Sum It Up!

Chemical reactions are processes whereby one chemical substance is converted into a different chemical substance. The rate of a chemical reaction can be increased by a catalyst, or enzyme. A normally functioning body requires a balance between acids and bases. Hydrogen ion concentration is measured by pH. As H⁺ increases, pH decreases; as H⁺ decreases, pH increases. Normal blood pH is 7.35 to 7.45 and is therefore slightly alkaline. When pH falls below 7.35, the person is said to be acidotic; when pH rises above 7.45, the person is said to be alkalotic. Blood pH is regulated within normal limits by three mechanisms: buffers, lungs, and kidneys.

? Re-Think

1. Describe what is happening in a neutralization reaction to cause pH to change.
2. What blood pH is indicative of acidosis? Of alkalosis?

ENERGY

Energy is the ability to perform work. The body depends on a continuous supply of energy. Even at rest, the body is continuously working and using up energy. Heart muscle, for example, is contracting and forcing blood throughout a large network of blood vessels. The cells of the pancreas are continuously making enzymes so that we can digest our food. Without energy, the body ceases to function.

FORMS OF ENERGY

There are six forms of energy, summarized in Table 2-3. Mechanical energy is expressed as movement. For example, when the leg muscles contract, you are able to walk. Chemical energy is stored within the chemical bonds holding the atoms together. When the chemical bonds are broken, chemical energy is released. The

Table 2-3 Forms of Energy

FORM OF ENERGY	DESCRIPTION	EXAMPLE
Mechanical	Energy that causes movement	Movement of legs in running, walking; contraction of heart muscle, causing movement of blood
Chemical	Energy stored in chemical bonds	Fuel to do work, such as running
Electrical	Energy released from the movement of charged particles	Electrical signal involved in transmission of information along nerves
Radiant	Energy that travels in waves	Light stimulates the eyes for vision; ultraviolet radiation from the sun causes tanning
Thermal	Energy transferred because of a temperature difference	Responsible for body temperature
Nuclear	Energy released during the decay of radioactive substances such as isotopes	Not useful physiologically

released energy can then be used to perform other types of work, such as digesting food. This process is similar to the running of a car's engine; the energy released from the burning, or breakdown, of the gas is used to turn the engine, and the running engine then moves your car.

CONVERSION OF ENERGY

Energy is easily converted from one form to another. For example, when a log burns, the chemical energy stored in it is converted to heat (thermal energy) and light (radiant energy). In a similar way, the chemical energy stored in the muscle is converted into mechanical energy when the muscle contracts and moves your leg.

The conversion of energy in the body is generally accompanied by the release of heat. For example, when muscles contract during strenuous exercise, chemical energy is converted into both mechanical energy and heat (thermal) energy. Consider how hot you get while exercising. (Body temperature is further described in Chapter 7.)

ENERGY TRANSFER: THE ROLE OF ADENOSINE TRIPHOSPHATE

The energy used to power the body comes from the food we eat (Figure 2-7, *A*). As the food is broken down, energy is released. This energy, however, cannot be used directly by the cells of the body. The energy must first be transferred to another substance, called **adenosine triphosphate (ATP)**. ATP is an energy transfer molecule.

ATP is composed of three parts: a base, a sugar, and three phosphate groups (see Figure 2-7, *B*). Note the phosphate groups of the ATP molecule; they have unique chemical bonds. The squiggly lines connecting the second and third phosphate groups indicate that these bonds are high-energy bonds. When these bonds are broken, a large amount of energy is released. More

importantly, the energy released from ATP can be used directly by the cell to perform its tasks.

The energy stored within the high-energy bonds is similar to the energy stored in a loaded mousetrap (see Figure 2-7, *C*). Energy is stored in the trap when you set the metal bar in its loaded position. When the trap is set off by the mouse, the metal bar snaps back into its original position, thereby releasing the stored energy. Similarly, when energy is needed by the body, ATP is split. The energy that was stored in ATP is released. In other words, the bond that holds the end phosphate group is broken, and energy is released. With the release of energy, the splitting of ATP also yields adenosine diphosphate (ADP) and phosphate (P). This process can be shown as follows:

$$ATP \rightarrow energy + ADP + P$$

ADP is almost identical to ATP, but the molecule now has one less phosphate group. ATP is replenished when energy, obtained from burning food, reattaches the end phosphate to ADP, as follows:

$$ADP + P + energy \rightarrow ATP$$

? Re-Think

Explain why ATP is an energy transfer molecule rather than an energy storage molecule.

MIXTURES, SOLUTIONS, SUSPENSIONS, AND PRECIPITATES

You will encounter several other chemical terms in clinical situations.

MIXTURES

Mixtures are combinations of two or more substances that can be separated by ordinary physical means. When separated, the substances retain their original properties. For example, imagine that you have a

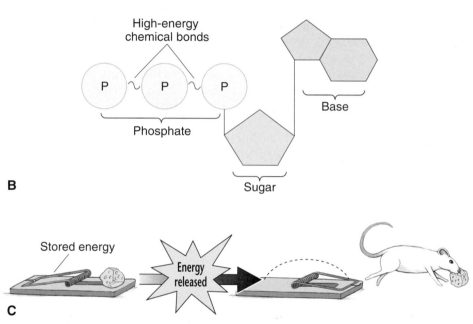

FIGURE 2-7 Energy. **A,** Source of energy. **B,** Storage of energy within the high-energy bonds of adenosine triphosphate (ATP). **C,** Release of energy.

mixture of sugar and little bits of iron. A magnet is then moved close to this sugar–iron mixture. The magnet pulls all the iron away from the sugar, thereby separating the two substances. Note that the two substances have retained their original properties. The sugar is still sugar, and the iron is still iron.

SOLUTIONS

Solutions are mixtures. In a solution, the particles that are mixed together remain evenly distributed. Salt water is an example of a solution. A solution has two parts, a solvent and a solute. The solute is the substance present in the smaller amount; it is the substance being dissolved. The salt in the salt water is the solute. The solute can be solid, liquid, or gas.

The solvent is the part of the solution present in the greater amount; it does the dissolving and is usually liquid or gas. Water is the solvent in salt water. If water is the solvent, the solution is referred to as an *aqueous solution*. If alcohol is the solvent, the solution is referred to as a *tincture*. A solution is always clear, and the solute does not settle to the bottom.

SUSPENSIONS

Suspensions are mixtures. In a suspension, the particles are relatively large and tend to settle to the bottom unless the mixture is shaken continuously. For example, if sand and water are shaken together and then allowed to sit undisturbed, the sand gradually settles to the bottom.

In a colloidal suspension, the particles do not dissolve, but they are so small that they remain suspended within the liquid, even when not being shaken. A colloid (KOL-oyd) is a gel-like substance that resembles egg whites. The body contains many colloidal suspensions. Blood plasma is a colloidal suspension because the proteins remain suspended within the plasma. Other examples of colloidal suspensions include mayonnaise and jelly.

PRECIPITATES

A precipitation reaction is the formation of a solid in a solution during a chemical reaction. The solid is called the *precipitate*. The formation of precipitates has several clinical consequences. For example, kidney stones are precipitates of salts in the urine and form especially when the salts are highly concentrated—hence, the direction to "drink plenty of fluids" as a preventive measure. Similarly, cholesterol-laden bile forms precipitates called *gallstones;* dietary teaching regarding cholesterol intake is provided in hopes of decreasing gallstone formation. Finally, you will be mixing

medications; some combinations of drugs form precipitates that, if administered intravenously, act as emboli (such as moving blood clots) that could kill a patient. Clinically, precipitates are very important.

2+2 Sum It Up!

Energy is the ability to do work. Without an adequate supply of energy, the body cannot work, and it dies. Energy is derived from food and transferred to high-energy bonds in ATP. When needed, the energy is released from ATP and used to power the body. Other chemical terms include mixtures, solutions, suspensions, and precipitates.

? Re-Think

1. Normal saline (0.9% NaCl) is a salt solution. Explain why it is a solution and not a colloid. What is the solute and what is the solvent?
2. What is meant by a precipitate?

Get Ready for Exams!

Summary Outline

Our bodies are made of different chemicals. To understand the body, you need to understand some general chemical principles.

   I. **Matter, Elements, and Atoms**
      A. Matter
         1. Anything that occupies space and has weight
         2. Exists in three states: solid, liquid, and gas
         3. Undergoes physical and chemical changes
      B. Elements
         1. Composed of atoms that have the same positive charge in their nuclei (same atomic number)
         2. Four elements (carbon, hydrogen, oxygen, and nitrogen) make up 96% of body weight.
      C. Atoms
         1. Composed of three subatomic particles: neutrons, protons, and electrons
         2. Atomic number: number of protons
         3. Atomic mass: number of neutrons and protons
         4. Isotope: atom with the same atomic number but a different atomic mass
         5. Radioisotope: an unstable isotope
  II. **Chemical Bonds**
      A. Ionic bond: involves donation and acceptance of electrons
      B. Covalent bond: shares electrons of interacting atoms
      C. Hydrogen bond: an example, intermolecular bonds formed by polar molecules
 III. **Ions**
      A. Ion: atom that carries an electrical charge
         1. Cation: positively charged ion
         2. Anion: negatively charged ion
      B. Electrolyte: substance that forms ions (ionization) when dissolved in water

  IV. **Molecules and Compounds**
      A. Molecule: substance formed by two or more atoms (e.g., O_2, H_2O)
      B. Compound: substance that forms when two or more different atoms bond (e.g., H_2O)
      C. Important molecules and compounds: include water, oxygen, and carbon dioxide
   V. **Acids and Bases**
      A. Acid: electrolyte that dissociates into hydrogen ion (H^+)
      B. Base: substance such as OH^- that combines with and eliminates H^+
      C. Neutralization reaction: acid and a base chemically react to form a salt and water
      D. pH scale: measures acidity and alkalinity. A pH of 7 is neutral. A pH less than 7 is acidic and a pH higher than 7 is basic, or alkaline.
      E. Normal pH of the blood: 7.35 to 7.45. A person with a pH less than 7.35 is acidotic, and a person with a pH higher than 7.45 is alkalotic.
      F. Regulation of blood pH: buffers, respiratory system, and kidneys
  VI. **Energy**
      A. Definition: ability to do work
      B. Forms of energy
         1. Six forms of energy: see Table 2-3
         2. Most energy released as heat
      C. Role of adenosine triphosphate (ATP)
         1. ATP: energy transfer molecule
         2. Energy stored in high-energy phosphate bonds
 VII. **Mixtures, Solutions, Suspensions, and Precipitates**
      A. Mixture: blend of two or more substances that can be separated by ordinary physical means
      B. Solutions, suspensions, and colloidal suspensions: types of mixtures
      C. Precipitate: solid formed during a chemical reaction

Review Your Knowledge

Matching: Atoms and Elements

Directions: Match the following words or symbols with their descriptions below.

a. atom
b. K
c. matter
d. Na
e. ion

1. ___ Composed of three particles: protons, neutrons, and electrons
2. ___ Symbol for potassium
3. ___ Symbol for sodium
4. ___ Exists in three states: liquid, solid, and gas
5. ___ Formed when sodium loses an electron

Matching: Structure of the Atom

Directions: Match the following words with their descriptions below. Some words may be used more than once, but others may not be used at all.

a. atomic mass
b. isotope
c. protons
d. electrons
e. neutrons
f. atomic number

1. ___ Number of protons in the nucleus
2. ___ Sum of number of protons and neutrons
3. ___ Same atomic number but different atomic mass
4. ___ Number of these in each atom equal to number of protons
5. ___ Circulate in orbits around the nucleus

Matching: Ions and Electrolytes

Directions: Match the following words with their descriptions below.

a. cation
b. ions
c. electrolyte
d. anion
e. ionization

1. ___ Classification of KCl
2. ___ Classification of K^+ and Cl^-
3. ___ K^+ is an ion classified as this
4. ___ Cl^- is an ion classified as this
5. ___ Dissociation of $KCl \rightarrow K^+ + Cl^-$

Matching: Acids and Bases

Directions: Match the following words or symbols with their descriptions below. Some words may be used more than once, but others may not be used at all.

a. alkalosis
b. pH
c. H^+
d. base
e. acid
f. acidosis

1. ___ Electrolyte that dissociates into H^+ and an anion
2. ___ Ion that makes a solution more acidic
3. ___ Measurement of hydrogen ion concentration $[H^+]$
4. ___ Condition characterized by pH lower than 7.35
5. ___ Condition caused by excess H^+

Multiple Choice

1. The ionization of salt (NaCl)
   a. is called a neutralization reaction.
   b. lowers pH.
   c. produces a cation (Na^+) and an anion (Cl^-).
   d. causes acidosis.

2. Which of the following is true of iodine and radioactive iodine?
   a. Both have the same atomic numbers.
   b. Both have the same atomic mass.
   c. Neither have electrons in their orbitals.
   d. Both create radiation hazards.

3. Which of the following is not true of Na^+?
   a. It is called the sodium ion.
   b. It has more protons than electrons.
   c. It is called a cation.
   d. It is measured by pH.

4. Which of the following is true of water?
   a. It is a molecule.
   b. It is an aqueous solvent.
   c. It is a compound.
   d. All of the above.

5. Which of the following best describes ATP?
   a. It is a buffer, removing H^+ from solution.
   b. It is an energy transfer molecule.
   c. It is a radioactive isotope of phosphate.
   d. It ionizes to H^+, thereby lowering pH.

6. Which of the following has donated an electron?
   a. H_2O
   b. Cl^-
   c. Na^+
   d. HCO_3^-

7. Which of the following is least descriptive of the nucleus of the atom?
   a. Its contents determine the atomic number.
   b. Its contents determine the atomic mass.
   c. It is the "home" of the electrons.
   d. It is the "home" of the protons.

8. Which of the following is descriptive of the patient with a blood pH of 7.28?
   a. The patient has a deficiency of H^+.
   b. The pH is within normal limits.
   c. The patient is acidotic.
   d. The patient is dehydrated.

Go Figure

1. According to Figure 2-3
   a. The stable inner shell of an atom contains eight electrons.
   b. The chloride ion has more electrons than protons.
   c. The sodium ion has more electrons than protons.
   d. Sodium and chlorine bond covalently.

2. According to Figure 2-3
   a. Hydrogen and oxygen bond ionically to form water.
   b. The oxygen atom has an unstable outer electron shell.
   c. The ionic bonding of sodium and chlorine changes the atomic number of the sodium and chlorine.
   d. The ionic bonding of sodium and chlorine changes the atomic mass of the sodium and chlorine.

3. According to Figure 2-4
   a. Ionization refers to the splitting of NaCl into Na^+ and Cl^-.
   b. Ionization refers to the formation of table salt from the sodium ion and chloride ion.
   c. NaCl cannot ionize in water.
   d. All of the above are true.

4. **According to Figure 2-5**
   a. The covalent bonding of two oxygen atoms yields an oxygen compound.
   b. Two hydrogen atoms bond ionically with one oxygen atom, yielding water.
   c. Water is formed as two hydrogen atoms share their electrons with one oxygen atom.
   d. A hydrogen atom can react with an oxygen atom but cannot react with another hydrogen atom.

5. **According to Figure 2-6**
   a. As $[H^+]$ decreases, the strip in the diagram becomes a deeper pink.
   b. As pH increases, the strip in the diagram becomes a deeper pink.
   c. The normal blood pH is slightly alkaline.
   d. All of the above are true.

6. **According to Figure 2-7**
   a. ATP means "all the power."
   b. The setting of the mouse trap represents the storage of energy in ATP.
   c. The release of the mouse trap is summarized as ADP + P + energy → ATP.
   d. The lucky mouse represents the source of the stored energy.

Cells

Key Terms

active transport (p. 36)
cell (p. 30)
cell cycle (p. 42)
cell membrane (p. 30)
cytoplasm (p. 32)
differentiate (p. 43)
diffusion (p. 36)
endocytosis (p. 41)

endoplasmic reticulum (ER) (p. 33)
equilibrium (p. 36)
exocytosis (p. 41)
facilitated diffusion (p. 37)
filtration (p. 40)
Golgi apparatus (p. 34)
lysosomes (p. 34)
mitochondria (p. 33)

mitosis (p. 42)
nucleus (p. 31)
organelles (p. 32)
osmosis (p. 38)
passive transport (p. 36)
ribosomes (p. 33)

Objectives

1. Label a diagram of the main parts of a typical cell, and do the following:
   - Explain the role of the nucleus.
   - Describe the functions of the main organelles of the cell.
   - Identify the components of the cell membrane.
2. Do the following regarding transport mechanisms:
   - Describe the active and passive movements of substances across a cell membrane.

- Define tonicity and compare isotonic, hypotonic, and hypertonic solutions.
3. Describe the phases of the cell cycle, including mitosis.
4. Explain what is meant by cell differentiation.
5. Explain the processes and consequences of uncontrolled and disorganized cell growth and apoptosis.

What do this monk and a cell have in common? While looking at a piece of cork under a microscope in the 1600s, Robert Hooke saw cube-like structures that resembled the rooms, or cells, occupied by monks in a monastery. Hooke thus called his structures "cells." The study of cellular structure and function is called *cytology*.

Microscope

Cells

The **cell** is the structural and functional unit of all living matter. Cells vary considerably in size, shape, and function. A red blood cell (RBC), for example, is

tiny, whereas a single nerve cell may measure 4 feet in length (Figure 3-1). The shapes and structures of the cells are also very different. The RBC is shaped like a Frisbee and is able to bend. The shape allows it to squeeze through tiny blood vessels and deliver oxygen and other nutrients throughout the body. Some nerve cells are very long, and many resemble bushes or trees. Their shapes enable them to conduct electrical signals quickly over long distances. Cell structure and function are closely related.

TYPICAL CELL

Despite the differences, cells have many similarities. Figure 3-2 is a typical cell with all known cellular components. Each specialized cell, such as a nerve cell, possesses some or all of the properties of the typical cell. Table 3-1 lists and summarizes the functions of the cellular components.

CELL MEMBRANE

The cell is encased by a **cell membrane**, also called the *plasma membrane*. The cell membrane separates intracellular (inside the cell) material from extracellular (outside the cell) material. In addition to physically holding the cell together, the cell membrane performs other important functions. One of its chief functions is the selection of substances allowed to enter or leave the cell. Because the membrane chooses the substances allowed to cross it, the membrane is said to be selectively permeable, or semipermeable.

What makes up a cell membrane? The cell membrane is composed primarily of phospholipids and protein, as well as a small amount of carbohydrates (Figure 3-3). The phospholipids are arranged in two layers. The protein molecules in the membrane perform several important functions; they provide structural support for the membrane, act as binding sites for hormones, and poke holes, or pores, through the lipid membrane. These pores form channels through which water and dissolved substances flow.

Substances move across the semipermeable membrane in two ways. They can dissolve in the lipid portion of the membrane, as do oxygen and carbon dioxide (lipid-soluble substances). Substances can also cross the membrane by flowing through the pores. Water and electrically charged substances such as sodium and chloride cannot penetrate the lipid membrane and must use the pores. These are called water-soluble substances. The size of the pores also helps select which substances cross the membrane. Substances larger than the pores cannot cross the membrane, whereas smaller substances such as sodium and chloride flow through easily. The solubility characteristics of the membrane also play an important role in pharmacology. Drugs are classified as lipid soluble or water soluble. Drug solubility determines its distribution throughout the body.

? Re-Think

1. What is meant by a semipermeable membrane?
2. How does a fat-soluble substance cross the cell membrane? How does a water-soluble substance cross the cell membrane?

INSIDE THE CELL

The inside of the cell is divided into two compartments: the nucleus and the cytoplasm. The inside of the cell resembles the inside of a raw egg; the "yellow yolk" is the nucleus, and the "white" is the cytoplasm.

NUCLEUS

The nucleus is the control center of the cell (see Figure 3-2). In particular, the nucleus contains the genetic information and controls all protein synthesis. Most adult cells have one nucleus; only mature RBCs have no nucleus. Surrounding the nucleus is a double-layered nuclear membrane. The nuclear membrane contains large pores that allow the free movement of certain substances between the nucleus and cytoplasm.

Blood vessel

Red blood cells

Nerve cell

FIGURE 3-1 Cells come in all shapes and sizes.

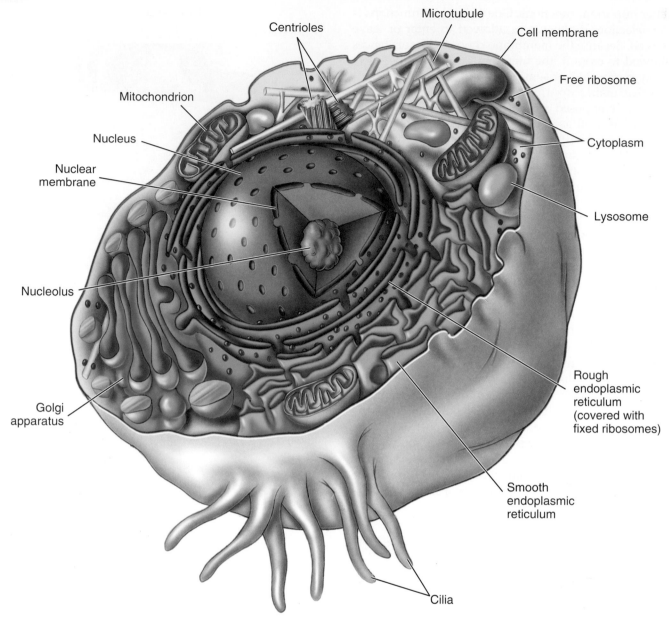

Centrioles

Microtubule

Cell membrane

Free ribosome

Mitochondrion

Nucleus

Cytoplasm

Nuclear
membrane

Lysosome

Nucleolus

Rough
endoplasmic
reticulum
(covered with
fixed ribosomes)

Golgi
apparatus

Smooth
endoplasmic
reticulum

Cilia

FIGURE 3-2 A typical cell.

The nucleus is filled with a fluid substance called *nucleoplasm*. Within the nucleoplasm are two other structures: the nucleolus and chromatin. The nucleolus, or little nucleus, synthesizes ribosomes that move through nuclear pores into the cytoplasm, where they play a role in protein synthesis. The nucleolus also produces a nucleotide necessary for protein synthesis.

Chromatin is composed mainly of strands of DNA (deoxyribonucleic acid), the carriers of the genetic code. In nondividing cells, chromatin appears as a tangled array of fine filaments. In dividing cells, however, chromatin strands coil tightly, forming DNA-containing structures called *chromosomes*. The genetic code and protein synthesis are described more fully in Chapter 4.

? Re-Think

Why is the nucleus called the control center of the cell?

CYTOPLASM

Cytoplasmic Gel

The **cytoplasm**, or the "gel in the cell," is found inside the cell but outside the nucleus (like the white of a raw egg). The cytoplasm contains the cytosol and organelles. The cytosol is the intracellular fluid and is composed primarily of water, electrolytes, proteins, and nutrients. The cytosol also contains inclusion bodies, insoluble materials such as glycogen granules and pigments such as melanin. The **organelles**, or little organs, are dispersed throughout the cytoplasm; each

Table 3-1 Cell Structure and Function

CELL STRUCTURE	DESCRIPTION AND FUNCTION
Cell Membrane	Contains the cellular contents; selects what enters and leaves the cell
Cilia	Hairlike projections that move substances across surface of cell membrane
Flagellum	Single long hair for swimming movement of the sperm
Microvilli	Accordion-like folds in the membrane; increase transport of water and dissolved solute
Nucleus	Control center of the cell; stores genetic information
Chromatin	Threadlike structures in the nondividing cell that contain DNA; chromatin threads form chromosomes in a dividing cell
Nucleolus	Synthesizes RNA and ribosomes
Nucleoplasm	Gel in the nucleus
Nuclear membrane	Separates the nucleoplasm from the cytoplasm
Cytoplasm	Gel located inside the cell but outside the nucleus
Cytosol	Medium composed of water and dissolved solute; organelles suspended in the cytosol
Organelles	Tiny organs suspended in the cytosol
Mitochondria	Site of ATP production; power plants of the cell
Endoplasmic reticulum (ER)	Membranes that form channels for the flow of cellular substances such as proteins
Rough ER	Contains ribosomes where protein is synthesized
Smooth ER	Site of lipid and steroid synthesis; synthesis of glycogen in liver and skeletal muscle
Golgi apparatus	Finishes and packages protein for export
Ribosomes	Site of protein synthesis
Free	Ribosomes that float within the cytosol; make protein used within the cell
Fixed	Ribosomes fixed to the ER, making it appear rough; concerned with the synthesis of protein that is exported
Lysosomes	Intracellular house cleaning, phagocytosis, removal of damaged organelles
Cytoskeleton	Microfilaments and microtubules that provide for intracellular shape, support, and movement
Centrioles	Paired, short, rod-shaped microtubules that form spindles and help separate the chromosomes during mitosis
Inclusion bodies	Temporary insoluble material such as glycogen granules and pigments such as melanin

ATP, Adenosine triphosphate.

organelle has a specific role. Locate the organelles in Figure 3-2 and Table 3-1.

CYTOPLASMIC ORGANELLES

Mitochondria

The mitochondria are tiny, slipper-shaped organelles. The number of mitochondria per cell varies, depending on the metabolic activity of the cell (how hard the cell works). The more metabolically active the cell, the greater the number of mitochondria. The liver, for example, is very active and therefore has many mitochondria per cell. Bone cells are less active metabolically and have fewer mitochondria.

The mitochondrial membrane has two layers (Figure 3-4); the outer layer is smooth, whereas the inner layer has many folds, referred to as *cristae*. The enzymes associated with ATP production are located along the cristae. Because the mitochondria produce most of the energy (ATP) in the body, they are referred to as the "power plants" of the cell. (See Chapter 2 for an

explanation of ATP and Chapter 4 for a description of ATP production.)

Ribosomes

Ribosomes are cytoplasmic organelles involved with protein synthesis. Some ribosomes are attached to the endoplasmic reticulum and are called *fixed ribosomes*. Fixed ribosomes are largely concerned with the synthesis of exportable protein—that is, protein secreted by the cell for use elsewhere in the body. Other ribosomes, called *free ribosomes,* float freely within the cytoplasm and generally synthesize proteins that are used within the cell.

Endoplasmic Reticulum

The endoplasmic reticulum (ER) is a network of membranes within the cytoplasm (see Figure 3-2). These long folded membranes form channels through which substances, especially newly synthesized protein, move. The two types of ER include the type containing

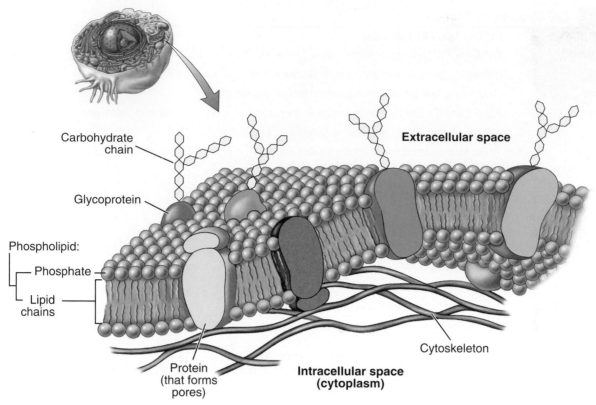

Carbohydrate chain

Glycoprotein

Phospholipid:

Phosphate

Lipid chains

Protein (that forms pores)

Extracellular space

Cytoskeleton

Intracellular space (cytoplasm)

FIGURE 3-3 Structure of the cell membrane.

ribosomes along its surface; it is called *rough endoplasmic reticulum (RER)* because of its rough, sandpaper-like appearance. The RER is primarily concerned with protein synthesis. Protein synthesized along the RER is transported through the channels, and delivered to the Golgi apparatus for further processing. The ER that does not contain ribosomes on its surface appears smooth; it is called *smooth endoplasmic reticulum (SER).* SER is primarily involved with the synthesis of lipids, steroids, glycerides, and glycogen in skeletal muscle and liver cells.

Golgi Apparatus

The Golgi apparatus is a series of flattened membranous sacs (Figure 3-5). Proteins synthesized along the RER are transported to the Golgi apparatus through channels formed by the ER. The Golgi apparatus puts the finishing touches on the protein. For example, a glucose molecule may be attached to a protein within the Golgi apparatus. A segment of the Golgi membrane then wraps itself around the protein and pinches itself off to form a secretory vesicle. In this way, the Golgi apparatus packages the protein. Note that many of the organelles, particularly the ribosomes, ER, and Golgi apparatus, are involved in protein synthesis. (Protein synthesis is described in Chapter 4.)

Lysosomes

Lysosomes are membranous sacs containing powerful enzymes. Lysosomal enzymes break down intracellular waste and debris, including damaged organelles,

and thus help "clean house." Lysosomal enzymes perform several other functions. They participate in the destruction of ingested bacteria, a process called *phagocytosis*. Lysosomes also break down the contractile proteins of inactive muscles. Retired athletes experience a decrease in muscle mass, as do chronically bedridden persons.

Cytoskeleton

The cytoskeleton is composed of threadlike structures called *microfilaments* and *microtubules*. The cytoskeleton helps maintain the shape of the cell and assists the cell in various forms of cellular movement. Cellular movement is particularly evident in muscle cells, which contain large numbers of microfilaments. Microtubules are the primary component of the cytoskeleton. In addition to making the cell strong and rigid, the microtubules anchor the position of the organelles within the cytoplasm. Microtubules also play a key role in cell division; they form the spindle apparatus that helps distribute the chromosomes to opposite ends of the dividing cell. (Cell division is explained in Chapter 4.)

Centrioles

Centrioles are paired, rod-shaped, and short microtubular structures that form the spindle apparatus in a dividing cell. Cells that have no centrioles are incapable of cell division; these include neurons, mature

Mitochondrion

FIGURE 3-4 Mitochondria are the "power plants" of the cells.

RBCs, skeletal muscle cells, and cardiac muscle cells. The cytoplasm surrounding the centrioles is called the *centrosome*. Microtubules of the cytoskeleton begin at the centrosome and spread throughout the cytoplasm.

 Re-Think

1. What is the primary function of the mitochondria?
2. What is the difference between fixed and free ribosomes?
3. What is the difference between the rough and smooth ER?

ON THE CELL MEMBRANE

MICROVILLI

For cells that are particularly involved with the movement of large amounts of water and its dissolved solute, the membrane forms accordion-like folds called *microvilli* (sing., microvillus). The folding of the cell membrane increases surface area, thereby increasing the amount of fluid absorbed. For example, some of the cells in the digestive tract have millions of foldings, called microvilli, to absorb water and the end products of digested food.

CILIA

Cilia are short hairlike projections on the outer surface of the cell membrane. Cilia use wavelike motions to move substances across the surface of the cell. For example, cilia are abundant on the cells that line the respiratory passages. The cilia help move mucus and trapped dust and dirt toward the throat, away from the lungs. Once in the throat, the mucus can be removed by coughing or swallowing. The cilia therefore help clear the respiratory passages. Cigarette smoking damages the cilia and thus deprives the smoker of this benefit.

FLAGELLA

Flagella (meaning whiplike) are similar to cilia in that both are hairlike projections of the cell membrane. Flagella, however, are thicker, longer, and fewer in number; they help move the cell. The tail of the sperm is an example of a flagellum; the tail enables the sperm to swim.

2+2 **Sum It Up!**

The cell is the structural and functional unit of all living matter. Although cells differ considerably, they also share many similarities. The "typical cell" illustrates these similarities. The cell is surrounded by a cell membrane. The inside of the cell is divided into the nucleus, the control center, and the cytoplasm, which contains the cytosol and many little organs, or organelles, each of which has a special task to perform. Table 3-1 lists the organelles and their functions.

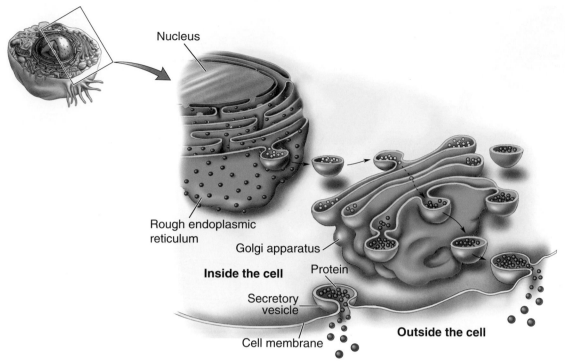

Nucleus

Rough endoplasmic
reticulum

Golgi apparatus

Inside the cell   Protein

Secretory
vesicle

Cell membrane

Outside the cell

FIGURE 3-5 The Golgi apparatus: packages the protein for export.

MOVEMENT ACROSS THE CELL MEMBRANE

Cells are bathed in an extracellular fluid that is rich in nutrients such as oxygen, glucose, and amino acids. These nutrients are needed in the cell and must therefore be able to cross the cell membrane. The cell's waste, which accumulates within the cell, must also be able to cross the cell membrane. Wastes are eventually eliminated from the body.

A number of mechanisms assist in the movement of water and dissolved substances across the cell membrane. The transport mechanisms can be divided into two groups: passive transport and active transport mechanisms. Table 3-2 summarizes both types of transport.

The passive transport mechanisms require no additional energy in the form of ATP. Passive transport is something like the downward movement of a ball (Figure 3-6, *A*). The ball is at the top of the hill. Once released, the ball rolls downhill. The ball does not need to be pushed; it moves passively, without any input of energy. Passive transport mechanisms cause water and dissolved substances to move without additional energy, like a ball rolling downhill.

Active transport mechanisms require an input of energy in the form of ATP. Active transport is like the upward movement of a ball (see Figure 3-6, *B*). For the ball to move uphill, it must be pushed, therefore requiring an input of energy.

PASSIVE TRANSPORT MECHANISMS

The passive mechanisms that move substances across the membrane include diffusion, facilitated diffusion, osmosis, and filtration.

DIFFUSION

Diffusion is the most common transport mechanism. Diffusion is the movement of a substance from an area of higher concentration to an area of lower concentration. For example, a tablet of red dye is placed in a glass of water (Figure 3-7, *A*). The tablet dissolves, and the dye moves from an area where it is most concentrated (glass 1) to an area where it is less concentrated (glasses 2 and 3). Diffusion continues until the dye is evenly distributed throughout the glass. The point at which no further net diffusion occurs (glass 3) is called equilibrium.

The scent of our pet skunk, Perfume, also illustrates diffusion (see Figure 3-7, *B*). Perfume's scent does not take long to permeate the area! Diffusion is involved in many physiological events. For example, diffusion causes oxygen to move across the membrane of an alveolus of the lung into the blood (see Figure 3-7, *C*). Oxygen diffuses from the alveolus because the concentration of oxygen is higher within the alveolus than within the blood. Conversely, carbon dioxide, a waste product that accumulates within the blood, diffuses in the opposite direction (carbon dioxide moves from

Table 3-2 Transport Mechanisms

MECHANISM	DESCRIPTION AND FUNCTION
Passive	
Diffusion	Movement of a substance from an area of high concentration to an area of low concentration
Facilitated diffusion	Helper molecule within the membrane assists movement of substances from area of high concentration to area of low concentration
Osmosis	Diffusion of water (solvent) from an area with more water to an area with less water. The water compartments are separated by a semipermeable membrane.
Filtration	The pushing of water and dissolved substances from an area of high pressure to an area of low pressure; the water and dissolved substances are pushed
Active	
Active transport pump	Moves a substance uphill (from an area of low concentration to an area of high concentration); requires an input of energy (ATP)
Endocytosis Phagocytosis Pinocytosis	Taking in or ingestion of substances by the cell membrane Engulfing of solid particles by the cell membrane (cellular eating) Engulfing of liquid droplets (cellular drinking)
Exocytosis	Secretion of cellular products (e.g., protein, debris) out of the cell

ATP, Adenosine triphosphate.

the blood into the alveolus). The lungs then exhale the carbon dioxide, thereby eliminating waste from the body. Thus, the process of diffusion moves oxygen into the blood and carbon dioxide out of the blood.

FACILITATED DIFFUSION

Facilitated diffusion is a form of diffusion that is responsible for the transport of many substances (*facilitate* means "to help"). As in diffusion, substances move from a higher concentration toward a lower concentration (Figure 3-8). In facilitated diffusion, however, the substance is helped across the membrane by a molecule within the membrane. The helper molecule increases the rate of diffusion. The transport of glucose by facilitated diffusion is illustrated in Figure 3-8 by a boy carrying the glucose. Note that he is moving downhill, indicating that facilitated diffusion is a passive transport process.

Passive (downhill)   Active (uphill)

A   **B**

FIGURE 3-6 Transport mechanisms. **A,** Passive transport mechanism. The ball rolls downhill on its own. **B,** Active transport mechanism. The ball must be pushed uphill using adenosine triphosphate (ATP).

FIGURE 3-7 Diffusion. **A,** Diffusion of a red dye. **B,** Diffusion of Perfume's "perfume." **C,** Diffusion of oxygen and carbon dioxide across the alveolar cell membrane in the lung.

OSMOSIS

Osmosis is a special case of diffusion. Osmosis is the diffusion of water through a selectively permeable membrane. A selectively permeable—or semipermeable—membrane allows the passage of some substances while restricting the passage of others. During osmosis, the water diffuses from an area with more water to one with less. The dissolved substances, however, do not move.

Two different solutions in the glass illustrate osmosis. The glass is divided into two compartments (A and B) by a semipermeable membrane (Figure 3-9). Compartment A contains a dilute glucose solution, whereas compartment B contains a more concentrated glucose solution. The membrane is permeable only to water. The glucose cannot cross the membrane and is therefore confined to its compartment.

During osmosis, the water moves from compartment A to compartment B (from the area where there is more water to the area with less). The following two effects occur: (1) the amount, or volume, of water in compartment B becomes greater than the volume in compartment A; and (2) the concentrations of the solutions in both compartments change. The solution in compartment A becomes more concentrated, whereas the solution in compartment B becomes more dilute.

FIGURE 3-8 Facilitated diffusion.

Because water moves toward the more concentrated solution, it appears to be "pulled" in that direction. Sometimes osmosis is described as a "pulling" pressure. For example, Na⁺ is said to pull or hold water. More correctly stated, water diffuses into the more concentrated saline solution.

Because osmosis causes water to move into a compartment, it can cause swelling. For example, tissue injury causes leakage and accumulation of proteins within the tissue space. The confined proteins act osmotically. Water diffuses toward the protein, causing the tissues to swell, a condition called *edema*.

 Re-Think

What are the driving forces for diffusion, facilitated diffusion, and osmosis?

TONICITY

Tonicity is the ability of a solution to affect the volume and pressure within a cell. Note what happens when a cell is placed in solutions of different concentrations (Figure 3-10). The following three terms are used to illustrate tonicity: *isotonic, hypotonic,* and *hypertonic.*

Isotonic Solution

An isotonic solution has the same concentration as intracellular fluid (*iso* means "same"). Consider an RBC placed in an isotonic solution. Because the solution is isotonic, no net movement of water occurs; the cell neither gains nor loses water.

Hypotonic Solution

If an RBC is placed in pure water (a solution containing no solute), then water moves into the cell by osmosis (from where there is more water to where there is less water). The pure water, being more dilute than the inside of the cell, is said to be

FIGURE 3-9 Osmosis. The effect of osmotically active particles on the movement of water.

hypotonic. Hypotonic solutions cause RBCs to burst, or lyse, in a process referred to as *hemolysis*. Because of hemolysis, pure water is not administered intravenously.

Do You Know...

Why a Blood Clot May Continue to "Grow," Even When the Bleeding Stops?

The components of the blood clot are osmotically active particles. Water therefore diffuses into the blood clot, causing it to enlarge. If the expanding blood clot is located within the brain, it presses on the brain tissue, causing a variety of life-threatening neurological deficits.

A boiled hot dog may also illustrate this bursting effect. The hot dog, which contains a lot of salt, is

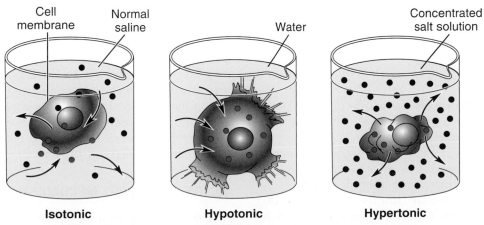

FIGURE 3-10 Effects of osmosis: isotonic, hypotonic, and hypertonic solutions.

boiled in plain water. Because the plain water is hypotonic relative to the hot dog, water diffuses into the hot dog, and it bursts.

Hypertonic Solutions

If an RBC is placed within a very concentrated salt solution, water diffuses out of the RBC into the bathing solution, causing the RBC to shrink, or crenate. The salt solution is referred to as a *hypertonic solution.*

Why is the tonicity of a solution important? If the cell gains water, the RBC membrane bursts. If the RBC loses water, the cell shrinks. In both cases, RBC function is impaired. Isotonic solutions do not cause cells to swell or shrink. While the RBC was used to explain tonicity, other cells respond in the same way. Clinically, isotonic solutions are frequently administered intravenously. Commonly used isotonic solutions include normal saline (0.9% NaCl), 5% D/W (5% dextrose or glucose in water, or D_5W), and Ringer's solution. Under special conditions, hypotonic or hypertonic solutions may be administered intravenously.

 Re-Think

1. Why does the exposure of an RBC to a hypotonic environment cause hemolysis?
2. What is the advantage of administering an isotonic IV solution?

Do You Know...

How to Shrink a Swollen Brain?

This can be done by administering a hypertonic solution (e.g., mannitol) intravenously. Because a hypertonic solution contains more solute than what is present in the interstitial or tissue fluid of the brain, water leaves the brain tissue in response to osmosis and moves into the blood. As the blood is carried away from the brain, brain swelling (cerebral edema) decreases.

FILTRATION

With diffusion and osmosis, water and dissolved substances move across the membrane in response to a difference in concentrations. With **filtration**, water and dissolved substances cross the membrane in response to differences in pressures. In other words, pressure pushes substances across the membrane.

A syringe can illustrate filtration (Figure 3-11). Syringe 1 is filled with water. If a force is applied to the plunger, the water is pushed out through the

FIGURE 3-11 Filtration. **A,** Water is forced through the needle. **B,** Water (H_2O) is forced through the holes in the barrel of the syringe. **C,** Water is forced out of the capillary through holes, or pores.

needle. The water moves in response to a pressure difference, with greater pressure at the plunger than at the tip of the needle. In the second syringe, tiny holes are made in the sides of the barrel. When force is applied to the plunger, water squirts out the sides of the syringe and out the tip of the needle.

Where does filtration occur in the body? The movement of fluid across the capillary wall can be compared with the movement of water in the syringe with holes in its side (syringe 2). A capillary is a tiny vessel that contains blood. The capillary wall is composed of a thin layer of cells with many little pores. The pressure in the capillary pushes water and dissolved substances out of the blood and through the pores in the capillary wall into the tissue spaces. This process is *filtration;* it is movement caused by pushing. (Capillary filtration is further explained in Chapter 19.)

ACTIVE TRANSPORT MECHANISMS

The active transport mechanisms include active transport pumps, endocytosis, and exocytosis.

ACTIVE TRANSPORT PUMPS

Active transport refers to a transport mechanism that requires an input of energy (ATP) to achieve its goal. It is necessary to pump certain substances because the amount of some substances in the cell is already so great that the only way to move additional substances into the cell is to pump them in. For example, the cell normally contains a large amount of potassium ions (K$^+$). The only way to move additional K$^+$ into the cell is to pump it in. To move the K$^+$ from an area of low concentration to an area of high concentration (uphill), energy is invested (Figure 3-12, *A*).

ENDOCYTOSIS

Endocytosis is a transport mechanism that involves the intake of food or liquid by the cell membrane (see Figure 3-12, *B*). In endocytosis, the particle is too large to move across the membrane by diffusion. Instead, the particle is surrounded by the cell membrane, which engulfs it and takes it into the cell. There are two forms of endocytosis. If the endocytosis involves a solid particle, it is called *phagocytosis* (fag-oh-sye-TOH-sis) (*phago-* means "eating"). For example, white blood cells eat, or phagocytose, bacteria, thereby helping the body defend itself against infection. If the cell ingests a water droplet, the endocytosis is called *pinocytosis* (pin-oh-sye-TOH-sis), or "cellular drinking."

EXOCYTOSIS

Whereas endocytosis brings substances into the cells, exocytosis moves substances out of the cells (see Figure 3-12, *C*). For example, the cells of the pancreas make proteins for use outside the pancreas. The pancreatic cells synthesize the protein and wrap it in a membrane. This membrane-bound vesicle moves toward and fuses with the cell membrane. The protein is then expelled from the vesicle into the surrounding space.

A

Endocytosis

B

Exocytosis

C

FIGURE 3-12 Active transport. **A,** The active pumping of potassium ions (K$^+$) into the cell. **B,** Endocytosis. **C,** Exocytosis.

 Sum It Up!

Water and dissolved substances must be able to move across cell membranes. This is achieved through passive and active transport mechanisms. Passive transport mechanisms require no investment of energy (ATP) and include diffusion, facilitated diffusion, osmosis, and filtration. Concentrations of solutions are expressed as tonicity: isotonic, hypotonic, and hypertonic. The active transport mechanisms require an input of ATP and include the active transport pumps, endocytosis (phagocytosis and pinocytosis), and exocytosis.

? Re-Think

Why does an active transport pump require an input of energy?

CELL DIVISION

Cell division is necessary for the body's growth, repair, and reproduction. The frequency of cell division varies considerably from one tissue to the next. Some cells reproduce very frequently, whereas other cells reproduce very slowly or not at all. For example, the cells that line the digestive tract are replaced every few days, and more than 2 million RBCs are replaced every second. Certain nerve cells in the brain and spinal cord, however, do not reproduce at all.

Two types of cell division are mitosis and meiosis. Meiosis occurs only in sex cells and will be discussed in Chapter 26. **Mitosis**, which is involved in bodily growth and repair, is the splitting of one mother cell into two identical "daughter cells." The key word is *identical*. In other words, an exact copy of genetic information, stored within the chromosomes, must be passed from the mother cell to the two daughter cells. Mitosis is described in more detail in the next section ("Cell Cycle").

 Do You Know...

Some Good News About the Aging Older Brain?

Neurons in the brain do not undergo mitosis and therefore do not replicate. Therefore, we have always assumed that there are no "new" brain neurons. Recently, however, new neurons in the brain have been identified, even in older brains. The neurons arise from newly discovered stem cells located in the brain. Brain cell replacement in the aging brain does happen!

CELL CYCLE

The **cell cycle** is the sequence of events that the cell goes through from one mitotic division to the next. The

FIGURE 3-13 Cell cycle: interphase and mitosis.

cell cycle is divided into two major phases: interphase and mitosis (Figure 3-13).

INTERPHASE

During interphase, the cell carries on with its normal functions and gets ready for mitosis through growth and DNA replication. Interphase is divided into three phases: first gap phase (G_1), phase (S), and second gap phase (G_2).

- First gap phase (G_1)—During this phase, the cell carries on its normal activities and begins to make the DNA and other substances necessary for cell division.
- Phase S—During the S phase, the cell duplicates its chromosomes, thereby making enough DNA for two identical cells.
- Second gap phase (G_2)—This phase is the final preparatory phase for cell division (mitosis); it includes the synthesis of enzymes and other proteins needed for mitosis. At the end of G_2, the cell enters the mitotic (M) phase.

MITOSIS

During the mitotic (M) phase, the cell divides into two cells in such a way that the nuclei of both cells contain identical genetic information. Mitosis consists of four phases: prophase, metaphase, anaphase, and telophase (Figure 3-14). During prophase, the chromosomes coil so tightly that they become visible under a light microscope. Each chromosome pair is composed of two identical strands of DNA called *chromatids;* each chromatid is attached at a point called the *centromere.* At the same time, two pairs of centrioles move to opposite poles of the nucleus. Late in prophase, the nuclear membrane disappears. During metaphase, the chromatids are aligned in a narrow central zone; spindle fibers connect the chromatids and centrioles. Anaphase begins when the centromere splits and the chromatids are pulled to opposite poles (end of anaphase). During telophase, each new cell reverts to the interphase state; the nuclear membrane reforms, the chromosomes uncoil, and the chromatin strands reappear. Telophase and cytokinesis mark the end of mitosis. Cytokinesis (sye-toh-kin-EE-sis), which begins in late anaphase, is the pinching of the cell membrane to split the cytoplasm into two distinct cells.

Repeat! Mitosis is a type of cell division that produces two genetically identical daughter cells. How can you remember the stages of mitosis? Think of "*Play Me A Tune*": *p*rophase, *m*etaphase, *a*naphase, *t*elophase.

At the end of mitosis, the daughter cells have two choices. They can enter G_1 and repeat the cycle (and divide again) or they can enter another phase, called *G zero* (G_0) (see Figure 3-13). Cells in G_0 "drop out" of the cell cycle and rest; they do not undergo mitosis. Cells may re-enter the cell cycle after days, weeks, or years. The inability to stop cycling and enter G_0 is

PROPHASE   **METAPHASE**   **ANAPHASE**

TELOPHASE   **DAUGHTER CELLS**

FIGURE 3-14 Stages of mitosis.

characteristic of cancer cells. Cancer cells constantly divide and proliferate. Anticancer drugs are more active against cells that are cycling than against cells resting in G_0. Thus, tumors that contain many cycling cells respond best to chemotherapy.

Anticancer drugs are classified according to the cell cycle phases that they affect. Some anticancer drugs are called *cell cycle phase–specific*. These drugs affect the cell when it is in a particular phase. With the use of this terminology, the anticancer drug methotrexate is considered cell cycle S phase–specific. Other drugs are cell cycle M phase–specific and cell cycle G_2 phase–specific. Some anticancer drugs can act at any phase of the cell cycle and are called *cell cycle phase–nonspecific*. By knowing the cell cycle terminology, you can understand anticancer drugs better.

 Re-Think

1. Explain how interphase prepares the cell for mitosis.
2. What happens during mitosis?

CELL DIFFERENTIATION

Mitosis assures us that the division of one cell produces two identical cells. How do we account for the differences in cells such as muscle cells, RBCs, and bone cells? In other words, how do cells differentiate or develop different characteristics?

An embryo begins life as a single cell, the fertilized ovum. Through mitosis, the single cell divides many times into identical cells. Then, at some time during their development, the cells start to specialize, or **differentiate** (Figure 3-15). One cell, for example, may switch on enzymes that produce RBCs. Other enzymes are switched on and produce bone cells. Regardless of the mechanism, you started life as a single adorable cell and ended up as billions of specialized cells!

What does it mean when a tissue biopsy (surgical removal of tissue for examination) shows many poorly differentiated cells? It means that the tissue cells have failed to differentiate or specialize. In other words, the poorly differentiated cells of a liver tumor do not resemble normal liver cells. Failure to differentiate is characteristic of cancer cells.

STEM CELLS

Stem cells are relatively undifferentiated or unspecialized cells whose only function is the production of additional unspecialized cells. Each time a stem cell divides, one of its daughter cells differentiates while the other daughter cell prepares for further stem cell division. The rate of stem cell division varies with the tissue type; the stem cells within the bone marrow and skin are capable of dividing more than once a day, whereas the stem cells in adult cartilage may remain inactive for years. Stem cell research is of particular interest because of the possibility of replacing damaged tissue and growing new organs. How amazing it would be if newly discovered stem cells could be used to repair a damaged spinal cord or restore the dopamine-secreting cells in the brains of persons with Parkinson's disease. Several years ago, an individual who was paralyzed after a spinal cord injury donated her own stem cells taken from deep within her nose. The stem cells were surgically placed within her spinal cord. The stem cells then differentiated into nerve cells. Although it is too early to claim success, some return of spinal cord function has been reported. Another advance in stem cell research is the development of a new technique that coaxes adult cells to regress to an embryonic state. These undifferentiated cells are called *induced pluripotent stem cells* (iPS cells). The iPS cells can then be induced to specialize into the desired cell type, such as bone, muscle, or blood cells. A major hurdle in

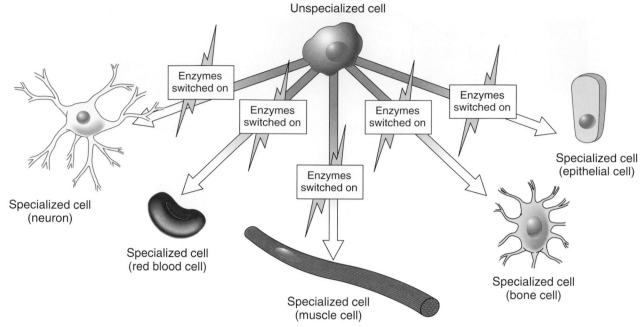

FIGURE 3-15 Cell differentiation.

stem cell research has been the use of embryos as stem cell donors. This technique required the destruction of the embryo, thereby creating an ethical dilemma for many. The development of iPS cells eliminates this issue and hopefully will hasten stem cell research.

? Re-Think

What is the relationship between stem cells and cellular differentiation?

ORDER, DISORDER, AND DEATH

Most cell growth is orderly. Cells normally reproduce at the proper rate and align themselves in the correct positions. At times, however, cell growth becomes uncontrolled and disorganized. Too many cells are produced. This process is experienced by the patient as a lump or tumor (tumor means swelling).

Tumors may be classified as benign (noncancerous) or malignant (cancerous). Cancer cells are appropriately named. *Cancer* means "crab"; cancer cells, like a crab, send out clawlike extensions that invade surrounding tissue. Cancer cells also detach from the original tumor (primary site) and spread throughout the body (secondary sites). Widespread invasion of the body by cancer cells often causes death. The spreading of cancer cells is referred to as *metastasis*.

There is also a programmed sequence of events that leads to cell death called *apoptosis,* or cell suicide. Apoptosis helps rid the body of old, unnecessary, and unhealthy cells. Because the body replaces a million cells per second, the elimination of some cells by apoptosis is necessary. Apoptosis, however, can go into overdrive, causing excessive cellular death and disease.

A Pap smear is a diagnostic procedure used to detect cancer. A sample of cells (a smear) is obtained, usually from around the cervix. The smear is then examined under a microscope for changes that could indicate cancer. A positive Pap smear can indicate cancer in its early stages. Early detection is associated with a very high cure rate.

Sometimes cells are injured so severely that they die, or necrose (from the Greek word *necros,* meaning "death"). For example, the cells may be deprived of oxygen for too long a period, be poisoned, be damaged by bacterial toxins, or suffer the damaging effects of radiation.

2+2 Sum It Up!

The union of the sperm and egg forms a single cell that divides by mitosis into billions of identical cells. The cell cycle is the sequence of events that the cell goes through from one mitotic division to the next. The cell cycle is divided into two phases: the interphase and the mitotic phase. Mitosis splits a cell into two genetically identical cells. There are four stages of mitosis: prophase, metaphase, anaphase, and telophase. The cells then specialize, or differentiate, into many different types of cells, all of which are needed to perform a wide variety of functions. Most cells grow in an orderly way. Cells can, however, grow abnormally. The result is sometimes a tumor, which may be benign or malignant (cancerous).

As You Age

1. All cells show changes as they age. The cells become larger, and their capacity to divide and reproduce tends to decrease.
2. Normal cells have built-in mechanisms to repair minor damage; this ability to carry out repair declines in aging cells.
3. When DNA is damaged, changes in membranes and enzymes occur in the cell. Changes in the transport of ions and nutrients occur at the cell membrane. The chromosomes in the nucleus undergo such changes as clumping, shrinkage, and fragmentation.
4. Certain genetic disorders such as Down syndrome are more common in children born to older women.
5. Organelles such as mitochondria and lysosomes are present in reduced numbers as a person ages. In addition, cells function less efficiently.

Note: The Medical Terminology and Disorders table appears in Chapter 4.

Get Ready for Exams!

Summary Outline

The cell is the structural and functional unit of all living matter.

I. A Typical Cell
- A. Cell membrane (plasma membrane)
  1. Composition: phospholipid bilayer and protein
  2. Semipermeable: selection of nutrients and waste that cross the membrane
  3. Structures on cell membrane: cilia, flagella, microvilli
- B. Structures inside the cell
  1. Nucleus: control center of the cell; stores genetic information and contains chromatin and the nucleolus
  2. Cytoplasm: gel-like substance inside the cell membrane but outside the nucleus; cytosol and organelles
  3. Organelles: in the cytoplasm
  4. Mitochondria: "power plants" of the cell
  5. Ribosomes (free and fixed): concerned with protein synthesis
  6. Endoplasmic reticulum (two types): rough endoplasmic reticulum (RER) and smooth endoplasmic reticulum (SER)
  7. Golgi apparatus: packages and puts the finishing touches on newly synthesized protein
  8. Lysosomes: intracellular "housekeepers"
  9. Cytoskeleton: (microfilaments and microtubules) provides shape and support to the cell
  10. Centrioles: play a role in cell reproduction

II. Movement Across the Cell Membrane: Passive and Active Mechanisms
- A. Passive transport mechanisms
  1. Passive transport mechanisms: require no input of energy (ATP)
  2. Diffusion: causes a substance to move from an area of greater concentration to an area of lesser concentration
  3. Facilitated diffusion: same as diffusion but uses a helper molecule to increase the rate of diffusion
  4. Osmosis: a special case of diffusion using a semipermeable membrane; involves diffusion of water from an area with more water to an area of less water
  5. Concentrations of a solution expressed as tonicity; solutions are isotonic, hypotonic, or hypertonic
  6. Filtration: movement of water and dissolved substances from an area of high pressure to an area of low pressure
- B. Active transport mechanisms
  1. Active transport: requires an input of energy (ATP)
  2. Active transport pumps: move substances from an area of low concentration to an area of high concentration
  3. Endocytosis: moves substances into a cell; pinocytosis: cellular "drinking"; phagocytosis: cellular "eating"
  4. Exocytosis: moves substances out of a cell

III. Cell Division
- A. Mitosis: produces two identical cells
- B. Meiosis: occurs only in sex cells

IV. Cell Cycle
- A. Interphase (G_1, S, and G_2 phases)
- B. Mitosis (M phase)
  1. The splitting of one mother cell into two identical daughter cells
  2. Four phases of mitosis: prophase, metaphase, anaphase, and telophase
  3. A cell can exit from the cell cycle and enter G_0 (resting).
- C. Cell cycle phase–specific and phase-nonspecific drugs
  1. Some drugs aim at specific phase of cell cycle.
  2. Some drugs are cell cycle phase–nonspecific.

V. Cell Differentiation: From Stem Cells to Specialized Cells

VI. Order, Disorder, and Death

Review Your Knowledge

Matching: Cell Structure
Directions: Match the following words with their descriptions below.

a. mitochondria
b. endoplasmic reticulum
c. ribosomes
d. cilia
e. lysosomes
f. nucleus
g. cytoplasm

1. ___ Control center of the cell; contains the DNA
2. ___ Short hairlike projections on the outer surface of the cell
3. ___ Power plants of the cell; most ATP made here
4. ___ Classified as rough and smooth
5. ___ These organelles are attached to the endoplasmic reticulum; involves protein synthesis
6. ___ Digestive organelles that engage in phagocytosis; intracellular "house cleaning"
7. ___ Gel in the cell (outside the nucleus)

Matching: Transport and Tonicity
Directions: Match the following words with their descriptions below. Some words may be used more than once.

a. hypotonic
b. diffusion
c. pinocytosis
d. isotonic
e. hypertonic
f. osmosis
g. filtration
h. facilitated diffusion
i. exocytosis

1. ___ Pressure gradient is the driving force for this type of passive transport.
2. ___ Passive transport mechanism whereby glucose is "helped" across the membrane by a helper molecule within the membrane
3. ___ Protein-containing vesicle within a cell fuses with the cell membrane and ejects the protein
4. ___ Called "cellular drinking"
5. ___ An example of this transport mechanism is the swelling of a blood clot as water is pulled into the clot.
6. ___ Describes a solution that is more concentrated than the inside of a cell
7. ___ Solution that causes a red blood cell to swell with water and burst
8. ___ Solution that has the same concentration as the inside of a red blood cell
9. ___ Drop of red dye is added to beaker of water; in 2 hours, the beaker of water is uniformly colored red.
10. ___ Because of its salt concentration, normal saline is considered this.

Multiple Choice

1. The selectively permeable membrane
   a. permits filtration but not diffusion or osmosis.
   b. determines which substances enter and leave the cell.
   c. allows for the unrestricted movement of water and electrolytes across the cell membrane.
   d. permits diffusion but not osmosis.

2. Which of the following is not true of the mitochondria?
   a. Numbers of mitochondria reflect the metabolic activity of the cell.
   b. Mitochondria are the organelles that make most of the body's ATP.
   c. Mitochondria are located in the cytoplasm.
   d. Mitochondria are the sites of protein synthesis.

3. Which of the following is an incorrect statement regarding the cellular organelles?
   a. Most ATP is produced in the mitochondria.
   b. Lysosomes contain potent enzymes that digest cellular waste and debris.
   c. Most DNA is located within the Golgi apparatus.
   d. The RER is concerned with protein synthesis.

4. A beaker contains two compartments. Compartment A contains a 20% glucose solution and compartment B contains a 5% glucose solution. The membrane is permeable to water, but impermeable to glucose. Which statement is true at equilibrium?
   a. The volume in A is greater than the volume in B.
   b. The volume in A is less than the volume in B.
   c. The volume remains the same in both compartments.
   d. Glucose diffuses from A to B.

5. With regard to the cell cycle,
   a. the M phase is the same as interphase.
   b. cells cannot enter phase G_0 when they complete the cycle.
   c. cell division occurs during the M phase.
   d. prophase, metaphase, anaphase, and telophase occur during phase G_1.

6. The blood pressure forces water and dissolved solute out of the capillaries into the tissue space. This process is called
   a. osmosis.
   b. active transport.
   c. pinocytosis.
   d. filtration.

7. What might happen if pure water were administered intravenously (directly into the blood via the veins)?
   a. The patient becomes dehydrated.
   b. The red blood cells undergo hemolysis.
   c. The red blood cells lose volume and shrink.
   d. The water dilutes the blood; water is "pulled" into the capillaries from the tissue spaces.

Go Figure

1. **According to Figures 3-1 and 3-2**
   a. All cells look like the "typical cell."
   b. The ER and Golgi apparatus are membranous cytoplasmic organelles.
   c. All ribosomes are attached to the ER and are concerned with protein synthesis.
   d. The nucleus is separated from the cytoplasm by an impermeable nuclear membrane.

2. **According to Figures 3-2, 3-3, and 3-4**
   a. Ribosomes are present on all endoplasmic reticulum.
   b. The Golgi apparatus is located within the nucleus; it "packages" protein for expulsion from the cell.
   c. The cell membrane is composed exclusively of phospholipids.
   d. Mitochondria are organelles that generate ATP.

3. **According to Figures 3-6 and 3-7**
   a. Gases cannot diffuse.
   b. Diffusion and facilitated diffusion are represented by Figure 3-6, *B*.
   c. Beaker 2 in Figure 3-7, *A*, represents equilibrium.
   d. Oxygen diffuses from the sacs (alveoli) in the lungs into the blood.

4. **According to Figures 3-6 and 3-9**
   a. Osmosis and filtration are represented by Figure 3-6, *B*.
   b. Equilibrium cannot be achieved if the volumes in the beaker are unequal.
   c. To achieve the results in Figure 3-9, the membrane must be impermeable to the solute.
   d. Solute concentration has no effect on osmosis.

5. **The transport in Figure 3-12**
   a. Occurs in a manner that is consistent with Figure 3-6, *A*.
   b. Is the same as the transport mechanism described in Figure 3-8.
   c. Only involves the movement of a substance into the cell.
   d. Can move a solute against its gradient.

6. **According to Figures 3-13 and 3-14**
   a. The cell rests when it enters interphase.
   b. The M phase consists of the G_1 phase, S phase, and G_2 phase.
   c. The cell divides during the M phase.
   d. The cell is most active during the G_0 phase.

Key Terms

aerobic catabolism (p. 50)
amino acids (p. 54)
anabolism (p. 48)
anaerobic catabolism (p. 50)
base pairing (p. 57)
base sequencing (p. 57)
carbohydrates (p. 48)

catabolism (p. 48)
deoxyribonucleic acid (DNA) (p. 56)
gluconeogenesis (p. 51)
glucose (p. 48)
glycogen (p. 50)
glycolysis (p. 50)
lipids (p. 52)

metabolism (p. 48)
monosaccharides (p. 48)
peptide bond (p. 55)
protein (p. 54)
ribonucleic acid (RNA) (p. 57)

Objectives

1. Define *metabolism*, *anabolism*, and *catabolism*.
2. Explain the use of carbohydrates in the body, and differentiate between the anaerobic and aerobic metabolism of carbohydrates.
3. Explain the use of fats in the body.

4. Explain the use of proteins in the body.
5. Describe the roles of DNA and RNA in protein synthesis, the structure of a nucleotide, and the steps in protein synthesis.

To carry on its function, the cell, like a factory, must bring in and use raw material. The raw material comes from the food we eat and includes carbohydrates, protein, and fat. Once inside the cell, the raw materials undergo thousands of chemical reactions. The cellular processing of the raw materials is called *metabolism*.

METABOLISM

Metabolism can be divided into two parts: anabolism and catabolism (Figure 4-1).

Anabolism (ah-NAB-oh-liz-em) includes reactions that build larger, more complex substances from simpler substances, such as the building of a large protein from individual amino acids. The process is similar to the building of a brick wall from individual bricks. Anabolic reactions generally require an input of energy in the form of adenosine triphosphate (ATP).

Catabolism (kah-TAB-oh-liz-em) includes reactions that break down larger, more complex substances into simpler substances, such as the breakdown of a large protein into individual amino acids. This process is similar to the knocking down of a brick wall. Catabolism releases energy that is converted into ATP and used to "run" the body.

CARBOHYDRATES

We have all eaten sugars and starchy food. Bread, potatoes, rice, pasta, and jelly beans are some of our favorite foods. These are all carbohydrates. **Carbohydrates** are organic compounds composed of carbon (C), hydrogen (H), and oxygen (O). Carbohydrates are classified according to size (Figure 4-2). **Monosaccharides** (mon-oh-SAK-ah-rides) are single (mono) sugar (saccharide) compounds. *Disaccharides* (dye-SAK-ah-rides) are double (di) sugars, and *polysaccharides* (pahl-ee-SAK-ah-rides) are many (poly) sugar compounds. The shorter monosaccharides and disaccharides are called *sugars*, and the longer chain polysaccharides are called *starches*. The carbohydrates are listed in Table 4-1.

MONOSACCHARIDES

Monosaccharides are sugars containing three to six carbons. The six-carbon simple sugars include glucose, fructose, and galactose. **Glucose** is the most important of the three and is used by the cells as an immediate source of energy.

There are also five-carbon monosaccharides; they include ribose and deoxyribose. These sugars are used in the synthesis of ribonucleic acid (RNA) and deoxyribonucleic acid (DNA).

FIGURE 4-1 Metabolism. **A,** Raw materials to run the factory. **B,** Anabolism. **C,** Catabolism.

DISACCHARIDES

Disaccharides are double sugars and are made when two monosaccharides are linked together. The disaccharides include sucrose (table sugar), maltose, and lactose; they are present in the food we eat. They must be digested, or broken down, into monosaccharides before they can be absorbed across the walls of the digestive tract and used by the cells.

POLYSACCHARIDES

Polysaccharides are made of many glucose molecules linked together. Some are linked together in straight

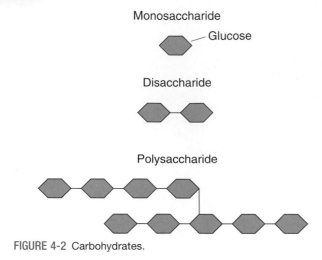

Monosaccharide

Glucose

Disaccharide

Polysaccharide

FIGURE 4-2 Carbohydrates.

chains, and others in branched chains. The three polysaccharides of interest to us are plant starch, animal starch (glycogen), and cellulose.

Starch is the storage polysaccharide in plants. It is a series of glucose molecules linked together in a branched pattern. Starchy foods such as potatoes, peas, grains, and pasta contain this type of starch and are part of our healthy diet.

Glycogen (GLYE-koh-jen) is also called animal starch and is a highly branched polysaccharide. Glycogen is the form in which humans store glucose; these glucose molecules are joined together in long branched chains called *glycogen*. Glycogen is stored primarily in the liver and skeletal muscle. Glycogen performs two important roles. First, glycogen stores help regulate blood sugar. When blood sugar levels become low, the glycogen in the liver is converted to glucose and released into the blood, where it restores normal blood sugar levels. When blood glucose increases after a meal, the excess glucose is converted in the liver to glycogen for storage. Second, glycogen acts as storage energy in skeletal muscle. When muscle contractile activity increases, as in running, glycogen is converted to glucose and burned as fuel.

Cellulose is a straight-chain polysaccharide found in plants. Although humans do not have the enzymes to digest cellulose as a source of nutrients, this polysaccharide plays an important role in our digestive process. The cellulose provides the fiber in our diet and improves digestive function.

? Re-Think

1. What is the relationship between glucose and glycogen?
2. Where is most glycogen stored?
3. How does glycogen help in the regulation of blood glucose levels?

USES OF GLUCOSE

What about that mound of jelly beans, those oval globs of sugar that you just ate? The jelly beans are eaten, digested, and absorbed. Then what? Glucose is used by the body in three ways: (1) it can be burned immediately as fuel for energy; (2) it can be stored as glycogen and burned as fuel at a later time; and (3) it can be stored as fat and burned as fuel at a later time. The "stored as fat" phrase is the most distressing!

THE BREAKDOWN OF GLUCOSE

Glucose is broken down under the following two conditions: (1) in the absence of oxygen (the process is called anaerobic catabolism); and (2) in the presence of oxygen (this process is called aerobic catabolism). In the absence of oxygen, glucose is broken down through a series of chemical reactions, first into pyruvic acid and then into lactic acid. This anaerobic process occurs in the cytoplasm and is called glycolysis (glye-KOHL-i-sis) (Figure 4-3, *A*). Because most of the energy is still locked up in the lactic acid molecule, glycolysis produces only a small amount of ATP.

If oxygen is available, glucose is completely broken down to form carbon dioxide, water, and ATP (see Figure 4-3, *B*). The glucose is first broken down to pyruvic acid in the cytoplasm. The pyruvic acid molecules then move into the mitochondria—the power plants of the cell. In the presence of oxygen and special enzymes in the mitochondria, the pyruvic acid

Table **4-1**	Carbohydrates
NAME	**FUNCTION**
Monosaccharides (Simple Sugars)	
Glucose	Most important energy source
Fructose	Converted to glucose
Galactose	Converted to glucose
Deoxyribose	Sugar in DNA
Ribose	Sugar in RNA
Disaccharides (Double Sugars)	
Sucrose	Splits into monosaccharides (glucose + fructose)
Maltose	Splits into monosaccharides (glucose + glucose)
Lactose	Splits into monosaccharides (glucose + galactose)
Polysaccharides (Many Sugars)	
Starches	Found in plant foods; digested to monosaccharides
Glycogen	Animal starch; excess glucose stored in liver and skeletal muscle
Cellulose	Nondigestible by humans; forms dietary fiber or roughage

DNA, Deoxyribonucleic acid; *RNA*, ribonucleic acid.

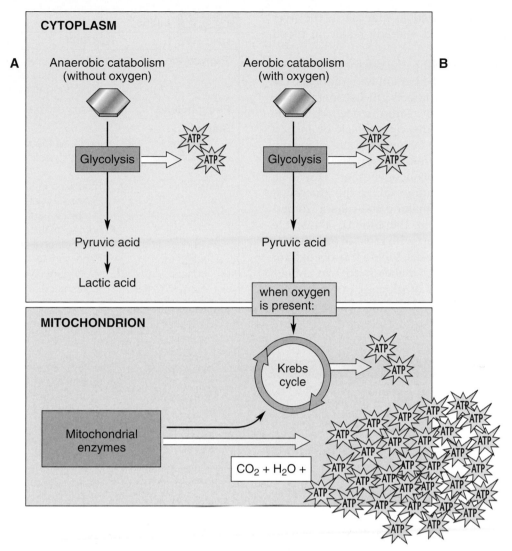

FIGURE 4-3 Breakdown of glucose. **A,** Anaerobic catabolism, to lactic acid and little ATP. **B,** Aerobic catabolism, to carbon dioxide, water, and lots of ATP.

fragments are completely broken down to carbon dioxide and water. This process is accompanied by the release of a large amount of energy (ATP). Two sets of enzymes exist in the mitochondria: the enzymes of the Krebs cycle and the enzymes of the electron transport chain. Both sets of enzymes work together to produce ATP aerobically.

Three important points about aerobic catabolism should be considered. First, the chemical reactions occurring in the mitochondria require oxygen. If the cells are deprived of oxygen, they soon become low in energy and cannot carry out their functions. This need for oxygen is the reason we need to breathe continuously—to ensure a continuous supply of oxygen to the cells. Second, when glucose is broken down completely to carbon dioxide and water, all the stored energy is released. Some of the energy is transferred to ATP, and the rest is released as heat. Thus, the aerobic breakdown of glucose produces much more ATP than the anaerobic breakdown of glucose. Third,

if oxygen is not available to the cell, the pyruvic acid cannot enter the mitochondria. Instead, the pyruvic acid is converted to lactic acid in the cytoplasm. The buildup of lactic acid is the reason that a lack of oxygen in a critically ill patient causes lactic acidosis.

THE MAKING OF GLUCOSE

As we have seen, glucose can be broken down in the cells as a source of energy. The body requires a constant supply of glucose for fuel. Dietary carbohydrates provide glucose, as does the conversion of glycogen into glucose. In addition, the body is capable of making glucose from noncarbohydrate substances. Protein, for example, can be broken down and the breakdown products used to make glucose. The making of glucose from nonglucose sources, especially protein, is called *gluconeogenesis*. **Gluconeogenesis** (gloo-koh-nee-oh-JEN-eh-sis) is an important mechanism in the regulation of blood sugar. For example, if blood sugar declines, protein is converted to glucose in the liver and released into the blood, thereby restoring blood sugar to normal.

Clinical conditions affecting glucose metabolism are common. For instance, in the person with diabetes, the lack of the insulin hormone affects glucose metabolism in two ways. First, because insulin is needed for the transport of glucose into the cell, a lack of insulin deprives the cells of glucose. Second, the lack of insulin causes body protein to be broken down and then converted into glucose (gluconeogenesis). However, because the diabetic cells cannot utilize the glucose, it accumulates in the blood, making the person hyperglycemic (excess glucose in the blood). Thus, the person with diabetes ends up with most of the glucose in the blood and not in the cells, where it is needed for energy. Drugs used to treat diabetes do two things: they increase the transport of glucose into the cells, and they suppress gluconeogenesis by the liver. Both effects lower blood glucose.

? Re-Think

Define gluconeogenesis. What purpose is served by gluconeogenesis?

2+2 Sum It Up!

The body, like a factory, requires raw material for growth, repair, and operation. The raw materials for the body come in the form of food: carbohydrates, proteins, and fats. Metabolism refers to the millions of chemical reactions that make the body run. Anabolic reactions are involved in the synthesis of complex substances from simpler substances. Catabolic reactions break down complex substances into simpler substances, generally in an effort to liberate energy stored within the food substances. Carbohydrates and fats are the body's primary fuel. Glucose can be broken down and used as fuel in two ways: anaerobically (glycolysis), yielding little ATP, and aerobically, within the mitochondria (Krebs cycle and electron transport chain enzymes), yielding large amounts of ATP. In addition to the consumption of dietary carbohydrates, glucose can also be made from the breakdown products of protein by a process called *gluconeogenesis*.

LIPIDS (FATS)

Lipids are organic compounds that are commonly called *fats* and *oils*. Fats are solid at room temperature whereas oils are liquid. Most of the lipids are eaten as fatty meats, egg yolks, dairy products, and oils. The lipids found most commonly in the body include triglycerides, phospholipids, and steroids. Other relatives of lipids, called *lipoid substances,* are listed in Table 4-2.

The building blocks of lipids are fatty acids and glycerol. The lipid illustrated in Figure 4-4, *A,* is a triglyceride (try-GLI-ser-ride). It has three (tri)

Table **4-2** Lipids	
LIPID TYPE	**FUNCTION**
Triglyceride	In adipose tissue: protect and insulate body organs; major source of stored energy
Phospholipid	Found in cell membranes
Steroid	
Cholesterol	Used in synthesis of steroids
Bile salt	Assist in digestion and absorption of fats
Vitamin D	Synthesized in skin on exposure to ultraviolet radiation; contributes to calcium and phosphate homeostasis
Hormones from adrenal cortex, ovaries, testes	Adrenal cortical hormones are necessary for life and affect every body system; ovaries and testes secrete sex hormones
Lipoid substances	
Fat-soluble vitamins (A, D, E, K)	Variety of functions (identified in later chapters)
Prostaglandins	Found in cell membranes; affect smooth muscle contraction
Lipoproteins	Help transport fatty acids; high-density lipoprotein (HDL) is "good cholesterol" and low-density lipoprotein (LDL) is "bad cholesterol"

long chains of fatty acids attached to one small glycerol molecule. A phospholipid is formed when a phosphorus-containing group attaches to one of the glycerol sites (see Figure 4-4, *B*). Phospholipids are important components of the cell membrane. (Do not confuse glycerol with glycogen.)

The steroid is a third type of lipid. The most important steroid in the body is cholesterol (see Figure 4-4, *C*).

Although cholesterol is consumed in the diet, the body can also synthesize cholesterol in the liver. In fact, most of our cholesterol is made by the liver from saturated fat. This observation raises an interesting point regarding the dietary control of cholesterol. The dietary intake of a healthy diet results in only a slight increase in blood cholesterol, whereas the dietary intake of saturated fats (meat, eggs, cheeses) accounts for a significant increase of blood cholesterol as it is used by the liver to synthesize cholesterol. Thus, the focus of dietary control of blood cholesterol is the restriction of saturated fats. Despite all the bad press about it, cholesterol performs several important functions. For example, cholesterol is found in all cell membranes and is necessary for the synthesis of vitamin D in the skin. It is also used in the ovaries and testes in the synthesis of the sex hormones.

A

Triglyceride

B **Phospholipid**

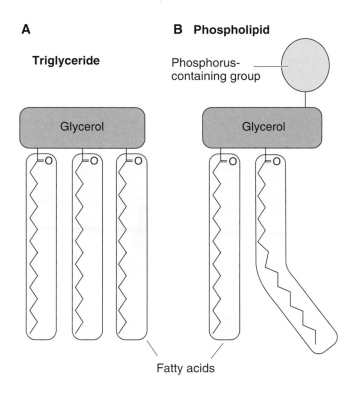

Phosphorus-
containing group

Fatty acids

C   **Steroid (cholesterol)**

FIGURE 4-4 Lipids.

Phospholipid
covering

Lipid core

Cholesterol
+
Triglycerides

Receptors

There are six major classes of lipoproteins, but we will describe only three: very low-density lipoprotein (VLDL), low-density lipoprotein (LDL), and high-density lipoprotein (HDL). This classification is based on the density, which is determined by the percentage composition of lipid and protein. Protein is more dense than lipid. Thus, lipoproteins that have a greater proportion of protein than lipid have a relatively high density. Conversely, lipoproteins with a lower percentage of protein have a lower density.

VERY LOW-DENSITY LIPOPROTEIN (VLDL)

VLDLs contain mostly triglycerides and little cholesterol as the core lipid; the triglycerides in VLDL account for almost all the triglycerides in the blood. The role of VLDLs is to transport triglycerides to adipose tissue and muscle. It is unclear about the role of VLDLs in heart disease, but marked elevations cause pancreatitis. The degradation of VLDLs produces LDLs.

LOW-DENSITY LIPOPROTEIN (LDL)

LDLs contain cholesterol as the core lipid and account for most (60%–70%) of the cholesterol in the blood. The role of LDLs is to deliver cholesterol to nonhepatic (nonliver) tissue. Cells of the target tissues have membrane receptors that recognize and bind to LDLs; on binding, the cholesterol is ingested by the cells by endocytosis. Of all lipoproteins, LDLs make the greatest contribution to atherosclerotic heart disease and are therefore called "bad" cholesterol. The goal of drug therapy for coronary heart disease is to decrease LDL levels.

There are a number of drugs that reduce LDLs. The most effective drugs are the "statins," such as lovastatin and pravastatin. The statins reduce LDLs by decreasing the hepatic synthesis of cholesterol and increasing the number of receptors on the liver cells (hepatocytes). The increased number of hepatic receptor sites increases the elimination of cholesterol into the bile. Because cholesterol synthesis is greater at night, the statins are generally administered at bedtime. Also, statins target the liver and hepatotoxicity may therefore develop as an adverse drug reaction. Other cholesterol- or triglyceride-lowering drugs do so by decreasing the formation of VLDLs, the producers of LDLs.

HIGH-DENSITY LIPOPROTEIN (HDL)

HDLs contain cholesterol as the primary core lipid and account for 20% to 30% of all cholesterol in the blood. HDLs carry cholesterol from the peripheral tissues to the liver for excretion into the bile. Thus, HDLs promote the removal of cholesterol from the blood. Unlike LDLs, which increase the risk of coronary heart disease, elevation of HDLs reduces the risk. Because HDLs are cardioprotective, they are called "good" cholesterol. Adherence to dietary guidelines, weight reduction, and exercise elevate HDLs.

Ramp It Up!

Cholesterol, Triglycerides, and Lipoproteins

Cholesterol and triglycerides are lipids that we love to hate, often for very good reason. Both have been implicated in coronary artery heart disease. Cholesterol and triglycerides are lipids and therefore are not soluble in water. Both, however, must be transported by the blood, a water (or aqueous) solution. How is the solubility problem solved? Enter the lipoproteins! They make the cholesterol and triglycerides soluble in water. Read on.

LIPOPROTEINS

A lipoprotein has a basic lipid-soluble core composed of cholesterol and triglycerides, surrounded by a single layer of phospholipid. It is the phospholipid coat that makes the lipid water-soluble. In addition to increasing the solubility of the lipid core, the phospholipid layer contains receptors. These receptors play a role in the delivery and excretion of cholesterol and triglycerides.

USES OF LIPIDS

What about the bacon you ate for breakfast? There is good news and bad news. The good news is that lipids are needed by the body (1) as a source of energy, (2) as a component of cell membranes and myelin sheath (coverings of nerve cells), and (3) in the synthesis of steroids. The bad news is that fat can be put into long-term storage. Fat can make you fat! It can also be deposited in areas where it is not wanted, such as inside your blood vessels. Many people develop hypercholesterolemia (excess cholesterol in the blood), a condition associated with the development of coronary artery disease. Cholesterol-related fatty plaques develop in the walls of the blood vessels (coronary arteries) that supply the heart. Over time, the plaques block the flow of blood to the heart, resulting in the death of heart muscle (commonly called a heart attack).

 Re-Think

1. What is a triglyceride?
2. Why is it unwise to feed an infant only "fat-free" milk?

METABOLISM OF LIPIDS

Like glucose, fatty acids and glycerol can be broken down in order to release the stored energy. Because the fatty acids are long structures, however, they must be chopped into tiny units before entering the mitochondria and being catabolized within the Krebs cycle. The aerobic burning of the fatty acid units in the mitochondria releases a huge amount of energy that is captured as ATP. Because the fatty acids are much longer than the glucose molecules, the amount of energy released in the burning of fatty acids is much greater than the amount released in the burning of glucose.

Do You Know...

That Griz Does Not Urinate during His Hibernating Months?

Nature encourages the grizzly bear ("Griz") to overeat and gain weight. By doing so, Griz is able to hibernate during the winter months because he can live off the fat stored during the summer feeding frenzy. While hibernating, the bear's fat is gradually broken down, and the energy that is released is sufficient to keep him alive.

What, then, about the waste produced by his metabolizing body? The bear has apparently developed the metabolic ability to convert his waste (urea) into a substance that can be used by the body. He literally recycles his urine. An understanding of this recycling process would certainly benefit the many persons who require dialysis because of kidney failure.

MAKING FAT

Like Griz, we too can go on a feeding frenzy and gain pound after pound! However, we do not hibernate and therefore do not easily shed those excess pounds. The extra donut eaten today is worn on your hip tomorrow. When excess calories are consumed, the hormones and enzymes that promote fat synthesis are stimulated. The fat is deposited in adipose tissue throughout the body.

PROTEINS

Protein is the most abundant organic matter in the body. Because proteins are present in so many physiologically important compounds, it is safe to say that they participate in every body function. For example, almost every chemical reaction in the body is regulated by an enzyme, which is a protein substance. Most hormones are proteins; they exert important widespread effects throughout the body. Hemoglobin, which delivers oxygen to every cell in the body, is a protein. Finally, muscles contract because of their contractile proteins. As you can see, proteins are essential to life.

AMINO ACIDS

The building blocks of protein are **amino acids**. About 20 amino acids are used to build body protein. Most amino acids come from protein foods, especially lean meat, milk, and eggs. More than half of the amino acids can be synthesized by the body. If the diet lacks the amino acid alanine, for example, alanine can be synthesized in the liver.

Some amino acids, however, cannot be synthesized by the body and must be obtained from dietary sources. Because dietary intake of these amino acids is essential, these amino acids are called *essential amino acids*. The amino acids that can be synthesized by the liver are called *nonessential amino acids*, meaning that these amino acids are not absolutely necessary in the diet. See Box 4-1 for a list of common amino acids.

Box 4-1	Common Amino Acids
Alanine	Leucine*
Arginine	Lysine*
Asparagine	Methionine*
Aspartic acid	Phenylalanine*
Cysteine	Proline
Glutamic acid	Serine
Glutamine	Threonine*
Glycine	Tryptophan*
Histidine*	Tyrosine
Isoleucine*	Valine*

*Essential amino acids.

NOTE: The word *nonessential* does not mean that these amino acids are not essential to the body. The term refers to the ability of the body to synthesize these amino acids when they are not included in the diet.

Like carbohydrates and lipids, amino acids are composed of carbon, hydrogen, and oxygen. In addition to these three elements, amino acids also contain nitrogen. The nitrogen appears as an amine group (NH_2). At the other end of the amino acid is the acid group (—COOH); hence, the name *amino acid*. Note the amine group and the acid group in Figure 4-5, *A*; the amino acid alanine is used as an example.

Amino acids are joined together by peptide bonds. A **peptide bond** is formed when the amine group (NH_2) of one amino acid joins with the acid group (—COOH) of a second amino acid. A peptide is formed when several amino acids are joined together by peptide bonds (see Figure 4-5, *B*). A polypeptide is formed when many amino acids are joined together. Proteins are very large polypeptides. Most proteins are composed of more than one polypeptide chain. The polypeptide chains are curly and coil around each other, creating a large and uniquely shaped protein. The amino acid sequence, and the size and shape of the protein are important to its function. If the amino acids are not assembled in the correct order, the shape of the protein changes and its function is impaired. For example, in sickle cell anemia, only one of the amino acids is "out of order " in the hemoglobin protein, the major component of a red blood cell. The improperly constructed hemoglobin causes the red blood cells to sickle and break apart.

Proteins can bond with other organic compounds. For example, the combination of a sugar and a protein forms a glycoprotein, whereas the combination of a lipid and protein creates a lipoprotein.

? Re-Think

1. What is the difference between an essential and nonessential amino acid?
2. Why do peptide bonds form between amino acids and not between glycogen molecules?

USES OF PROTEINS

Proteins are used in three ways. The most important use is in the synthesis of hormones, enzymes, antibodies, plasma, muscle proteins, hemoglobin, and most cell membranes. In one way or another, proteins play a key role in every physiological function. The various types of proteins and their functions are listed in Table 4-3. With such a large demand for protein, most of the amino acids are carefully conserved by the body and used in the synthesis of protein.

Proteins have two less common uses. First, protein can be broken down and used as fuel, as a source of energy for ATP production. This process, however, is not desirable. The preferred energy sources are glucose and fat. Second, protein can be broken down and converted to glucose (gluconeogenesis). This mechanism is used by the body to ensure that the blood glucose level does not become too low to sustain life. In severe starvation, the body catabolizes its own protein, including the heart muscle, in order to survive.

? Re-Think

What is the most important use of amino acids?

BREAKDOWN OF PROTEIN AND THE PROBLEM WITH AMMONIA

Because amino acids contain nitrogen, as well as carbon, hydrogen, and oxygen, the breakdown of

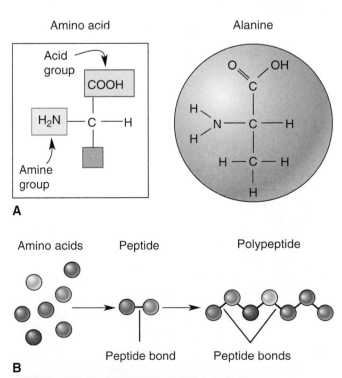

FIGURE 4-5 Amino acids and proteins. **A,** The structure of an amino acid (alanine). **B,** The assembly of amino acids to form a polypeptide. Note the peptide bonds.

protein poses a special problem. Carbon, hydrogen, and oxygen can be broken down into carbon dioxide and water and eliminated from the body. The nitrogen part of the amino acid, however, must be handled in a special way, primarily by the liver. Nitrogen is either recycled and used to synthesize different amino acids or converted to urea and excreted.

Formation of Urea

Some of the nitrogen released by the breakdown of amino acids is converted to urea by the liver (Figure 4-6). Note the nitrogen in the structural formula of urea. Blood then carries the urea, a nitrogenous waste, from the liver, where it is made, to the kidneys, where it is eliminated in the urine. This is important clinical information and forms the basis for several diagnostic tests.

Worrying About Ammonia. Why does the liver "worry" about ammonia? Under normal conditions, the liver extracts ammonia (NH_3) from the blood and converts it to urea. Why? Ammonia is toxic to brain cells and causes disorientation and a diminished level of consciousness. In liver failure, the extraction of ammonia from the blood is diminished, so blood levels of ammonia rise. The toxic effect of ammonia on the brain is called *hepatic encephalopathy* (heh-PAT-ik en-sef-al-OP-eh-thee). A diagnostic test called the *blood urea nitrogen* (BUN) test measures the amount of urea in the blood. A change in BUN can be caused from either poor liver function (cannot make urea) or poor kidney function (cannot excrete it).

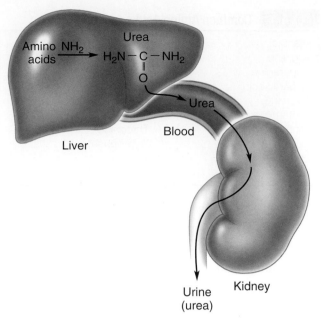

FIGURE 4-6 Urea: formation in the liver and excretion by the kidney.

? Re-Think

1. Why is urea production so important?
2. What happens if a damaged liver is unable to make urea?
3. Why may an elevated BUN indicate poor kidney function?

2+2 Sum It Up!

There are three types of lipids: triglycerides, phospholipids, and steroids. Cholesterol is the most important steroid. Lipids are used in the synthesis of cell membranes and steroids and in the storage of energy; they are catabolized as fuels. Amino acids are used primarily in the synthesis of body proteins: hormones, enzymes, antibodies, plasma proteins, and structural components of cells. Amino acids join together by peptide bonds, whereby the amine group ($-NH_2$) of one amino acid joins with the acid group ($-COOH$) of a second amino acid. In addition to carbon, hydrogen, and oxygen, the catabolism of proteins produces nitrogen that is toxic to the brain. The hepatic (liver) production and renal (kidney) excretion of the nitrogenous waste, urea, is the biochemical solution to ammonia (NH_3) toxicity.

PROTEIN SYNTHESIS AND DNA

Proteins play a crucial role in every body function. Protein synthesis involves the arrangement of amino acids in a specific sequence. Because the sequencing of amino acids is so precise, there is an elaborate protein-synthesizing mechanism in each cell. How does the cell know the exact pattern of amino acid assembly? The pattern of amino acid assembly is coded and stored in the **deoxyribonucleic** (de-OX-see-rye-boh-noo-KLAY-ik) **acid (DNA)** in the nucleus. In fact, the essential role of DNA is to serve as a code for the structure of protein.

Table 4-3   Proteins

TYPE	FUNCTION
Structural proteins	
Components of cell membranes	Perform many functions: determine pore size; allow hormones to "recognize" cell
Collagen	Structural component of muscle and tendons
Keratin	Part of skin and hair
Peptide hormones	Many hormones are proteins; have widespread effects on many organ systems (e.g., insulin, growth hormone)
Hemoglobin	Transports oxygen
Antibodies	Protect body from disease-causing microorganisms
Plasma proteins	Used in blood clotting, fluid balance, and defense against disease
Muscle proteins	Enable muscles to contract
Enzymes	Regulate the rates of chemical reactions

DNA STRUCTURE

DNA is a nucleic acid. Nucleic acids are composed of smaller units called *nucleotides* (Figure 4-7, *A*). A nucleotide has three parts: a sugar, a phosphate group, and a base. Nucleotides are joined together to form long strands. Two strands of nucleotides are arranged in a twisted ladder formation (the double helix) to form DNA (see Figure 4-7, *B*). The two sides of the DNA ladder are composed of sugar and phosphate molecules. The rungs, or steps, of the ladder are composed of bases, one base from each side. The names of the bases in DNA are adenine (A), cytosine (C), guanine (G), and thymine (T). Note the different shapes of the bases in the rungs of the ladder. Note also that the bases have a particular arrangement. Adenine can pair only with thymine, and cytosine can pair only with guanine. Adenine and thymine are base pairs, as are cytosine and guanine. This system is called **base pairing**.

THE GENETIC CODE

The protein-synthesizing code is stored within the DNA. More specifically, the information is stored, or encoded, within the sequence of bases along one strand (one side of the ladder) of DNA (Figure 4-8). Because the DNA is arranged in hereditary units called *genes*, the code is called the *genetic code*. (Genes and heredity are discussed further in Chapter 27.)

Reading the Code

A single strand of DNA (see Figure 4-8) reads vertically (according to the bases in the rungs), such as GAC-GCCCAA. GAC (a sequence of three bases) codes for a particular amino acid, GCC codes for another amino acid, and CAA codes for a third amino acid. The list of bases in triplicate is called **base sequencing**. In this way, DNA codes for the proper sequence of amino acids and therefore the synthesis of protein.

NOTE: Do not confuse base pairing with base sequencing. *Base pairing* describes the way in which two strands of DNA are linked together by the bases. *Base sequencing* describes the sequence, or order, of the bases along a single strand of DNA. The code is stored within the sequence of bases.

Copying the Code: mRNA

The code for protein synthesis is stored in the nucleus in the DNA. DNA does not leave the nucleus because it is too large to fit through the pores of the nuclear membrane. Protein synthesis, however, occurs along the ribosomes in the cytoplasm. The big question? How does the code get out of the nucleus and into the cytoplasm? The copying and delivery of the code is done by a second nucleic acid called **ribonucleic** (rye-boh-noo-KLAY-ik) **acid (RNA)**.

A

FIGURE 4-7 **A,** Nucleotide. **B,** The ladder structure of DNA. Note the base pairing of the DNA strands.

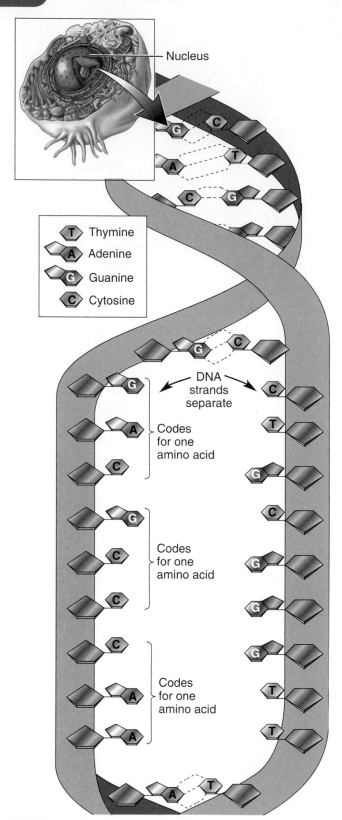

FIGURE 4-8 DNA: genetic code and base sequencing.

| Thymine |
| Adenine |
| Guanine |
| Cytosine |

Legend symbols: **T** Thymine, **A** Adenine, **G** Guanine, **C** Cytosine

Nucleus

DNA strands separate

Codes for one amino acid

Codes for one amino acid

Codes for one amino acid

Table **4-4**	Comparison of DNA and RNA Structures	
	DNA	**RNA**
Sugar	Deoxyribose	Ribose
Base	Adenine	Adenine
	Guanine	Guanine
	Cytosine	Cytosine
	Thymine	Uracil
Strands	Double (two)	Single (one)

RNA is a nucleic acid composed of nucleotides and resembles the structure of DNA. RNA differs from DNA in three ways:

1. The sugars are different. The sugar in DNA is deoxyribose, whereas the sugar in RNA is ribose.
2. DNA has two strands, whereas RNA has only one strand.
3. There is a difference in one of the bases. Both DNA and RNA contain cytosine (C), guanine (G), and adenine (A). The fourth base differs. DNA contains thymine (T), whereas RNA contains uracil (U). The uracil in RNA forms a base pair with adenine. The differences between DNA and RNA are summarized in Table 4-4.

There are three types of RNA, but we are concerned only with messenger RNA (mRNA) and transfer RNA (tRNA). Messenger RNA copies the code from DNA in the nucleus and then carries the code, or message, to the ribosomes in the cytoplasm. Because this type of RNA acts as a messenger, it is called *mRNA*.

Transfer RNA (tRNA) is found attached to individual amino acids within the cytoplasm and, through its own base sequencing, can "read" the code on the mRNA sitting on the ribosome. Each individual amino acid is carried by tRNA to its proper site on the mRNA. The amino acids are assembled in the proper sequence as the polypeptide (protein) is formed.

mRNA as Copycat

Refer to Figure 4-8 as we see how mRNA copies the code. DNA separates and exposes the base sequences, GACGCCCAA. A strand of mRNA reads the base sequence by forming base pairs. The strand of mRNA has this code: CUGCGGGUU. (The mRNA is not shown.) The copying of the code by mRNA is called *transcription*.

NOTE: Transcription is a base-pairing event. Following transcription, the mRNA takes the code to the ribosomes in the cytoplasm, where the amino acids will be assembled.

? Re-Think

1. List three differences between DNA and RNA.
2. What is the difference between base pairing and base sequencing?

Do You Know...

What Are Purines and Pyrimidines, and Why Are Cancer Drugs Aimed at Them?

The bases in the nucleotides that make up DNA and RNA are classified as either purines or pyrimidines. Adenine and guanine are purines, and cytosine, thymine, and uracil are pyrimidines. This terminology is important to know because some anticancer drugs are called *purine analogs* and others *pyrimidine analogs*. This means that the drugs resemble purines and pyrimidines. When incorporated in the DNA or RNA molecules, the drugs introduce errors into the genetic code, impair protein synthesis, and kill the cancer cell. Unfortunately, the drugs are also incorporated into many normal cells, thereby causing their death and producing many of the toxic effects of cancer therapy. No wonder these anticancer drugs are classified as cytotoxic agents; they are toxic to both cancer and normal cells.

STEPS IN PROTEIN SYNTHESIS

How do DNA and RNA control protein synthesis? See Figure 4-9 and identify the following five steps in protein synthesis:

1. When a particular protein is to be synthesized, the strands of DNA in the nucleus separate. The exposed sequence of bases on the separated DNA strand is copied onto a strand of mRNA (transcription).
2. The mRNA leaves the nucleus and travels to the ribosomes in the cytoplasm.
3. The code on the mRNA (now sitting on a ribosome) determines which amino acids can attach to it. For example, the code may specify that only the amino acid alanine can bind to site 1 and only the amino acid cysteine can bind to site 2.

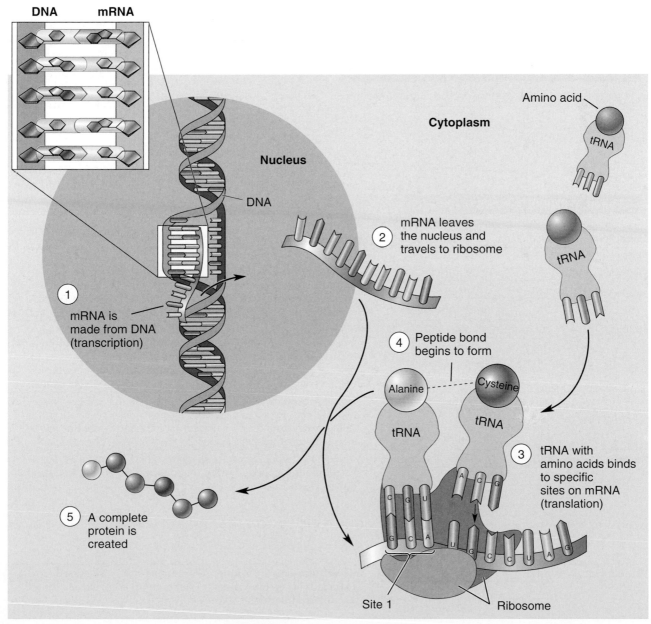

FIGURE 4-9 Steps (1 to 5) in protein synthesis.

How does alanine (located in the cytoplasm) know that it should move to the ribosome for protein assembly? Alanine is attached to tRNA. The tRNA contains bases, a sequence called its *anticodon*, that can recognize and pair with the bases on mRNA. For example, if mRNA contains the base sequence GCA, then only a tRNA with the base sequence (anticodon) of CGU can attach to that site. The reading of the mRNA code by tRNA is called *translation*. Like transcription (nucleus), translation (cytoplasm–ribosomes) is a base-pairing event.

4. The amino acids are lined up in proper sequence along the ribosome. A peptide bond forms between each amino acid, creating a growing peptide chain.

5. When all the amino acids have been assembled in the exact sequence dictated by the code, the protein chain is terminated. A complete protein has been created. The protein is now ready for use in the cell or for export to another site outside the cell.

? Re-Think

What is the difference between transcription and translation?

2+2 Sum It Up!

Body structure and function are largely determined by the specific proteins synthesized by the cells. Because of the crucial roles played by proteins, an elaborate cellular mechanism guides the assembly of the amino acids into proteins. Your protein blueprint, or genetic code, is stored in the DNA in the nucleus. When there is need for protein synthesis, the code must be transferred to the ribosome by mRNA, where amino acid assembly takes place. Protein synthesis occurs in five steps (see Figure 4-9).

🍂 As You Age

1. Age brings a decrease in the number and function of organelles such as mitochondria. Because mitochondria play a key role in metabolism, a decrease in mitochondrial function affects metabolism.

2. In general, metabolism slows with aging. This effect is a result of a decrease in hormonal secretion, particularly the thyroid hormones. A decreased metabolism has several effects: less tolerance to cold, a tendency to gain weight, and metabolic effects, such as a decreased efficiency in using glucose.

3. The rate of protein synthesis decreases. Tissue growth and repair slow down, as does the synthesis of other proteins, such as digestive enzymes.

👤 MEDICAL TERMINOLOGY AND DISORDERS   Cell Function and Disorders of the Cell

Medical Term	Word Parts	Word Part Meaning or Derivation	Description
Words			
anaerobic	an-	without	An **anaerobic** reaction occurs in the absence of oxygen. For example, lactic acid is produced by the anaerobic metabolism of glucose. **Aerobic** (with oxygen) catabolism of glucose is more efficient with regard to energy (ATP) production.
	-aer/o-	air or gas	
	-ic	pertaining to	
cytology	cyt/o-	cell	Broadly, **cytology** is *a branch of biology concerned with the study of cell structure and function.* From the medical perspective, cytology is a branch of pathology that is concerned with the diagnosis of disease and disorders through examination of tissue samples. The Pap smear is a **cytological** examination used to detect cancer.
	-logy	study of	
endocytosis	endo-	within	"Cellular drinking" is a type of **endocytosis** that moves water into the cell. *The ejection of a digestive enzyme from a pancreatic cell* is called **exocytosis** (ex/o = outside), or the movement of the enzyme out of the cell.
	-cyt/o-	cell	
	-osis	condition of	
gluconeogenesis	gluc/o-	sugar, glucose	A diabetic is hyperglycemic (elevated blood glucose), in part, because of **gluconeogenesis,** the making of new glucose from a nonglucose source.
	-neo-	new	
	-gen/o-	origin, production	
glycolysis	glyc/o-	sugar, glucose	**Glycolysis** is *the anaerobic breakdown (catabolism) of glucose to lactic acid.*
	-lysis	break down, dissolution	
intracellular	intra-	within	**Intracellular** (intra = within) refers to *the space inside a cell.* **Extracellular** (extra = outside) refers to *the space outside the cell.* The **intercellular** (inter = between) space is *the space between the cells.*
	-cell-	cell	
	-ar	pertaining to	

MEDICAL TERMINOLOGY AND DISORDERS   Cell Function and Disorders of the Cell—cont'd

Medical Term	Word Parts	Word Part Meaning or Derivation	Description
isotonic	iso-	*same* with regard to stretch of the membrane	An **isotonic** (same stretch) **solution** is *a solution that does not cause a change in cell volume or pressure.*
	-ton/o-	tension	
	-ic	pertaining to	
metabolism	meta-	beyond	**Metabolism** includes all of the enzymatic reactions needed to run the body. It includes **anabolism** (ana = up, and a Greek word meaning "to throw") and **catabolism** (cat = down, and a Greek word meaning "to throw").
	-bol-	From a Greek word, *ballein,* meaning "to throw"	
	-ism	condition of	
monosaccharide	mono-	one	Glucose is a **monosaccharide,** or *a simple sugar.* Sucrose is table sugar, or a **disaccharide** (di = two). Glycogen is a **polysaccharide** (poly = many).
	-saccharide	From a Greek word meaning "sugar"	
synthesis	syn-	together, with	**Synthesis** means *the putting together of simpler substances to make a larger, more complex substance.*
	-thesis	From a Greek word meaning "to put"	
transport	trans-	across	**Transport** means *to carry from one place to another.* Most water and dissolved solute is transported by diffusion.
	-port	From a Latin word meaning "to carry"	

Disorders
Adaptive Cellular Changes

atrophy	a-	without	*A cellular adaptive process that results in a decrease in the size of a tissue or organ caused by a decrease in the number of cells or a reduction in cell size.* Numerous causes: resulting from a disease such as muscular dystrophy; diminished blood supply, muscle inactivity, nutritional deficiency, and the natural aging process.
	-troph-	development; nourishment	
	-y	condition of	
hypertrophy	hyper-	excessive	*An increase in the size (not number) of cells.* **Hypertrophy** is *a response to increased workload.* Lifting weights hypertrophies arm and shoulder muscles.
	-troph-	development	
	-y	condition of, process	
hyperplasia	hyper-	excessive	*An increase in the number of cells caused by an increase in cell division.* There is compensatory and hormonal hyperplasia. An increase in the number of liver cells subsequent to the removal of part of the liver is an example of **compensatory hyperplasia.** The uterine response to estrogen is an example of **hormonal hyperplasia.**
	-plasia	formation	
metaplasia	meta-	beyond, after, change	*A reversible cellular transformation (from one cell type to another).* Cigarette smoking can cause the transformation of columnar epithelium into squamous epithelium; cessation of smoking can reverse the cellular change.
	-plasia	formation	

Maladaptive Cellular Changes

dysplasia	dys-	faulty	*A maladaptive cellular disorder in which the cells show evidence of abnormal differentiation, resulting in changes in cell size, shape, and appearance.* Dysplasias, such as cervical dysplasia, are considered malignant precursors.
	-plasia	formation	
anaplasia	ana-	up; apart	*A serious maladaptive (mal = bad) cellular change.* Cells are poorly differentiated (immature and embryonic). Anaplastic cell growth is characteristic of malignant (cancerous) cells.
	-plasia	formation	

Get Ready for Exams!

Summary Outline

To carry on its functions, the cell must metabolize carbohydrates, proteins, and fats.

I. Metabolism
  A. Anabolism: chemical reactions that build more complex substances from simpler substances
  B. Catabolism: chemical reactions that break down complex substances into simpler substances

II. Carbohydrates: Structure and Function
  A. Carbohydrates: composed of carbon, hydrogen, and oxygen; classified as monosaccharides, disaccharides, and polysaccharides
  B. Glucose: the primary source of energy
  C. Glucose: can be stored as glycogen or converted to and stored as fat
  D. Glucose: can be catabolized anaerobically and aerobically. Anaerobically, glucose is incompletely broken down (glycolysis) into lactic acid and small amounts of ATP. Aerobically, glucose is broken down completely (Krebs cycle) into carbon dioxide (CO_2) and water (H_2O) and large amounts of energy (ATP).
  E. Glucose: can be synthesized from nonglucose substances such as protein; called gluconeogenesis

III. Lipids
  A. Most common lipids are triglycerides, phospholipids, and steroids.
  B. Cholesterol: the most important steroid; made soluble by lipoprotein; called "good" and "bad"
  C. Lipids: used primarily in the synthesis of membranes and fuel
  D. Long fatty acid chains: broken down into two-carbon units and metabolized by the enzymes of Krebs cycle and electron transport chain enzymes to CO_2 and H_2O, releasing large amounts of energy (ATP)

IV. Proteins
  A. Proteins: composed of amino acids linked together by peptide bonds in a specific sequence
  B. Proteins: used primarily in the synthesis of hormones, enzymes, antibodies, plasma proteins, muscle proteins, hemoglobin, and cell membranes; also used as fuel and for gluconeogenesis
  C. Urea synthesis: special handling of protein nitrogen by enzymes in the liver

V. Protein Synthesis and DNA
  A. DNA (deoxyribonucleic acid)
    1. DNA: stores the code for protein synthesis
    2. DNA: double-stranded series of nucleotides, arranged in a twisted ladder formation
    3. Nucleotide: composed of a sugar, a phosphate group, and a base. For DNA, the sugar is deoxyribose; the bases are adenine, thymine, cytosine, and guanine.
    4. Genetic code: stored in a sequence of three bases
    5. Base pairs with DNA and RNA

  B. RNA
    1. Ribonucleic acid (RNA): similar structure to DNA, with the following differences. In RNA, the sugar is ribose, RNA is single-stranded, and the RNA bases are adenine, uracil, cytosine, and guanine.
    2. Two types of RNA: messenger RNA (mRNA) and transfer RNA (tRNA)
    3. Transcription: DNA and mRNA (occurs within nucleus)
    4. Translation: mRNA and tRNA (occurs within cytoplasm/ribosomes)
  C. Protein synthesis: five steps, summarized in Figure 4-9

Review Your Knowledge

Matching: Carbohydrates, Proteins, and Fats
Directions: Match the following words with their descriptions below. Some words may be used more than once.
  a. glycogen
  b. amino acids
  c. lipids
  d. urea
  e. monosaccharides
  f. glucose
  g. disaccharides
  h. fatty acids and glycerol

  1. ___ Nitrogen-containing waste product
  2. ___ Building blocks of proteins
  3. ___ Classification of steroids and triglycerides
  4. ___ Sucrose, maltose, and lactose
  5. ___ Monosaccharide that is chief fuel for the body
  6. ___ Building blocks held together by peptide bonds
  7. ___ Building blocks of lipids
  8. ___ Storage form of glucose
  9. ___ Glucose, fructose, and galactose
  10. ___ Animal starch stored in the liver and skeletal muscles

Matching: Biochemistry Terms
Directions: Match the following words with their descriptions below. Some words may be used more than once.
  a. glycolysis
  b. Krebs cycle and electron transport chain enzymes
  c. gluconeogenesis
  d. enzyme
  e. ketone bodies

  1. ___ Series of aerobic reactions that occur within the mitochondria
  2. ___ Series of anaerobic reactions that occur within the cytoplasm
  3. ___ Process of converting protein to glucose
  4. ___ Catalyst
  5. ___ Series of reactions that convert glucose to lactic acid
  6. ___ Metabolic consequence of rapid and incomplete breakdown of fatty acids

Matching: Genetic Code and Protein Synthesis

Directions: Match the following words with their descriptions below.

a. mRNA
b. ribose
c. base pairing
d. DNA
e. base sequencing

1. ___ Double-stranded nucleotide that stores the genetic code
2. ___ The manner in which the genetic code is stored
3. ___ The manner whereby one strand of a nucleotide interacts with another
4. ___ Single-stranded nucleotide that brings the code from the nucleus to the ribosomes
5. ___ A sugar used in the formation of a nucleotide

Multiple Choice

1. Which of the following is true of the Krebs cycle and electron transport chain enzymes?
   a. Are located within the mitochondria
   b. Function anaerobically
   c. Result in lactic acid production
   d. Are responsible for glycolysis
2. Which of the following is not characteristic of glycolysis?
   a. Occurs within the cytoplasm
   b. Operates anaerobically
   c. Forms lactic acid
   d. Completely metabolizes glucose to CO_2, H_2O, and energy
3. Which of the following is not characteristic of urea?
   a. Formed in the liver
   b. Contains nitrogen
   c. Characterized as an essential amino acid
   d. Excreted by the kidneys
4. Which of the following is not true of amino acids?
   a. Joined together by peptide bonds
   b. The building blocks of protein
   c. Classified as monosaccharides, disaccharides, and polysaccharides
   d. Classified as essential and nonessential
5. Monosaccharides
   a. include glucose, fructose, and galactose.
   b. include sucrose, lactose, and maltose.
   c. are classified as saturated and unsaturated.
   d. are the building blocks of protein.
6. Which of the following is descriptive of glycogen?
   a. Can be converted to glucose, thereby elevating the blood glucose level
   b. Combines with three fatty acids to form a lipid
   c. Contains nitrogen
   d. Is a disaccharide

Go Figure

1. **According to Figure 4-3**
   a. Most ATP is generated by glycolysis.
   b. Glycolysis is an aerobic catabolic pathway.
   c. Under aerobic conditions, the end products of glycolysis enter the mitochondria where they are completely metabolized to CO_2, water, and ATP.
   d. Figure 4-3, *A*, illustrates glycolysis, whereas Figure 4-3, *B*, illustrates gluconeogenesis.

2. **According to Figure 4-3, *A***
   a. Pyruvic acid is aerobically metabolized to lactic acid.
   b. Lactic acid is generated under anaerobic conditions.
   c. Lactic acid is produced within the mitochondrion under aerobic conditions.
   d. Mitochondrial ATP production is dependent on the production of lactic acid.

3. **According to Table 4-2 and Figure 4-4**
   a. Cholesterol and adrenal cortical hormones are steroids.
   b. All lipoid substances are steroids.
   c. All cholesterol is "bad."
   d. Glycerol, an alcohol, can only combine with long-chain fatty acids.

4. **According to Box 4-1 and Figure 4-5**
   a. All amino acids in Box 4-1 contain an $-NH_2$ and $-COOH$ group.
   b. All amino acids in Box 4-1 are essential.
   c. The only amino acids that form peptide bonds are alanine and phenylalanine.
   d. Peptide bonds form when the $-COOH$ group of one amino acid combines with the $-COOH$ group of a second amino acid.

5. **According to Figure 4-6**
   a. Urea is a nitrogen-containing waste product produced in the kidney.
   b. Urea is transported from the kidneys to the liver, where it is excreted into the bile and eliminated from the body.
   c. Urea is produced in the liver and excreted by the kidneys in the urine.
   d. Urea is produced in the blood and excreted by both the liver and the kidneys.

6. **According to Figures 4-7 and 4-8 and Table 4-4**
   a. mRNA is double-stranded.
   b. The base sequence codes for an amino acid.
   c. The rung of the DNA ladder is formed by sugar–phosphate bonds.
   d. The base sequence CAA codes for the entire hemoglobin protein.

7. **According to Figures 4-7 and 4-8**
   a. Cytosine can base-pair with thymine.
   b. Adenine can base-pair with thymine.
   c. Structurally, adenine resembles thymine more than it resembles guanine.
   d. Thymine can base-pair with both adenine and guanine.

8. **According to Figure 4-9**
   a. mRNA is transcribed from DNA in the nucleus.
   b. DNA is transcribed from mRNA in the nucleus.
   c. mRNA cannot leave the nucleus.
   d. The assembly of amino acids into peptide strands occurs in the nucleus.

9. **According to Figure 4-9**
   a. The assembly of amino acids occurs along the ribosomes in the cytoplasm.
   b. mRNA carries the genetic code from the nucleus to the ribosomes in the cytoplasm.
   c. Translation involves the base pairing between mRNA and tRNA in the cytoplasm.
   d. All of the above are true.

Microbiology Basics

Key Terms

bacteria (p. 65)
carrier (p. 72)
fungus (p. 67)
helminths (p. 68)
infection (p. 64)

normal flora (p. 65)
nosocomial infection (p. 71)
parasites (p. 67)
pathogens (p. 64)
protozoa (p. 67)

rickettsia (p. 67)
spores (p. 66)
sporozoa (p. 67)
vector (p. 68)
viruses (p. 67)

Objectives

1. Define *disease* and *infection*.
2. List the characteristics of the different types of pathogens, including the types of bacteria by shape.
3. Describe the types of bacteria by staining characteristics.

4. Define portals of exit and portals of entry.
5. List common ways by which infections are spread.
6. Identify the microbiological principles described in Five Germ-Laden Stories.

For as long as humans have roamed the earth, we have been plagued by disease, especially infectious disease. A long and colorful history of medicine relates many tales of how we learned to dose, purge, lance, and incant. Sometimes we managed to arrest and cure the disease, but many times we killed the patient long before we killed the germs. The battle against disease is far from over. The microbial warriors are tough; they mount a great offensive and are very persistent! Although we may not tremble at the thought of the Black Death that terrorized Europe in the 1300s, we tremble at the thought of other plagues around today, as well as those that can erupt tomorrow. We are living through the terror of acquired immunodeficiency syndrome (AIDS), and we dread an outbreak of avian or swine flu, the contamination of a minor abrasion with flesh-eating streptococcus, and the possibility of contracting mad cow disease, of all things! What about the new generation of life-threatening "super bugs" that are resistant to all antibiotics? This chapter provides background information about microbiology—the world of microorganisms, those tiny critters that keep scientists glued to their microscopes. Chapter 21 describes the body's response to this microbial challenge.

diseases, diseases caused by nutritional deficiencies, tumors, and diseases related to trauma and environmental toxins. This chapter focuses on infectious disease. Although most microorganisms are harmless or even beneficial to the body, some are harmful, causing disease and sometimes death. A leading cause of disease in humans is the invasion of the body by pathogens, or disease-producing microorganisms. The invasion of the body by a pathogen and the symptoms that develop in response to this invasion are called an infection. A localized infection is restricted to a small area, whereas a systemic infection is more widespread throughout the body. A systemic infection is spread by the blood; it affects the entire body and generally makes you feel sick. With regard to a wound, there is often an attempt to differentiate between colonization and infection. Colonization means that the microorganism is present but is not causing illness. Infection means that the microorganism is present and is causing illness. Obviously, a wound that is colonized may eventually become infected. Table 5-1 describes several key terms used in discussing microbiology.

? Re-Think

Differentiate between a local and systemic infection.

WHAT IS DISEASE?

Disease is a failure of the body to function normally. There are many types of diseases, not all caused by germs. These include inherited diseases, diseases caused by birth defects, age-related degenerative

TYPES OF PATHOGENS

The groups of microorganisms (some of which are pathogens) are bacteria, viruses, fungi, and protozoa. Other larger, disease-causing organisms include worms and arthropods (Figure 5-1).

Table 5-1	Key Microbiological Terms
TERM	**DEFINITION**
Antibiotic	Chemical used to treat bacterial infections. A broad-spectrum antibiotic destroys many different types of bacteria, whereas a narrow-spectrum antibiotic destroys only a few types.
Communicable disease	Any disease that can be spread from one host to another. A noncommunicable disease is an infectious disease that cannot be transmitted directly or indirectly from host to host. For example, a bladder infection caused by *Escherichia coli* cannot be spread from the infected person to another person. A contagious disease is a communicable disease that is easily spread from one person to another. Measles and chickenpox are contagious diseases because they are easily spread.
Commensal	Organisms living in a harmonious and beneficial relationship with each other. The organisms derive nutritional or other environmental benefits from the other. Commensal bacteria are part of the normal flora.
Epidemic disease	A disease acquired by many people in a given area over a short period. An endemic disease is always present in a population. A pandemic is a worldwide epidemic.
Epidemiology	The study of the occurrence and distribution of a disease in a population.
Incubation period	The lapsed period of time from the exposure of a person to a pathogen to the development of the symptoms of the disease.
Normal flora	A group of microorganisms that colonize a host without causing disease. Normal flora colonize the mouth, intestinal tract, vagina, nasal cavities, and other areas of the body. Microorganisms that are not pathogenic in one area may become pathogenic when transferred to another area. For example, when the *E. coli* bacterium that is part of the normal flora of the large intestine is unintentionally transferred to the urinary bladder, it causes a bladder infection. Some body fluids such as blood, urine, and cerebrospinal fluid are sterile and do not have a normal flora.
Nosocomial infection	A hospital-acquired infection.
Reservoir of infection	A continual source of infection. A reservoir of infection can be living organisms such as humans and other animals; nonliving objects are substances that are contaminated with the pathogen. A contaminated nonliving object is called a *fomite*, such as a dirty glass and used needles. Contaminated soil and water also serve as inanimate reservoirs of infection.
Resistance	The ability to ward off diseases. A lack of resistance is called *susceptibility*.
Sterilization	A process that destroys all living organisms.
Vector	A carrier of pathogens from host to host. The mosquito is the animal vector carrying the plasmodium (malaria) to humans. A contaminated syringe is a nonliving vector (fomite).

MICROORGANISMS (MICROBES)

Bacteria (sing., bacterium) are single-celled organisms found everywhere. They were first observed under the microscope by van Leeuwenhoek, who called them "little beasties." Most bacteria consider living conditions within the human body to be ideal, so they move right in. The good news is that many bacteria perform useful roles. For example, **normal flora** (organisms that normally and harmoniously live in or on the human body without causing disease) prevents the overgrowth of other organisms, keeping them under control. Some bacteria synthesize needed substances such as vitamin K. The bad news is that bacteria can also cause disease; in fact, bacteria make up the largest group of pathogens. When bacteria successfully invade the human body, they cause damage in two ways: (1) by entering and growing in the human cell; and (2) by secreting toxins that damage the cells.

Bacteria are classified into three groups based on shape: (1) coccus (round); (2) bacillus (rod-shaped); and (3) curved rod. Rickettsiae and chlamydiae are also classified as bacteria, although they differ in several important ways from cocci, bacilli, and curved rods.

The cocci are round cells and are arranged in patterns. Cocci that are arranged in pairs are called diplococci (dip-loh-KOHK-eye). Streptococci (strep-toh-KOHK-eye) are arranged in chains, like a chain of beads. Staphylococci (staf-il-oh-KOHK-eye) look like bunches of grapes and are arranged in clusters. The cocci cause many diseases, including gonorrhea, meningitis, and pneumonia. The bacilli (bah-SIL-ee) are long and slender and are shaped like a cigar. Diseases caused by bacilli include tetanus, diphtheria, and tuberculosis. The curved rods include the vibrio, the spirillum (spy-RIL-um), and the spirochete (SPY-ro-keet). The vibrios have a slight curve and resemble a comma. Cholera is caused by a vibrio (*Vibrio cholerae*). The spirillum is a long cell that coils like a corkscrew. Tightly coiled spirilla that are capable of waving and

FIGURE 5-1 Pathogens: microorganisms and larger disease-causing organisms.

twisting motions are called spirochetes. The most famous spirochete, *Treponema pallidum*, causes syphilis. Syphilis has been around for centuries. Its origin, if nothing else, is colorful. The French called syphilis the Italian disease and, of course, the Italians reciprocated, calling it the French disease. The Polish referred to it as the German disease and—you guessed it—the Germans called it the Polish disease! Regardless of its origin, syphilis is well traveled.

Do You Know...

What Maria, Sophia, and Leah Have in Common?

"Hey! Maria, Sophia, and Leah ... y'all got gonorrhea," shouts their main squeeze. Mr. Busy has just been informed that he has gonorrhea, a sexually transmitted infection caused by *Neisseria gonorrhoeae*. As the girls now know, gonorrhea is highly contagious. Today has been hectic for our carrier, Mr. B. He began treatment with the antibiotic ciprofloxacin and is currently burning up the phone lines informing his sexual partners (called *contacts* in public health jargon) of probable and almost certain infection. It is crucial that all four be treated for gonorrhea to prevent the "ping-pong effect": treatment and cure, followed by reexposure and reinfection. By this time next week, Maria, Sophia, and Leah should also be taking ciprofloxacin and sitting at home in front of the flat-screen contemplating the definition of "safe sex."

No one is "clapping," as in days of old, when the infected were welcomed home by the clapping sounds of their shipmates (hence the nickname "clap" for gonorrhea).

Do You Know...

That Lues, Lues Is Not a Hit Tune?

"Lues, Lues" sounds like an oldie-but-goody hit tune. In fact, it is an oldie, but definitely not a goody. Lues refers to syphilis. Lesions associated with syphilis are referred to as *luetic lesions*. Got lues? "Singin' nothing but the blues ..."

There are two clinically important characteristics of bacteria: (1) the presence of a cell wall and (2) the ability to form spores. Although the human cell is surrounded by the cell membrane, the bacterial cell is surrounded by two structures: a cell membrane and an outer cell wall. The bacterial cell wall is a rigid wall that protects the underlying cell membrane from bursting. If the cell wall is damaged, the cell membrane of the bacterium bursts, killing the bacterium. Enter penicillin! Penicillin prevents cell wall synthesis in the bacterium, causing the cell membrane to burst and the bacterium to die. Because human cells do not have a cell wall, they are not damaged by penicillin; penicillin is therefore relatively safe when administered to humans. Because a virus does not have an outer cell wall, it is not affected by penicillin. So, do not take penicillin for a viral infection—it does not work.

Many bacteria form **spores** that allow them to survive harsh environmental conditions such as drying, heating, and exposure to certain disinfectants. Spores enable the bacteria to exist in a "sleepy," or dormant, state until conditions improve. Then the bacteria wake up, grow, and resume their usual activities. For example, *Clostridium botulinum*, the organism that causes a deadly form of food poisoning (botulism), is a spore former and can withstand several hours of exposure to boiling water. Obviously, spore-forming microorganisms have great survival skills and present a challenge in infection control procedures.

Rickettsia (ri-KET-see-ah) and chlamydia (cla-MID-ee-uh) are classified as bacteria. However, they are smaller than most bacteria and must reproduce within the living cells of a host. Because they require a living host, they are called **parasites**. The rickettsiae are often carried by fleas, ticks, and body lice. For example, the rickettsia that causes Rocky Mountain spotted fever is carried by the tick. Body lice carry the rickettsia responsible for epidemic typhus. The chlamydiae are smaller than rickettsiae and cause several major human diseases. One of the most prevalent sexually transmitted diseases in the United States today is caused by *Chlamydia trachomatis*. Chlamydial infection is also responsible for trachoma, a serious eye infection that is a leading cause of blindness in the world. Like other bacterial infections, rickettsial and chlamydial infections are treated with antibiotics.

 Do You Know...

Who Russ T. Nale Is?

By stepping on his namesake, Russ T. Nale accomplished two things. First, he allowed a potentially lethal pathogen, *Clostridium tetani,* to enter his body. Second, he had a deep puncture wound that encouraged the growth of the pathogen. Because little bleeding is associated with a puncture wound, the pathogen was not washed out of the wound. More importantly, however, a deep puncture wound prevents air (oxygen) from entering the wound. Because this pathogen grows anaerobically (without oxygen), the conditions associated with a puncture wound are ideal. Sure hope Russ is up to date on his tetanus shots!

Viruses (from the Latin *virus,* meaning "poison") are the smallest of the infectious agents. They are not cells and consist of either ribonucleic acid (RNA) or deoxyribonucleic acid (DNA) surrounded by a protein shell. Because viruses can only reproduce within the living cells of a host, they are parasites. Examples of viral diseases are measles, mumps, influenza, poliomyelitis, and AIDS. Because of the intimacy of the virus–host relationship, the development of nontoxic antiviral agents has been slow and difficult. This point is well illustrated by the drug zidovudine (AZT), used in the treatment of AIDS. While exerting antiviral effects, the drug also causes widespread damage to the host cells. Most upper respiratory infections are viral and are not responsive to antibiotic therapy.

Fungus is a plantlike organism, such as a mushroom, that grows best in dark, damp places. Yeasts and molds (such as bread mold) are types of fungi. Pathogenic fungi cause mycotic infections (*myco* means "fungus"). Mycotic infections are usually localized and include athlete's foot, ringworm, thrush, and vaginitis. *Candida albicans* is a yeastlike fungus that normally inhabits the mouth, digestive tract, and vagina. When *Candida* overgrows, it can cause an infection in the mouth (thrush), intestinal symptoms, or vaginitis. Systemic fungal infections are rare, but when they occur, they are life-threatening and difficult to cure.

 Do You Know...

About the Ring of Ringworm?

Ringworm is an infection of the skin caused not by worms, but a fungus. Why the circular or ring shape? The fungus grows outward from the center. The fungi in the center of the lesion die before the outer circle of fungi die. This type of fungal growth pattern leaves a clear or healed center surrounded by living fungi.

NOTE: There is a ringworm bush (*Cassia alata*) whose leaves produce a juice that is used as a cure for ringworm and poisonous bites. The two explanations for the name *ringworm* are as follows: (1) an ancient and mistaken belief existed that worms caused the infection; and (2) it was named after the ringlike or circular appearance of the lesion. Both theories have a "ring" of truth.

Protozoa (pro-toe-ZO-ah) are single-celled, animal-like microbes. The four main types of protozoa are amebas (ah-MEE-bah-z), ciliates (SIL-ee-atz), flagellates (FLAH-jel-atz), and **sporozoa** (spor-uh-ZOH-uh). Protozoa are found in the soil and in most bodies of water. Amebic dysentery and giardiasis are caused by protozoan parasites. The parasites are ingested in contaminated water and food and cause severe diarrhea. Malaria is caused by a sporozoan called a plasmodium. *Plasmodium malariae* is carried by a mosquito, which is capable of spreading malaria over a wide region. Indeed, malaria still causes more than 3 million deaths per year in the more tropical regions of the world. Two other members of the sporozoa group pose a serious health threat to those persons with impaired immune systems. *Pneumocystis jiroveci* and *Cryptosporidium* cause infections in persons with AIDS and other immunocompromised persons.

 Re-Think

What is a normal flora? What is the consequence of disturbing the intestinal normal flora?

OTHER (MULTICELLULAR) DISEASE-CAUSING ORGANISMS

Other disease-causing organisms that are larger than microorganisms include multicellular organisms such as parasitic worms and arthropods.

Parasitic worms, called **helminths**, are multicellular animals that are parasitic and pathogenic to humans. In other words, worms can be germs. The identification of most worm infestations requires microscopic examination of body samples (usually stool) and reveals the presence of the adult worms or the larval forms. The worms are classified as roundworms or flatworms. Roundworms include ascarides, pinworms, hookworms, trichinae, and the tiny worms that cause filariasis (fi-LAR-eye-ah-sys) or elephantiasis. Infestation by pinworms is common in children and is very hard to control. The pinworms live in the intestinal tract but lay their eggs on the outer perianal area. The deposition of the eggs causes itching (pruritus). A child may then scratch the anal area and transfer the eggs to his or her mouth and onto others. The eggs are swallowed and the newly hatched pinworms grow into adulthood in the intestine. Most worm infestations are transmitted by the fecal–oral route (in which hands contaminated by feces introduce the worms, eggs, or larvae into the mouth). Trichinosis is transmitted by ingestion of undercooked contaminated pork, and filariasis is transmitted by biting insects.

The flatworms include the tapeworms and the flukes. Tapeworms that live in the intestines may grow from 5 to 50 feet in length. Imagine hosting a 50-foot tapeworm! Flukes are flat, leaf-shaped worms that invade the blood and organs such as the liver, lungs, and intestines. Because these large flatworms feed on the human host, infestation causes weight loss, anemia, and generalized debilitation. Infestation by worms is treated with drugs called *anthelmintics* (which means "against worms").

Arthropods are animals with jointed legs and include insects. They are of concern for two reasons. Arthropods such as mites and lice are ectoparasites, meaning that they live on the surface of the body, skin, and mucous membranes. Ectoparasites cause itching and discomfort but are not life-threatening. More seriously, arthropods such as mosquitoes, biting flies, fleas, and ticks act as vectors of disease. (A **vector** is an object, living or nonliving, that transfers a pathogen from one organism to another.) The bite of the arthropod vector introduces pathogens into the host (the person or organism that is infected by a pathogen), causing infection. For example, the mosquito (arthropod vector) can carry the pathogens for malaria and encephalitis. The tick can carry the pathogens that cause Lyme disease and Rocky Mountain spotted fever.

? Re-Think

What is meant by the fecal–oral route? How would you prevent the spread of an organism that is spread by this route of transmission?

LABORATORY IDENTIFICATION OF PATHOGENS

Many laboratory procedures and techniques are used to identify pathogens. One of these techniques is called *staining* and involves the use of dyes. A second technique is a culture.

Many bacteria are classified according to staining characteristics using the Gram stain (a dye). A gram-positive bacterium is one that stains purple or blue. *Streptococcus* is an example of a gram-positive bacterium. A gram-negative bacterium such as *Escherichia coli* does not absorb the purple Gram stain. Instead, a gram-negative bacterium picks up a pink or red stain. Because most bacteria are gram-positive or gram-negative, Gram staining is an important first step in the identification of the causative organism of an infection.

Another stain is called the *acid-fast stain*. The bacterium is first stained with a red dye and then washed with an acid. Most bacteria lose the red stain when washed with acid. However, several bacteria retain the red stain and are therefore called *acid-fast*. The most famous of the acid-fast bacteria is the *Mycobacterium tuberculosis*, the causative organism of tuberculosis (TB). This organism is commonly called the *acid-fast bacillus*. Some bacteria do not stain with any of the commonly used dyes. Thus, spirochetes and rickettsiae must be stained with special dyes and techniques.

Sometimes the physician wants to identify the specific pathogen growing in an infected wound and orders a wound culture to be done. A sample of the wound exudate (pus) is placed on culture medium (food that supports the growth of the pathogens). The pathogens are incubated and allowed to grow and multiply. The pathogens can then be stained and identified. The growth of pathogens in a culture medium is called a *culture*. The cultured pathogens can also be tested for their susceptibility to various antibiotics (culture and sensitivity test). For example, if an antibiotic is placed in the same culture and stops the growth of the pathogen, the pathogen is assumed to be responsive or sensitive to the effects of the antibiotic. The antibiotic is given to the patient to treat the infection. Other antibiotics may have no effect on the growth of the pathogens in the culture and therefore would not be used in the treatment of the infection.

You will often be asked to collect samples for laboratory analysis. Specific rules must be followed for each specimen. For example, in collecting a urine specimen that will be analyzed for the presence of pathogens, you must be careful not to contaminate the urine with microorganisms from your hands or unsterile containers. The proper identification of the pathogen depends on correct technique.

FIGURE 5-2 Spread of infection: portals of entry, portals of exit, and modes of transmission.

Re-Think

What does it mean to say that a bacterium is gram-positive or gram-negative?

THE SPREAD OF INFECTION

To understand how infection is spread, we must know how germs move—in, out, and about (Figure 5-2).

PORTALS OF ENTRY AND EXIT

How do pathogens enter the body? Pathogens enter the body by portals of entry, which include the respiratory, gastrointestinal, and genitourinary tracts, eye, skin, and parenteral route. The parenteral route includes those injuries that penetrate the skin or mucous membrane, such as bites, cuts, and surgery. A break in the skin is an excellent way for pathogens to enter the body. This is the reason that health care workers wear gloves when handling blood or other body fluids. In the event that the body fluids are contaminated (with, say, the AIDS or hepatitis viruses), the gloves prevent the entrance of the virus through tiny cuts or abrasions. Most pathogens enter the body through the respiratory tract (inhaled droplets of water and dust) and the gastrointestinal tract (by eating spoiled food or placing contaminated hands in the mouth).

How do pathogens leave the body of an infected person? Pathogens leave an infected body by portals of exit, which include the respiratory, gastrointestinal, or genitourinary tracts, the skin (intact and broken), eyes (tears), and breasts (milk). The most common portals of exit are the respiratory and gastrointestinal tracts. For example, the common cold virus is often sneezed or coughed into room air from the respiratory passages of the infected person, whereas the *Salmonella* organism in a person with typhoid fever exits the body in the stool. Discharge from the urogenital tract is also an important means of spreading infection (sexually transmitted diseases). By knowing the portal of exit of each pathogen, one can set up procedures for preventing the spread of the infection. For example, by knowing that *Salmonella typhi* is excreted in the stool, we know that the patient's underwear and bed linens are contaminated with the pathogens. We can then take measures to clean the soiled clothing and linens, thereby preventing the spread of the disease. By far, the most important procedure in preventing the spread of infection is handwashing!

Re-Think

Give an example of a portal of entrance and portal of exit. Explain in terms of the fecal–oral route. Work the term *handwashing* into your answer!

HOW PATHOGENS SPREAD

We know how pathogens enter and leave the body—but how do they move about, or "spread"? Pathogens are spread from person to person, environment to person, and from "tiny animals" (insects) to persons (see Figure 5-2).

PERSON-TO-PERSON CONTACT

Suppose you have a cold and go to work. Within a week, everyone in the office has your cold. What happened? First, whenever you sneezed, the cold virus was sprayed into the room air in little droplets of nasal discharge. These droplets were then inhaled by your coworkers. The virus was spread by droplet contact. Second, your hands were contaminated with the virus, and you touched many objects in the office (e.g., doorknobs, desktops, other people's hands after handshaking), thereby contaminating these objects. Others touched the contaminated objects and eventually introduced the virus into their own bodies. The spread of infection from person to person is effective. One of the best ways to prevent respiratory infections is to avoid crowds during cold and flu season. Another way is to avoid contact with a fomite or vector. The doorknob is considered to be both a vector and a fomite. Remember that a vector is an object, living or nonliving, that transfers a pathogen from one organism to another. A *fomite* is a nonliving vector. Other fomites include soiled handkerchiefs and eating utensils.

ENVIRONMENT-TO-PERSON CONTACT

This mode of transmission includes contact with contaminated water, air, food, or soil. For example, you can develop typhoid fever if you drink a glass of water contaminated by *S. typhi*. Similarly you can develop food poisoning if you eat food contaminated with *E. coli*.

"TINY ANIMAL"-TO-PERSON CONTACT

This mode of transmission includes the use of insects (and other "crawling critters") in the spread of disease; these tiny animals are living vectors. For example, a mosquito bites a person with malaria. The malaria-causing plasmodium matures in the stomach of the mosquito. The plasmodium-loaded mosquito then bites another person and voila!—malaria. You can understand why the eradication of mosquitoes is key in malaria control. A final stomach-churning example is flies hopping from dog feces to food on a picnic table. The pathogens from the dog feces are transferred by the fly feet to the food, which is then eaten by you.

Note that the mosquito and fly both spread disease. The mosquito, however, plays a more complicated and biological role. The plasmodium (causative organism of malaria) requires the mosquito as part of its life cycle; it matures in the stomach of the mosquito. Because of this role, the mosquito is called a *biological*

vector. The lowly fly does not participate in the life cycle of the pathogen; it merely walks on the dog feces and the germs stick to the feet of the fly. The fly then flies onto your food and deposits the germs on your food. The fly is only a *mechanical vector* but a very effective germ spreader.

? Re-Think

1. Explain how a doorknob can act both as a vector and fomite during flu season.
2. Describe why the malaria-causing mosquito acts as a biological vector whereas the common housefly usually acts as a mechanical vector.

FIVE GERM-LADEN STORIES

The following five stories illustrate important microbiological principles and introduce you to the language of microbiology. "Wash Those Mitts!" is a tragic story of handwashing, nosocomial infection, and the arrogance of the scientific community. "Flora and Her Vaginal Itch" addresses the normal flora and superinfection. "Rick, Nick, and the Sick Tick" describes disease transmission by an arthropod vector and differentiates between a communicable and contagious disease. "Why Typhoid Mary Needed to Lose Her Gallbladder" describes the carrier state and the efficiency of the fecal–oral route in disease transmission. Finally, "A Pox News Alert!" focuses on the pox throughout history and some of the current concerns. As you read the stories, refer to Table 5-1 for the definitions of unfamiliar terms; the table defines and expands the microbiological principles illustrated in the stories.

DR. SEMMELWEIS SCREAMS, "WASH THOSE MITTS!"

Dr. Ignaz Semmelweis was an assistant at the First Obstetrical Clinic in Vienna (circa 1850). At that time, an alarmingly high mortality rate was associated with puerperal fever or childbirth fever. Puerperal fever begins as an infection of the uterus after childbirth and is commonly caused by a strain of beta-hemolytic streptococcus. Puerperal fever progresses from an infection of the uterus to peritonitis and to generalized septicemia, ending in an agonizing death.

Semmelweis made the following two keen observations while caring for his patients:

1. A woman became ill immediately after being examined by a medical student who had previously examined a woman dying of puerperal fever.
2. If a medical student cut himself while attending a woman with puerperal fever, his wound became infected, and he subsequently died of puerperal sepsis.

Dr. Semmelweis concluded that puerperal fever is caused by conveyance to the pregnant woman of "putrid particles derived from living organisms through the agency of the examining fingers." This conclusion was impressive because he linked the disease to the putrid particles—tiny disease-producing critters that would not be discovered and linked to disease officially for another 25 years.

As a result of his observations, Semmelweis demanded that his medical students wash their hands with a disinfectant before examining each patient. "Wash those mitts!" he screamed, and wash they did. Mortality rates in his clinic decreased from 18% to 1%. You might conclude that Semmelweis eliminated puerperal fever and was honored by his colleagues. Not so! They ridiculed him for his insistence on hand-washing. He eventually became so distraught that he deliberately cut his finger and contaminated his injury with the vaginal discharge of a woman with puerperal fever. Ranting and raving, he was committed to the Budapest Insane Asylum, where he quickly died of the disease that he had worked so hard to eradicate.

With the passing of Semmelweis, the practice of handwashing was discontinued and the mortality rate from puerperal fever again soared. Puerperal fever, although rarely seen today, is a great example of a nosocomial infection. A **nosocomial** (noh-soh-CO-mee-al) **infection** is a hospital-acquired infection that is most often transmitted from patient to patient by direct contact (through the agency of the examining finger, according to Semmelweis). Today, a nosocomial infection is transmitted by health professionals who *do not wash their hands*. We go from patient to patient, carrying germs from one to another. Historically, nosocomial infections have been a tremendous problem. Today, 15% of hospitalized patients develop a nosocomial infection. "Wash those mitts!" echoes through the centuries but generally falls on deaf ears.

 Re-Think

Explain why the same problem dealt with by Semmelweis is the same as today's issue with nosocomial infection.

FLORA AND HER VAGINAL ITCH

Stuffed up and miserable, Flora went to her physician. She was given an antibiotic for a sinus infection. Within a week, the sinus infection was cured; the misery, however, had headed south. Flora now had an antibiotic-induced vaginal discharge.

The vagina is normally inhabited by a population of diverse microbes. These microbes are permanent residents and, when present in normal amounts, do not produce disease. This population of microbes within the vagina is called the *normal flora*. Other body cavities or areas such as the skin, large intestine, mouth, and respiratory tract contain their own diverse populations of microbes and therefore have their own normal flora.

The presence of a normal flora within the vagina prevents the overgrowth of yeast called *Candida albicans* that is present in small numbers within the vagina. If the normal flora is destroyed by an antibiotic, the yeast grows uncontrollably and causes candidiasis, a vaginal yeast infection, characterized by discharge, odor, and itching. Candidiasis is an example of a superinfection. Organisms that do not cause disease in their normal habitat become pathogenic when allowed to overpopulate the area. What was the cause of Flora's itch? Flora's normal flora had become abnormal. Watch those antibiotics!

? **Re-Think**

Why may antibiotic therapy cure one infection but cause a superinfection in the same patient?

RICK, NICK, AND THE SICK TICK

One week after returning from a camping trip with his friend Nick, Rick went to his physician feeling awful. He had chills, a high fever, headache, muscle pain, and a red, measles-like spotted rash that was prominent on the palms of his hands and the soles of his feet. On examination, the physician removed a tick from Rick's back. He was diagnosed with Rocky Mountain spotted fever (RMSF) and treated with the antibiotic tetracycline. Microbiologically speaking, Rick had become the perfect host (an organism who had become infected with a pathogen).

Enough about Rick! What's with the tick? The tick that bit Rick was sick; it was infected with the pathogen called *Rickettsia rickettsii*, the causative organism of RMSF. When the tick bit Rick, the infected saliva was injected into the bite site. The rickettsia then feasted on Rick's blood by growing, multiplying, and eventually causing the signs and symptoms that sent Rick to the doctor.

The tick acts as an arthropod vector for RMSF. An animal vector is an organism that transmits a pathogen such as rickettsia. An arthropod is a class of tiny animals that have jointed legs. In this case, the arthropod is the sick tick. The rickettsia is transmitted by saliva (the bite of the tick) or the feces of the tick that are rubbed into the bite. The tick also serves as a reservoir of infection, which harbors pathogens; in this case, the tick is the reservoir.

The tick is not killed by the rickettsia. Mama tick coexists with the rickettsia and passes the rickettsia through her eggs to her baby ticks, thereby perpetuating and expanding generations of sick ticks.

Why didn't Nick catch Rick's infection? RMSF is considered a communicable disease inasmuch as the infection can be spread (through the bite of a tick). RMSF, however, is not considered a contagious disease—that is, one easily spread from host to host like a common cold or impetigo. Thus, Nick remained well, despite his close association with Rick.

One last thing about RMSF: it is an example of zoonosis, an animal disease that is transmissible to humans. Other zoonotic diseases include malaria and endemic typhus.

? Re-Think

Explain the role of the arthropod vector in Rocky Mountain spotted fever.

WHY TYPHOID MARY NEEDED TO LOSE HER GALLBLADDER

Mary Mallon (Typhoid Mary) lived in New York in the early 1900s. While employed as a cook, she unintentionally infected many persons with typhoid fever. Hearing several rumors of Mary's unfortunate associations with this disease, her wealthy employer hired a sanitary engineer, George Soper, to investigate the sudden outbreak of typhoid fever within the former's home. Soper soon informed Mary that she was a carrier of the germ that caused typhoid fever. Mary vehemently denied that she was the infecting culprit, because she herself did not feel ill. Understandably, she chased Soper from her kitchen with a carving fork. But Soper was correct—Mary was indeed a carrier of typhoid fever.

The *S. typhi* bacterium, the causative organism of typhoid fever, is transmitted by the fecal–oral route through contaminated food or water. Mary's vocation as a cook was a perfect way to spread the salmonella organism via her contaminated hands touching food. Carriers of typhoid fever never rid their systems of *Salmonella;* instead, they harbor the organisms in the bile stored within the gallbladder. Salmonella-laden bile then enters the intestine and contaminates the feces. Removal of the gallbladder rids the body of the salmonella, thereby eliminating the carrier state. Surgical removal of the gallbladder would have made an enormous difference in Mary's life. Unfortunately, surgery was not an option and Mary was forced into isolation on a coastal island, where she lived unhappily for 26 years.

? Re-Think

How may a cholecystectomy (gallbladder removal) and antibiotics have rendered Mary "safe"?

A POX NEWS ALERT!

Pox News, responding to an ancient medieval curse "A pox be upon you," has issued an update on the pox. Here it is, fair and balanced!

- There has been much confusion about the pox throughout history. The ancients referred to any infectious disease as a "dose of the pox." (Because pox infection was so ugly and visible, the ancients commonly invoked pox curses on their enemies.) Later, the term *pox* was restricted to any disease characterized by a vesicular skin lesion. The term *pox* focuses only on the skin lesion and does not address its cause or treatment. Today, the medical focus is placed on the type of virus that causes a pox.

- Pox diseases are not limited geographically, nor are they restricted to humans. There are "flocks of pox": monkey pox, parrot pox, camel pox, squirrel pox, goat pox, fox pox, ox pox—even plants have pox (plum pox).

- What about chickenpox? Chickenpox is caused by the varicella-zoster virus, a member of the Herpesvirus group. It is characterized by a vesicular pox, accompanied by severe pruritus, and capable of causing pock marks. Why the name *chickenpox?* Explanations abound. In England, children were often called "chicken." Because chickenpox is primarily a disease of children, the pox was dubbed "childrenpox." Others suggest that the name is derived from the appearance of the pock mark; it looks like the skin has been pecked by a chicken. Others observe the pox as resembling chick peas. There's no telling what it means.

- Think that's strange? Pox News has just learned that some parents are throwing "pox parties" in which they are deliberately exposing their unvaccinated children to those who currently have chickenpox! Some parents are convinced that the chickenpox vaccine is unsafe and that the only safe way to build up immunity is to "get" a real case of chickenpox. When a child contracts chickenpox, their friends are invited to a party. The infected child is told to blow a whistle and to then pass the whistle to the friends. The whistle, acting as a vector, then spreads the virus from child to child. The practice is effective but dangerous; whereas most children recover uneventfully from chickenpox, some develop serious complications. In particular, children who are immunocompromised may develop a lethal multiple organ infection by the virus; this carries a 17% mortality. Pox parties are probably not the best approach to infectious disease control.

- Poxes come in different sizes. There is the dreaded lethal smallpox and the infamous Great Pox. Pox News, however, has just learned that the Great Pox is no pox at all; its pocky lesion is a chancre and is caused by a spirochete called *Treponema pallidum.* Yikes! The Great Pox is syphilis, the source of untold misery. Just ask Beethoven, Hitler and his lovely bunker mate Eva B, Henry VIII and his tower ladies, to mention a few. As for the "Chief of Grief" (syphilis), its cause was accurately described by the ancients: "It is taken when one pocky person doth synne (sin) in lechery with one another." Prevention is obvious: "Sin thou not with a pocky person."

Do You Know...

That Dr. Herbie Zoster Hung Out His Shingle?

Meet Dr. Herbie Zoster, a herpes specialist according to his newly hung shingle. Today, he is seeing his first patient, Ms. Vera Cella. Ms. Cella is miserable; she has a string of painful skin lesions around her waist. Dr. Zoster makes an immediate diagnosis: It is shingles, medically known as *herpes zoster*. Shingles is an acute infection of the peripheral nervous system caused by the varicella-zoster virus, the same virus that causes chickenpox. After a person recovers from chickenpox, the virus hides in a posterior root ganglion. Later in life, often in response to stress or immunosuppressive therapies, the virus leaves the ganglion and travels along the sensory neurons to the skin. This results in a line of skin blisters along the infected nerve and severe pain. As a complication, some persons develop a postherpetic neuralgia (pain that lingers long after the skin lesions have cleared). Yes, shingles can be triggered by exposure to a child with chickenpox.

 Re-Think

What is the relationship between chickenpox and shingles?

2+2 Sum It Up!

Infectious disease has plagued us forever. Today the battle continues against the tiny but tough disease-producing organisms called pathogens. Pathogens include bacteria, viruses, fungi, protozoa, parasitic worms, and arthropods. To understand the transmission of an infection, one should know the portals of entry (how the pathogen enters the body), the portals of exit (how the pathogen leaves the body), and how the pathogen is spread (person-to-person, environment-to-person, or "tiny animal"-to-person). Important microbiological principles are illustrated in Five Germ-Laden Stories.

Table 5-2   Disorders Caused by Pathogens

PATHOGEN	DISORDER
Cocci	
Neisseria	*N. gonorrhoeae* causes gonorrhea and inflammation of the mucous membranes of the reproductive and urinary tracts. May cause sterility and pelvic inflammatory disease (PID). Infants of infected mothers may develop ophthalmia neonatorum. *N. meningitidis* causes meningitis, or inflammation of the membranes covering the brain and the spinal cord.
Staphylococcus	*S. aureus* causes skin infections such as boils and impetigo, pneumonia, kidney and bladder infections, osteomyelitis, septicemia, and food poisoning. *S. aureus* is a leading cause of nosocomial (hospital-acquired) infections.
Streptococcus	*S. pneumoniae* causes pneumonia, middle ear infection, and meningitis. *S. pyogenes* causes septicemia, strep throat, middle ear infection, scarlet fever, pneumonia, and endocarditis. An immunological response can cause rheumatic fever with permanent damage to the heart valves, and glomerulonephritis (kidney damage).
Bacilli	
Bordetella pertussis	*Bordetella* causes pertussis (whooping cough), a severe infection of the trachea and bronchi characterized by episodes of violent coughing. The "whoop" is an effort to inhale after the coughing bouts.
Clostridium	*C. botulinum* causes botulism, a potentially fatal form of food poisoning caused by improper processing of foods. *C. perfringens* causes gas gangrene, in which death of the tissue is accompanied by the production of a gas. *C. tetani* causes tetanus, or lockjaw.
Escherichia coli	*E. coli* is part of the normal flora of the intestines. *E. coli* causes local and systemic infections, food poisoning, diarrhea, septicemia, and septic shock; it is a leading cause of nosocomial infection.
Haemophilus	*H. aegyptius* causes conjunctivitis, a highly contagious infection that occurs in areas where there are many young children. *H. influenzae* causes meningitis in children and upper respiratory infection in older adults.
Helicobacter pylori	*H. pylori* causes gastritis and ulceration of the stomach and duodenum.
Legionella pneumophila	*L. pneumophila* is responsible for legionnaires' disease, a type of pneumonia. The organism contaminates water supplies, as in air-conditioning units.

Continued

Table 5-2   Disorders Caused by Pathogens—cont'd

PATHOGEN	DISORDER
Mycobacterium tuberculosis	*M. tuberculosis* causes tuberculosis (TB). The organism, also called the tubercle bacillus, causes primary lesions called *tubercles*. The bacillus most commonly affects the lungs. The incidence of TB is high in the homeless population, persons with AIDS, and closed populations such as in prisons. Formerly called the "white plague," TB is making a comeback in a more virulent and drug-resistant strain.
Pseudomonas aeruginosa	*P. aeruginosa* is the common cause of wound and urinary tract infections in debilitated patients, such as patients with severe burns, cancer, and other chronic conditions.
Salmonella	*S. enteritidis* causes salmonellosis, food poisoning characterized by severe diarrhea. *S. typhi* causes typhoid fever, an intestinal infection. Typhoid fever is rare in the United States because of the chlorination of the water supply, but the incidence increases during periods of flooding when the water supply is contaminated with sewage.
Shigella dysenteriae	*S. dysenteriae* causes dysentery.
Curved Rods	
Borrelia burgdorferi	*B. burgdorferi* causes Lyme disease and is characterized by a rash, palsy, and joint inflammation. It is transmitted by a small deer tick.
Treponema pallidum	*T. pallidum* causes syphilis.
Vibrio cholerae	*V. cholerae* causes cholera.
Rickettsia* and *Chlamydia	
Rickettsia	*R. prowazekii* causes epidemic typhus, which is transmitted to humans by lice. *R. rickettsii* causes Rocky Mountain spotted fever, which is transmitted to humans by ticks. *R. typhi* causes endemic or murine typhus, which is transmitted to humans by fleas.
Chlamydia	*C. trachomatis* causes trachoma, the leading cause of blindness in the world. Another form causes nongonococcal urethritis, the most common sexually transmitted disease in the United States.
Viruses	
Encephalitis viruses	Encephalitis is the inflammation of the brain.
Hepatitis viruses	Several forms of hepatitis exist, causing inflammation of the liver, as follows: Hepatitis A is spread by the fecal–oral route. Hepatitis B is spread by sexual activity or contact with contaminated blood and body fluids. Hepatitis C is caused by contaminated blood transmitted via transfusions, through needles in drug abuse, and to health care workers on the job. Hepatitis can become chronic, develop into a carrier state, or deteriorate to hepatic failure.
Herpes simplex viruses	*Type 1:* Cold sores or fever blisters appear on the lip, in the oral cavity, or in the nose. The virus lies dormant in the nerves between attacks. *Type 2:* Genital herpes is a common sexually transmitted disease characterized by painful lesions in the genitalia.
Herpes varicella-zoster	Chickenpox (varicella) is a mild infection characterized by generalized skin lesions. On remission of the infection, the virus becomes dormant and may reactivate in later years as shingles (herpes zoster).
Human papillomavirus (HPV)	HPV causes genital warts, which are transmitted sexually.
Influenza viruses	Influenza ("flu") is caused by different strains of the influenza viruses.
Measles virus	Measles (rubeola) is an acute respiratory inflammation characterized by fever, sore throat, skin rash, and Koplik's spots (white spots in the mouth).
Mumps virus	Mumps is epidemic parotitis (inflammation of a salivary gland).
Polio virus	Poliomyelitis (infantile paralysis) is an acute infection that may destroy nerve cells in the spinal cord, causing paralysis.
Rhabdovirus	Rabies is a fatal disease characterized by headache, fever, seizures, and spasm of the throat muscles while swallowing (hydrophobia). It is spread by the saliva of infected animals such as dogs and other wild animals (e.g., bats, raccoons).
Rhinoviruses	Rhinoviruses are responsible for the common cold (coryza).
Rubella virus	Causes German measles. The virus causes severe teratogenic birth defects that occur during the first trimester, such as blindness, deafness, brain damage, and heart defects.

Table 5-2 Disorders Caused by Pathogens—cont'd	
PATHOGEN	**DISORDER**
Fungi	
Tinea	Tinea causes ringworm, a highly contagious fungal infection of the skin. One form of ringworm (tinea pedis) is found on the foot and is called *athlete's foot*. Other forms of ringworm are found on the scalp (tinea capitis) and on the bearded areas of the face and neck (tinea barbae). (Ringworm is not caused by a worm, nor is the lesion always ring-shaped.)
Protozoa	
Entamoeba histolytica	*E. histolytica* causes amebic dysentery.
Giardia lamblia	Giardiasis is characterized by gastrointestinal discomfort and diarrhea.
Trichomonas vaginalis	Trichomoniasis is a sexually transmitted disease.
Worms	
Ascaris	These are long worms that live in the small intestine.
Hookworm (*Necator*)	Larval worms burrow their way through the skin of a bare foot, migrate to the intestine, and hook on to the intestinal wall. The worms feed on the blood of the host, causing anemia, fatigue, and wasting.
Pinworm (*Enterobius*)	Pinworm is the most common worm infestation in the United States.
Tapeworms (*Taenia,* others)	Tapeworms are acquired by eating poorly cooked contaminated food such as beef, fish, and pork.

Get Ready for Exams!

Summary Outline

The human body is often invaded by disease-producing organisms; these pathogens disrupt normal structure and function and are a common cause of disability and death.

I. Disease and Pathogens
  A. Disease is a failure of the body to function normally.
  B. Infections are diseases caused by pathogens.

II. Types of Pathogens
  A. Microorganisms
    1. Bacteria (cocci, bacilli, curved rods, chlamydia, rickettsia)
    2. Viruses
    3. Fungi
    4. Protozoa (amebas, ciliates, flagellates, sporozoa)
  B. Other larger pathogens
    1. Worms
    2. Arthropods

III. Laboratory Identification
  A. Staining (Gram stain, acid-fast stain)
  B. Culture

IV. Spread of Infection
  A. Portals of entry (most pathogens enter the body through the respiratory tract and the gastrointestinal tract).
  B. Portals of exit (the most common portals of exit are the respiratory and gastrointestinal tracts).
  C. Modes of transmission
    1. Person-to-person
    2. Environment-to-person
    3. "Tiny animals"-to-person

V. Five Germ-Laden Stories
  A. "Wash Those Mitts!"
  B. "Flora and Her Vaginal Itch"
  C. "Rick, Nick, and the Sick Tick"
  D. "Why Typhoid Mary Needed to Lose Her Gallbladder"
  E. "Pox News Alert!"

Review Your Knowledge

Matching: Microorganisms and Other Pathogens
Directions: Match the following words with their descriptions below. Some words are used more than once.

a. virus
b. bacteria
c. arthropods
d. worms
e. fungi
f. protozoa

1. ___ Coccus, bacillus, curved rods
2. ___ RNA or DNA surrounded by a protein shell; parasitic
3. ___ Yeasts and molds
4. ___ Ascarides, trichinae, flukes
5. ___ Helminths
6. ___ Ectoparasites
7. ___ Mycotic infections
8. ___ Chlamydia and rickettsia
9. ___ Animals with jointed legs
10. ___ Arranged in pairs, chains, and bunches of grapes
11. ___ Amebas, ciliates, flagellates, and sporozoa

Multiple Choice

1. A vaginal yeast infection *(Candida albicans)* is most apt to develop
   a. as a consequence to antibiotic therapy.
   b. in response to eating contaminated food.
   c. as an allergic response to penicillin.
   d. in response to being bitten by a "sick tick."
2. The plasmodium
   a. is pathogenic to mosquitoes.
   b. causes malaria.
   c. is an arthropod.
   d. is a biological vector.
3. Cocci, bacilli, and curved rods
   a. are eradicated by anthelmintics.
   b. cause mycotic infections.
   c. are types of bacteria.
   d. always act as pathogens.
4. Which of the following is most descriptive of *Staphylococcus?*
   a. Viral
   b. Parasitic
   c. Gram-positive
   d. Chainlike arrangement

5. Spores
   a. allow the bacterium to stain blue (gram-positive).
   b. only develop in parasites.
   c. are characteristic of arthropods.
   d. make a bacterium heat-resistant and hard to kill.

Go Figure

1. **According to Figures 5-1 and 5-2**
   a. Cocci are classified as viruses.
   b. Strep and staph are classified as bacilli.
   c. Worms can be pathogenic.
   d. A virus is classified as an arthropod vector.

2. **According to Figures 5-1 and 5-2, and Table 5-1**
   a. The normal flora in the large intestine differs from the normal flora in the nose.
   b. A nosocomial infection is hospital-acquired.
   c. Fungi can be pathogenic.
   d. All of the above are true.

Tissues and Membranes

Key Terms

adipose tissue (p. 82)
areolar tissue (p. 82)
chondrocytes (p. 84)
columnar epithelium (p. 78)
connective tissue (p. 81)
cuboidal epithelium (p. 78)
endocrine glands (p. 81)

epithelial tissue (p. 77)
exocrine glands (p. 81)
ligaments (p. 83)
mucous membranes (p. 88)
muscle tissue (p. 85)
nervous tissue (p. 85)
osseous tissue (p. 85)

parietal layer (p. 88)
serous membranes (p. 88)
squamous epithelium (p. 78)
tendons (p. 83)
visceral layer (p. 88)

Objectives

1. List the four major types of tissues.
2. Do the following regarding epithelial tissue:
   - Describe the characteristics and functions of epithelial tissue.
   - Explain how epithelial tissue is classified.
   - List the types of epithelial tissue membranes.
   - Differentiate between endocrine and exocrine glands.
3. Describe the characteristics and functions of connective tissue, and list the types of connective tissue membranes.
4. Describe the characteristics and functions of nervous and muscle tissues.
5. Explain the process of tissue repair after an injury.
6. Differentiate between mucous and serous membranes.

In Chapter 3, we studied a typical cell. We explained how it divides into millions of identical cells and how they differentiate into cells with unique shapes, sizes, and functions. In this chapter, we see how these cells are arranged to perform specific functions.

Tissues are groups of cells that are similar to each other in structure and function. Four major types of tissues are epithelial, connective, nervous, and muscular. The study of tissues is called *histology*.

EPITHELIAL TISSUE

WHERE IS IT FOUND?

Epithelial (ep-i-THEE-lee-al) tissue, also called *epithelium*, forms large continuous sheets. Epithelial tissue helps form the skin and covers the entire outer surface of the body. Sheets of epithelium also line most of the inner cavities such as the mouth, respiratory tract, and reproductive tract. Types of epithelial tissue are listed in Table 6-1.

WHAT DOES IT DO?

Epithelial tissue is primarily concerned with protection, absorption, filtration, and secretion (see Table 6-1). The skin, for example, protects the body from

sunlight and from invasion by disease-producing bacteria. The epithelial tissue lining the respiratory passages helps clean inhaled air. The epithelium of the respiratory tract secretes mucus and is lined with cilia. The mucus traps the dust inhaled in the air, and the constantly waving cilia move the dust and mucus toward the throat. The dust and mucus are then either coughed up or swallowed and eliminated in the stools.

Epithelial tissue also functions in the transport of substances across membranes. Epithelium is abundant in organs like those in the digestive tract, which must absorb large amounts of water and digested food. Finally, epithelial tissue forms glands that secrete a variety of hormones and enzymes.

WHAT IS IT LIKE?

Epithelial tissue has the following characteristics:
- Epithelial tissue forms continuous sheets (Figure 6-1). The cells fit together snugly like tiles.
- Epithelial tissue has two surfaces. One surface is always unattached, like the surface of the outer skin or the inner lining of the mouth. The undersurface of the epithelium is attached to a basement membrane, which is a very thin material that anchors the epithelium to the underlying structure.

Table 6-1 Types of Epithelial Tissue

TYPE	LOCATION	FUNCTION
Simple		
Simple squamous	Walls of blood vessels (capillaries) Alveoli (air sacs in lungs) Kidneys	Permits the exchange of nutrients and wastes Allows diffusion of oxygen and carbon dioxide Filtration of water and electrolytes
Simple cuboidal	Lining of kidney tubules Various glands (thyroid, pancreas, salivary glands)	Absorption of water and electrolytes Secretion of enzymes and hormones
Simple columnar	Digestive tract	Protection, absorption, and secretion of digestive juice; often contains goblet cells (mucus)
Pseudostratified columnar	Lining of respiratory tract Lining of reproductive tubes (fallopian tubes)	Protection and secretion; cleans respiratory passages; sweeps egg toward uterus
Stratified		
Stratified squamous	Outer layer of skin Lining of mouth, esophagus, anus, and vagina	Protects body from invading microorganisms; withstands friction
Transitional	Urinary bladder	Permits expansion of an organ

- Epithelial tissue has no blood supply of its own; it is avascular. For its nourishment, it depends on the blood supply of underlying connective tissue.
- Because epithelial tissue is so well nourished from the underlying connective tissue, it is able to regenerate, or repair itself, quickly if injured.

> **? Re-Think**
>
> 1. List four types of tissue.
> 2. List three words that describe epithelial tissue.

CLASSIFICATION

Epithelial tissue is classified according to its shape and the numbers of layers. It has three shapes: squamous,

Floor tiles

A Floor

Cells

B Tissue

FIGURE 6-1 **A,** A tile floor. **B,** Tight-fitting cells of epithelial tissue.

cuboidal, and columnar (Figure 6-2 and Table 6-1). The **squamous** (SKWAY-muss) **epithelium** cells are thin and flat, like fish scales. (The word "squamous" comes from *squam,* meaning "scale.") The **cuboidal epithelium** cells are cubelike and look like dice. The **columnar epithelium** cells are tall and narrow and look like columns.

Epithelial cells are arranged in a single layer or multiple layers (see Figure 6-2). One layer of cells is a simple epithelium. Two or more layers of cells are a stratified (STRAT-i-fyed) epithelium.

Both the shape and the number of layers describe the various types of epithelium. For example, simple squamous epithelium refers to a single layer of squamous cells. Stratified squamous epithelium contains multiple layers of squamous cells. Note that Figure 6-2 shows stratified squamous epithelium but not stratified cuboidal or columnar tissue. Stratified cuboidal and stratified columnar epithelia are found in very few organs.

SIMPLE EPITHELIA

Because simple epithelia are so thin, they are concerned primarily with the movement, or transport, of various substances across the membranes from one body compartment to another (Figure 6-3).

Simple squamous epithelium is a single layer of squamous cells with an underlying basement membrane. Because this tissue is so thin, simple squamous epithelium is found where substances move by rapid diffusion or filtration. For example, the walls of the capillaries (the smallest blood vessels) are composed of simple squamous epithelium. The walls of the alveoli (air sacs of the lungs) are also composed of simple squamous epithelium. This tissue allows the

Looks like: **Cell shapes:**

**Types of
cell layers:**

FIGURE 6-2 Classification of epithelial tissue: shapes and layers of cells.

rapid diffusion of oxygen from the alveoli into the blood.

Simple cuboidal epithelium is a single layer of cuboidal cells resting on a basement membrane. This epithelial layer is most often found in glands and in the kidney tubules, where it functions in the transport and secretion of various substances.

Simple columnar epithelium refers to a single layer of columnar cells resting on its basement membrane. These tall, tightly packed cells line the entire length of the digestive tract and play a major role in the absorption of the products of digestion. Lubricating mucus is produced by goblet cells, which are modified columnar cells.

Pseudostratified (SOOD-oh-STRAT-i-fyed) columnar epithelium is a single layer of columnar cells. Because the cells are so irregularly shaped, they appear multilayered; hence the term *pseudostratified,* meaning "falsely stratified." Their function is similar to that of

simple columnar cells: They facilitate absorption and secretion.

STRATIFIED EPITHELIA

Stratified epithelia are multilayered (from 2 to 20 layers) and are therefore stronger than simple epithelia. They perform a protective function and are found in tissue exposed to everyday wear and tear, such as the mouth, esophagus, and skin. Stratified squamous epithelium is the most widespread of the epithelial tissue.

Transitional epithelium is found primarily in organs that need to stretch, such as the urinary bladder. This epithelium is called *transitional* because the cells slide past one another when the tissue is stretched. The cells appear stratified when the urinary bladder is empty (unstretched) and simple when the bladder is full (stretched).

Epithelial Tissue

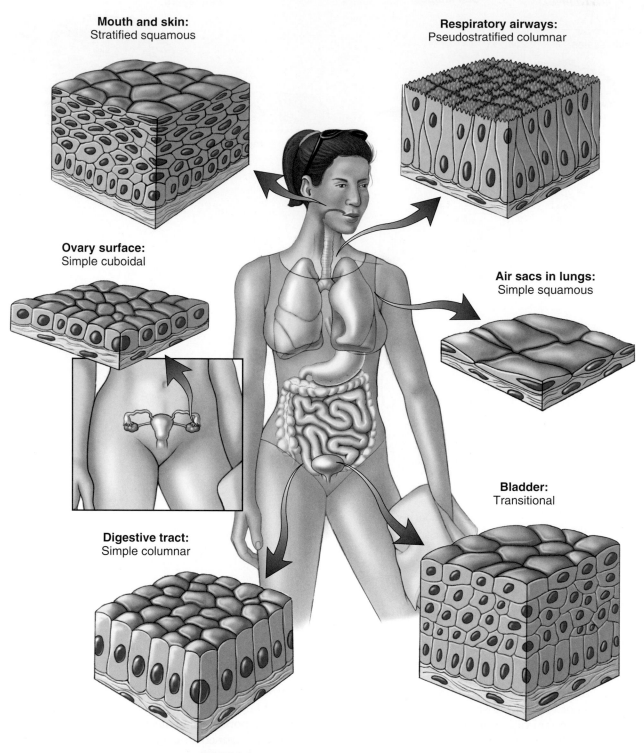

Mouth and skin:
Stratified squamous

Respiratory airways:
Pseudostratified columnar

Ovary surface:
Simple cuboidal

Air sacs in lungs:
Simple squamous

Digestive tract:
Simple columnar

Bladder:
Transitional

FIGURE 6-3 Types and location of epithelial tissue.

Do You Know...

What Causes a Pressure, or Decubitus ("Lying Down"), Ulcer?

A decubitus ulcer is another name for a bedsore or a pressure ulcer. The ulcer is caused by an interruption of the blood supply to a tissue. Decubitus ulcers often develop in patients who have been bedridden or confined to a wheelchair for long periods. Decubitus comes from a Latin word meaning to lie down. The ulcers are caused by the weight of the body on the skin overlying a bony area (e.g., elbow, heel, hip). The weight of the body compresses the blood vessels, cutting off the supply of blood to the tissues. Deprived of its blood supply, the tissue dies, forming an ulcer.

GLANDULAR EPITHELIA

The function of glandular epithelium is secretion. A gland is made up of one or more cells that secrete a particular substance. Much of the glandular tissue is composed of simple cuboidal epithelium.

Two types of glands are the exocrine glands and the endocrine glands. The **exocrine glands** have ducts, or tiny tubes, into which the exocrine secretions are released before reaching body surfaces or body cavities. The exocrine secretions include mucus, sweat, saliva, and digestive enzymes. The ducts carry the exocrine secretions outside the body. For example, sweat flows from the sweat glands through ducts onto the surface of the skin for evaporation (Figure 6-4).

The **endocrine glands** secrete hormones, such as insulin. Endocrine glands do not have ducts and are therefore called *ductless glands*. Because endocrine glands are ductless, the hormones are secreted directly into the blood. The blood then carries the hormones to their sites of action.

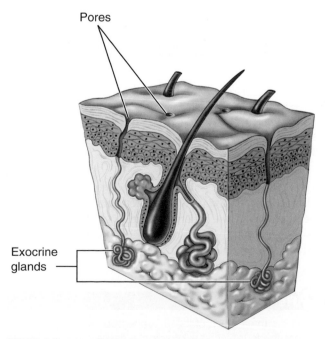

FIGURE 6-4 Exocrine gland, a sweat gland.

? Re-Think

1. With regard to classification, what are two differences between simple columnar epithelial tissue and stratified squamous epithelial tissue?
2. What is the primary function of simple squamous epithelium?

2+2 Sum It Up!

Tissues are groups of cells that are similar to each other in structure and function. The four types of tissues are epithelial, connective, nervous, and muscle. Epithelial tissue covers the body (as the skin) and lines cavities that open to the outside; it is primarily concerned with protection, secretion, filtration, and absorption. The shape of epithelial tissue is described as squamous, cuboidal, and columnar. Depending on the number of layers, epithelial tissue is described as simple or stratified.

CONNECTIVE TISSUE

WHERE IS IT FOUND?

Connective tissue is the most abundant of the four tissue types and is widely distributed throughout the body. Connective tissue is found in blood, under the skin, in bone, and around many organs. As the name suggests, connective tissue connects, or binds together, the parts of the body. Other functions include support, protection, fat storage, and transport of substances.

WHAT DOES IT LOOK LIKE?

Although connective tissue types may not resemble each other very closely, they share two characteristics. First, most connective tissue, with the exception of ligaments, tendons, and cartilage, has a good blood supply. Ligaments, tendons, and cartilage have a poor blood supply. As any athlete knows, an injury to these structures usually heals very slowly. The second characteristic shared by most connective tissue is an abundance of intercellular matrix.

CONNECTIVE TISSUE CELLS

Each major type of connective tissue contains immature or "blast" cells. Fibroblasts are cells found in loose and dense fibrous tissue. Chondroblasts (KON-droh-blasts) are found in cartilage and osteoblasts are found in bone. Blast cells secrete matrix that is characteristic of the tissue. In addition to fibroblasts, connective tissue contains other types of cells, such as macrophages, adipocytes, and cells that fight infection and inflammation.

The intercellular matrix is what makes the various types of connective tissue so different. Matrix is composed of fibrous protein and ground substance. The hardness of the matrix varies from one cell type to the next. The intercellular matrix may be liquid as in blood, gel-like as in fat tissue, rubbery as in cartilage, or hard as in bone. The amount of matrix also varies from one cell type to the next. In fat tissue, the cells are close together, with little intercellular matrix. Bone and cartilage, however, have few cells and large amounts of intercellular matrix.

Also found in the matrix of most connective tissue are protein fibers. These fibers are secreted by fibroblasts, and the fiber types include collagen, elastin, and reticular fibers (fine collagen). Collagen fibers are strong and flexible but are not easily stretched. Elastin fibers are not very strong, but they are stretchy, like a rubber band.

Injections of collagen are used cosmetically to remove unwanted lines and wrinkles. Collagen is obtained from cattle or, more often, from the patient's own hips, thighs, and abdomen. The collagen is then injected under the patient's skin. Acting as filler, the collagen smoothes out unwanted wrinkles, creating a surgical "fountain of youth." Tex, here, could use some collagen filler.

? Re-Think

Compare the amount of intercellular material of epithelial tissue with the amount of intercellular matrix of connective tissue.

TYPES OF CONNECTIVE TISSUE

The many types of connective tissue are loose connective tissue, dense fibrous connective tissue, cartilage, bone, and the "liquid" connective tissue (blood and lymph; Figure 6-5). Table 6-2 describes these types.

LOOSE CONNECTIVE TISSUE

Loose connective tissue contains fibers that are loosely arranged around cells. There are three types of loose connective tissue: areolar tissue, adipose tissue, and reticular connective tissue (see Figure 6-5).

Areolar (ah-REE-oh-lar) **tissue** is made up of collagen and elastin fibers in a gel-like intercellular matrix. Areolar tissue is soft and surrounds, protects, and cushions many of the organs, acting as "tissue glue." It is the most widely distributed type of connective tissue.

Adipose (AD-i-pohs) **tissue** or fat is composed primarily of adipocytes, or cells that store fat (see Figure

6-5). The more fat that is stored, the larger the adipocyte. Fat performs several important functions:

- Fat serves as the body's reservoir of energy. When the body needs energy, the fat is broken down and the energy is released. Unfortunately, fat storage often exceeds energy requirements.
- Fat assists in body temperature regulation. Adipose tissue forms the tissue layer underlying the skin (the subcutaneous layer). Because of its location, adipose tissue can insulate the body from extremes of outside temperature. For example, in a cold environment, adipose tissue prevents the loss of heat from the body. This protection is best appreciated in observing the fat content of animals living in arctic conditions. The walrus, for example, has huge layers of fat tissue (blubber). Because of the insulating qualities of the blubber, the walrus can swim in deep cold waters without freezing to death. Think of how long you could sit on an iceberg, even if you had a few extra pounds.
- Fat acts as a cushion. For example, a pad of fat behind the eyeball protects the eye from the hard bones of the eye socket.
- Fat protects some organs by anchoring them in place. The kidney, for example, has a layer of fat tissue that helps hold it in place. In extremely thin individuals, this fat tissue may be absent, allowing the kidney to move around (a "floating kidney").

📝 Do You Know...

Why a Too-Tight Tourniquet Is "Bad News"?

A too-tight tourniquet can cut off the flow of blood to a limb. If the blood supply to an area is stopped for too long, the tissue distal to the tourniquet is deprived of oxygen and dies. Tissue damage caused by diminished blood supply, called *ischemia*, often results in gangrene and necrosis.

Reticular tissue is characterized by a network of delicately interwoven cells and reticular (fine collagen) fibers. It forms the internal framework for lymphoid tissue such as the spleen, lymph nodes, and bone marrow.

? Re-Think

1. List the three types of loose connective tissue.
2. Describe four functions of adipose tissue.

Connective Tissue

Dense fibrous

Ligaments

Bone

Cartilage

Reticular

Bone marrow

Adipose

Skin

Basement membrane

Areolar

FIGURE 6-5 Types and location of connective tissue. (Blood and lymph are not shown.)

DENSE FIBROUS CONNECTIVE TISSUE

Dense fibrous connective tissue is composed of fibroblasts and an intercellular matrix that contains many collagen and elastic fibers. Collagen is the main type of fiber in dense fibrous tissue. The fibers form strong, supporting structures such as tendons, ligaments, capsules, fascia, and the dermal layer of skin.

Tendons are cordlike structures that attach muscles to bones. **Ligaments** cross joints and attach bones to each other. Because ligaments contain more elastic fibers than tendons, they stretch more easily. The ability to stretch is important; it prevents tearing of the ligaments when the joints bend. Dense fibrous connective tissue also forms tough capsules around certain organs (kidney and liver) and forms sheets of tissue

Table **6-2**   Types of Connective Tissue

TYPE	LOCATION	FUNCTION
Loose Connective		
Areolar	Beneath skin and most epithelial layers; between muscles	Binds together, protects, cushions; "tissue glue"
Adipose	Beneath skin (subcutaneous) Around kidneys and heart Behind eyeballs	Cushions, insulates, stores fat
Reticular	Lymphoid tissue such as lymph nodes, spleen, and bone marrow	Forms internal framework of lymphoid organs
Dense Fibrous Connective		
	Tendons, ligaments, capsules, and fascia Skin (dermis)	Binds structures together
Cartilage		
Hyaline	Ends of long bone at joints Connects ribs to sternum Rings in trachea of respiratory tract Nose Fetal skeleton	Supports, protects, provides framework
Fibrocartilage	Intervertebral discs (in backbone) Pads in knee joint Pad between pubic bones (symphysis pubis)	Cushions, protects
Elastic cartilage	External ear and part of larynx	Supports, provides framework
Bone		
	Bones of the skeleton	Supports, protects, provides framework
Blood		
	Blood vessels throughout the body	Transports nutrients, hormones, respiratory gases (oxygen and carbon dioxide), waste
Lymph		
	Lymphatic vessels throughout the body	Drains interstitial fluid; involved in immune response

called *fascia* (FASH-uh) that covers, supports, and anchors organs to nearby structures.

If stretching is excessive, as with athletic injuries, tendons and ligaments can tear, causing severe pain and impaired mobility. A ruptured Achilles tendon, for example, is a serious injury. The Achilles tendon attaches the leg muscles to the heel of the foot. If excessive force is exerted on the tendon, it may snap or rupture, causing loss of foot movement.

 Do You Know...

About Cooper's Droop?

As we age, the effects of gravity take over and some parts of the anatomy "head south." Breast tissue is anchored to the underlying structures by strands of connective tissue called *suspensory ligaments* (Cooper's ligaments). As we age, the tissue weakens and, sadly, sagging happens. The sorry saga of the sagging breasts is called *Cooper's Droop*.

 Re-Think

What is the difference between a tendon and a ligament? Between fascia and a capsule?

CARTILAGE

Cartilage is formed by chondroblasts that eventually mature into chondrocytes, or cartilage cells. The chondroblasts secrete a protein-containing intercellular matrix that becomes firm, smooth, and rubbery. Although the matrix of cartilage is solid, it is not as hard as that of bone. Except for fibrocartilage, most cartilage is covered by perichondrium (pair-i-KON-dree-um), a layer of connective tissue that carries blood vessels to the cartilage. The blood vessels supply oxygen and nutrients to the cartilage. Located between the perichondrium and the cartilage is a storage supply of chondroblasts. The stored chondroblasts provide for cartilage growth throughout life.

Types of Cartilage

Three types of cartilage are hyaline cartilage, elastic cartilage, and fibrocartilage. Hyaline cartilage is found in (1) the larynx, or voicebox, (2) the ends of long bones at joints, (3) the nose, and (4) the area between the breastbone and the ribs. Figure 6-5 illustrates the attachment of the ribs to the breastbone by hyaline cartilage. Hyaline cartilage is found in larger quantities in the fetal skeleton. As the fetus matures, however, most of the cartilage is converted to bone.

 Do You Know...

Why Overweight Men and Women "Round Out" into Different Shapes?

Overeating results in the storage of fat in adipose tissue. Because fat metabolism is affected by the sex hormones estrogen and testosterone, storage sites differ for males and females. In the male, excess fat is stored primarily in the abdominal region, whereas in the female, excess fat is stored around the breasts and hips. Excess adipose tissue, especially that which deposits in the abdominal region, becomes metabolically active and secretes hormones that adversely affect metabolism. The "spare tire" hormones increase blood glucose, increase resistance to insulin, and increase blood pressure, none of which is healthy.

BONE

Bone tissue is also called **osseous** (OS-ee-us) **tissue**. Immature bone cells are called *osteoblasts*. Osteoblasts secrete an intercellular matrix that includes collagen, calcium salts, and other minerals. The collagen provides flexibility and strength; the mineral-containing matrix as a whole makes the bone tissue hard. The hardness of the bone enables it to protect organs such as the brain and to support the weight of the body for standing and moving. Bone also acts as a storage site for mineral salts, especially calcium (see Chapter 8). Osteoblasts mature into osteocytes.

When mineralization of bone tissue is diminished, as in osteoporosis, the bone is weakened and tends to break easily. Adequate dietary intake of calcium is essential for strong bones. Calcium is needed throughout the life cycle but is especially important during childhood and pregnancy, when bones are growing, and after menopause, when estrogen levels in women decline. Estrogen normally encourages the deposition of calcium in bone tissue, as does exercise and weight-bearing activity.

BLOOD AND LYMPH

Blood and lymph are two types of connective tissue that have a liquid intercellular matrix. Blood consists of blood cells surrounded by a fluid intercellular matrix called *plasma*. Unlike other connective tissues, which contain collagen and elastin fibers in the intercellular matrix, plasma contains nonfibrous plasma proteins (see Chapter 15). Lymph is the fluid that is found in lymphatic vessels (see Chapter 20).

 Re-Think

What is the difference in the intercellular matrix of cartilage, bone, and blood?

NERVOUS TISSUE

Nervous tissue makes up the brain, spinal cord, and nerves. Nervous tissue consists of two types of cells: neurons and neuroglia (Figure 6-6).

NEURONS

Neurons are nerve cells that transmit electrical signals to and from the brain and spinal cord. The neuron has three parts: (1) the dendrites, which receive information from other neurons; (2) the cell body, which contains the nucleus and is essential to the life of the cell; and (3) the axon, which transmits information away from the cell body.

Neuroglia (noo-ROG-lee-ah), or glia, are cells that support and take care of the neurons. The word *glial* means "gluelike" and refers to the ability of these cells to support, or bind together, the vast network of neurons. (Nervous tissue is described more fully in Chapters 10 to 13.)

MUSCLE TISSUE

Muscle tissue is composed of cells that shorten, or contract. In doing so, they cause movement of a body part. Because the cells are long and slender, they are called *fibers* rather than *cells*. The three types of muscle are skeletal, smooth, and cardiac (Figure 6-7).

Nervous Tissue

Neuron

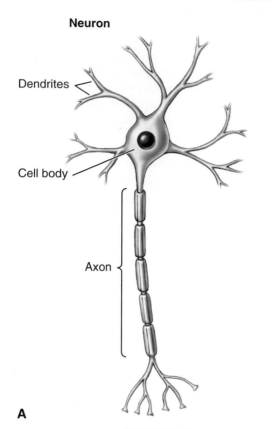

Dendrites

Cell body

Axon

A

Neuroglia (glia)

B

FIGURE 6-6 Two types of nervous tissue. **A,** Neuron. **B,** Neuroglia.

SKELETAL MUSCLE

Skeletal muscle is generally attached to bone (the skeletal system). Because of the appearance of striations (STRYE-ay-shuns) or stripes, *skeletal muscle* is also called *striated muscle*. Skeletal muscles move the skeleton, maintain posture, and stabilize joints.

SMOOTH MUSCLE

Smooth muscle, also called *visceral muscle,* is generally found in the walls of the viscera, or organs, such as the stomach, intestines, and urinary bladder. It is also found in tubes such as the bronchioles (breathing passages) and blood vessels. The function of smooth muscle is related to the organ in which it is found. For example, smooth muscle in the stomach helps mash and churn food, whereas the smooth muscle in the urinary bladder helps expel urine.

CARDIAC MUSCLE

Cardiac muscle is found only in the heart, where it functions to pump blood into a vast network of blood vessels. Cardiac muscle fibers are long branching cells

that fit together tightly at junctions; this arrangement promotes rapid conduction of coordinated electrical signals throughout the heart.

[?] Re-Think

List the four types of tissue and state the general function of each type.

2+2 Sum It Up!

Connective tissue is the most widespread and diverse of the tissue types; its abundant intercellular matrix can be solid, rubbery, gel-like, or liquid. Connective tissue generally connects and binds together parts of the body. Nervous tissue is found in the brain, spinal cord, and nerves and is concerned with the transmission of information throughout the entire body. Muscle tissue is composed of cells that can contract and thus produce movement of body parts. The three types of muscle are skeletal, smooth, and cardiac.

TISSUE REPAIR

How does tissue repair itself after an injury? Two types of tissue repair are regeneration and fibrosis. Regeneration refers to the replacement of tissue by cells that

Muscle Tissue

Skeletal

Cardiac

Smooth

FIGURE 6-7 Types of muscle tissue: skeletal, cardiac, and smooth.

are identical to the original cells. Regeneration occurs only in tissues whose cells undergo mitosis, such as the skin.

Fibrosis is the replacement of injured tissue by the formation of fibrous connective tissue, or scar tissue. The fibers of scar tissue pull the edges of the wound together and strengthen the area. Damaged skeletal muscle, cardiac muscle, and nervous tissue do not undergo mitosis and must be replaced by scar tissue. The steps involved in tissue repair are illustrated and described in Figure 6-8. The injured skin of some persons exhibits excessive fibrosis, leading to the formation of keloids. Keloid (KEE-loyd) scars develop most often on the upper trunk and earlobes and are of concern cosmetically. Unfortunately, they tend to recur when surgically removed. Some tribespeople practice scarification during which the skin is sliced in hopes of inducing keloid scar formation. The keloid scar pattern reflects a significant event or rite of passage in the person's life.

Do You Know...

What a Confederate Medical Officer Observed about a Maggot-Infested Battle Wound?

He observed that the wound was "cleaner" than wounds not infested with maggots. The incidence of septicemia (blood poisoning) was also lower in patients with maggot-infested wounds. Maggots are fly larvae; in the battlefield, the infected wound attracted flies that promptly laid their eggs, producing the larvae. Hungry maggots feasted on dead and infected tissue, thereby débriding the wound. (Débridement is the process of removing necrotic tissue from a wound to promote growth of healthy tissue.) Despite our disgust at such dining practices, maggots have recently been re-employed in the hospital setting to clean up infected wounds. Maggots, hatched and dispatched under sterile conditions, perform their duties under a new fancy name: biodébridement. Maggots are placed in the infected wound and allowed to "do their thing." New name, same old maggot.

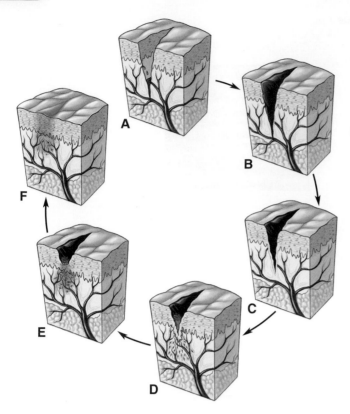

FIGURE 6-8 Steps in tissue repair. **A,** A deep wound to the skin severs blood vessels, causing blood to fill the wound. **B,** A blood clot forms and, as it dries, it forms a scab. **C, D,** The process of tissue repair begins. Scar tissue forms in the deep layers. **E,** At the same time, surface epithelial cells multiply and fill the area between the scar tissue and the scab. **F,** When the epithelium is complete, the scab detaches. The result is a fully regenerated layer of epithelium over an underlying area of scar tissue.

MEMBRANES

CLASSIFICATION OF MEMBRANES

Membranes are thin sheets of tissue that cover surfaces, line body cavities, and surround organs. Membranes are classified as epithelial or connective tissue (Table 6-3). (The connective tissue membranes are described in Chapters 8 and 10.)

EPITHELIAL MEMBRANES

The epithelial membranes include the cutaneous membrane (skin), the mucous membranes, and the serous membranes (Figure 6-9). Although called *epithelial,* these membranes contain both an epithelial sheet and an underlying layer of connective tissue.

Cutaneous Membrane

The cutaneous membrane is the skin. The outer layer of skin (epidermis) is stratified squamous epithelium. The underlying layer (dermis) is composed of dense fibrous connective tissue (see Chapter 7).

Mucous Membranes

Mucous membranes line all body cavities that open to the exterior of the body (see Figure 6-9). They include the digestive, urinary, reproductive, and respiratory tracts. For example, the digestive tract opens to the exterior of the body at the mouth and anus, whereas the respiratory tract opens to the exterior at the nose and mouth. Mucous membranes usually contain stratified squamous epithelium or simple columnar epithelium. Most mucous membranes are adapted for absorption and secretion. Mucous membranes secrete mucus, which keeps the membrane moist and also lubricates it. For example, in the digestive tract, the mucus allows food to move through the tract with little friction.

Serous Membranes

Serous membranes line the ventral body cavities that are not open to the exterior of the body. If you were to enter the abdominal or thoracic cavity surgically, you would be looking at serous membranes. Serous membranes secrete a thin, watery, serous fluid. The fluid allows the membranes to slide past one another with little friction.

A serous membrane is composed of simple squamous epithelium resting on a thin layer of loose connective tissue. Serous membranes line a cavity and then fold back onto the surface of the organs within that cavity. Thus, part of the membrane lines the wall of the cavity, and the other part covers the organ or organs within that cavity. The part of the membrane that lines the walls of the cavity (like wallpaper) is the **parietal layer**, and the part of the membrane that covers the outside of an organ is the **visceral layer**.

The three serous membranes are the pleura, pericardium, and peritoneum (see Figure 6-9):

1. Pleurae are found in the thoracic cavity. The parietal pleurae line the wall of the thoracic cavity, and the visceral pleurae cover each lung. The space between the pleural layers is called the *pleural cavity;* the membranes are lubricated by pleural fluid. Why is pleurisy so painful? Pleurisy refers to an inflammation of the pleurae and a decrease in serous fluid. As the inflamed and "dry" pleural membranes slide past one another during breathing movements, the person experiences pain.

2. The pericardium is found in the thoracic cavity and partially surrounds the heart. There is a parietal and visceral pericardium that offers slinglike support to the heart. The space between the pericardial membranes is called the *pericardial cavity;* the membranes are lubricated by pericardial fluid. Pericardial structure is described further in Chapter 16.

3. The peritoneum is found within the abdominal cavity. The parietal peritoneum lines its walls, and the visceral peritoneum covers some of the abdominal organs (see Chapter 23).

Infection in the abdominal cavity often involves the peritoneum. For example, a ruptured appendix allows the escape of intestinal contents, loaded with bacteria, into the peritoneal cavity. This leakage causes a life-threatening infectious condition called *peritonitis*.

 Re-Think

1. List the two classifications of membranes.
2. List and locate three epithelial membranes.

 Sum It Up!

Membranes are sheets of tissue. Membranes cover surfaces, line body cavities, and surround organs. Membranes are classified as epithelial membranes or connective tissue membranes. The epithelial membranes include cutaneous (skin), mucous, and serous membranes. The location and functions of the epithelial and connective tissue membranes are summarized in Table 6-3.

 As You Age

1. Because tissues consist of cells, cellular aging alters the tissues formed by the cells. Alterations in tissues, in turn, affect organ function. For example, by age 85, lung capacity has decreased by 50%, muscle strength has decreased by about 45%, and kidney function has decreased by 30%.
2. Collagen and elastin decrease in connective tissue. Consequently, tissues become stiffer, less elastic, and less efficient in their functioning.
3. Lipid and fat content of tissues change. In men, a gradual increase in tissue lipids and fat occurs until age 60, and then a gradual decrease follows. In women, lipids and fats accumulate in the tissues continuously; no decline occurs as in men.
4. The total amount of water in the body gradually decreases. The change in body fat and the decrease in water are major reasons why older adults respond differently to drugs than the younger population.
5. Tissue atrophy causes a decrease in the mass of most organs.

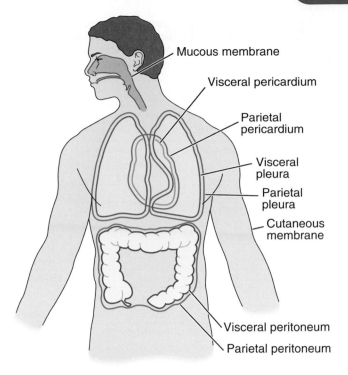

FIGURE 6-9 Epithelial membranes.

Table 6-3	Types of Membranes
TYPE	**LOCATION**
Epithelial Membranes	
Cutaneous membrane	Skin (outer layer)
Mucous membrane	Digestive tract lining Urinary tract lining Reproductive tract lining Respiratory tract lining

Serous membrane
  Pleurae
  Pericardium
 	
  Peritoneum
	
	Thoracic cavity; pleural cavity
	Thoracic cavity around the
	  heart; pericardial cavity
	Abdominopelvic cavity

Connective Tissue Membranes	
Synovial	Lines joint cavities; secretes synovial fluid
Periosteum	Covers bone; contains the blood vessels that supply the bone
Perichondrium	Covers cartilage; contains capillaries that nourish the cartilage
Meninges	Covers brain and spinal cord
Fascia (various kinds)	Appears throughout body

MEDICAL TERMINOLOGY AND DISORDERS			Disorders of Tissues and Membranes
Medical Term	**Word Parts**	**Word Part Meaning or Derivation**	**Description**
Words			
biopsy	bi/o-	life	A **biopsy** is *the removal and examination of tissue from a living body for diagnostic purposes.*
	-opsy	view of	
diagnosis	dia-	apart	**Diagnosis** is *the process of identifying a disease or disorder by examination of the patient and all relevant data.* A correct diagnosis allows the physician to give the patient his **prognosis** (pro = before; gnos/o = knowing), *a forecast of the probable course of the disease.*
	-gnos/o-	distinguishing, learning, knowing	
endocrine	endo-	within	An endocrine gland secretes hormones that circulate through the blood and function within the body. For example, insulin is secreted by a gland called the *pancreas* and is carried throughout the body in the blood. An exocrine (exo = outside) gland secretes substances into ducts that carry the secretion to the outside of the body, as in sweat and sebum.
	-crin/o-	secrete	
histology	hist/o-	tissue	**Histology** is *the study of tissues.*
	-logy	study of	
necrosis	necr/o-	death	**Necrosis** refers to *the process of death of the cells or tissues, especially in a localized area.* Tissue that is deprived of its blood supply necroses, or dies.
	-osis	condition of	
Disorders			
adhesions	ad-	to, toward, or near	**Adhesions** are *bands of "internal scar tissue" that bind or constrict organs.* Surgery and infection are common causes. As part of the healing process, fibrin and other tissue repair cells penetrate the fibrous bands, contributing to the formation of the adhesion. Adhesions are particularly common in the abdominopelvic cavity. An example of an adhesion-related consequence is intestinal obstruction.
	-hension	From a Latin word meaning "sticking to"	
connective tissue diseases			*A group of diseases that attack the connective tissues of the body.* The connective tissues are composed of two major structural proteins: collagen and elastin. *Diseases that affect collagen specifically* are also referred to as *collagen diseases.* Many connective tissue diseases are associated with abnormal immune system activity. A wide variety of symptoms occur depending on the location of the connective tissue. Systemic autoimmune connective tissue diseases include systemic lupus erythematosus (SLE) and scleroderma.
gangrene		From a Greek word meaning "to gnaw"	**Gangrene** is *a condition in which an insufficient blood supply causes tissue necrosis.* Two types of gangrene are dry and wet gangrene. Dry gangrene is caused by ischemia (poor blood supply). Wet gangrene involves infection of a wound that impairs both arterial and venous blood flow and cell function.
neoplasm	neo-	new	A **neoplasm** is *an abnormal proliferation of cells, the growth being excessive and uncoordinated with surrounding cells.* The excessive growth most often forms a lump or a solid tumor. Neoplasms may be benign, premalignant, or malignant. Examples of benign (meaning "well," as opposed to malignant) neoplasms include fibromas, adenomas, lipomas, and skin moles. They are localized, do not become malignant, and do not metastasize. An example of a premalignant neoplasm is carcinoma-in-situ; it remains localized for a while but becomes cancerous, given enough time. Hence, the urgency for early diagnosis and treatment. Malignant (from a Latin word meaning "acting from malice") neoplasms are called *cancers.* Because they are invasive and metastatic (spreading), they eventually kill the host. The primary neoplasm is *the original or first tumor;* untreated, it spreads or metastasizes throughout the body. A **secondary neoplasm** refers to *a cancerous tumor that is the result of metastasis (metastatic lesion).* Carcinomas and sarcomas are malignant tumors. A **carcinoma** is *a malignant tumor that arises from epithelial tissue.* A **sarcoma** is *a malignant tumor that arises from connective tissue.*
	-plasm	formed material	

Get Ready for Exams!

Summary Outline

Tissues are groups of cells similar to each other in structure and function. Membranes are thin sheets of tissue that cover surfaces, line body cavities, and surround organs.

I. **Types of Tissue**
   A. Epithelial tissue
      1. Covers surfaces, lines cavities, and engages in secretion/absorption and protective functions
      2. Classified according to cell shape (squamous, cuboidal, and columnar) and layers (simple and stratified)
      3. Types and functions are summarized in Table 6-1.
   B. Connective tissue
      1. Primary function of connective tissue is to bind together the parts of the body. Other functions include support, protection, storage of fat, and transport of substances. See Table 6-2.
      2. Has an abundant intercellular matrix that may be liquid, gel-like, or hard; often contains protein fibers that are secreted by the cells
      3. Types of loose connective tissue: areolar, adipose, and reticular
      4. Dense fibrous connective tissue forms tendons, ligaments, capsules, fascia, and the dermal layer of skin.
      5. Types of cartilage: hyaline, elastic, and fibrocartilage
      6. Bone (osseous tissue) has a hard intercellular matrix that includes collagen, calcium salts, and other minerals.
      7. Blood and lymph have a watery intercellular matrix.
   C. Nervous tissue
      1. Nervous tissue: found in the nerves, brain, and spinal cord
      2. Two types of nervous tissue: neurons (transmit electrical signals) and neuroglia (support and take care of the neurons)
   D. Muscle tissue
      1. Muscle cells contract, thereby causing movement.
      2. Three types of muscle: skeletal, smooth, and cardiac
II. **Tissue Repair**
   A. Tissue repair by regeneration: replacement of tissue by cells that undergo mitosis
   B. Tissue repair by fibrosis: formation of scar tissue
III. **Membranes**
   A. Epithelial membranes (see Table 6-3)
      1. Cutaneous membrane: the skin
      2. Mucous membrane: lines all body cavities that open to the exterior of the body
      3. Serous membranes: line the ventral body cavities, which are not open to the exterior of the body
      4. Layers of serous membranes: a parietal layer that lines the wall of the cavity and a visceral layer that covers the outside of an organ
      5. Three serous membranes: pleurae, pericardium, and peritoneum

   B. Connective tissue membranes (see Table 6-3): includes synovial, periosteum, pericardium, meninges, and fascia

Review Your Knowledge

Matching: Tissues
Directions: Match the following words with their descriptions below. Some words may be used more than once.
a. epithelial
b. connective
c. muscle
d. nervous

1. ___ Important functions: secretion, absorption, excretion, and protection
2. ___ Blood, bone, cartilage, and adipose tissue
3. ___ Classified as squamous, cuboidal, or columnar
4. ___ Endocrine and exocrine glands arise from this type of tissue
5. ___ Binds together parts of the body; examples include tendons, ligaments, and fascia
6. ___ Skeletal, cardiac, and smooth
7. ___ Has the greatest amount of intercellular matrix
8. ___ Chondrocytes and osteocytes are included in this tissue
9. ___ Intercellular matrix may be liquid, gel, or rigid
10. ___ Dendrites, axons, and glia

Matching: Membranes
Directions: Match the following words with their descriptions below.
a. visceral pleura
b. parietal peritoneum
c. connective tissue membranes
d. mucous membranes
e. parietal pleura

1. ___ Membranes lining all body cavities that open to the outside of the body
2. ___ Serous membrane that lines the walls of the thoracic cavity
3. ___ Serous membrane that lines the walls of the abdominopelvic cavity
4. ___ Serous membrane that covers each lung
5. ___ Synovial membranes: periosteum, perichondrium, and meninges

Multiple Choice
1. Which of the following is not characteristic of epithelial tissue?
   a. Arranged like floor tiles
   b. Simple, cuboidal, and columnar
   c. Large amount of mineral-containing intercellular matrix
   d. Gives rise to endocrine and exocrine glands
2. Adipose tissue is
   a. a type of connective tissue that stores fat.
   b. described as striated and voluntary.
   c. classified as endocrine and exocrine.
   d. classified as skeletal, cardiac, and smooth.

3. Osseous tissue
   a. contains hard mineral-containing intercellular matrix.
   b. contains osteocytes.
   c. is a type of connective tissue.
   d. All of the above.
4. With regard to the pleural membranes,
   a. there is a visceral and parietal pleural membrane.
   b. they are connective tissue membranes.
   c. they are mucous membranes.
   d. they are located in the dorsal cavity.
5. The pleurae and peritoneum
   a. are serous membranes.
   b. are located within the thoracic cavity.
   c. are located within the abdominal cavity.
   d. surround the lungs and the heart.
6. Epithelial tissue is avascular, meaning that it
   a. is shaped like a fish scale.
   b. contains no blood vessels.
   c. has no intercellular matrix.
   d. cannot repair itself.
7. The intercellular matrix of connective tissue
   a. is less apparent than the intercellular matrix of epithelial tissue.
   b. is absent in blood and lymph.
   c. is classified as squamous, cuboidal, and columnar.
   d. can be hard, liquid, or gel-like in consistency.

Go Figure

1. **According to Figures 6-1, 6-2, and 6-3**
   a. Only squamous epithelial tissue forms large continuous sheets.
   b. Epithelial tissue has a superabundance of intercellular matrix.
   c. Epithelial tissue is confined to the thoracic cavity.
   d. Epithelial tissue is described as squamous, cuboidal, columnar, simple, or stratified.

2. **According to Figure 6-5 and Table 6-2**
   a. The air sacs in the lungs are lined with adipose tissue.
   b. Cartilage, bone, and adipose tissue are classified as connective tissue.
   c. All connective tissue has a hard intercellular matrix.
   d. *Pseudostratified* and *transitional* are descriptive terms most associated with connective tissue.

3. **According to Figures 6-6 and 6-7**
   a. Dendrites, cell bodies, and axons are parts of neuroglial cells.
   b. *Skeletal, cardiac,* and *smooth* are terms that describe visceral muscle.
   c. Both skeletal and cardiac muscle are striped or striated.
   d. Smooth muscle is striped or striated, like skeletal muscle.

4. **According to Figure 6-9**
   a. The terms *parietal* and *visceral* only refer to serous membranes located within the thoracic cavity.
   b. Pleural membranes surround the lungs and heart.
   c. The visceral and parietal peritoneal membranes are located in the abdominopelvic cavity.
   d. The cutaneous membrane lines the mouth and digestive tract.

Integumentary System and Body Temperature

Key Terms

apocrine glands (p. 99)
ceruminous glands (p. 100)
conduction (p. 101)
convection (p. 101)
cutaneous membrane (p. 94)
dermis (p. 94)
eccrine glands (p. 100)

epidermis (p. 94)
evaporation (p. 101)
integument (p. 94)
keratin (p. 94)
melanin (p. 96)
radiation (p. 101)
sebaceous glands (p. 99)

stratum corneum (p. 94)
stratum germinativum (p. 94)
subcutaneous layer (p. 95)
sudoriferous glands (p. 99)
thermoregulation (p. 101)

Objectives

1. List seven functions of the skin.
2. Discuss the structure of the skin, including:
   - Describe the two layers of skin: the epidermis and the dermis.
   - Define *stratum germinativum* and *stratum corneum*.
   - List the two major functions of the subcutaneous layer.
3. List the factors that influence the color of the skin.

4. Describe the accessory structures of the skin: hair, nails, and glands.
5. Discuss heat production in the body, including:
   - Explain four processes whereby the body loses heat.
   - Describe how the skin helps regulate body temperature.
   - Describe how burns are classified and list ways to protect the skin.

Oh no, a zit! How many times have you looked in the mirror only to see a pimple, rash, wrinkle, or unwanted hair? No other organ in the body is so scrutinized, scrubbed, lifted, and painted over as the skin. Yet, year after year, the skin withstands the effects of harsh weather, the burning rays of the sun, constant bathing, friction, injury, and microorganisms that are constantly trying to penetrate its surface.

Oh no ... a zit!

The skin, its accessory structures (sweat glands, oil glands, hair, and nails), and the subcutaneous tissue below the skin form the integumentary system.

FUNCTIONS OF THE INTEGUMENTARY SYSTEM

The integumentary (in-teg-yoo-MEN-tar-ee) system is a complex organ that performs many different functions:

- Acts as a mechanical barrier. It keeps harmful substances out of the body and helps retain water and electrolytes. The acid pH of the skin surface serves as a protective chemical barrier.
- Protects the internal structures and organs from injuries caused by blows, cuts, harsh chemicals, sunlight, burns, and pathogenic microorganisms.
- Participates in the immune response against invading microbes by housing specialized cells, called *dendritic* or *Langerhans' cells*. When the skin is broken, the dendritic cells alert the immune system so that it can ward off infection.
- Performs an excretory function. Although excretion is a minor role, the skin is able to excrete water, salt, and small amounts of waste, such as urea.
- Acts as a gland by synthesizing vitamin D when exposed to sunlight. Vitamin D is necessary for the absorption of calcium from the digestive tract.
- Performs a sensory role by housing the sensory receptors for touch, pressure, pain, and temperature. In this way, the skin helps detect information about the environment.
- Plays an important role in the regulation of body temperature.

 Re-Think

What does the integumentary system do for the body?

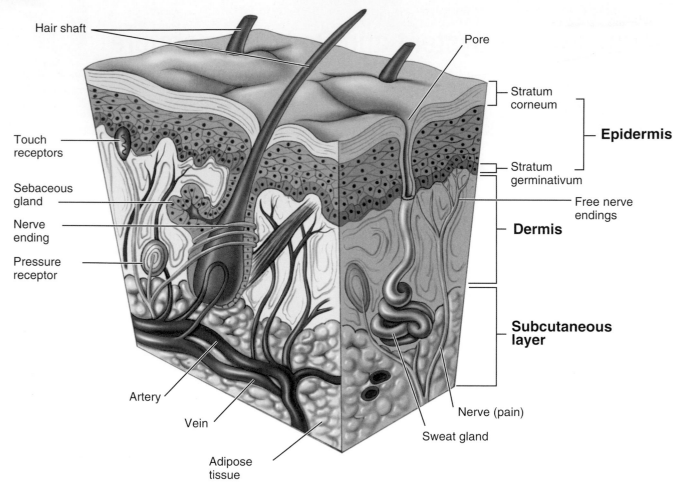

FIGURE 7-1 The skin.

STRUCTURE OF THE SKIN

The skin is called the integument or cutaneous membrane and is considered an organ; it is the largest organ in the body. The skin has two distinct layers—the outer, or surface, layer is the epidermis and the inner layer is the dermis. The dermis is anchored to a subcutaneous layer (Figure 7-1). The study of skin and skin disorders is referred to as *dermatology*.

LAYERS OF THE SKIN

EPIDERMIS

The epidermis (ep-i-DER-mis) is the thin outer layer of the skin and is composed of stratified squamous epithelium. Like all epithelial tissue, the epithelium is avascular; it has no blood supply of its own. Oxygen and nutrients, however, diffuse into the lower epidermis from the rich supply of blood in the underlying dermis. The epidermis can be divided into five layers. Two of the layers are the deeper stratum germinativum and the more superficial stratum corneum.

The stratum germinativum (jer-mi-nah-TIV-um) lies on top of the dermis and thus has access to a rich supply of blood. The cells of this layer are continuously dividing, producing millions of cells per day. As the cells divide, they push the older cells up toward the surface of the epithelium. As the cells move away from the dermis, two changes take place. First, as they move away from their source of nourishment, the cells begin to die. Second, the cells undergo a process of keratinization, whereby a tough protein, keratin (KER-ah-tin), is deposited within the cell. The keratin hardens and flattens the cells as they move toward the surface of the skin. In addition to hardening the cells, the keratin makes the skin water-resistant. Have you ever noticed that your hand does not dissolve when you place it in water?

The stratum corneum is the surface layer of the epidermis and is composed of about 30 layers of dead, flattened, keratinized cells. The dead cells are continuously sloughed off, exfoliated (eks-FOH-lee-a-tid), or desquamated (des-kwah-MAY-tid) through wear and tear. The dead sloughed cells are called *dander;* when dander is clumped together by the oil on the skull, it is called *dandruff*. The sloughed cells are replaced by other cells that are constantly moving up from the deeper layers. You shed about 40,000 skin cells each minute; each month you have a new layer of epithelium.

If Toad Did It?

Did Toad have anything to do with the wart on Helga's nose? No. A wart is an epidermal growth on the skin and is caused by a virus. Although Toad is innocent of this charge, there are several other health concerns. Toad skin can harbor and therefore transmit *Salmonella*, and some toad skins secrete toxins that are harmful to pets and humans. However, from Toad's perspective, handling can damage his skin.

DERMIS

The dermis is located under the epidermis and is the largest portion of the skin; it is composed of dense fibrous connective tissue. It contains numerous collagen and elastin fibers surrounded by a gel-like substance. The fibers make the dermis strong and stretchable; note how well the skin stretches during pregnancy and weight gain. Sometimes, however, excessive stretching of the skin causes small tears in the skin producing white lines. These lines are called stretch marks, or striae (STRYE-ay). The thickness of the epidermis and dermis varies according to the location on the body. Look at the skin on the palms of your hands and the soles of your feet; it is much thicker here than it is over your inner arm or eyelids.

 Do You Know...

What's in That Bathtub Ring and What Are You Dusting?

The bathtub ring: What's in it? Dirt, grime...and, yes, a piece of yourself—dead skin (stratum corneum). How much dead skin? A person sheds about 1.5 lb per year, or about 105 lb over a lifetime. This means that you will scrape the equivalent of your entire body from the sides of your tub and watch it go down the drain. Also, about 75% of household dust is human skin flakes. What doesn't wash down the drain gets sucked up by a vacuum cleaner.

Dead skin on your furniture? Dust not only looks nasty but also feeds critters such as the house dust mite (*Dermatophagoides*). Those who have been diagnosed as having house dust allergy will be relieved to know that they are really allergic to the inhaled feces of the dust mite.

The wavy boundary between the epidermis and dermis resembles the ridges of corrugated cardboard.

The interlocking ridges prevent the slippage of the skin layers. More importantly, for you forensic sleuths, the ridges form the fingerprints.

Although derived from the epidermis, the accessory structures such as the hair, nails, and certain glands are embedded within the dermis. Located within the dermis are blood vessels, nervous tissue, and some muscle tissue. Many of the nerves have specialized endings called *sensory receptors* that detect pain, temperature, pressure, and touch.

? Re-Think

1. What "happens" in the stratum germinativum?
2. Describe two changes that the cells undergo as they "ascend" to the stratum corneum.

THE SKIN TELLS A STORY

- The skin reflects disease processes in the body. For example, a person with herpes zoster (shingles)—an inflammation of nerves caused by the chickenpox virus—develops painful skin lesions along the path of the nerve. A person with a severe generalized staphylococcal infection may develop scalded skin syndrome, a condition in which the skin appears scalded and peels off in layers. Many clinical disorders present initially with skin rashes; the rashes offer clues to the underlying problems.
- Drug reactions are often revealed by skin changes. For example, a person allergic to penicillin may develop hives, or urticaria (er-ti-KAIR-ee-ah). Similarly, a person allergic to sulfa drugs may develop a generalized rash that can progress to a lethal syndrome called *Stevens-Johnson syndrome*.
- The skin responds to chronic irritation. Epidermal cell growth increases in response to certain stimuli. For example, constant irritation or rubbing of an area causes the rate of epidermal cell division to increase, producing a thickened area called a *callus*. Constant rubbing of a toe by a poorly fitting shoe can also produce an overgrowth of epidermal cells arranged in a conical shape. This overgrowth is called a *corn*.
- The skin mirrors your stress level. How many times have you become stressed out and then broke out? The skin truly reveals on the outside what is going on inside!

SUBCUTANEOUS LAYER

The dermis lies on the subcutaneous layer. This layer is not considered part of the skin; it lies under the skin and is therefore called the **subcutaneous layer**, or the hypodermis. The subcutaneous layer is composed primarily of loose connective and adipose tissue. The subcutaneous tissue performs two main roles: it helps insulate the body from extreme temperature changes in the external environment, and it anchors the skin to the underlying structures. A few areas of the body have no subcutaneous layer and the skin anchors directly to the bone. Look at the skin over your knuckles. It is wrinkled and creased because it attaches directly to bone. Imagine what you would look like if all your skin were anchored directly to underlying bone.

 Do You Know...

How You Inject a Medication into the Subcutaneous Layer?

When injecting medication subcutaneously, you need to use a correctly sized needle and insert the needle at the proper angle. The needle penetrates the epidermis and dermis so that the tip of the needle is located in the subcutaneous layer, where the medication is deposited.

THE SKIN, DRUGS, AND CHEMICALS

The skin can absorb many chemicals; this is good news and bad news. The good news is concerned with drug absorption. Drugs can be placed on the surface of the skin and absorbed transdermally (across the skin) in order to achieve a systemic effect (throughout the body). For example, nitroglycerin can be applied using an adhesive patch on the skin. The drug penetrates the skin, is absorbed by the dermal blood vessels, and is transported by the blood throughout the body where it exerts its effects. The skin can also be used to detect allergies by injecting antigens (possible allergic substances) intradermally. An allergic response will appear as a skin reaction (redness, swelling, and itching). Drugs can also be applied topically; the drug is meant to exert its effect on the surface of the skin. Lastly the subcutaneous route is a common way to inject drugs.

The bad news? Skin can absorb toxins; these include pesticides, cleaning fluids, the acetone in nail polish remover, mercury, and many other toxic chemicals that we encounter daily. Farm workers, exposed to chemical sprays, are commonly treated for pesticide poisoning. Are your hands in household chemicals? Wear gloves, and do not underestimate the ability of the skin to absorb toxins!

? Re-Think

Describe the role of the skin in drug administration (i.e., four routes of administration).

SKIN COLOR

Why are there different colors of skin? Skin color is determined by many factors: some genetic, some physiological, and some caused by disease. When we think of skin color, we generally think of black, brown, yellow, and white, as well as the many shades in between! These skin colors are genetically determined.

Deep within the epidermal layer of the skin are cells called *melanocytes*. Melanocytes (meh-LAN-oh-sytes) secrete a skin-darkening pigment called **melanin**; the melanin stains the surrounding cells, causing them to darken. The more melanin secreted, the darker the skin color. Interestingly, we all have the same numbers of melanocytes. What determines our skin color is not the numbers of melanocytes but the amount of melanin secreted. The following factors play a role in changes in skin color:

- *Melanin.* Can melanocytes increase their secretion of melanin? Yes! When exposed to the ultraviolet radiation of sunlight, the melanocytes secrete more melanin. The skin darkens in an attempt to protect the deeper layers from the harmful effects of radiation. This effort creates the famous summer tan. A number of conditions involve malfunctioning melanocytes. If the melanocytes completely fail to secrete melanin, the skin, hair, and the colored part of the eye (iris) are white. This condition is referred to as *albinism*. Other persons develop a condition called *vitiligo* (vit-i-LYE-go). This condition involves a loss of pigment (melanin) in certain areas of the skin, creating patches of white skin. Melanin can also stain unevenly. Freckles and moles are examples of melanin that becomes concentrated in local areas.
- *Carotene.* The yellowish tint of carotene in most persons is hidden by the effects of melanin. Because people of Asian descent have little melanin in their skin, the carotene gives their skin a yellow tint.
- *Blood.* What accounts for the pinkish color of fair-skinned people? So little melanin is produced that the blood in the dermal blood vessels is visible, thereby providing a pinkish tinge to the skin. Poorly oxygenated blood causes the skin to look blue. This condition is called *cyanosis* (sye-ah-NO-sis). Embarrassment causes the blood vessels in the skin to dilate. This condition increases blood flow to the skin, causing the person to blush or flush. What about the saying, "He was white as a sheet"? A person who is scared experiences a constriction of the blood vessels in the skin and a decrease in the amount of oxygenated blood. The resulting pale or ashen color is called *pallor*. A black and blue discoloration (bruise) indicates that blood has escaped from the blood vessels into the injured tissue. A black and blue area is called an *ecchymosis* (ek-ih-MOH-sis).
- *Bilirubin.* Skin color may also change in response to disease processes. A person with liver disease is

unable to excrete a pigment called *bilirubin* (bil-ih-ROO-bin). This pigment is instead deposited in the skin, causing it to turn yellow—a condition known as *jaundice.*

- *Diet.* Finally, skin color may also change in response to diet. For example, it is possible to impart a yellow tint to the skin by overeating carotene-rich vegetables such as carrots.

2+2 Sum It Up!

The integumentary system is composed of the skin and accessory organs (hair, nails, and glands). It is a complex organ that performs many functions. It affords protection for the entire body, acts as a barrier, regulates temperature, detects sensations (e.g., touch, pressure, temperature, and pain), synthesizes vitamin D, participates in the immune response, and acts as an excretory organ. The skin is composed of two layers: the epidermis and dermis. The dermis sits on a subcutaneous layer called the *hypodermis.* There are different colors of skin. Our natural skin color is genetically determined; we are light-skinned, dark-skinned, and many shades in between. Our skin color changes in response to certain stimuli or underlying conditions; these changes include tanning, blushing, cyanosis, and jaundice. The skin can also reveal certain disease states, such as allergic responses, infections, and liver disease. The skin often announces on the outside what is happening on the inside.

? Re-Think

Describe the underlying causes of the following color changes: cyanosis, flushing, pallor, jaundice, tanning, and vitiligo.

ACCESSORY STRUCTURES OF THE SKIN

The skin is the home of several accessory structures, including the hair, nails, and glands.

HAIR

Thousands and thousands of years ago, we humans were a hairy lot. Like our furry pets, we depended on a thick crop of hair to keep us warm. Today, most of the hair covering our bodies is sparse and very fine, with the exception of the hair on our heads (and for some, that too is sparse). The main function of our sparse body hair is to sense insects on the skin before they can sting us. Some body parts are hairless. These include the palms of the hands, soles of the feet, lips, nipples, and parts of the external reproductive organs.

Some areas of hair perform other functions. For example, the eyelashes and eyebrows protect the eyes from dust and perspiration. The nasal hairs trap dust and prevent it from being inhaled into the lungs. The hair of the scalp helps keep us warm and, of course, plays an important cosmetic role.

Hair growth is influenced by the sex hormones estrogen and testosterone. The onset of puberty is heralded by the growth of hair in the axillary and pubic areas in males and females. In the man, the surge of testosterone also produces a beard and hairy chest. Estrogen, of course, does not have this effect. When a woman has too much testosterone, excessive hair growth occurs, including facial hair. The excessive growth of hair is called *hirsutism* (HER-soo-tiz-em), from a Greek word meaning "shaggy." One more thing: apparently, hair growth responds rather well to mind–body signals. The beards of men who have been at sea for an extended period experience a growth spurt of hair when told that they are going ashore.

The chief parts of a hair are the shaft (the part above the surface of the skin) and the root (the part that extends from the dermis to the surface) (Figure 7-2). Each hair arises from a group of epidermal cells that penetrate down into the dermis. This downward extension of epithelial cells forms the hair follicle. The epidermal cells of the hair follicle receive a rich supply of blood from the dermal blood vessels. As these cells divide and grow, the older cells are pushed toward the surface of the skin. As they move away from their source of nourishment, the cells die. Like other cells that compose the skin, the hair cells also become keratinized. The hair that we brush, blow-dry, and curl every day is a collection of dead, keratinized cells.

Hair color is determined by the type and amount of melanin secretion. An abundance of melanin produces dark hair, whereas less melanin produces blond hair. With age, the melanocytes become less active; the absence of melanin produces white hair. Gray hair is caused by a mixture of pigmented and nonpigmented hairs. Interestingly, red hair is caused by a modified type of melanin that contains iron.

Curly, wavy, or straight—this is determined by the shape of the hair shaft. A round shaft produces straight hair, whereas an oval shaft produces wavy hair. Curly and kinky strands of hair are the result of flat hair shafts. Hair can be curled by chemically flattening the hair shafts.

How does Frightened Kitty get her hair to stand on end? Attached to the hair follicle is a group of smooth muscle cells called the *arrector pili* (ah-REK-tor PYE-lye) muscles (see Figure 7-2). Contraction of these muscles causes the hair to stand on end. When frightened, the cat's brain sends its panic message along the nerves to these muscles. The muscles then contract and pull the hair into an upright position. Kitty looks more ferocious with her fur standing on end, and the spiked look helps frighten off her attackers. Her fur also

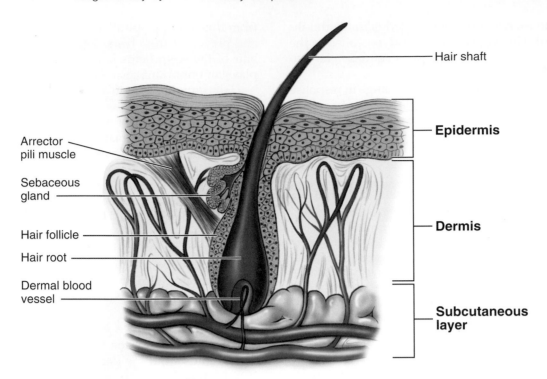

FIGURE 7-2 Hair follicle and parts of the hair.

stands on end when she is cold; the raised fur traps heat and helps keep her warm.

Although humans may not benefit as much from hair as do our furry friends, we respond to fear and cold in the same way. Contraction of the arrector pili muscles also causes our hair to stand on end. As the hair stands, it pulls the skin up into little bumps. This reaction is the basis of goose flesh, or goose bumps. Unlike Kitty, the erect human hair does not do much to trap heat.

Cosmetically, hair is important. Hair loss to the point of baldness is distressing—enter the comb-over. Loss of hair is called *alopecia* (al-o-PEE-sha), which comes from a word meaning "fox mange." The most common type of baldness is male pattern baldness, which is a hereditary condition characterized by a gradual loss of hair with aging—hair today, gone tomorrow! A second common cause of hair loss is related to drug toxicity, as with chemotherapy or radiation therapy. Anticancer drugs are so cytotoxic that they often destroy hair-producing epithelial cells. When drug therapy is terminated, the cells regenerate and start to grow hair again. Interestingly, the new hair

may be a different color or texture from the original (pre-drug) hair.

Forensically, hair is a gold mine. For example, arsenic is called *inheritance powder*, because it is a long-time favorite for dispatching wealthy family members. Chronic arsenic poisoning is difficult to detect medically, but analysis of the hair not only detects the presence of arsenic—it can also detect the time course of the poisoning.

? Re-Think

1. What is the function of the hair follicle?
2. Differentiate between hirsutism and alopecia.

NAILS

Nails are thin plates of stratified squamous epithelial cells that contain a very hard form of keratin (Figure 7-3). The nails are found on the distal ends of the fingers and toes and protect these structures from injury.

Each nail has the following structures: a free edge, a nail body (fingernail), and a nail root. The cells of the nail body develop and are keratinized in the nail root. The extent of nail growth is represented by the half-moon–shaped lunula (LOO-nyoo-lah), located at the base of the nail. As the nail body grows, it slides over a layer called the *nailbed*, a part of the epidermis. The pink color of nails is caused by the blood vessels in the underlying dermal layer beneath the nail. The cuticle is a fold of stratum corneum that grows onto the proximal portion of the nail body.

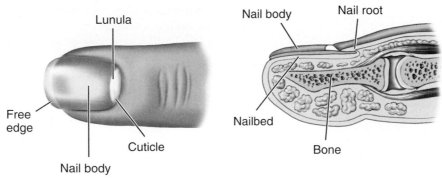

FIGURE 7-3 Nail.

Like the skin, the nails also tell stories. The condition of the nails provides important diagnostic information regarding systemic disease. Nails should be examined for shape, dorsal curvature, adhesion to the nail bed, color, and thickness. Some clinical observations include the following:

- *Clubbing*. Chronic lung and heart disease cause clubbing, a condition that indicates that the fingertips have received an insufficient supply of oxygenated blood over a period of time. Clubbing involves changes in the fingertips and nails; the fingertips enlarge and the nails become thick, hard, shiny, and curved at the free end. With severe clubbing, the nail may detach from its base.
- *In the pink...or not*. Nail color should be pink. Poor oxygenation makes the blood appear bluish-red (cyanosis), which in turn makes the nails appear bluish. Other color changes include pigment bands; these dark bands are normally seen in dark-skinned individuals. When present in light-skinned persons, the bands may indicate melanoma.
- *Brittle*. Nails may also be described as brittle; this is generally caused by poor oxygenation, thyroid gland dysfunction, and nutritional anemia.

? Re-Think

What is clubbing and why is it indicative of heart and/or lung disease?

GLANDS

Two major exocrine glands are associated with the skin: the sebaceous glands and the sweat glands (Figure 7-4).

Most sebaceous (seh-BAY-shus) glands, or oil glands, are associated with hair follicles and are found in all areas of the body that have hair. They secrete an oily substance called *sebum* that flows into the hair root and then out onto the surface of the skin. A small number of sebaceous glands open directly onto the surface of the skin. The sebum lubricates and helps waterproof the hair and skin, as well as inhibits the growth of bacteria on the surface of the skin. With aging, sebum production gradually decreases. This change accounts, in part, for the dry skin and brittle hair seen in older persons. The sebaceous glands play a unique role in the fetus. Babies are born with a covering that resembles cream cheese. The covering is called the *vernix caseosa* (VERN-iks kay-see-OH-sah) and is secreted by the sebaceous glands. The vernix caseosa protects the skin of the fetus from the macerating effects of amniotic fluid.

Sometimes, the sebaceous glands become blocked by accumulated sebum and other debris. When the sebum is exposed to the air and dries out, it turns black, forming a blackhead. When the blocked sebum becomes infected with staphylococci, it is a pimple (pustule). You have seen the contents of a pimple. Blackhead and pimple formation is common among adolescents, because sebaceous gland activity responds to the hormonal changes associated with puberty. Babies may also have a problem with their sebaceous glands. The sebaceous glands on the scalp can oversecrete sebum, producing oily scales. Because this condition occurs during infancy, the cradle period, it is called *cradle cap*.

Do You Know...

About Blackheads, Pimples, and Worms?

There is a long history of persons squeezing (not a good idea!) or expressing the contents (sebum) of a blackhead or comedo. The expressed sebum resembles a long worm. The ancients concluded that the skin was being eaten into by a worm—hence, the word *comedo* (from a Latin word meaning "to eat into").

The sweat glands, or sudoriferous (soo-dor-IF-er-us) glands, are located in the dermis (see Figure 7-4). As the name implies, these glands secrete sweat; the sweat is secreted into a duct that opens onto the skin as a pore. An individual has approximately 3 million sweat glands.

Two types of sweat glands are the apocrine and eccrine sweat glands. The apocrine (AP-oh-krin) glands are usually associated with hair follicles and are found in the axillary and genital areas. The apocrine glands

Sebaceous gland

- **Epidermis**
- **Dermis**
- **Subcutaneous layer**

Apocrine gland (sweat gland)

Eccrine gland (sweat gland)

FIGURE 7-4 Skin glands: sebaceous glands and sweat glands.

respond to emotional stress and become active when the person is frightened, upset, in pain, or sexually excited. Because the development of these glands is stimulated by the sex hormones, they become more active during puberty. The sweat produced by these glands does not have a strong odor. If allowed to accumulate on the skin, however, the substances in sweat are degraded by bacteria into chemicals with a strong unpleasant odor. This is called *body odor* and is the reason we use deodorant.

 Do You Know...

'Bout Them "Apples"?

In some species of animals, the olfactory area of the brain, the "smell brain," is the largest part of the brain. The survival of these animals depends heavily on the sense of smell. Humans also have a smell brain that, although very small, plays a powerful role in our emotional responses and is responsible for some very strange responses. For example, in Elizabethan times, lovers exchanged "love apples." And where did you get them? You made them. A woman peeled a common apple and placed it in her armpit until it was saturated with her perspiration (thanks to the apocrine glands). The sweat-soaked apple was then given to her lover to smell—for his pleasure, at his leisure.

Some of these secretions act as sex attractants. Watch how eagerly Rover sniffs when a potential mate is in the immediate area. These sex attractants are called *pheromones* (FAIR-o-mohns). The vaginal secretions of an ovulating female contain pheromones called *copulines*. The copulines can cause a testosterone surge (and an urge to merge) in the male.

The **eccrine** (EK-rin) **glands** are the more numerous and widely distributed of the sweat glands. They are located throughout the body and are especially numerous on the forehead, neck, back, upper lip, palms, and soles. Unlike apocrine glands, the eccrine glands are not associated with hair follicles.

The sweat secreted by the eccrine glands plays an important role in body temperature regulation. As sweat evaporates from the skin surface, heat is lost. These are the glands that sweat profusely on hot days or during periods of strenuous exercise. Unlike the apocrine glands, which become active during puberty, the eccrine glands function throughout an entire lifetime. Eccrine secretion is composed primarily of water and a few salts.

Modified sweat glands include the mammary glands and ceruminous (ser-ROO-mi-nus) glands. The mammary glands are located in the breasts and secrete milk. (The secretion of milk is discussed further in Chapter 27.) The **ceruminous glands** are found in the external auditory canal of the ear. They secrete cerumen (seh-ROO-men), or ear wax. This yellow, sticky, waxlike secretion repels insects and traps foreign material. Silkworms and spiders use modified sweat glands to secrete silk and weave intricate webs.

Think all sweat looks the same? Not so! Some dyes, foods, and drugs are excreted in the sweat and may color the sweat in a variety of bright hues. This condition is called *chromhidrosis*.

 Re-Think

State the most important roles of the sebaceous, apocrine, and eccrine glands.

 Do You Know...

Why Perspiration Is Sensible...or Insensible?

About 500 mL/day of water is normally lost through the skin and is called *insensible perspiration*. If the epidermis is damaged, as in severe burns, the rate of insensible perspiration increases enormously; fluid loss is so great that the untreated patient may die from shock because of low blood volume. The eccrine glands are largely responsible for sensible perspiration. As body temperature rises, as in exercise, the eccrine glands increase the secretion of sweat, thereby cooling the body. When operating maximally, the eccrine glands can secrete 1 gallon of sweat per hour in an attempt to cool the body.

[handwritten: 36.1 - 37.8°C (ideal = 37°C)]

The skin is the home of several accessory structures, including the hair, nails, and glands. There are two major exocrine glands: the sebaceous glands and the sweat glands (also called sudoriferous glands). There are two types of sweat glands: the eccrine glands and the apocrine glands. Modified sweat glands include the ceruminous glands, which secrete ear wax, and the mammary glands, which secrete milk.

BODY TEMPERATURE   *[handwritten: 37.0°C]*

Normal body temperature is said to be 98.6°F, although it can range from 97° to 100°F. The temperature, however, fluctuates about 1.8°F in a 24-hour period, being lowest in the early morning and highest in the late afternoon. Body temperature also differs from one part of the body to another. The inner parts of the body (cranial, thoracic, and abdominal cavities) reflect the higher core temperature. The more surface areas (skin and mouth) reflect the cooler shell temperature. For example, the rectal temperature measures core temperature and ranges between 99° to 99.7°F, whereas the oral temperature is about 1°F lower.

Body temperature is maintained by balancing heat production and heat loss. The mechanism whereby the body balances heat production and heat loss is called **thermoregulation**. Failure to thermoregulate causes body temperature to fluctuate; an excessive decrease in body temperature is called *hypothermia* and an excessive increase is called *hyperthermia*. Extreme changes in body temperature are often fatal.

Do You Know...

Why You Shouldn't Offer a Hypothermic Individual a Rum Punch?

Although this is a thoughtful gesture, the alcohol in the rum causes dilation of the blood vessels in the skin, thereby increasing blood flow and the loss of heat. Mr. Hypothermia needs his heat. He may prefer the rum punch, but he is better served with a cup of hot tea.

HEAT PRODUCTION

Heat is thermal energy and is produced by the millions of chemical reactions occurring in the cells of the body. The heat is distributed throughout the body by the blood. The heat produced by metabolizing cells is the basis of body temperature. In the resting state, the greatest amount of heat is produced by the muscles, liver, and endocrine glands. The resting brain produces only about 15% of the heat. Interestingly, the studying brain does not produce much more heat.

The amount of heat produced can be affected by many factors, such as food consumption, the amounts and types of hormones secreted, and physical activity. With exercise, the amount of heat produced by the muscles may increase enormously. The hormonal effects on heat production are dramatically illustrated by persons with thyroid gland disease. The hypothyroid person generally has a lower-than-normal body temperature, but the hyperthyroid person has an elevated temperature. In fact, an extreme hyperthyroid state (thyroid storm) can elevate body temperature into a range that is potentially lethal.

HEAT LOSS

Most heat loss (80%) occurs through the skin. The remaining 20% is lost through the respiratory system (lungs) and in the excretory products (urine and feces). Heat loss occurs by four means: radiation, conduction, convection, and evaporation.

The amount of blood in the dermal blood vessels influences the amount of heat that can be lost or dissipated by radiation, conduction, and convection. **Radiation** means that heat is lost from a warm object (the body) to the cooler air surrounding the warm object. Thus, a person loses heat in a cold room. **Conduction** is the loss of heat from a warm body to a cooler object in contact with the warm body. For example, a person (warm object) becomes cold when sitting on a block of ice (cooler object). Clinically, a cooling blanket may reduce a dangerously high fever. **Convection** is the loss of heat by air currents moving over the surface of the skin. For example, a fan moves air across the surface of the skin, thereby constantly removing the layer of heated air next to the body.

Finally, heat may be lost through evaporation. **Evaporation** occurs when a liquid becomes a gas. For example, when liquid alcohol is rubbed on the skin, it evaporates and cools the skin. Similarly, during strenuous exercise, sweat on the surface of the skin evaporates and cools the body. Note that the evaporation of water is associated with a loss of heat. On a hot humid day, water cannot evaporate from the surface of the skin. Hence, heat loss is diminished. This is why we feel the heat so intensely on a hot humid day.

Check out some of the thermoregulatory mechanisms of some of our animal friends. Squirrels cool off by waving their bushy tails, and elephants flap their wonderful ears. And we all know that Rover pants. On a less appealing note, the vulture cannot sweat and cools itself by excreting waste along its own legs. The vulture? Not a house-friendly pet.

? Re-Think

1. Differentiate between core and shell temperature.
2. What is the origin of body temperature?
3. List three factors that can change heat production.

REGULATION

Normal body temperature is regulated by several mechanisms. The thermostat of the body is located in a part of the brain called the *hypothalamus*. The

FIGURE 7-5 Temperature regulation.

hypothalamus (hye-poh-THAHL-ah-mus) senses changes in body temperature and sends information to the skin (blood vessels and sweat glands) and skeletal muscle.

With exercise and temperature elevation, the blood vessels dilate, thereby allowing more blood to flow to the skin. This activity transfers heat from the deeper tissues to the surface of the body. Note how flushed our jogger is because of the blood coming to the surface (Figure 7-5). Temperature elevation also stimulates the activity of the sweat glands. As the sweat evaporates from the surface of the body, heat is lost. Under extreme conditions of heat, 12 L of sweat can be secreted in a 24-hour period. These two activities lower body temperature.

What about Mr. Ear Muffs in Figure 7-5? How does his body respond as his temperature decreases? First, the blood vessels constrict, reducing blood flow to the skin. This response traps the blood and heat in the deeper tissues, preventing heat loss. Second, the sweat glands become less active, also preventing heat loss. Third, skeletal muscles contract vigorously and involuntarily, causing shivering and an increase in the production of heat. These three activities raise body temperature. Contraction of the arrector pili muscles causes goose bumps, indicating a decline in body temperature, but contributes minimally to heat production. In furry animals the story is a little different;

contraction of the arrector pili muscles pulls the fur upright, thereby trapping warm air. So, it's not good to shave Rover in the winter.

NEWBORNS AND BODY TEMPERATURE

In the delivery room everyone is relieved when Baby (neonate) takes her first breath and delivers her first wail, waa waa waa. Next to establishing respiratory activity, however, is the infant's need to regulate body temperature. In short, the neonate produces only about two thirds of the heat produced by an adult, but loses twice as much. Several factors contribute to the excess heat loss:

- The neonate generally has a large surface area that increases heat loss. (The curled-up position of the infant decreases surface area and conserves heat.) Interestingly, considerable heat is lost from the head area; hence, the use of caps in the newborn nursery.
- The neonate generally has only a thin layer of subcutaneous fat. (Fat acts as an insulator, thus preventing heat loss.)
- The neonate cannot shiver. (Shivering produces heat.)

The neonate, like a squirrel, produces heat by a process called *nonshivering thermogenesis*. A neonate has brown adipose tissue (BAT), or brown fat, scattered throughout its body, especially around the neck and shoulder area. Metabolism of BAT generates more heat than the metabolism of ordinary adipose tissue (white fat). The heat produced by BAT is picked up by the blood and dispersed throughout the body.

Although we are generally concerned about excessive heat loss in the neonate, we must also be concerned about excess heat. An infant has a very limited capacity to dissipate heat and is therefore at risk for hyperthermia. Do not leave Baby in a hot car!

 Re-Think

1. Explain why shivering and vasoconstriction increases body temperature.
2. Explain how the body cools itself.

WHEN SKIN IS BURNED

Large areas of skin are often lost because of burns. Burns are classified according to the depth of the burn and the extent of the surface area burned (Figure 7-6, *A*). On the basis of depth, burns are classified as partial-thickness burns or full-thickness burns. Partial-thickness burns are further divided into first-degree and second-degree burns. A first-degree burn is red, painful, and slightly edematous (swollen). Only the epidermis is involved. Sunburn is an example of a first-degree burn. A second-degree burn involves damage to both the epidermis and dermis. With little damage to the dermis, the symptoms of a second-degree burn include redness, pain, edema, and blister formation. With greater damage to the dermis, the skin may appear red, tan, or white.

Full-thickness burns are also called *third-degree burns*. With a burn this severe, both the epidermis and dermis are destroyed, often with destruction of the deeper underlying layers. Although first- and second-degree burns are painful, third-degree burns are painless because the sensory receptors have been destroyed.

 Ramp It Up!

Temperature Terms and the Body Thermostat

Unlike your cold-blooded pet boa, you are warm-blooded and therefore maintain your body temperature within a narrow range. Body temperature, however, changes under many clinical conditions and gives rise to several confusing terms. Refer to the diagram of the thermometer as we define these terms. The temperatures on the thermometer were recorded orally; temperatures recorded by other techniques (rectal or axillary) are higher or lower.

- *Normothermia.* This refers to the normal range of body temperature from 97° to 99.6°F (36.1° to 37.6°C).
- *Fever (pyrexia).* The right side of the thermometer illustrates an increase in temperature that is called a *fever*, or *pyrexia*. Pyrogenic cytokines, often secreted by pathogens, increase the hypothalamic set point (thermostat). Then, vasoconstriction (to conserve heat) and shivering (to produce heat) cause the body temperature to reach the elevated set point. The set point can be lowered, usually by resolving its cause (often infection) or by the use of a fever-lowering drug (e.g., aspirin), called an *antipyretic*. Then the body loses heat through vasodilation and sweating. Laypersons often describe this late phase as the "fever has broken." A very high, life-threatening fever is called *hyperpyrexia* (105.8°F [41°C]).
- *Hyperthermia.* The left side of the thermometer illustrates hyperthermia and hypothermia. Hyperthermia refers to an elevation of body temperature caused by the inability of the body to get rid of excess heat; the body simply cannot cool itself. The cause of hyperthermia is most often environmental; the person is subjected to prolonged exposure to high temperatures, as in an infant being left in a car during the hot weather. Unlike fever, hyperthermia is not caused by resetting the thermostat; the set point is normal. Treatment measures focus on cooling the body; antipyretics are not effective because the set point is normal. In the advanced state (104°F [40°C]), hyperthermia is called *heat stroke* or *sunstroke* and represents thermoregulatory failure. Death ensues without immediate treatment.

- *Hypothermia.* This refers to a decrease in body temperature and is usually caused by prolonged exposure to cold, as in falling through ice into cold water. Body temperature becomes too low for the body to sustain body metabolism. Death usually ensues when the body temperature drops below 95°F (35°C).

	C°		F°	
	42		107.6	
	41		105.8	Fever (pyrexia)
Hyperthermia	40		104.0	
	39		102.2	
	38		100.4	
	37		98.6	Normothermia
	36		96.8	
	35		95.0	
Hypothermia	34		93.2	

Ranges   Temperature recorded orally
C = Celsius
F = Fahrenheit

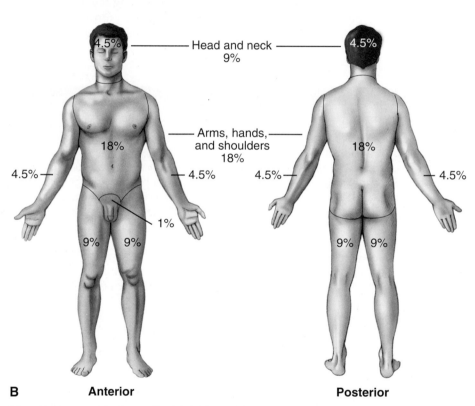

FIGURE 7-6 A, Parts of the skin damaged by burns. Partial-thickness (first- and second-degree burns) and full-thickness burns (third-degree burns). **B,** The rule of nines.

Third-degree burns may appear white, tan, brown, black, or deep cherry red.

The extent of the burn injury is initially evaluated according to the rule of nines (see Figure 7-6, *B*). In this system, the total body surface area is divided into regions. The assigned percentages are related to the number 9. For example, the head and neck are considered to be 9% of the total body surface area. Each upper limb is 9%, whereas each lower limb is 18% (9 × 2). Note the percentages assigned to each specific body region. To determine proper treatment, the clinician needs to evaluate the depth and extent of the burn injury.

ESCHAR

Severe burns are associated with eschar (ESS-kahr) formation. Eschar is dead burned tissue that forms a thick, inflexible, scablike layer over the burned surface. Eschar is a problem for two reasons. First, it may surround an area, such as a leg, and act like a tourniquet, thereby cutting off the flow of blood to the extremity. More seriously, if the eschar surrounds the chest, it prevents chest expansion and breathing. Second, eschar, which is initially sterile, becomes a breeding ground for bacteria and secretes toxins into the blood. These toxins adversely affect various organs in the body, such as the lungs and kidneys. Because eschar can have such serious consequences, it is often slit (escharotomy) to allow expansion of the burned area or removed to rid the body of a source of toxin.

 Re-Think

Explain why an extensive body burn causes fluid and electrolyte imbalance.

A NOTE ABOUT SKIN CARE

The skin is constantly exposed to all sorts of insults, such as the drying effects of soap and water, the damaging effects of the ultraviolet radiation of the sun, friction, numerous bumps, and exposure to sharp objects. Although we cannot avoid normal wear and tear, we can protect the skin in several ways. For example, we can lessen exposure of the skin to ultraviolet radiation. Sunbathing is deadly to the skin. Sun exposure both dries and irreversibly damages the skin. It also makes the skin leather-like and increases the risk of skin cancer and malignant melanoma.

 Do You Know...

What "Vagabond Syndrome" Is and Why It Makes You "Feel Lousy"?

The skin of people who continuously harbor body lice becomes hardened and darkly pigmented; this condition is known as *vagabond syndrome*. Chronic infestation of lice also causes the person to feel tired and irritable, hence the term *feeling lousy*.

Skin care is particularly important in older adults. The skin of an older person is normally drier, more easily injured, and slower to heal. Because the skin is so dry, excessive use of soap should be discouraged. Limiting the use of soaps and excessive bathing can help prevent additional drying of the skin. Moreover, maintaining the acid surface of the skin discourages the growth of bacteria. In addition to becoming drier with aging, the skin changes in another important way. Both the dermis and underlying subcutaneous layer become thinner. As a result, older people bruise more easily because the blood vessels are not as well protected. In addition, heat is lost from the blood vessels so that older people often feel cold.

2+2 Sum It Up!

Body temperature is caused by metabolizing cells. Metabolism, in turn, is affected by several factors: food consumption, hormones, exercise, and disease states. Thermoregulatory mechanisms balance heat production and heat loss. These mechanisms include the coordinated activities of the hypothalamus, blood vessels, and sweat glands. Because the skin performs so many vital functions, burns severely compromise many organ systems, often causing death.

As You Age

1. Aging causes a generalized thinning of the epidermis; the epidermal cells reproduce more slowly and are larger and more irregular. These changes result in thinner, more translucent skin.
2. Melanocyte activity decreases, resulting in decreased protection from ultraviolet light and greater susceptibility to sunburn and skin cancer. Selected melanocytes increase melanin production, resulting in brown spots, or age spots, especially in areas exposed to the sun.
3. The dermis becomes thinner, with a decreased amount of collagen and decreased number of elastin fibers. The result is increased fragility of the skin, as well as increased wrinkles. The skin also heals more slowly.
4. There is a decreased number of dermal blood vessels with a slower rate of repair. This change causes the skin to become more susceptible to small hemorrhages and pressure ulcers.
5. Blood vessels in the subcutaneous tissue decrease, so that drugs administered subcutaneously are absorbed more slowly.
6. The amount of adipose tissue in the subcutaneous layer decreases, resulting in increased and wrinkled skin that has a decreased ability to maintain body temperature. The person tends to feel cold.
7. Sebaceous gland activity decreases, resulting in dry, coarse, itchy skin.
8. Sweat gland activity decreases, resulting in decreased ability to regulate body temperature and intolerance to cold.
9. The rate of melanin production by the hair follicle decreases. As a result, hair may become lighter in color, turning gray or white. Hair does not replace itself as often and becomes thinner.
10. Blood supply to the nailbed decreases. Consequently, the nails can become dull, brittle, hard, and thick; their growth rate also slows.

MEDICAL TERMINOLOGY AND DISORDERS — Disorders of the Integumentary System

Medical Term	Word Parts	Word Part Meaning or Derivation	Description
Words			
cutaneous	cutane/o-	skin	**Cutaneous** means "relating to the skin," which is comprised of two layers: the epidermis and the dermis.
	-ous	pertaining to	
dermis	derm/o-	skin	The **dermis** is *the thick layer of skin under the epidermis. Drugs may be administered using the skin.*
epidermis	epi-	upon	The **epidermis** is *the layer that lies upon the dermis and forms the outer layer of skin.*
	derm/o-	skin	
melanocyte	melan/o-	black	A **melanocyte** is *an epidermal cell that secretes melanin, a pigment that darkens the skin.*
	-cyte	cell	
thermogenesis	therm/o-	heat	**Thermogenesis** refers to *the production of heat by physiological processes, as in shivering.*
	-genesis	production	
xeroderma	xer/o-	dry	**Xeroderma** refers to *dry skin.*
	-derm/a	skin	
Disorders			
Cancers of the Skin			
nonmelanomas	non-	not	**Nonmelanomas** are *neoplasms that arise from epithelial tissue and most commonly occur on sun-exposed areas of the body.* **Actinic keratosis** (kerat/o- = hard), or **solar keratosis,** is *a premalignant form of squamous cell carcinoma.* **Basal cell carcinoma (BCC)** is *the most common skin cancer and arises from epidermal basal cells that fail to mature and keratinize.* **Squamous cell carcinoma (SCC)** arises from squamous epithelial cells.
	-melan/o-	black	
	-oma	tumor	
malignant melanoma	melan/o-	From the Greek *melas-*, for "dark"	**Malignant melanoma** is *a malignant neoplasm of the melanocytes.* Because of its tendency to metastasize extensively, it is the most deadly form of skin cancer. All moles should be monitored. Remember the **ABCD**s of "mole watch": **A**symmetry, **B**order irregularity, **C**olor, **D**iameter.
	-oma	tumor	
Cutaneous Lesions			
macule	-ule	-ule means "little one"	A **macule** is a flat lesion, also called a blemish. Macules include **freckles, flat mole (nevus), vitiligo, port-wine stains,** the rash of **measles** and **smallpox,** some **drug-induced reactions,** and **petechiae** (pinpoint hemorrhages under the skin). A congenital nevus is a **birthmark.** There are many types of nevi, including **hemangiomas (strawberry mark),** a vascular nevus.
papule		From a Latin word meaning "pustule"	*An elevated lesion that looks like a solid blister.* Examples of a papule include elevated moles **(nevi), lichen planus, insect bites,** some **skin cancers,** and **verrucae** (wart). A **wart** is *a contagious viral infection caused by one of the many human papillomaviruses (HPVs). A **nodule** is a firm papule that extends into the dermis or subcutaneous tissue. Nodules include cysts, lipomas, and fibromas.*
pustule		From a Latin word meaning to "swell up" or "blow up"	*A small pus-containing elevation of the skin that is seen in conditions such as acne and impetigo. A **pimple** is a small pustule.*
wheal		From an Old English word meaning "to go round," as a wheel	Also called a **hive.** Multiple hives are called **urticaria,** a pruritic or itchy skin eruption. Urticaria is usually an allergic response to medication, food, and insect venom.
vesicle	vesic/o-	From a Latin word meaning "little bladder" vesic/o- refers to *bladder,* -icle refers to *small*	Also called a **blister.** *A vesicle is a round lesion filled with serous fluid.* Vesicular lesions characterize herpes zoster (shingles), herpes simplex infection, and contact dermatitis. A larger vesicle is called a **bulla.**
	-icle		

MEDICAL TERMINOLOGY AND DISORDERS   Disorders of the Integumentary System—cont'd

Medical Term	Word Parts	Word Part Meaning or Derivation	Description
ulcer		From a Latin word meaning "wound"	*A crater-like lesion formed by the loss of the epidermis and dermis.* Examples include a decubitus ulcer and a chancre. A **decubitus ulcer** is *a pressure-induced ulcer.* A **chancre,** meaning "little ulcer," is *the lesion that develops in response to infection by* Treponema pallidum *(syphilis).*

Disorders of Pigmentation

Medical Term	Word Parts	Word Part Meaning or Derivation	Description
hypopigmentation	hypo-	insufficient	**Vitiligo** and **albinism** are conditions of **hypopigmentation,** in which *the melanocytes fail to secrete melanin.*
	-pigment-	pigment	
	-a/tion	state or condition	
hyperpigmentation	hyper-	more than normal	**Hyperpigmentation** is *a condition wherein there is an abnormally high amount of pigment in the skin.* **Dermal melanocytosis (mongolian spots)** is congenital; the spots appear as a blue-gray pigmentation in the sacral area. **Melasma,** related to hormone sensitivity, occurs during pregnancy **("mask of pregnancy")** and with the use of oral contraceptives. **Lentigo** refers to brown to black flat lesions, called **"liver spots,"** often seen in older persons **(senile lentigo).** The spots may occur in sun-exposed areas **(solar lentigo).** Infections, allergic reactions, and trauma can also induce a **post-inflammatory hyperpigmentation.**
	-pigment-	coloring matter	
	-a/tion	state or condition	

Infections of the Skin

Medical Term	Word Parts	Word Part Meaning or Derivation	Description
bacterial	bacteri-	Derived from New Latin, from Greek baktērion, for "staff"	**Impetigo** (from a word meaning "to attack") is *a bacterial infection that appears most often on the face and is caused by beta-hemolytic streptococci or staphylococci.* It is characterized by vesiculopustular lesions that are itchy and have a thick, honey-colored crust. A **furuncle** is *a deep staphylococcal infection around a hair follicle.* A **carbuncle** is *a group of interconnecting furuncles.* **Cellulitis** is *an inflammation of the subcutaneous tissue and is most commonly caused by* S. aureus *or streptococci.*
	-al	pertaining to	
viral		From a Latin word meaning "poison"	The most common viral infections of the skin are herpes simplex, herpes zoster, and warts. Herpes comes from a word meaning "to creep along," a reference to the progression of the vesicular development. The *herpes varicella* virus causes **chickenpox** (see Chapter 5), a highly contagious infection characterized by pruritic crusty vesicles. **Warts (veruccae)** are hyperkeratotic papular growths caused by the human papillomavirus (HPV).
fungal infections		From a Latin word meaning "mushroom," in reference to the appearance of fungi	**Dermatophytosis,** or **"ringworm,"** refers to *infection by a group of fungi called dermatophytes and occurs primarily in the skin, nails, and hair.* Ringworm conditions are named according to location: **tinea pedis (athlete's foot), tinea cruris ("jock itch"), tinea capitis (scalp), tinea corporis (body), tinea faciei (face), tinea manuum (hands).** **Candidiasis,** also called **moniliasis,** is a yeast infection caused by *Candida albicans.* **Cutaneous candidiasis** appears primarily in moist areas such as the thigh and beneath the breasts. Other common sights of infection are the mouth and vagina.
infestations and insect bites			There are numerous possibilities with regard to insect bites and infestations. The physiological response is due to a reaction to the venom, or to a reaction to the ova, body parts, or feces of the invading organism. *Infestation with lice* is called **pediculosis** (head, body, and pubic). **Scabies** develops in response to a parasitic mite that seeks out skin creases or folds in which to deposit eggs.

Continued

MEDICAL TERMINOLOGY AND DISORDERS Disorders of the Integumentary System—cont'd

Medical Term	Word Parts	Word Part Meaning or Derivation	Description
Disorders of the Hair and Nails			
onychocryptosis	onych/o-	nail	An **onychocryptosis** is *an ingrown nail, usually on the big toe.* It is most often caused by improper cutting of the toenails or the wearing of tight shoes.
	-crypt/o-	hidden, secret	
	-osis	condition of	
onychomycosis	onych/o-	nail	**Onychomycosis** is called *"ringworm of the nail," a fungal infection.*
	-myc/o-	fungus	
	-osis	condition of	
paronychia	para-	alongside of	A **paronychia** is *a skin infection around the nail usually at the site of a hangnail or cuticle.*
	-onych/o-	nail	
	-ia	condition of	
trichotillomania	trich/o-	hair	**Trichotillomania** is *an impulse control disorder in which the person compulsively twists strands of hair until it breaks off.*
	-tilo-	From a Latin word meaning "I pull out"	
	-mania	abnormal impulse	
Skin Diseases			
acne		From a Latin word meaning "point," as in the point of a pimple	**Acne vulgaris**—*common acne*—is characterized by scaly red skin, comedones (whiteheads and blackheads), papules, nodules, and pustules. These changes are due to sebaceous ducts that are plugged by sebum and dead skin cells.
dermatitis	dermat/o-	skin	**Dermatitis** is *a general term referring to inflammation of the skin.* There are different forms of dermatitis, including contact, seborrheic, and atopic dermatitis. Contact dermatitis may be allergic or irritant dermatitis. Allergic contact dermatitis is a skin allergy to something that touches the skin, as in poison ivy. Irritant contact dermatitis is dermatitis that develops in response to repeated exposure to an irritating substance. Atopic dermatitis, also called *eczema,* from a Greek word meaning "to erupt," is often associated with allergies and asthma. Atopic refers to the genetic predisposition to the allergen. Seborrheic dermatitis is a greasy (skin oil, or sebum), white to yellow scaling on the face (forehead, side of nose), scalp, or genitals.
	-itis	inflammation	
psoriasis	psor-	From a Greek word meaning "to have the itch"	An autoimmune disease often confused with eczema. Psoriasis affects the life cycle of skin cells, causing them to build up on the surface of the skin. The accumulation of skin cells forms thick silvery scales and itchy and painful red patches.

Get Ready for Exams!

Summary Outline

The integumentary system includes the skin, accessory structures, and subcutaneous tissue that covers the body, protects the internal organs, and plays an important role in the regulation of body temperature.

I. Structures: Organs of the Integumentary System

    A. Skin

        1. Called the *cutaneous membrane* or *integument*

        2. Functions: acts as mechanical barrier, protects internal organs, performs immune function, excretes waste, synthesizes vitamin D, houses sensory receptors, contributes to temperature regulation

        3. Has two layers: an outer layer called the *epidermis* and an inner layer called the *dermis*

        4. The epidermis has five layers. The stratum germinativum is the layer in which cell division takes place. The outer layer is the stratum corneum and consists of flattened, dead, keratinized cells.

        5. The dermis is the largest part of the skin and contains blood vessels, nerves, and sensory receptors.

6. The dermis lies on the subcutaneous tissue.
7. Skin color is determined by many factors, some genetic, some physiological, and some caused by disease. Melanin causes skin to darken. Carotene causes skin to appear yellow. The amount of blood in the skin affects skin color (e.g., flushing) as does the appearance of abnormal substances such as bilirubin (jaundice) and a low blood oxygen content (cyanosis).

B. Accessory structures of the skin
1. The location of the hair determines its function. Eyebrows and eyelashes protect the eyes from dust and perspiration.
2. Main parts of a hair: shaft, root, and follicle
3. Hair color: determined by the amount and type of melanin
4. Nails are thin plates of stratified squamous epithelial cells that contain a hard form of keratin.
5. Two major exocrine glands: sebaceous glands and sweat glands
6. Sebaceous glands secrete sebum (lubricates hair and skin). In the fetus, these glands secrete vernix caseosa, a cheeselike substance that coats the skin of a newborn.
7. Two types of sweat glands (sudoriferous glands): apocrine glands and eccrine glands (especially important in temperature regulation)
8. Modified sweat glands: Mammary glands secrete milk and the ceruminous glands secrete ear wax.

C. Subcutaneous tissue (hypodermis)
1. Anchors the dermis to underlying structures
2. Acts as an insulator; it prevents heat loss.

II. Regulation of Body Temperature (Thermoregulation)

A. Heat production
1. Heat produced by metabolizing cells constitutes the body temperature.
2. Shivering and nonshivering thermogenesis

B. Heat loss
1. Most of the heat (80%) is lost through the skin.
2. Heat loss occurs through radiation, conduction, convection, and evaporation.
3. Normal body temperature: set by the body's thermostat in the hypothalamus
4. Heat: lost through sweating and vasodilation. Heat is conserved by vasoconstriction and produced by shivering.

III. When Skin Is Burned

A. Physiological effects
1. Short-term effects (e.g., fluid and electrolyte losses, shock, inability to regulate body temperature, infection)
2. Long-term effects (e.g., scarring, loss of function, and cosmetic and emotional problems)

B. Classification of burns
1. Classified according to the thickness of the burn (partial, full); also first-, second-, and third-degree burns
2. The rule of nines is a way to evaluate burns.

Review Your Knowledge

Matching: Skin
Directions: Match the following words with their descriptions below. Some words may be used more than once.

a. keratin
b. dermis
c. subcutaneous layer
d. epidermis

1. ___ Thin outer layer of skin
2. ___ Layer that sits on the hypodermis and supports the epidermis
3. ___ A protein that flattens, hardens, and makes the skin water-resistant
4. ___ A layer of insulation
5. ___ Contains the stratum germinativum and stratum corneum
6. ___ Contains blood vessels that nourish the stratum germinativum

Matching: Glands
Directions: Match the following words with their descriptions below. Some words may be used more than once.

a. eccrine
b. sebaceous
c. ceruminous
d. mammary

1. ___ Oil glands
2. ___ Glands that secrete vernix caseosa
3. ___ Glands that play a crucial role in body temperature regulation
4. ___ Modified sweat glands that secrete ear wax
5. ___ Modified sweat glands that secrete milk
6. ___ Classified as sudoriferous
7. ___ Most related to blackhead, pimple, and cradle cap
8. ___ Pours sweat during intense exercise

Matching: Colors
Directions: Match the following words with their descriptions below. Some words may be used more than once.

a. jaundice
b. cyanosis
c. melanin
d. vitiligo
e. ecchymosis

1. ___ Tanning pigment
2. ___ Condition in which the skin has a bluish tint because of poor oxygenation
3. ___ Yellowing of the skin because of bilirubin
4. ___ Patches of white skin caused by loss of pigmentation
5. ___ Black and blue mark; bruising

Multiple Choice
1. Which of the following is most apt to increase body temperature?
   a. Dilation of the blood vessels in the skin
   b. Shivering
   c. Secretion of the eccrine glands
   d. Secretion of sebum
2. The stratum germinativum
   a. is a dermal layer.
   b. gives rise to epidermal cells.
   c. contains the blood vessels that nourish the epidermis.
   d. is part of the hypodermis.

3. The epidermis is nourished by the
   a. air in the environment that diffuses into the pores.
   b. blood vessels in the hair shafts.
   c. blood vessels in the underlying dermis.
   d. oxygen and glucose in the sebum.
4. Which of the following is true of the stratum corneum?
   a. Continuously produces epidermal cells
   b. Secretes keratin for making the skin water-resistant
   c. Is the dead layer that is sloughed off
   d. Continuously secretes bilirubin
5. Which word best describes the function of the stratum germinativum?
   a. Desquamation
   b. Mitosis
   c. Keratinization
   d. Shivering thermogenesis
6. Secretion of the eccrine glands
   a. "oils" the hair shafts.
   b. produces vernix caseosa that protects the skin of the fetus.
   c. lowers body temperature.
   d. tans the skin.
7. Cyanosis occurs when
   a. the blood in the cutaneous blood vessels is unoxygenated.
   b. bilirubin deposits in the skin and mucous membrane.
   c. cutaneous blood vessels dilate.
   d. sebum is exposed to air and changes color.
8. Which word pertains to all the following: apocrine, sudoriferous, eccrine, and sebaceous?
   a. Sweat glands
   b. Vernix caseosa
   c. Sebum
   d. Exocrine glands
9. Shivering thermogenesis
   a. is due to metabolism of brown fat.
   b. increases body temperature.
   c. is primarily due to the contraction of the arrector pili muscles.
   d. is triggered by hypoxemia and cyanosis.

Go Figure

1. **According to Figures 7-1 and 7-2**
   a. There is a rich supply of blood vessels within the epidermis.
   b. The dermis sits on the epidermis.
   c. Blood vessels, touch receptors, and free nerve endings are located within the dermis.
   d. The stratum corneum and the stratum germinativum are dermal layers.

2. **According to Figures 7-1 and 7-2**
   a. The stratum germinativum sits on the hypodermis.
   b. The hair arises within the cells of the epidermis.
   c. The arrector pili muscles attach the epidermis to the hypodermis.
   d. Dermal cells arise within the stratum germinativum.

3. **According to Figures 7-1 and 7-2**
   a. All glands arise from cells at the base of the hair shaft.
   b. All touch and pressure receptors are located within the epidermis.
   c. Some epidermal cells are imbedded within the dermis.
   d. All sensory receptors are located in the hypodermis.

4. **Which of the following is not consistent with Figure 7-4?**
   a. Sweat glands are located in the dermis.
   b. The sebaceous gland is associated with the hair root.
   c. Apocrine, sebaceous, and eccrine glands are sweat glands.
   d. Eccrine glands secrete sweat into ducts that carry it to the surface of the skin.

5. **According to Figure 7-5**
   a. Blood vessel constriction and shivering increase body temperature.
   b. The thermostat is located in the brain.
   c. Blood vessel dilation and sweating lower body temperature.
   d. All of the above are true.

Skeletal System

Key Terms

abduction (p. 137)
adduction (p. 137)
appendicular skeleton (p. 117)
articulation (p. 115)
axial skeleton (p. 117)

diaphysis (p. 115)
epiphysis (p. 115)
extension (p. 137)
flexion (p. 137)
fontanels (p. 121)

haversian system (p. 114)
osteoblasts (p. 113)
osteoclasts (p. 116)
periosteum (p. 115)
synovial joint (p. 133)

Objectives

1. List the functions of the skeletal system and the classification of bones by size and shape.
2. Differentiate between the composition and location of compact and spongy bone.
3. Describe the structure of a long bone.
4. Describe the roles of osteoblasts and osteoclasts, and how bones grow in length and width.

5. List the bones of the axial skeleton and label important landmarks on selected bones.
6. List the bones of the appendicular skeleton and label important landmarks on selected bones.
7. List the main types and functions of joints and describe the types of joint movement.

The skeletal system consists of the bones, joints, and cartilage and ligaments associated with the joints. Bone tissue is living and metabolically active, but because it contains so much nonliving material, such as calcium and phosphorus, it appears dead or dried up. In fact, the word *skeleton* comes from a Greek word meaning "dried-up body."

The skeletal system, however, is anything but dead. It contains 206 bones that are very much alive and perform a number of important functions.

Do You Know...

About Growing Down with Osteoporosis?

Osteoporosis is a common bone disorder, especially in postmenopausal women. Osteoporosis is characterized by a decline in bone-making activity and the loss of bone tissue. As tissue is lost, the bones weaken and break. Common sites of fracture caused by osteoporosis are the hip, wrist, and vertebrae. Osteoporosis may also affect the vertebral column. As the vertebrae collapse, nerves may be pinched, causing severe pain. The collapsed vertebrae also cause a shortening of the vertebral column (growing down) and a change in its curvature. This change in shape, in turn, often impairs the functioning of organs such as the lungs.

ARRANGEMENT AND FUNCTIONS OF BONES

The bones of the skeletal system are arranged to provide a framework for our bodies (Figure 8-1). The skeletal system gives us our basic shape. Imagine what you would look like without bones!

THE SKELETAL SYSTEM: WHAT IT DOES

In addition to shaping us up, the skeletal system performs other functions:
• The bones of the lower extremities support the weight of the body.

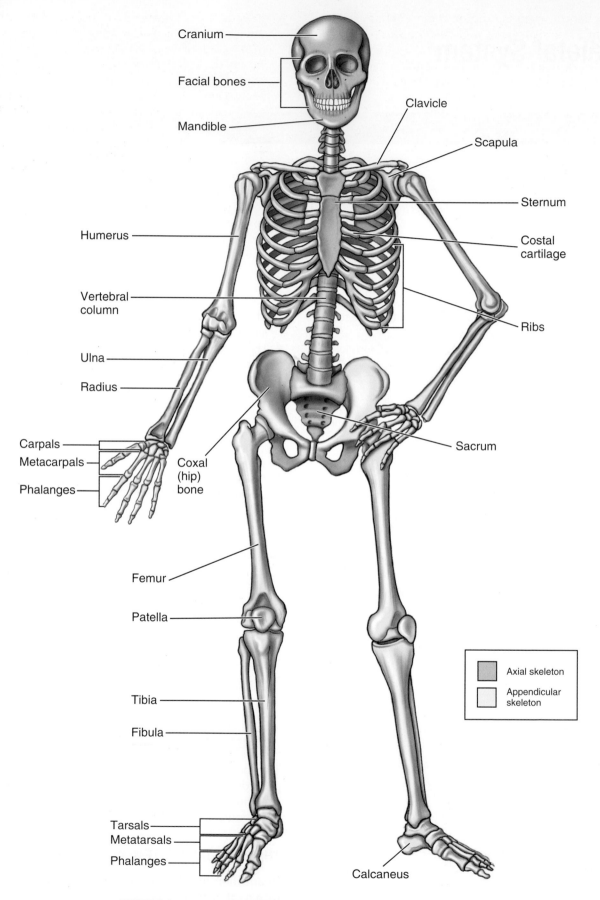

FIGURE 8-1 Skeleton. Axial skeleton *(red)* and appendicular skeleton *(tan)*.

- The bones support and protect the soft body organs.
- With the assistance of muscles, the skeletal system enables the body to move about.
- Bones store a number of minerals, the most important being calcium and phosphorus. The calcium makes the bones strong and is a readily available source of the mineral for the regulation of calcium in the blood.
- Red bone marrow produces blood cells.

MANY SIZES AND SHAPES OF BONES

Bones come in many sizes and shapes, from the pea-sized bones in the wrist to the 24-inch femur in the thigh. The size and shape of a bone reflect its function (Figure 8-2). The long strong femur in the thigh, for example, supports a great deal of weight and can withstand considerable force. Some of the skull bones, on the other hand, are thin, flat, and curved. Their function is to encase and protect the brain.

Bones are classified as follows:

- *Long bones.* Long bones are longer than they are wide. They are found in the arms, forearms, palms, fingers, thighs, legs, and instep. Although it is obvious that the femur (thigh) and the humerus (arm) are long bones, even small bones such as the metacarpals and finger bones are considered long bones.
- *Short bones.* Short bones are shaped like cubes and are found primarily in the wrists and ankles.
- *Flat bones.* Flat bones are thin, flat, and curved. They form the ribs, breastbone, cranium, and bones of the shoulder girdle.
- *Irregular bones.* Irregular bones are differently shaped and are not classified as long, short, or flat. They include the hip bones, vertebrae, and various bones in the skull.

BONE TISSUE AND BONE FORMATION

Bone is also called *osseous tissue* and the process of bone formation is called *ossification*. Bone cells, called **osteoblasts**, secrete an intercellular matrix, containing calcium, other minerals, and protein fibers. The osteoblasts mature into osteocytes that sit within the hard bone matrix and maintain the bone.

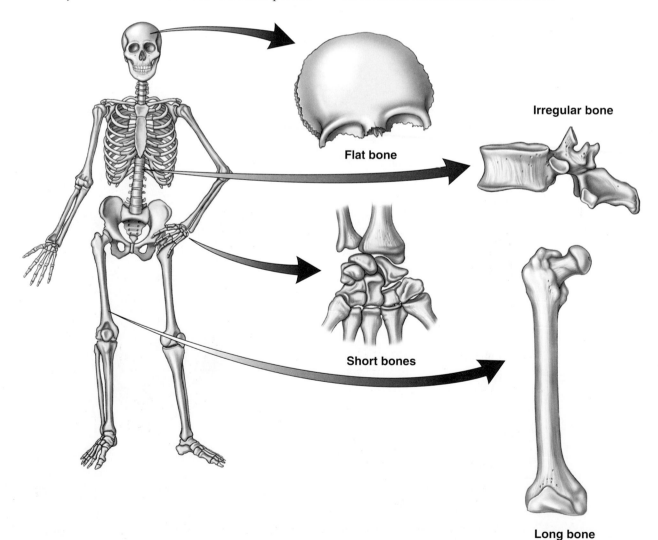

Irregular bone

Flat bone

Short bones

Long bone

FIGURE 8-2 Types of bones.

COMPACT AND SPONGY BONE

There are two types of bone: compact and spongy (Figure 8-3). Compact bone refers to dense, hard bone tissue found primarily in the shafts of long bones and on the outer surfaces of other bones. Spongy, or cancellous, bone is less dense. Spongy bone is located primarily at the ends of long bones and in the center of other bones.

Compact and spongy bone look different under the microscope. Compact bone is tightly packed, so that its density can provide a great deal of strength (see Figure 8-3, *B*). The microscopic unit of compact bone is the osteon, or **haversian** (hah-VER-shun) **system**. Each haversian system consists of mature osteocytes arranged in concentric circles around large blood vessels. The area surrounding the osteocytes is filled with protein fibers, calcium, and other minerals. The protein fibers provide elasticity, and the minerals make bone tissue hard and strong. Each haversian system looks like a long cylinder.

Compact bone consists of many haversian systems running parallel to each other. Communicating blood vessels run laterally and connect the haversian systems with each other and with the periosteal lining that surrounds the bone. The network of blood vessels ensures

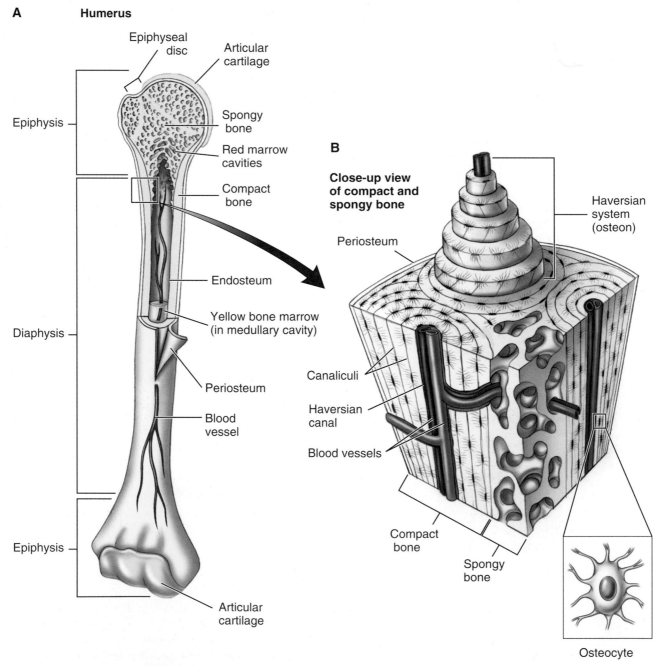

A **Humerus**

- Epiphyseal disc
- Articular cartilage
- Epiphysis
- Spongy bone
- Red marrow cavities
- Compact bone
- Endosteum
- Diaphysis
- Yellow bone marrow (in medullary cavity)
- Periosteum
- Blood vessel
- Epiphysis
- Articular cartilage

B

Close-up view of compact and spongy bone

- Periosteum
- Haversian system (osteon)
- Canaliculi
- Haversian canal
- Blood vessels
- Compact bone
- Spongy bone
- Osteocyte

FIGURE 8-3 Bone. **A,** Anatomy of a long bone. **B,** Compact and spongy bone.

that the bone tissue receives an adequate supply of blood. Blood supplies tissues with oxygen and nutrients.

Spongy, or cancellous, bone has a much different structure than compact bone (see Figure 8-3, *B*). Unlike compact bone, spongy bone does not contain haversian systems. In spongy bone, the bone tissue is arranged in plates called *trabeculae* (trah-BEK-yoo-lay). These bony plates are separated by holes that give spongy bone a punched-out Swiss cheese appearance. The holes are important for two reasons: (1) they decrease the weight of the bone, and (2) they contain red bone marrow. The red bone marrow richly supplies the spongy bone with blood and also produces blood cells for use throughout the body. Spongy bone is located in the short, flat, and irregular bones. It is also found in the ends of long bones.

 Re-Think

1. What are two types of bones?
2. What is the structure of an osteon, or haversian system?

LONG BONES

The arrangement of the compact and spongy tissue in a long bone accounts for its strength. Long bones also contain sites of growth and reshaping and structures associated with joints. Locate the parts of a long bone in Figure 8-3, *A:*

- *Diaphysis.* The **diaphysis** (dye-AF-i-sis) is the long shaft of the bone. It is composed primarily of compact bone and therefore provides considerable strength.
- *Epiphysis.* The enlarged ends of the long bone are the epiphyses. The **epiphysis** (eh-PIF-i-sis) of a bone articulates, or meets, with a second bone at a joint. Each epiphysis consists of a thin layer of compact bone overlying spongy bone. The epiphyses are covered by cartilage.
- *Epiphyseal disc.* A growing long bone contains a band of hyaline cartilage located near the proximal and distal ends of long bones. This band of cartilage is the epiphyseal disc, or growth plate. It is here that longitudinal bone growth occurs.
- *Medullary cavity.* The medullary cavity is the hollow center of the diaphysis. In infancy, the cavity is filled with red bone marrow for blood cell production. In the adult, the medullary cavity is filled with yellow bone marrow and functions as a storage site for fat. The inside of the medullary cavity is lined with connective tissue called the *endosteum* (en-DOS-tee-um).
- *Periosteum.* The **periosteum** is a tough, fibrous, connective tissue membrane that covers the outside of the diaphysis. It is anchored firmly to the outside of the bone on all surfaces except the articular cartilage. The periosteum protects the bone, serves as a

point of attachment for muscle, and contains the blood vessels that nourish the underlying bone. Because the periosteum carries the blood supply to the underlying bone, injury to this structure has serious consequences to the health of the bone. Like any other organ, the loss of blood supply can cause its death.
- *Articular cartilage.* The articular cartilage is found on the outer surface of the epiphysis. It forms a smooth shiny surface that decreases friction within a joint. Because a joint is also called an **articulation**, this cartilage is called *articular cartilage.*

OSSIFICATION

The process of bone formation is called *ossification.* Ossification begins in the late embryonic period with the formation of fibrous connective tissue and hyaline cartilage that is shaped like a miniskeleton (Figure 8-4). As the fetus matures, the cartilage and connective tissue change into bone. Ossification occurs in two ways: intramembranous ossification and endochondral ossification.

OSSIFICATION OF FLAT BONES: INTRAMEMBRANOUS OSSIFICATION

In the fetus, the flat bones (those in the skull) consist of thin connective tissue membranes. Ossification begins when osteoblasts, or bone-forming cells, migrate to the region of the flat bones. The osteoblasts secrete calcium and other minerals into the spaces between the membranes, thereby forming bone. This type of ossification involves the replacement of thin membrane with bone.

OSSIFICATION OF LONG BONES: ENDOCHONDRAL OSSIFICATION

Most bones are formed by endochondral ossification as bone tissue replaces cartilage. The fetal skeleton is composed largely of cartilage, and the layout of the cartilage in the fetus provides a model for bone formation (see Figure 8-4). As the fetus matures, osteoblasts invade the cartilage and gradually replace the cartilage with bone. This process continues in each long bone until all but the articular cartilage and epiphyseal disc have been replaced by bone. By the time the fetus has fully matured, most cartilage of the body has been replaced by bone. Only isolated pieces of cartilage remain, such as the bridge of the nose and parts of the ribs.

GROWING BONES

Maturation from infancy to adulthood is characterized by two types of bone growth: (1) bones grow longitudinally and determine the height of an individual, and (2) bones grow thicker and become wider to support the weight of the adult body.

Ossification of connective tissue membrane

Ossification of cartilage

FIGURE 8-4 Ossification.

GROWING TALLER

Longitudinal bone growth occurs at the epiphyseal disc (also called the growth plate; see Figure 8-3, *A*). The cartilage adjacent to the epiphysis continues to multiply and grow toward the diaphysis. The cartilage next to the diaphysis, however, is invaded by osteo-blasts and becomes ossified. As long as the cartilage continues to form within the epiphyseal disc, the bone continues to lengthen. Longitudinal bone growth ceases when the epiphyseal disc becomes ossified and fused.

The epiphyseal disc is sensitive to the effects of certain hormones, especially growth hormone and the sex hormones. Growth hormone stimulates growth at the epiphyseal disc, making the child taller. The sex hormones estrogen and testosterone, however, cause the epiphyseal disc to fuse, thereby inhibiting further longitudinal growth. Because the epiphyseal disc is especially sensitive to the effects of the female hormone estrogen, girls tend to be shorter than boys. After puberty, which is associated with increasing plasma levels of sex hormones, longitudinal growth eventually ceases.

The "What-Ifs" of the Epiphyseal Disc
- What if there is an oversecretion or undersecretion of growth hormone? Giantism occurs with hyperse-cretion, whereas a type of dwarfism develops with hyposecretion.

- What if the epiphyseal disc is injured? Longitudinal bone growth is impaired in the injured bone. A child who injures the epiphyseal disc in a leg bone, for example, may end up with that leg considerably shorter than the noninjured leg.
- What if a young athlete uses anabolic steroids to enhance performance? Steroids induce premature fusion of the epiphyseal plate, thereby permanently stunting growth.

GROWING THICKER AND WIDER

During and long after longitudinal bone growth has ceased, bones continue to increase in thickness and width. The bones are continuously being reshaped. Bone remodeling is accomplished by the combined actions of osteoblasts, which are bone-forming cells, and osteoclasts, which are bone-destroying cells. Osteoblasts on the undersurface of the periosteum continuously deposit bone on the external bone surface.

Figure 8-5 shows how osteoblastic activity works like a bricklayer. Whereas osteoblasts build new bone, osteoclasts, found on the inner bone surface surround-ing the medullary cavity, break down bone tissue, thereby hollowing out the interior of the bone. Osteo-clastic activity is like sculpting. The bricklayer and the sculptor gradually create a large, wide hollow bone that is strong but not too heavy.

The process whereby osteoclasts break down bone matrix is called *bone resorption* (not to be confused with *reabsorption*). Bone resorption not only widens bone, but also moves calcium from the bone to the blood. In this way, bone resorption also plays a crucial role in the regulation of blood calcium levels. The influence of parathyroid hormone on bone resorption is described in Chapter 14.

Factors that stimulate bone growth are weight-bearing and exercise; both keep calcium in the bone and increase bone mass. The bones of bedridden or sedentary people tend to lose bone mass and are easily broken when stressed. The weightlessness experienced by astronauts similarly causes a loss of bone mass and easily broken bones. The beneficial effects of exercise on bone strength cannot be overemphasized.

? Re-Think
1. Differentiate between the functions of osteoblasts and osteoclasts.
2. Describe how a bone grows in length and in width, using the term *bone resorption*.

BUMPS AND GROOVES

The surface of bone appears irregular and bumpy as a result of numerous ridges, projections, depressions, and grooves called *bone surface markings*. The project-ing bone markings (the markings that stick out) serve as points of attachment for muscles, tendons, and liga-ments. The grooves and depressions form the routes

FIGURE 8-5 Bone remodeling.

traveled by blood vessels and nerves as they pass over and through the bones and joints. The projections and depressions also help form joints. The rounded head of the proximal arm bone, for example, fits into a round depression in a shoulder bone, forming the shoulder joint. The specific bone markings are summarized in Table 8-1. Note the various markings on individual bones as they are described.

BROKEN BONES

Occasionally, a bone breaks, or fractures (Figure 8-6). A simple fracture is a break in which the overlying skin remains intact; local tissue damage is minimal. A compound fracture is a broken bone that has also pierced the skin. The ends of the broken bone usually cause extensive tissue damage. The risk of infection is a concern with a compound fracture.

A greenstick fracture is an incomplete break in the bone and usually occurs in children. Why is it called a greenstick fracture? If you were to bend a branch of a young tree, the branch would not snap and break apart completely. It would, instead, bend and perhaps break incompletely. The branch responds this way because it is young and pliable, much like a child's bone. Children's bones still contain enough cartilaginous material to make them flexible.

There are many other types of bone fractures. For example, there is a spiral fracture in which the line of the fracture extends in a spiral direction along the diaphysis. It is caused when the bone is subjected to a twisting type of force. There is a comminuted fracture in which there are more than two bone fragments; the small fragments seem to be floating. An impacted fracture is a comminuted fracture in which the two parts of the broken bone have been jammed into each other. The list of fractures goes on.

2+2 Sum It Up!

The skeletal system consists of bones, joints, cartilage, and ligaments found in and around the joints. Bones are composed of two types of osseous tissue: compact (dense bone) and spongy (cancellous bone). Bones come in a variety of sizes and shapes and are classified as long, short, flat, or irregular. We begin life in the womb as a skeleton-like frame made of cartilage and thin connective tissue membrane. With maturation, the process of ossification changes most of the cartilage and certain connective tissue membranes into bone. As a person matures, the skeleton enlarges as the bones grow longer, wider, and thicker.

DIVISIONS OF THE SKELETAL SYSTEM

The skeleton is divided into the axial skeleton and appendicular skeletons (see Figure 8-1). The **axial** (AK-see-all) **skeleton** includes the bones of the cranium, face, middle ear bones, hyoid bone, vertebral column, and bony thorax. The **appendicular skeleton** includes the bones of the pelvic girdles, the upper extremities (arms, forearms, wrist, palms, and fingers), and lower extremities (thighs, legs, ankles, instep, and toes). The names of the 206 bones of the skeleton are listed in Table 8-2.

AXIAL SKELETON

SKULL

The skull sits on top of the vertebral column and is formed by two groups of bones: the cranium and the facial bones (Figure 8-7).

Table 8-1 Bone Markings	
BONE MARKINGS	**DEFINITION**
Projections or Processes	
Condyle	A large rounded knob that usually articulates with another bone
Epicondyle	An enlargement near or above a condyle
Head	An enlarged and rounded end of a bone
Facet	A small flattened surface
Crest	A ridge on a bone
Process	A prominent projection on a bone
Spine	A sharp projection
Tubercle (tuberosity)	A knoblike projection
Trochanter	A large tubercle (tuberosity) found only on the femur
Depressions or Openings	
Foramen	An opening through a bone; usually serves as a passageway for nerves, blood vessels, and ligaments
Fossa	A depression or groove
Meatus	A tunnel or tubelike passageway
Sinus	A cavity or hollow space

Closed (simple)   **Open (compound)**

Incomplete (greenstick)

FIGURE 8-6 Common types of fractures.

Cranium

The cranium is a bony structure that encases and protects the brain. The cranium is composed of eight bones, most of which are curved and flat.

- *Frontal bone.* The frontal bone forms the forehead and the upper part of the bony structure surrounding the eyes.
- *Parietal bones.* The two parietal (pah-RYE-i-tal) bones form the upper sides of the head and the roof of the cranial cavity (top of the head).
- *Temporal bones.* The two temporal bones are on the sides of the head, close to the ears (commonly called the *temples*). Several important bone markings are found on the temporal bones. They include the external auditory meatus (mee-AY-tus), an opening for the ear; the zygomatic (zye-goh-MAT-ik) process, which articulates with the cheekbone (not to be confused with the zygomatic bones); the styloid process, a sharp projection used as a point of attachment for several muscles associated with the tongue and larynx; and the mastoid process, which forms a point of attachment for some of the muscles of the neck.

Here's an interesting note about the temporal bone. *Tempor* is a Latin word meaning "time." As

men age, over time, they usually develop their first grey hairs over the temple area. So, the name of the temporal bone is a reference to aging.

- *Occipital bone* (see Figure 8-7, *C*). The occipital (ok-SIP-it-al) bone is located at the back and base of the cranium. The large hole in the occipital bone is called the *foramen magnum*. The foramen allows the brain stem to extend downward and become the spinal cord. On either side of the foramen magnum are bony projections, called *occipital condyles* (KON-dylz), that sit on the first vertebra of the vertebral column. Unfortunately, the foramen magnum can act as a deathtrap, because it provides the only escape hatch in the cranium in the event that the brain swells. The increased intracranial pressure created by the swollen brain pushes the brain through the foramen magnum into the spinal region. The downward displacement or herniation of the brain exerts pressure on the brain stem, causing respiratory arrest and death.
- *Sphenoid bone.* The sphenoid (SFEE-noyd) bone is a butterfly-shaped bone that forms part of the floor and sides of the cranium (see Figure 8-7, *C*). The sphenoid bone also helps form the orbits

Table 8-2   Bones of the Adult Skeleton

BONES	NUMBER	BONES	NUMBER
Axial Skeleton (80)		**Thoracic Cage (25)**	
Skull (28)		True ribs	14
Cranium (8)		False ribs	10
Frontal	1	Sternum	1
Parietal	2	**Appendicular Skeleton (126)**	
Temporal	2	**Pectoral Girdle (4)**	
Occipital	1	Scapula	2
Sphenoid	1	Clavicle	2
Ethmoid	1	**Upper Limbs (60)**	
Facial (14)		Humerus	2
Maxilla	2	Radius	2
Zygomatic	2	Ulna	2
Palatine	2	Carpals	16
Mandible	1	Metacarpals	10
Lacrimal	2	Phalanges	28
Nasal	2	**Pelvic Girdle (2)**	
Inferior concha	2	Coxal	2
Vomer	1	**Lower Limbs (60)**	
Middle Ear Bones (6)		Femur	2
Malleus	2	Tibia	2
Incus	2	Fibula	2
Stapes	2	Patella	2
Hyoid Bone (1)		Tarsals	14
Vertebral Column (26)		Metatarsals	10
Cervical vertebrae	7	Phalanges	28
Thoracic vertebrae	12	**Total Number of Bones**	**206**
Lumbar vertebrae	5		
Sacrum	1		
Coccyx	1		

surrounding the eyes. In the midline of the sphenoid bone is a depression called the *sella turcica* (Turk's saddle); it forms the seat for the pituitary gland (not shown).

- *Ethmoid bone.* The ethmoid (ETH-moyd) bone is an irregularly shaped bone located between the eye orbits; it is the major supporting bony structure of the nasal cavity. A projection of the ethmoid bone forms a point of attachment for the meninges, or the membranes that surround the brain and contain cerebrospinal fluid. The location and shape of the ethmoid bone has important clinical implications. A sharp blow to the ethmoid bone can drive the pointed bone into the brain, causing severe brain injury and death. Because the shattered bone tears the meninges, cerebrospinal fluid leaks into the nasal passages. This type of injury also creates a direct opening into the brain for pathogens and subsequent infections of brain tissue, so watch that

karate chop to the face. The impact of the face with the steering wheel during a car wreck can also drive the shattered ethmoid bone into the brain. Slow down!

Facial Bones

The face has 14 facial bones, most of which are paired (see Figure 8-7, *B*). Only the mandible and the vomer are single bones.

- *Mandible.* The mandible (MAN-di-bal), the lower jaw bone, carries the lower teeth. The anterior portion of the mandible forms the chin. The mandible forms the only freely movable joint in the skull. Two posterior upright projections on the mandible have bony processes that articulate with the temporal bones at the temporomandibular joint (TMJ). The TMJ can be felt as the depression immediately in front of the ear. Tension or stress often causes pain in the TMJ. This condition is often

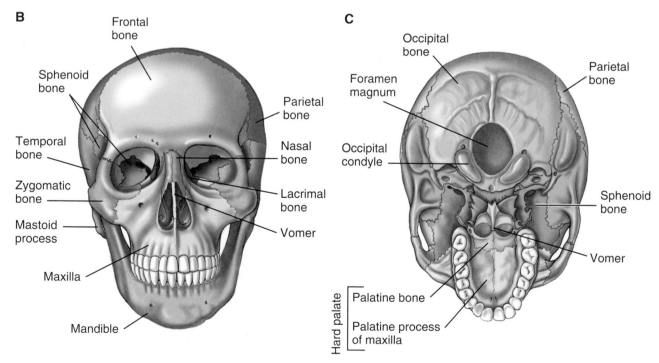

FIGURE 8-7 Bones of the skull. **A,** Side view. **B,** Front view. **C,** Base of the skull.

associated with tooth grinding (bruxism) during sleep. Bony processes on the mandible serve as points of attachment for chewing muscles.

• *Maxilla.* Two maxillary bones fuse to form the upper jaw. The maxilla (mak-SIH-lah) carries the upper teeth. An extension of the maxilla, the palatine process, forms the anterior portion of the hard palate (roof) of the mouth (see Figure 8-7, C). These bones also form parts of the nasal cavity and the eye orbits.

- *Palatine bones.* Two palatine (PAL-ah-tine) bones form the posterior part of the hard palate and the floor of the nasal cavity. Failure of the palatine and/ or maxillary bones to fuse causes a cleft palate, making suckling very difficult for an infant. Fortunately, a cleft palate can be surgically repaired.
- *Zygomatic bones.* The zygomatic bones are the cheekbones. They also form a part of the orbits of the eyes.
- *Other facial bones.* Several other bones complete the facial structure, including the lacrimal bones, nasal bones, vomer, and inferior nasal conchae.

 Do You Know...

About Two Drug-Induced Jaw-Breaking Events?

The mandible often takes it on the chin! A rather common mandibular event is the alcohol-fueled Saturday night brawl that often culminates in a broken jaw. Unlike a broken leg bone, which can be immobilized by a cast, the mandible (lower jaw) can be immobilized only by wiring it to the maxilla (upper jaw). Can't talk, can't eat, can't expel vomit. In fact, people with wired jaws must have access to wire cutters in case they vomit. What about nutrition? Puréed food is delivered through a straw.

A second mandibular malady is a drug-induced "Fossy jaw." Alendronate (Fosamax), which belongs to a group of drugs called *bisphosphonates*, is used in the prevention and treatment of osteoporosis in postmenopausal women. It works by inhibiting bone resorption by osteoclasts. A rare but distressing side effect of Fosamax is osteonecrosis of the jaw, characterized by loose teeth and crumbling jaw bone; hence the term *dead jaw*, or *Fossy jaw*. In addition to osteonecrosis, a small group of patients treated with bisphosphonates also experiences a distinctive type of low-energy fracture of the femur. One theory has suggested that by suppressing bone turnover (diminished osteoclastic activity), normal wear-and-tear microscopic bone cracks are not repaired daily, and ultimately progress to bone weakening and fracture.

 Re-Think

1. List the cranial bones that articulate with the parietal bone.
2. What are the functions of the foramen magnum and occipital condyles?
3. With regard to head injury, why is the foramen magnum called a "death trap"?

Sinuses

Sinuses are air-filled cavities located in several of the bones of the skull. They perform two important functions: (1) they lessen the weight of the skull, and (2) they modulate the sound of the voice.

The four sinuses are called the *paranasal sinuses* because they surround and connect with the nasal structures (Figure 8-8). The names of the four sinuses reflect their location within the various skull bones: frontal sinus, ethmoidal sinuses, sphenoidal sinus, and maxillary sinuses.

Because the sinuses connect with the nasal passages and the throat, infections may spread from the nose and throat into the sinuses. An inflammation of the

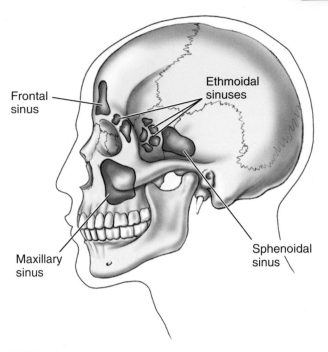

FIGURE 8-8 Sinuses.

sinus is called *sinusitis* and is characterized as stuffiness and pain in the overlying facial regions. Why do allergies sometimes make your face hurt? Allergies often cause the membranes that line the facial sinuses to oversecrete mucus. The mucus forms an excellent medium for bacterial growth. As the mucus accumulates and the membranes swell, pressure and discomfort are often experienced in the facial region, which overlies the sinuses (around the eyes and nose).

How the Skull Bones Are Held Together

The bones of the adult skull form a unique type of joint called a *suture* (see Figure 8-7, *A*). The sutures join together the bones of the skull, much like a zipper. The major sutures include the coronal suture, the lambdoidal suture, and the squamosal suture. Unlike other joints in the body, no significant movement occurs between cranial bones.

The Infant Skull

The two major differences between the infant and adult skulls are the fontanels and unfused sutures in the infant skull.

The infant skull has areas that have not yet been converted to bone. Instead, they are covered by fibrous membrane. Because these areas are soft to touch, they are called a baby's *soft spots*. Also, the rhythm of the baby's pulse can be felt in these soft spots, and so they are called **fontanels** (FON-tah-nels), meaning "little fountains."

The two major fontanels are the larger, diamond-shaped anterior fontanel and the smaller, posterior occipital fontanel. Two smaller fontanels are located more laterally—the anterolateral and posterolateral fontanels (Figure 8-9). By the time a child reaches 2

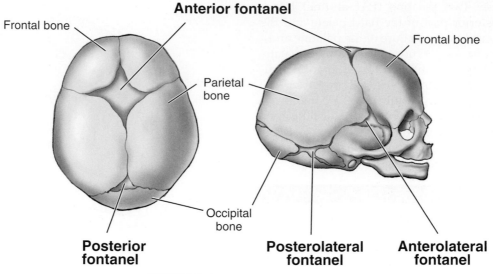

Frontal bone
Anterior fontanel
Frontal bone
Parietal bone
Occipital bone
Posterior fontanel
Posterolateral fontanel
Anterolateral fontanel

FIGURE 8-9 Fontanels in the infant skull.

years of age, these fontanels have been gradually converted to bone and can no longer be felt.

The fontanels are one reason why infant skull bones are more movable than those of the adult skull. Another reason is that the sutures of the infant skulls are not fused. Unfused sutures allow the skull to be compressed during birth. They also allow for the continued growth of the brain and skull after birth and throughout infancy. It also explains why your adorable newborn may look like a "conehead." The fetal skull is too large to fit through the birth canal, so the movable bones overlap, thereby decreasing the diameter of the head. Fortunately, the pointy skull reshapes shortly after birth.

Occasionally, the sutures of the infant skull fuse too early, preventing the growth of the brain. This condition is called *microcephalia* and is characterized by a small cranium, restricted brain growth, and impaired intellectual functioning. Sometimes the skull expands too much. For example, if excessive fluid accumulates within the brain of an infant, the bones are forced apart, and the skull enlarges. This condition is called *hydrocephalus* (or "water on the brain").

Observation of the fontanels can provide valuable information regarding brain swelling. What does a bulging or sunken fontanel indicate? If an infant suffers a head injury or infection, the brain may swell. Because the fontanel is soft tissue, it will bulge outward in response to increasing pressure within the skull. Conversely, the fontanels may become sunken in the presence of dehydration.

? Re-Think

1. What are fontanels?
2. In what sense does the fontanel indicate a state of dehydration? Of increased intracranial pressure?
3. Why is it important that the infant sutures are unfused?

Hyoid Bone

The hyoid (HYE-oyd) bone is a U-shaped bone located in the upper neck. It anchors the tongue and is associated with swallowing. The hyoid bone is often fractured during strangulation. Watch for this during an autopsy, you forensic sleuths!

Bones of the Middle Ear

Each ear contains three small bones called *ossicles* (see Chapter 13 for the role of the ossicles in hearing).

VERTEBRAL COLUMN

The Back and Its Stack of Bones

The vertebral column, also called the backbone, extends from the skull to the pelvis (Figure 8-10). The vertebral column consists of 26 bones, called *vertebrae* (VER-teh-bray), stacked in a column. Sitting between each vertebra is a cartilaginous disc. The vertebral column performs four major functions:

- Forms a supporting structure for the head and thorax
- Forms an attachment for the pelvic girdle
- Encases and protects the spinal cord
- Provides flexibility for the body

The vertebrae are named according to their location. Seven cervical vertebrae (C1 to C7) are located in the neck region. If you bend your head forward and run your hand down the cervical vertebrae, you will feel a large bump; this large vertebra is C7, which is called the *vertebra prominens* (VER-teh-bra PRAH-meh-nenz) and is used as a landmark in assessing surface anatomy. Twelve thoracic vertebrae (T1 to T12) are located in the chest region; and the five lumbar vertebrae (L1 to L5) are located in the lower back region. If you place your hands on your hips, you are at the level of L4. In addition, five sacral vertebrae fuse into one sacrum. The sacrum forms the posterior wall of the pelvis. Four small vertebrae fuse into the tailbone. How did the

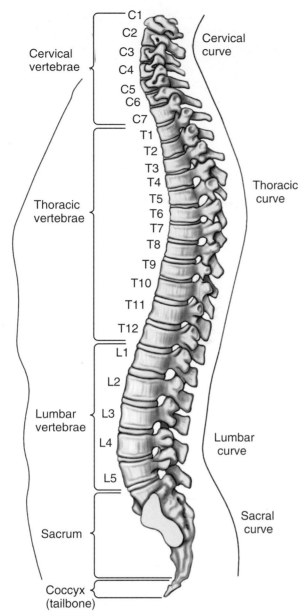

Cervical vertebrae
C1
C2
C3
C4
C5
C6
C7

Cervical curve

Thoracic vertebrae
T1
T2
T3
T4
T5
T6
T7
T8
T9
T10
T11
T12

Thoracic curve

Lumbar vertebrae
L1
L2
L3
L4
L5

Lumbar curve

Sacrum

Sacral curve

Coccyx (tailbone)

FIGURE 8-10 Vertebral column: cervical vertebrae (7), thoracic vertebrae (12), lumbar vertebrae (5), sacrum, and coccyx. Vertebral curves are the cervical, thoracic, lumbar, and sacral curves.

atlas supports the skull and allows you to nod "yes." The atlas is named after a figure in Greek mythology, Atlas, who carried the earth on his shoulders.

The second cervical vertebra (C2) is called the *axis*. The axis has a projection, called the *dens* (nicknamed for the toothlike odontoid process), which fits into the atlas and acts as a pivot or swivel for the atlas. The axis allows your head to rotate from side to side as you say "no." A strong blow to the top of the head can force the dens through the foramen magnum and into the base of the brain, causing sudden death. Not good! In children, the fusion between the dens and the axis is incomplete. Shaking a child can easily dislocate the dens, causing injury to the spinal cord.

Characteristics of Vertebrae

The vertebra is an irregular bone that contains several distinct structures (see Figure 8-11). The body of the vertebra is padded by a cartilaginous disc and supports the weight of the vertebra sitting on top of it. Some processes provide sites of attachment for ligaments, tendons, and muscles; other processes articulate with bones such as the ribs. The vertebral foramen is the opening for the spinal cord; the vertebral foramen of all vertebrae form the vertebral canal. The vertebrae are aligned so that if you run your hand down your back, you will feel the spinous processes. For this reason, the vertebral column is also called the *spine*. Note that the vertebrae become larger as the vertebral column descends. The larger lower vertebrae support a heavier load.

The bodies of the vertebrae are padded and separated by cartilaginous discs. The intervertebral discs act as shock absorbers. They also act as "spacers" between vertebrae, allowing peripheral nerves to connect to the spinal cord without being squashed. (Ouch!)

❓ Re-Think

1. How does the structure and function of C1 and C2 differ from that of other vertebrae?
2. What is the function of the vertebral foramen?
3. Why is the vertebral column called the spine?

SOME VERTEBRAL COLUMN CONCERNS

- The vertebra has a barlike lamina. Spina bifida refers to the failure of the lamina to fuse during fetal development. The vertebral defect allows the spinal cord to protrude onto the surface of the back. Depending on the level of the defect, compression of the spinal cord then causes paralysis and loss of bladder and bowel control.
- A surgical procedure called a *laminectomy* may be performed to access the intervertebral disc; the opening allows the surgeon to remove a damaged, or "slipped," disc. Occasionally, several vertebrae are fused together to stabilize a part of the vertebral column. This procedure is called *spinal fusion*.

sacrum get its name? The ancients thought that the seat of the soul was located at the base of the spine and therefore called the sacred area the "sacrum." The tailbone is called the *coccyx* (KOHK-iks) because it resembles the beak of a cuckoo bird.

Two Special Vertebrae: Atlas (C1) and Axis (C2)

The first and second cervical vertebrae have several special features and names (Figure 8-11). The first cervical vertebra (C1) is called the *atlas*. The atlas has no body but does have depressions into which fit the bony projections of the occipital bone of the skull. The

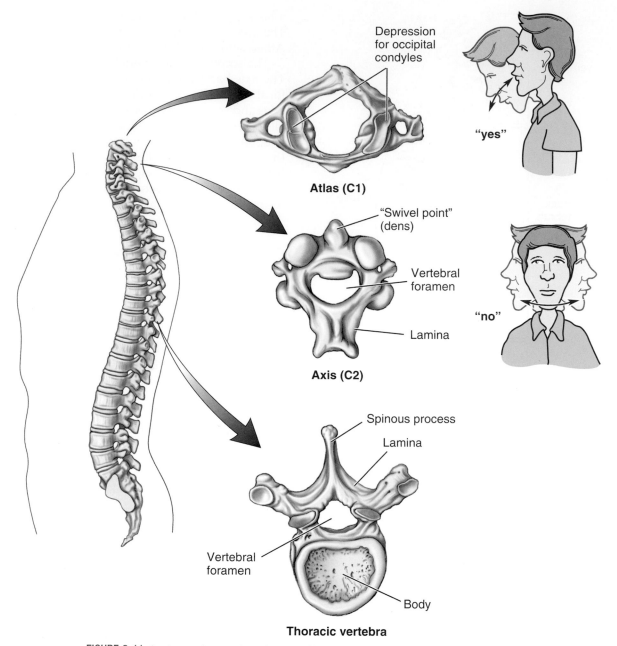

FIGURE 8-11 Anatomy of a vertebra: the atlas (C1) and axis (C2), and a thoracic vertebra.

- Note that the spinal cord descends from the base of the brain through the vertebral foramen of the stack of vertebrae. Injury to the vertebral column at any point can compress or sever the spinal cord, causing paralysis. You must use extreme caution while treating or moving a person with a spinal cord injury. Immobility is a key term in the first-aid treatment of suspected spinal cord injury.

Curvatures

When viewed from the side, the vertebral column has four normal curvatures (see Figure 8-10): the cervical, thoracic, lumbar, and sacral curves. The directions of the curvatures are important. The cervical and the lumbar curvatures bend toward the front of the body.

The thoracic and sacral curvatures bend away from the front of the body. These curves center the head over the body, thereby providing the balance needed to walk in an upright position.

The curvature of the fetal spine is different. Its single C-shaped curvature bends away from the front of the body. Its shape reflects the curled-up position of the fetus during the 9 months in the cozy, but cramped, uterine living quarters. The cervical curvature develops about 3 to 4 months after birth as infants start to hold up their heads. The lumbar curvature develops at about 1 year of age, when children begin standing and walking.

Figure 8-12 illustrates several abnormal curvatures of the spine. Scoliosis (skoh-lee-OH-sis) refers to a

Scoliosis   **Kyphosis**   **Lordosis**

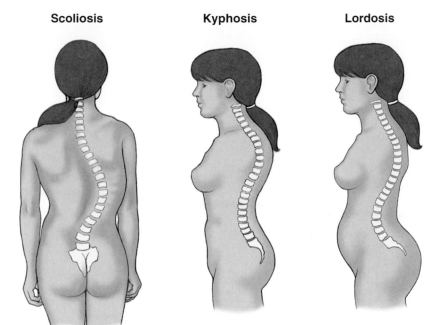

FIGURE 8-12 Abnormal curvatures of the vertebral column.

lateral curvature, usually involving the thoracic verte-brae. If severe, a lateral curvature can compress abdominal organs. It can also diminish expansion of the rib cage and therefore impair breathing. Kyphosis (kye-FOH-sis) is an exaggerated thoracic curvature; it, too, can impair breathing and is sometimes called *hunchback*. Lordosis is an exaggerated lumbar curvature and is sometimes called *swayback*. These abnormalities may be caused by a genetic defect or may develop in response to disease or poor posture.

THORACIC CAGE

The *thorax* (THOH-raks) is a term that refers to the chest region. The thoracic cage is the skeletal part of the chest; it is a bony, cone-shaped cage that surrounds and protects the lungs, heart, large blood vessels, and some of the abdominal organs, such as the liver, spleen, and kidneys (Figure 8-13). It plays a crucial role in breathing and helps support the bones of the shoulder. The thoracic cage is composed of the sternum, ribs, and thoracic vertebrae.

Sternum

The sternum, or breastbone, is a dagger-shaped bone located along the midline of the anterior chest. The three parts are the manubrium (man-OO-bree-ahm), body, and xiphoid (ZYE-foyd) process. The xiphoid process is the tip of the sternum and serves as a point of attachment for some abdominal muscles. It is also a landmark for cardiopulmonary resuscitation (CPR). Note the suprasternal notch (also called the jugular notch), a depression on the upper part of the manubrium between the two clavicles; it is used as a landmark to locate other structures.

Ribs

Twelve pairs of ribs attach posteriorly to the thoracic vertebrae. Anteriorly, the top seven pairs of ribs attach directly to the sternum by costal cartilage and are called *true ribs*. The next five pairs attach indirectly to the sternum by cartilage or do not attach at all and are called *false ribs*. The bottom two pairs of false ribs lack sternal attachment and are therefore called *floating ribs*. Because of their location and lack of sternal support, the floating ribs are easily broken. Note that the ribs are numbered, which allows us to describe the location of thoracic structures. The spaces between the ribs (intercostal spaces) are also numbered. For example, the heart is located between the second rib and fifth intercostal space (the space between the fifth and sixth ribs). You will spend a lot of time counting ribs and intercostal spaces as part of your clinical practice.

Other Thoracic Cage Structures

Located between the ribs are the intercostal muscles. Contraction of these muscles helps move the thoracic cage during breathing. If you put your hand on your chest and take a deep breath, you will feel your thoracic cage move up and out. The costal margins are the edges of the cartilage that form an angle as they converge near the xiphoid process. The costal angle should be less than 90 degrees. The costal angle can change size; for example, during pregnancy the angle increases. It also increases when the chest diameter expands with certain lung diseases, such as emphysema. Another sternal landmark is the sternomanubrial joint, also called the *angle of Louis*. This landmark is used in counting ribs and is at the level of the second rib.

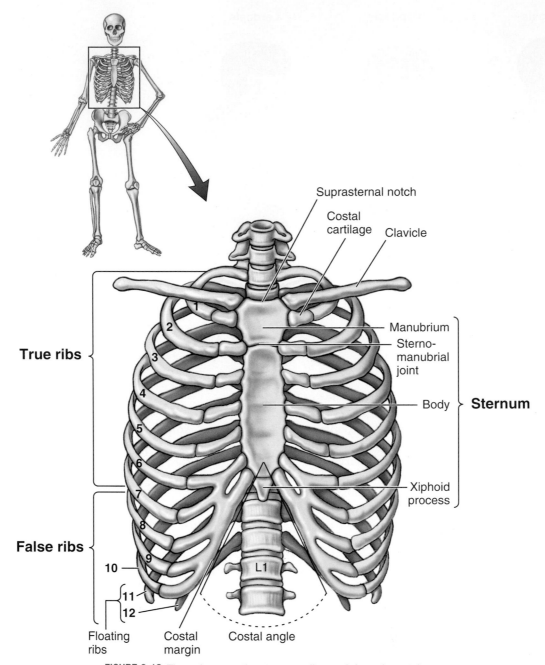

FIGURE 8-13 Thoracic cage: the sternum, ribs, and thoracic vertebrae.

APPENDICULAR SKELETON

The appendicular skeleton is composed of the bones of the shoulder girdle, upper limbs, pelvic girdle, and lower limbs (see Figure 8-1).

FIGURE 8-14 Bones of the upper limb. **A,** Shoulder girdle, arm, forearm, and hand. **B,** Position of the radius and ulna during supination and pronation.

SHOULDER GIRDLE

The shoulder girdle is also called the *pectoral girdle*. Each shoulder girdle contains two bones: one clavicle (KLAV-i-kul) and one scapula (SKAP-yoo-lah) (Figure 8-14). The shoulder girdle supports the upper limbs and serves as a place of attachment for muscles. The shoulder girdle is designed for great flexibility; move your shoulder and arm around and note how many different movements you can make. Compare this with the limited movement you have at the elbow and the knee.

Clavicle

The clavicle is also called the *collarbone*. It looks like a long, slender, S-shaped rod and articulates with both the sternum and scapula. The clavicle helps stabilize the shoulder. The attachment, however, is weak and easily dislocated or broken. The clavicle is the most frequently broken bone in the body.

Scapula

The scapula, also called the *shoulder blade* or *wing bone*, is a large flat bone shaped like a triangle. The two scapulae are located on the posterior thorax. Two large processes on the scapula allow it to articulate with the clavicle and serve as points of attachment for arm and chest muscles. The glenoid cavity on the scapula is the site where the head of the humerus (arm bone) fits, thereby allowing you to rotate your arm at the shoulder. Note the acromion process and coracoid process on the scapula near the glenoid cavity. Both processes serve as points of attachment for ligaments and muscles. The acromion process forms the "pointy" part of the shoulder and articulates with the clavicle.

 Do You Know...

About Xtreme Modeling and Toe Cleavage?

The saying, "You can never be too thin" (or off-balance) has taken on a new meaning. In addition to a starvation diet, Xtreme Modeling has taken surgical aim at the skeletal system. It's called "remodeling the model." How so? Surgeons have successfully shortened or removed toes, thereby allowing the foot to fit into stylish "pointy" shoes. More importantly, toe removal also creates revealing toe cleavage. The toe is not the only osseous victim of this skeletal redesign. Removal of the lower floating ribs further slims the slim. When accompanied by high colonic irrigations (enemas), our remodeled model easily slips into the elusive size 0. Of obvious concern: the risk of general anesthesia, the loss of ribs that normally protect the kidneys, and the loss of toes that assist in walking, balance, and overall comfort! Go figure!

UPPER LIMBS

The upper limbs contain the bones of the arm (humerus), forearm (ulna and radius), and hand (carpals, metacarpals, and phalanges).

Humerus

The humerus is the arm bone. The proximal humerus contains a head, which fits into the glenoid cavity of the scapula, allowing the arm to rotate at the shoulder joint. At the distal end of the humerus are several processes that allow it to articulate with the bones of the forearm. The olecranon (oh-LEK-rah-non) fossa is a depression of the humerus that holds the olecranon process of the ulna when the elbow is extended (not bent).

Radius

The radius is one of two bones of the forearm. It is located on the lateral or thumb side when the palm of the hand is facing forward. The head of the radius articulates with the humerus and proximal ulna, whereas the distal end articulates with the distal ulna and the carpal or wrist bones. The radial tuberosity at the proximal end of the radius is the site of attachment for one of the muscles responsible for bending the forearm at the elbow.

 Do You Know...

Why Hitting My Funny Bone Doesn't Feel Funny?

When you hit your elbow and get that sharp pain that is associated with the "funny bone," you are actually hitting the ulnar nerve. The unprotected ulnar nerve lies over the distal end of the humerus and is therefore vulnerable to being bumped. Why do we call it funny? Maybe because of its location near the humerus, a "humorous" name for a bone.

Ulna

The ulna is the second bone of the forearm. The longer of the two bones, the ulna, is located on the medial or little finger side of the forearm. It has processes and depressions that allow it to articulate with the humerus and radius proximally and with the radius distally. The olecranon process of the ulna is what you feel as the bony point of the elbow. Note that the distal ends of both the ulna and radius have a pointed styloid process; the styloid processes can be felt at the wrist.

Also note the relationship of the radius to the ulna when the hand moves from a palm-up (supination) to a palm-down (pronation) position. When the palm is up, the two bones are parallel. When the palm is down, the two bones cross to achieve this movement.

Hand

The hand is composed of a wrist, palm, and fingers. The wrist contains eight bones called *carpal bones*, which are tightly bound by ligaments. Five metacarpal bones form the palm of the hand; each metacarpal bone is in line with a finger. Feel your metacarpal bones on the back of your hand; note how each aligns with your fingers. The 14 finger bones are called *phalanges* (fah-LAN-jeez), or digits. Note that each digit has three bones except the thumb (called the *pollex*), which has only two bones. The heads of the phalanges are prominent as the knuckles when a fist is made.

 Re-Think

1. List the bones of the pectoral girdle.
2. What happens at the glenoid cavity?
3. What bones form the elbow? What is the olecranon process?

Pelvic Girdle

The pelvic girdle is composed of two coxal bones that articulate with each other anteriorly and with the sacrum posteriorly (Figure 8-15, *A*). The pelvic girdle performs three functions: (1) it bears the weight of the body; (2) it serves as a place of attachment for the thighs; and (3) it protects the organs located in the pelvic cavity, including the urinary bladder and reproductive organs.

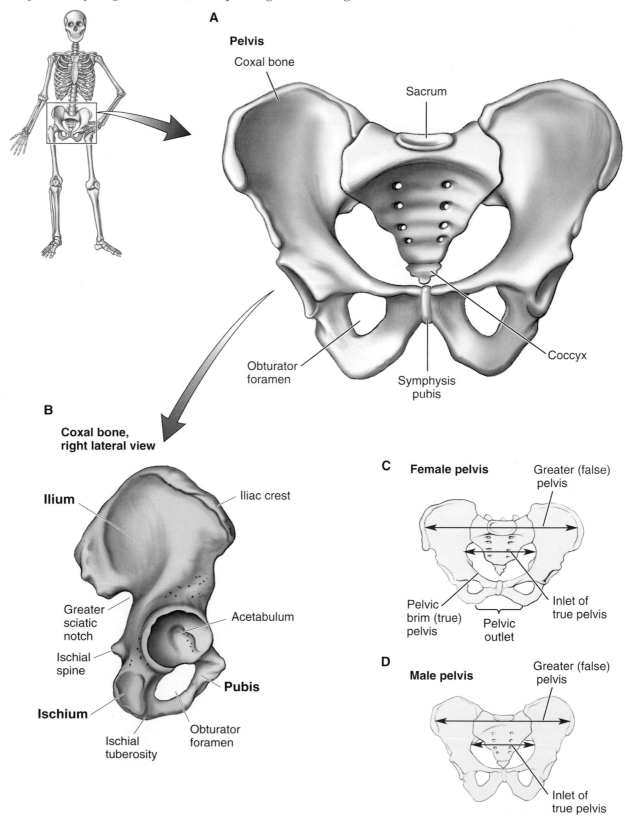

A

Pelvis

Coxal bone

Sacrum

Coccyx

Obturator foramen

Symphysis pubis

B

Coxal bone, right lateral view

Ilium

Iliac crest

Greater sciatic notch

Acetabulum

Ischial spine

Pubis

Ischium

Ischial tuberosity

Obturator foramen

C   **Female pelvis**

Greater (false) pelvis

Pelvic brim (true) pelvis

Pelvic outlet

Inlet of true pelvis

D

Male pelvis

Greater (false) pelvis

Inlet of true pelvis

FIGURE 8-15 Pelvic cavity. **A,** Bones that make up the pelvic cavity. **B,** Coxal bone (ilium, ischium, and pubis). **C,** Female pelvis. **D,** Male pelvis.

Pelvis

The pelvis is formed by the pelvic girdle, sacrum, and coccyx.

Male and Female Differences. The differences between the female and male pelvis are related to the childbearing role of the female. In general, the female pelvis is broader and shallower than the male pelvis. The male pelvis is narrow and funnel-shaped (see Figure 8-15, *C* and *D*).

Do You Know...

About Dr. Pollex and Mr. Blackberry's Thumb?

Mr. Blackberry went to his family physician, Dr. Pollex, with a chief complaint of extreme pain in his left thumb. He writhed in pain and sobbed uncontrollably as he punched numbers into his cell and frantically sent text messages to everyone he had ever met. Dr. Pollex, however, was all over it. "Thumb abuse!" he roared. He explained to Mr. Blackberry. "Your thumb (pollex) was not designed to click away 24/7; it's aching for relief. The sheath around your thumb is inflamed and swollen." The digit doc assured Mr. Blackberry that with rest and retraining, he would soon be clicking away again. Other digits could be trained to share the clicking load. Thumb pain resulting from repetitive thumb-clicking marathons is called *Blackberry thumb,* a reference to the popular handheld device.

Coxal Bone

The coxal bone is the hip bone (see Figure 8-15, *B*). Each coxal bone is composed of three parts: the ilium, ischium, and pubis. The three bones join together to form a depression called the *acetabulum* (ass-it-TAH-buhl-um). The acetabulum is important because it receives the head of the femur and therefore enables the thigh to rotate at the hip joint.

Ilium. The ilium (IL-ee-um) is the largest part of the coxal bone. The ilium is the flared upper part of the bone and can be felt at the hip. The outer edge of the ilium is called the *iliac crest*. The ilium connects in the back with the sacrum, forming the sacroiliac joint. The greater sciatic notch is the site where blood vessels and the sciatic nerve pass from the pelvic cavity into the posterior thigh region. Like the sternum, the ilium produces blood cells and is a site for bone marrow biopsy.

Ischium. The ischium (ISH-ee-um) is the most inferior part of the coxal bone. The ischium contains three important structures: the ischial tuberosity, ischial spine, and lesser sciatic notch. The ischial tuberosity is the part of the coxal bone on which you sit. The ischial spine projects into the pelvic cavity and narrows the outlet of the pelvis. If the spines of a woman's two ischial bones are too close together, the pelvic outlet becomes too small to allow for the birth of a baby. The measurement of the distance between the two spines therefore provides valuable information about the adequacy of the pelvis for childbearing.

Pubis. The pubis is the most anterior part of the coxal bone. The two pubic bones meet in front as the symphysis (SIM-fi-sis) pubis. A disc of cartilage separates the pubic bones at the symphysis pubis. In women, the disc expands in response to the hormones of pregnancy, thereby enlarging the pelvic cavity to provide a bigger space for the growing fetus.

A large hole called the *obturator foramen* is formed as the pubic bone fuses with a part of the ischium. The obturator is the largest foramen in the body.

What is meant by the true pelvis and false pelvis? The false pelvis is the area surrounded by the flaring parts of the two iliac bones (see Figure 8-15, *C*). The true pelvis lies below the false pelvis and is much smaller. The true pelvis is a ring formed by the fusion of the pelvic bones; it is also called the *pelvic brim*. The true pelvis has an inlet and outlet area. In women, the dimensions of these areas are important because they must be large enough to allow for the passage of an infant during childbirth.

Re-Think

1. Name the three bones that form the coxal bone.
2. What is the function of the acetabulum?
3. Locate the symphysis pubis. Explain how it affects the size of the pelvis during pregnancy.

LOWER LIMBS

The lower limb includes the bones of the thigh, kneecap, leg, and the foot (Figure 8-16).

Femur

The femur is the thighbone; it is the longest and strongest bone in the body. The femur articulates with the coxal bone to form the hip joint and with the bones of the leg to form the knee joint. The head of the femur sits in the acetabulum of the coxal bone and allows the thigh to rotate at the hip joint. The head of the femur attaches to the rest of the femur by the neck. A number of bony processes are on the femur. The most important are the greater and lesser trochanters (tro-KAN-ters). These trochanters provide sites of attachment for many muscles.

In older persons, the neck of the femur is easily broken during a fall and is known as a broken hip. Forced immobility (bed rest) often results in serious complications. For example, because of the weight of the injured leg, an immobile bedridden person may experience an outward rotation of the hip. If allowed to develop, this outward rotation makes walking very difficult and therefore delays rehabilitation. Other hazards of immobility, such as blood clots and pneumonia, contribute to the seriousness of a fractured hip.

Patella

The patella is the kneecap. It is a triangular bone located within a tendon that passes over the knee. The patella articulates with both the femur and tibia. An infant is born without kneecaps; somewhere between the ages of 2 and 6 years, in response to weight bearing, a small sesamoid bone (one that looks like a sesame seed) in the patellar region enlarges, thereby forming the kneecap.

Tibia and Fibula

The tibia and the fibula form the leg. The tibia is the shinbone and articulates with the distal femur at the knee. The tibia is the larger weight-bearing bone of the leg. A protuberance called the *tibial tuberosity* is the site of attachment for the muscles and ligaments from the thigh. At the distal end of the tibia, a protuberance called the *medial malleolus* (mah-LEE-oh-lis) articulates with the inner ankle bones (tarsals).

The fibula (FIB-yoo-lah) is a long, thin bone positioned laterally alongside the tibia in the leg. The proximal end of the fibula articulates with the tibia. It does not articulate with the femur, is not part of the knee, and does not bear any weight. The distal end forms the lateral malleolus, which articulates with the outer ankle bones (tarsals). Skiers often twist their ankles and break the fibula at the lateral malleolus. You don't need snow, however, to hobble. Just roll the ankle and you too can be on crutches!

How do we remember the positions of the leg bones? The **tib**ia is the *T*hick *I*nner *B*one; the fibu**la** is *LA*teral to the tibia.

Foot

Each foot (Figure 8-17) has an ankle, instep, and five toes. Seven tarsal bones form the ankle. The most proximal of the tarsal bones, the talus, articulates with the tibia and fibula. Most of the weight of the body is supported by another tarsal bone, the calcaneus (kal-KAY-nee-us), or heel bone. The instep of the foot is formed by five metatarsal bones. The ball of the foot is formed by the distal ends of the metatarsals. The tarsals, metatarsals, and associated tendons and ligaments form the arch of the foot. If the ligaments and tendons weaken, the arches can fall, and the person is said to have flat feet. The toes contain 14 phalanges. The great toe is called the *hallux*.

Foot Notes: We all know about the thrill of victory (looking great in heels and flaunting the latest in toe

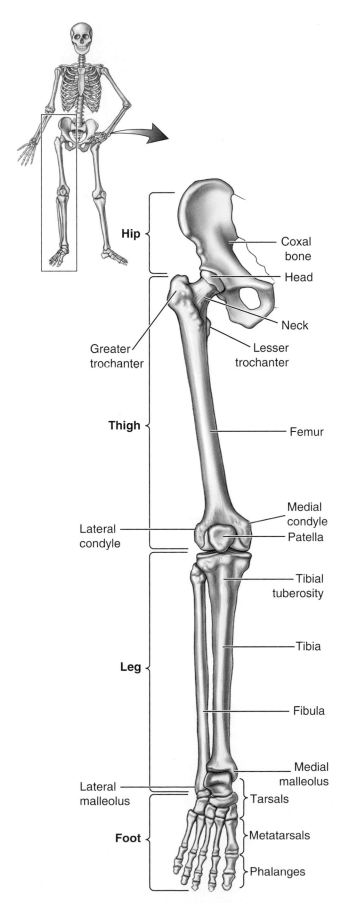

FIGURE 8-16 Bones of the lower limb: thigh, leg, and foot.

FIGURE 8-17 Bones of the foot: tarsals, metatarsals, and phalanges. Arches support the structure of the foot.

cleavage). What about the "agony of de-feet"? Think about it. Sometimes we jam our square feet into pointy shoes, creating an unnatural, uncomfortable, and crippling tiptoe gait. The entire weight of the body is pushed forward to the balls of the feet. What do we get for this stylish effort?

- *Bunions.* Bunions develop in response to excessive force, whereby the big toe is compressed and forced toward the second toe. The joint becomes distorted, inflamed, and painful.
- *Neuromas.* The shift of body weight to the balls of the feet causes painful and debilitating nerve growths (neuromas) between the toes.
- *Metatarsalgia.* The shift of body weight causes metatarsalgia, or pain in the ball of the foot.
- *Shortening of the Achilles tendon.* The tiptoe position causes contraction of the Achilles tendon; the shortened tendon makes the use of flat shoes uncomfortable.

- *Pump bump.* Excess pressure of the heel of the shoe on bone causes an enlargement (bump) on the heel bone. Pump bump is so common that it has its own medical name: Haglund's deformity.
- *Knee pain.* The shift in weight adds unnatural stress to the knee joint; knee joint replacement is more common in women and is often related to wearing abusive footwear.
- *Last but not least.* There have been several documented cases of death associated with falling while wearing platform shoes.

What to do? Although it can be performed, the surgical removal of toes is not the answer. Instituting a fashion change is certainly less painful than redesigning the foot. In any event, heels are definitely an anatomical step in the wrong direction!

? Re-Think

1. List the bones that articulate with the femur.
2. What bones articulate at the knee?
3. What bones form the foot?

JOINTS (ARTICULATIONS)

A joint, or articulation, is the site where two bones meet. Joints perform two functions: they hold the bones together, and they provide flexibility to a rigid skeleton. Without joints, we would move around stiffly like robots. Think of how awkward a basketball player would look if the entire skeleton were rigid. There is a branch of science that studies joints, called *arthrology;* the branch of medicine that studies disease of the joints is called *rheumatology.*

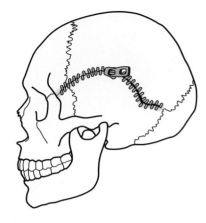

2+2 Sum It Up!

The appendicular skeleton includes bones of the pectoral girdle (clavicle, scapula), upper extremities (humerus, radius, ulna, carpals, metacarpals, phalanges), pelvic girdle (coxal bone), and lower extremities (femur, patella, tibia, fibula, tarsals, metatarsals, phalanges).

Do You Know...

What Dripping "Humours" Have to Do with Gout?

The typical cartoon of a person experiencing gout is that of an older, red-faced, obese, well-off man. His elevated, throbbing big toe fits the picture perfectly. Gout is caused by an increase of uric acid in the blood. The uric acid deposits in joints, where it forms tiny sharp crystals (called *tophi*) that inflame the joint and cause intense pain. Foods high in uric acid can bring on an attack of gout. A diet of meat and alcohol (the rich man's diet) can cause it; hence, the caricature of a glutton—wealthy, obese, and red-faced—comes to mind. The term *gout* comes from *gutta*, a Latin word meaning "to drop." It was originally believed that gout was caused by unhealthy humours (fluids) or poisons that dropped or dripped into the joints, particularly the joint of the great toe. This disease was so common that the pubs often had gout stools for their portly porkers. Remember this:

G	**g**reat toe
O	**o**ne joint, usually the great toe
U	**u**ric acid
T	**t**ophi
Y	**Y**ikes, that hurts!

Joints can be classified into three groups according to the amount of movement: immovable, slightly movable, and freely movable (Table 8-3). Joints can also be classified according to the types of tissues—fibrous, cartilaginous, or synovial—that bind the bones at the joint.

JOINT CLASSIFICATION

IMMOVABLE JOINTS

Immovable joints permit no movement. The sutures in the skull are immovable joints. The sutures are formed as the irregular edges of the skull bones interlock and are bound by fibrous connective tissue. When fused, they look like zippers.

SLIGHTLY MOVABLE JOINTS

Slightly movable joints permit limited movement. Limited movement is usually achieved by bones connected by a cartilaginous disc. For example, movement of the spinal column occurs at the intervertebral discs. Also, during pregnancy, the symphysis pubis allows the pelvis to widen.

FREELY MOVABLE JOINTS

Freely movable joints provide much more flexibility and movement than the other two types of joints. Most of the joints of the skeletal system are freely movable. All freely movable joints are known as **synovial** (si-NO-vee-all) **joints** (Figure 8-18).

A typical synovial joint includes the following structures:

- *Articular cartilage.* The articulating surface of each of the two bones is lined with articular cartilage, forming a smooth surface within the joint.
- *Joint capsule.* The joint capsule is made of fibrous connective tissue. It encloses the joint in a strong sleevelike covering.
- *Synovial membrane.* Lining the joint capsule is the synovial membrane. This membrane secretes synovial fluid into the joint cavity.
- *Synovial fluid.* Synovial fluid lubricates the bones in the joint, thereby decreasing the friction within the joint. Synovial fluid gets its name from an ovum or egg, because the thick consistency of the synovial fluid resembles the consistency of an egg white.

Table 8-3 Types of Joints

TYPE	DESCRIPTION	EXAMPLES
Immovable	Suture, or "zipper"	Cranial bones
Slightly movable	Disc of cartilage between two bones	Intervertebral discs; symphysis pubis
Freely movable	Ball-and-socket	Shoulder (scapula and humerus): hip (pelvic bone and femur)
	Hinge	Elbow (humerus and ulna): knee (femur and tibia); fingers
	Pivot	Atlas and axis; allows for rotation (side-to-side movement) of the head, indicating "no"
	Saddle	Thumb (carpometacarpal joint); sternoclavicular joint
	Gliding	Carpals
	Condyloid	Temporal bone and mandible (jaw); knuckles

FIGURE 8-18 Synovial joint (knee), structure, and contents.

- *Bursae.* Many synovial joints contain bursae (sing., bursa). Bursae are small sacs of synovial fluid between the joint and the tendons that cross over the joint. Bursae permit the tendons to slide as the bones move. Excessive use of a joint may cause a painful inflammation of the bursae, called *bursitis*. Tennis elbow is bursitis caused by excessive and improper use of the elbow joint.
- *Supporting ligaments.* Surrounding the joint are supporting ligaments. These ligaments join the articulating bones together and stabilize the joint. Sometimes a ligament is stretched or torn, causing pain and loss of mobility.

NAMING JOINTS

The joints of the body are named so as to provide information about the articulating bones. The joints are named according to the bones they connect. Refer to Figure 8-19 as we identify several joints. The temporomandibular joint connects the temporal bone in the skull with the mandible (lower jaw). The tibiofemoral joint is the articulation between the tibia and the femur—the knee. The knuckles refer to the metacarpophalangeal joints. The name indicates that the metacarpal bone articulates with a phalange (finger). Some names specify the bony process rather than the bone.

For example, the glenohumeral joint names the glenoid cavity of the scapula and humerus, the arm bone that fits into the glenoid cavity. The acromioclavicular joint is the articulation between the acromion process of the scapula and the clavicle. Finally, locate the sternomanubrial joint (breastbone); it is a landmark used to count ribs.

MOVING SYNOVIAL JOINTS

The body contains many types of freely movable synovial joints. The type of motion and the degree of flexibility vary with each type of joint. For example, if you move your elbow, your forearm will move like two boards joined by a hinge. This motion is very different from the arm-swinging motion at the shoulder joint. Both the elbow and shoulder joints are freely movable, but the types of movement differ.

Six types of freely movable joints are classified according to the type of movement allowed by the joint (Figure 8-20; see Table 8-3).

HINGE JOINT

The hinge joint allows movement similar to the movement of two boards joined together by a hinge. The hinge allows movement in one direction, where the angle at the hinge increases or decreases. Hinge joints

FIGURE 8-19 Naming joints.

(Figure labels:)
Temporomandibular
Sternoclavicular
Sternomanubrial
Acromioclavicular
Glenohumeral
Humeroulnar
Proximal and distal radioulnar
Radiocarpal
Metacarpophalangeal
Tibiofemoral
Proximal tibiofibular
Distal tibiofibular

include elbows, knees, and fingers. Move each of these joints to clarify the movement described here.

BALL-AND-SOCKET JOINT

A ball-and-socket joint is formed when the ball-shaped end of one bone fits into the cup-shaped socket of another bone, so that the bones can move in many directions around a central point. The shoulder and hip joints are ball-and-socket joints. The head of the humerus fits into the glenoid cavity of the scapula in the shoulder joint. The head of the femur fits into the acetabulum of the coxal bone in the hip joint.

Move your shoulder all around (as in pitching a softball) and note the freedom of movement. Compare this movement with the limited movement at the elbow or knee joints. Although the ball-and-socket joint allows for a wide range of movement, it also predisposes the joint to easy displacement. When a strong force (as in falling) is applied to the shoulder, for example, a dislocation may occur.

PIVOT JOINT

A pivot joint allows for rotation around the length of a bone. The pivot joint allows only for rotation. An example is the side-to-side movement of the head indicating "no." This rotation occurs as the atlas (first cervical vertebra) swivels around, or pivots, on the axis (second cervical vertebra). This joint is called the *atlantoaxial joint*.

SADDLE JOINT

A saddle joint is formed when the surfaces of both articulating bones are saddle shaped; the saddle shape of one bone is concave whereas the saddle shape of the second bone is convex. The position of the articulating bones is like a rider in a saddle. The clearest example of a saddle joint is the carpometacarpal joint at the base of the thumb, which allows the thumb a wide range of motion. Move your thumb all around to check out its versatility. Now, touch the tip of each finger with your thumb, a movement referred to as opposition. Interestingly, having an opposable thumb is one of the bragging points for being classified as human!

GLIDING JOINT

A gliding joint is formed by the interaction of the flat surfaces of the articulating bones. A gliding joint allows for a limited but complex gliding movement. Gliding joints are found in the wrist (intercarpal joints), ankle (intertarsal joints), and vertebral column.

CONDYLOID JOINT

A condyloid (KON-di-loyd) joint is formed when the oval articular surface of one bone fits into the oval depression of the second articulating bone. The radiocarpal joint (wrist) and the metacarpophalangeal joints (knuckles) at the bases of the fingers are examples of condyloid joints.

CLINICALLY "BIG" SYNOVIAL JOINTS

KNEE

The knee joint, called the *tibiofemoral joint*, is a hinge joint. In addition to all the structures contained in a synovial joint, the knee joint contains extra cushioning in the form of pads of cartilage. These pads absorb the shock of walking and jumping. Two crescent-shaped pads of cartilage, the medial meniscus (min-ISS-kiss) and lateral meniscus, rest on the tibia. Like other synovial joints, the knee joint is reinforced and aligned by supporting ligaments, the cruciate (KROO-she-ate) ligaments in particular. There is an anterior cruciate ligament (ACL) and a posterior cruciate ligament (PCL). All athletes are very aware of these joint-stabilizing structures.

PEAS FOR THE KNEES AND MORE DISEASE

- Knees are frequently sprained and strained. As every soccer mom or dad knows, a bag of frozen peas is good first aid for injured knees and is consistent with the first-aid treatment of strains and sprains, or RICE (*R*est, *I*ce, *C*ompression, and *E*levation).
- The cruciate ligaments, especially the ACL, are frequent victims of athletic events. The ACL prevents hyperextension of the knee and is torn when the knee is forcibly hyperextended. Torn cartilage is

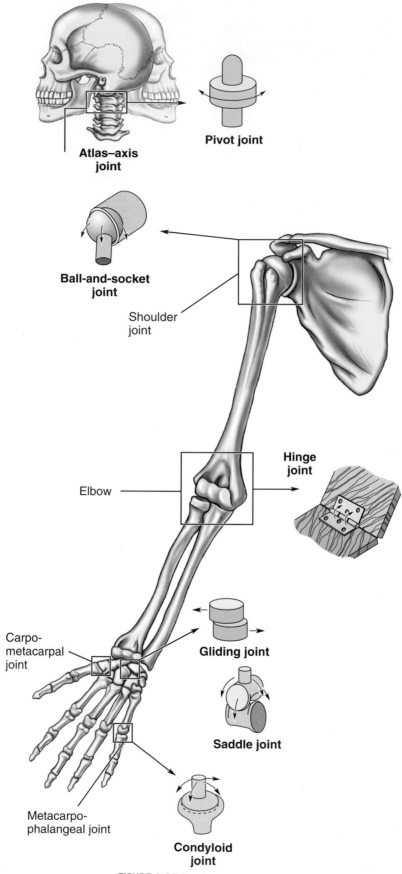

Pivot joint

Atlas–axis joint

Ball-and-socket joint

Shoulder joint

Hinge joint

Elbow

Carpo-metacarpal joint

Gliding joint

Saddle joint

Metacarpo-phalangeal joint

Condyloid joint

FIGURE 8-20 Freely movable joints.

removed by arthroscopic surgery. An arthroscope is a viewing tube that allows the surgeon to see into the knee joint.

- As any football player knows, being tackled at the sides of the knees can put a fast end to one's career. A clipping penalty attests to the seriousness of knee injuries and is fully deserving of a 15-yard penalty.

SHOULDER

The shoulder joint is called the *glenohumeral joint,* indicating that the head of the humerus fits into the glenoid cavity of the scapula. The shoulder joint is a ball-and-socket joint that permits the greatest range of motion. The joint is stabilized by surrounding skeletal muscles, tendons, and ligaments. The rotator cuff muscles and tendons, in particular, hold the head of the humerus in the glenoid cavity. The shoulder joint is the most frequently dislocated joint.

ELBOW

The elbow is called the *humeroulnar joint.* A lesser component of the elbow is the humeroradial joint. The olecranon process of the ulna forms the pointy part of the elbow when it is flexed. The elbow is a hinge joint that is very stable; nonetheless, it can be injured. For example, "nursemaid's elbow" is caused by an impatient parent dragging a toddler by the arm. The upward twisting pull causes a partial dislocation of the child's elbow and possible damage to the growth plate (epiphyseal disc).

HIP

The hip, called the *coxal joint,* is a ball-and-socket joint formed where the head of the femur articulates with the acetabulum, the depression formed by the three coxal bones. The hip is strengthened by surrounding muscles, tendons, and ligaments. A fractured hip refers to a break in the neck of the femur.

? Re-Think

Classify each of the following freely movable joints: tibiofemoral, humeroulnar, glenohumeral, atlas-axis joint, and hip joints.

Types of Joint Movements

Movements at freely movable joints occur when the muscles that lie across the joints contract and exert pressure on the attached bone. These movements are illustrated in Figure 8-21 and defined as follows:

- **Flexion.** This is the bending of a joint that decreases the angle between the bones (bending the leg at the knee or the fingers).
- **Extension.** This is the straightening of a joint so that the angle between the bones increases (e.g., straightening the leg at the knee or the fingers to open the hand).

- *Plantar flexion.* This is bending the foot down, as in toe dancing.
- *Dorsiflexion.* This is bending the foot up toward the leg.
- *Hyperextension.* This is overextending the joint beyond its normally straightened position, as in moving the hand toward the upper surface of the wrist.
- **Abduction.** This is movement away from the midline of the body (move your leg sideways, away from your body).
- **Adduction.** This is movement toward the midline of the body (return your leg toward your body).
- *Inversion.* This is turning the sole of the foot inward so that it faces the opposite foot.
- *Eversion.* This is turning the sole of the foot outward.
- *Supination.* This is turning the hand so that the palm faces upward.
- *Pronation.* This is turning the hand so that the palm faces downward.
- *Circumduction.* This is a combination of movements, as in the circular arm movement that a softball pitcher makes while pitching the ball.

? Re-Think

Refer to Figure 8-19 and describe the type of joint movements of the following parts: left hand at the wrist, right leg at the knee, right forearm at the elbow, left forearm at the elbow, and right hand at the wrist.

2+2 Sum It Up!

A joint, or articulation, is the place where two or more bones meet. The three types of joints are immovable joints, slightly movable joints, and freely movable joints. Freely movable joints are synovial joints. Types of freely movable joints include hinge, ball-and-socket, pivot, gliding, saddle, and condyloid joints. Because of the diverse types of joints, the skeleton is capable of a variety of movements.

❧ As You Age

1. Because of loss of calcium and organic material, bones are less strong and more brittle. Many older women develop osteoporosis. As a result, bones fracture more easily. Moreover, fractured bones heal incompletely and more slowly.
2. As sex hormones in the blood decrease, there is a decrease in new bone growth and in bone mass, thus increasing the susceptibility to osteoporosis.
3. Tendons and ligaments are less flexible. As a result, joints have a decreased range of motion. A thinning of the articular cartilage and bony overgrowths in the joints contributes to joint stiffness.
4. The intervertebral discs shrink. Because of the compressed discs and the loss of bone mass, body height decreases and the thoracic spine curves (causing kyphosis).

Note: The Medical Terminology and Disorders table appears in Chapter 9.

FIGURE 8-21 Types of movements at joints.

Get Ready for Exams!

Summary Outline

The skeletal system supports the weight of the body, supports and protects body organs, enables the body to move, acts as a storage site for minerals, and produces blood cells.

I. Bones: An Overview
  A. Sizes, shapes, and markings
    1. Bones are classified as long, short, flat, and irregular.
    2. Bone markings: projections and depressions; function as sites of muscle attachments and passages for nerves and blood vessels
    3. Composed of compact (dense) bone and spongy (cancellous) bone
  B. Parts of a long bone
    1. Diaphysis (shaft)
    2. Epiphyses (ends), covered by articular cartilage
    3. Other components: medullary cavity, periosteum, bone marrow, epiphyseal disc, endosteum, and articular cartilage
  C. Ossification
    1. Intramembranous
    2. Endochondral
  D. Bone growth
    1. Bones grow longitudinally at the epiphyseal disc to determine height.
    2. Bones grow thicker and wider to support the weight of the body.

II. Divisions of the Skeletal System
The names of the 206 bones of the skeleton are listed in Table 8-2.
  A. Axial skeleton
    1. The axial skeleton includes the bones of the skull (cranium and face), hyoid bone, bones of the middle ear, bones of the vertebral column, and thoracic cage.
    2. The skull of a newborn contains fontanels, which are membranous areas that allow brain growth.
    3. The skull contains air-filled cavities called *sinuses*.
    4. The vertebral column is formed from 24 vertebrae, one sacrum, and one coccyx. The vertebrae are separated by cartilaginous discs. The vertebral column of the adult has four curvatures: cervical, thoracic, lumbar, and sacral.
    5. The thoracic cage is a bony cone-shaped cage formed by the sternum, 12 pairs of ribs, and thoracic vertebrae.
  B. Appendicular skeleton
    1. The appendicular skeleton includes the bones of the extremities (arms and legs) and the bones of the hip and pectoral (shoulder) girdles.
    2. The pectoral (shoulder) girdle consists of the scapula and the clavicle.
    3. The pelvic girdle is formed by the two coxal bones and is secured to the axial skeleton at the sacrum.

III. Joints
A joint or articulation is the site where two bones meet.
  A. Types of joints (based on the degree of movement)
    1. Immovable joints
    2. Slightly movable joints
    3. Freely movable joints or synovial joints. Structures within a synovial joint (knee) are the articular cartilage, joint capsule, synovial membrane, synovial fluid, bursae, and supporting ligaments.
    4. The types of freely movable joints include hinge, ball-and-socket, pivot, gliding, saddle, and condyloid joints.
  B. Joint movement
    1. Flexion, extension, and hyperextension
    2. Abduction and adduction
    3. Inversion and eversion
    4. Supination and pronation
    5. Circumduction
    6. Plantar flexion and dorsiflexion

Review Your Knowledge

Matching: Long Bone
Directions: Match the following words with their descriptions below.

a. epiphysis
b. spongy bone
c. epiphyseal disc
d. diaphysis
e. medullary cavity
f. haversian system
g. osteoblast
h. osteoclast
i. red bone marrow
j. periosteum

1. ____ Shaft of a long bone
2. ____ Site of longitudinal bone growth
3. ____ Bone-building cell
4. ____ Site of blood cell production
5. ____ Tough outer covering of the bone
6. ____ Enlarged end of a long bone
7. ____ Cancellous bone
8. ____ Osteon
9. ____ Bone-eroding cell that helps in bone remodeling
10. ____ Hollow center of a long bone

Matching: Names of Bones
Directions: Match the following words with their descriptions below.

a. femur
b. scapula
c. mandible
d. ulna
e. sternum
f. coxal bone
g. tibia
h. calcaneus
i. frontal
j. phalanges

1. ____ Manubrium, body, xiphoid process
2. ____ Acetabulum formed by parts of this bone
3. ____ Contains the glenoid cavity that holds the head of the humerus
4. ____ Contains the "pointy" olecranon process
5. ____ The thick inner bone of the leg
6. ____ Heel bone
7. ____ Fingers and toes
8. ____ The head of this bone that articulates with the acetabulum
9. ____ Lower jaw bone
10. ____ Forms the forehead

Matching: Joints and Joint Movement

Directions: Match the following words with their descriptions below. Some words may be used more than once.

a. ball-and-socket
b. adduction
c. flexion
d. pronation
e. dorsiflexion
f. circumduction
g. extension
h. plantar flexion
i. abduction
j. supination

1. ____ Type of joint movement at the elbow (angle decreases)
2. ____ Turning the forearm so that the palm of the hand "looks" at the sky
3. ____ Movement away from the midline of the body
4. ____ Toe dancing
5. ____ Movement of the ulna toward the humerus
6. ____ Type of joint at the shoulder and hip
7. ____ Shoulder movement, as in pitching a softball
8. ____ Movement toward the midline of the body
9. ____ Turning the forearm so that the hand "looks" at the floor
10. ____ Straightening the bended knee

Multiple Choice

1. The epiphyseal disc is
   a. located in the medullary cavity.
   b. composed of cartilage and is involved in the growth of long bones.
   c. composed exclusively of osteoclasts.
   d. the site of blood cell formation.
2. Osteoclastic activity
   a. is responsible for longitudinal bone growth.
   b. lowers blood calcium levels.
   c. stimulates bone breakdown.
   d. regulates the production of blood cells.
3. Which of the following is not true of the acetabulum?
   a. Formed by the ilium, ischium, and pubis
   b. Receives the head of the femur
   c. Articulates with the greater trochanter
   d. Forms a ball-and-socket joint
4. The atlas and axis
   a. are pelvic bones.
   b. are processes located on the posterior scapula.
   c. form the glenoid cavity.
   d. are vertebrae that allow the head to move.
5. To determine the approximate length of the humerus, you would measure from the
   a. olecranon process to the styloid process of the radius.
   b. acromion to the olecranon process.
   c. suprasternal notch to the xiphoid process.
   d. greater trochanter to the medial malleolus.
6. Depression of the red bone marrow
   a. causes a life-threatening decline in blood cells.
   b. stunts longitudinal bone growth.
   c. causes arthritis.
   d. causes loss of bone mineralization and osteoporosis.

7. Identify the movement at the elbow that decreases the angle at the humeroulnar joint.
   a. Extension
   b. Adduction
   c. Pronation
   d. Flexion
8. Which of the following is not true of the skull?
   a. The joint between the frontal and parietal bones is called the *coronal suture*.
   b. The lambdoidal suture is an immovable joint.
   c. Cranial bones include zygomatic, frontal, occipital, and temporal bones.
   d. Facial bones include maxilla, mandible, and ethmoid bones.
9. Which of the following is true of the foramen magnum? It is
   a. a large hole through which the brain exits the cranium.
   b. located within the frontal bone.
   c. part of C1, the atlas.
   d. a suture between the frontal and parietal bones.
10. C1 to C7, T1 to T12, and L1 to L5 are
    a. responsible for the lumbar curve.
    b. vertebrae.
    c. cranial sutures.
    d. part of the appendicular skeleton.

Go Figure

1. **According to Figures 8-2 and 8-3**
   a. The osteon is the structural unit for compact bone.
   b. The bone marrow is part of the haversian system.
   c. The diaphysis is composed exclusively of cancellous bone.
   d. The upper extremity is composed of all long bones.

2. **According to Figure 8-5**
   a. The bricklayer represents osteoclastic activity.
   b. Osteoclasts stimulate bone synthesis.
   c. Osteoblasts are bone-building cells (as in the bricklayer).
   d. Osteoclasts only work on the external surface of the bone.

3. **According to Figures 8-7, 8-8, and 8-9**
   a. The suture is the only type of joint found in the skull.
   b. Fontanels are most evident in the side view of the adult skull.
   c. The frontal, zygomatic, and sphenoid bones help form the eye socket.
   d. The anterior fontanel is located between the occipital and parietal bones.

4. **According to Figures 8-10, 8-11, and 8-12**
   a. The structure of all cervical vertebrae resemble C1.
   b. Intervertebral discs are located between all vertebrae.
   c. The atlas and axis are cervical vertebrae.
   d. Kyphosis refers to a lateral curvature of the vertebral column.

5. **According to Figures 8-13 and 8-14**
   a. The clavicle articulates with the scapula at the coracoid process.
   b. The pectoral girdle refers to the humerus, clavicle, and scapula.
   c. The costal angle is formed by the true ribs.
   d. The second rib is at the level of the sternomanubrial joint.

6. **According to Figure 8-15**
   a. The symphysis pubis is cartilage that lines the acetabulum.
   b. The symphysis pubis stretches across both obturator foramen.
   c. The sacrum does not articulate with the coxal bone.
   d. The acetabulum is formed by all three parts of the coxal bone.

7. **According to Figures 8-16 and 8-17**
   a. The patella articulates with the distal femur, proximal tibia, and lateral malleolus.
   b. The lateral malleolus is located on the distal tibia.
   c. The calcaneus articulates with the proximal fibula.
   d. The talus articulates with the distal tibia and fibula.

8. **According to Figures 8-19 and 8-20**
   a. The humeroulnar joint is a hinge joint that is known as the elbow.
   b. The glenohumeral joint is formed by the scapula and the clavicle.
   c. Both the proximal and distal tibiofibular joints are ball-and-socket joints.
   d. All of the above are true.

9. **According to Figures 8-19 and 8-21**
   a. Movement at the tibiofemoral joint is called *abduction* and *adduction*.
   b. Movement at the hip joint allows for adduction and abduction of the thigh; it also allows for flexion, extension, and hyperextension of the thigh.
   c. Plantar flexion and dorsiflexion occurs at the glenohumeral joint.
   d. All of the above are true.

Key Terms

acetylcholine (ACh) (p. 147)
actin (p. 145)
antagonists (p. 152)
aponeurosis (p. 145)
belly (p. 143)
cardiac muscle (p. 143)
fascia (p. 144)
insertion (p. 152)

motor unit (p. 147)
myosin (p. 147)
neuromuscular junction (NMJ) (p. 147)
origin (p. 152)
prime mover (p. 152)
recruitment (p. 147)
sarcomere (p. 145)

sarcoplasmic reticulum (SR) (p. 145)
skeletal muscle (p. 142)
smooth muscle (p. 142)
synergists (p. 152)
tetanus (p. 151)
tonus (p. 151)
twitch (p. 150)

Objectives

1. Identify three types of muscle tissue.
2. Compare the structure of the whole muscle and the structure of a single muscle fiber.
3. Describe the sliding filament mechanism of muscle contraction.
4. Explain the role of calcium and adenosine triphosphate (ATP) in muscle contraction.
5. Describe the relationship between skeletal muscles and nerves, including the motor unit and its relationship to

recruitment and the events that occur at the neuromuscular junction.
6. Discuss the force of muscle contraction, including:
   • Define *twitch* and *tetanus*.
   • Identify the sources of energy for muscle contraction.
   • Trace the sequence of events from nerve stimulation to muscle contraction.
7. Define muscle terms and state the basis for naming muscles.
8. Identify and list the actions of the major muscles.

The word *muscle* comes from the Latin word *mus*, meaning "little mouse." As muscles contract, the muscle movements under the skin resemble the movement of mice scurrying around—thus the name *mus*, or *muscle*. Muscle tissue makes up 40% to 50% of body weight.

TYPES AND FUNCTIONS OF MUSCLES

The three types of muscles are skeletal, smooth, and cardiac (Figure 9-1). Smooth muscle is discussed throughout the book and cardiac muscle in Chapters 16 and 17. In this chapter, the focus is on skeletal muscle.

SKELETAL MUSCLE

Skeletal muscle is generally attached to bone. Because skeletal muscle can be controlled by choice (I choose

to move my arm), it is also called *voluntary muscle*. The skeletal muscle cells are long, shaped like cylinders or tubes, and composed of proteins arranged to make the muscle appear striped, or striated (STRYE-ay-ted). Skeletal muscles produce movement, maintain body posture, and stabilize joints. They also produce considerable heat and therefore help maintain body temperature. If damaged, skeletal muscle has a limited capacity for regeneration.

SMOOTH MUSCLE

Smooth muscle is generally found in the walls of the viscera, such as the stomach, and is called *visceral muscle*. It is also found in tubes and passageways such as the bronchioles (breathing passages) and blood vessels. Because smooth muscle functions automatically, it is called *involuntary muscle*. Unlike skeletal muscles, smooth muscle does not appear striped, or striated, and is therefore called *nonstriated muscle*.

Smooth muscle contraction has two unique characteristics in comparison with skeletal muscle contraction. First, smooth muscle contraction is slower and continues for a longer period. This characteristic allows

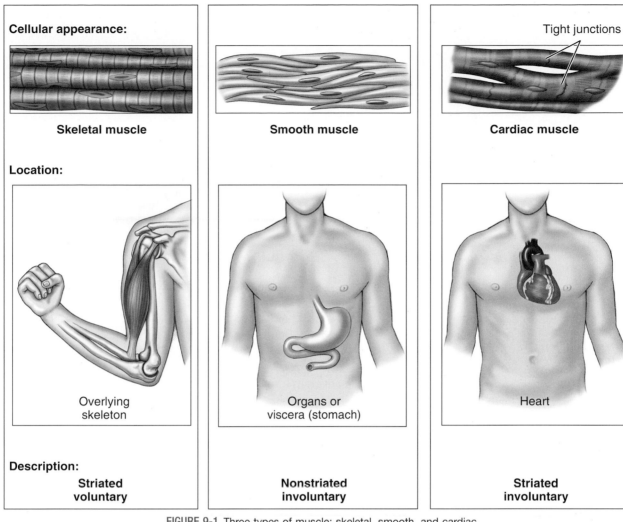

Cellular appearance:

Skeletal muscle

Smooth muscle

Cardiac muscle

Tight junctions

Location:

Overlying
skeleton

Organs or
viscera (stomach)

Heart

Description:

**Striated
voluntary**

**Nonstriated
involuntary**

**Striated
involuntary**

FIGURE 9-1 Three types of muscle: skeletal, smooth, and cardiac.

for a continuous partial contraction of the smooth muscle, called *smooth muscle tone*. Smooth muscle tone plays an important role physiologically. For example, the muscle tone of the smooth muscle in blood vessels helps maintain blood pressure. If the muscle tone were to decrease, the person might experience a life-threatening decline in blood pressure. In addition to its contractile ability, smooth muscle has a greater degree of stretchiness as compared with skeletal muscle. This allows the walls of organs such as the uterus, urinary bladder, and stomach to expand to store their contents temporarily. Contraction of the smooth muscle of the organ then expels its content. For example, the urinary bladder expands to store urine. When the bladder fills, the smooth muscle of the urinary bladder contracts, thereby expelling the urine. Similarly, contraction of the smooth muscles of the stomach mixes solid food into a paste and then pushes it forward into the intestine. If injured, smooth muscle has a better capacity for regeneration than does skeletal muscle.

CARDIAC MUSCLE

Cardiac muscle is found only in the heart, where it functions to pump blood throughout the body. Cardiac muscle cells are long branching cells that fit together tightly at junctions called *intercalated discs*. These tight-fitting junctions promote rapid conduction of electrical signals throughout the heart. Cardiac muscle is classified as striated and involuntary muscle. If damaged, as in a heart attack, cardiac muscle has no capacity for regeneration.

STRUCTURE OF THE WHOLE MUSCLE

MUSCLE

If you touch your anterior thigh, you will feel a large muscle. What you are actually feeling are thousands of elongated muscle fibers (cells) packaged together by various layers of connective tissue. The **belly** refers to the enlarged fleshy body of the muscle between the slender points of attachment.

A The whole muscle

Triceps muscle (cut)

Bone

Tendon

Perimysium

Blood vessels

Epimysium (fascia)

Endomysium

B Muscle fiber (cell)

Sarcoplasmic reticulum

Cell membrane (sarcolemma)

T tubule

Muscle fiber (cell)

Myofibrils

Ca^{2+} Ca^{2+} Ca^{2+} Ca^{2+} Ca^{2+} Ca^{2+}

Fascicle

C Sarcomere

Myosin head

Cross-bridge

Z   Z

Thin   Thick

Z   Z

Thin   Thick

Relaxed sarcomere

Contracted sarcomere

FIGURE 9-2 Muscle structure. **A,** Structure of a whole muscle attached to the bone by a tendon. **B,** Structure of a muscle fiber (muscle cell). **C,** Sarcomeres, relaxed and contracted.

LAYERS OF CONNECTIVE TISSUE

A large skeletal muscle is surrounded by layers of tough connective tissue called **fascia** (FASH-uh) (Figure 9-2, *A*). This outer layer of fascia is called the *epimysium*. Another layer of connective tissue, called the *perimysium,* surrounds smaller bundles of muscle fibers. The bundles of muscle fibers are called *fascicles* (FAS-i-kuls). Individual muscle fibers are found within

the fascicles and are surrounded by a third layer of connective tissue called the *endomysium*. The epimysium, perimysium, and endomysium extend toward and attach to the bone as a tendon, a long cordlike structure.

In the limbs, the extensive amount of fascia separates the muscles into isolated compartments. Each muscle compartment also receives blood vessels and nerves necessary for muscle function. With a severe crush injury, the muscle is damaged; it becomes inflamed and leaks fluid into the compartment. Pressure within the compartment increases and compresses the nerves and blood vessels. Deprived of its oxygen and nourishment, the muscle and nerves begin to die—condition called *compartment* or *crush syndrome*. Immediate treatment involves reduction of the compartment pressure by surgically slicing the fascia lengthwise. Failure to restore blood flow to the muscle results in permanent muscle and nerve damage.

MUSCLE ATTACHMENTS

Muscles form attachments to other structures in three ways: (1) the tendon attaches the muscle to the bone, (2) muscles attach directly (without a tendon) to a bone or to soft tissue, and (3) a flat sheetlike fascia called **aponeurosis** (ap-oh-nyoo-ROH-sis) connects muscle to muscle or muscle to bone.

 Re-Think

1. List the three types of muscles.
2. With regard to muscle types, what is meant by striated/nonstriated and voluntary/involuntary?
3. How does the connective tissue of muscle relate to the development of compartment syndrome?

STRUCTURE AND FUNCTION OF A SINGLE MUSCLE FIBER

The muscle cell is an elongated muscle fiber (see Figure 9-2, *B*). The muscle fiber has more than one nucleus and is surrounded by a cell membrane called a *sarcolemma*. At several points, the cell membrane penetrates deep into the interior of the muscle fiber, forming transverse tubules (T tubules). Within the muscle fiber is a specialized endoplasmic reticulum called the **sarcoplasmic reticulum (SR)**.

Each muscle fiber is composed of long cylindrical structures called *myofibrils* (my-oh-FYE-brils). Each myofibril is made up of a series of contractile units called **sarcomeres** (SAR-koh-meers) (see Figure 9-2, *C*). Each sarcomere extends from Z line to Z line and is formed by a unique arrangement of contractile proteins, referred to as thin and thick filaments. The thin filaments extend toward the center of the sarcomere from the Z lines. The thin filament is composed of two proteins called **actin** and the *troponin-tropomyosin* (troh-POH-nin–troh-poh-MY-oh-sin) *complex*. The actin contains binding sites for the **myosin**. The thicker myosin filaments sit between the thin filaments. Extending from the thick myosin filaments are structures called *myosin heads*. The arrangement of the thin and thick filaments in each sarcomere gives skeletal and cardiac muscle their striated appearances.

Do You Know...

Why Beef Is Red and Chicken Meat is White?

Certain muscle fibers contain a reddish-brown protein called *myoglobin*. The myoglobin stores oxygen in the muscle and gradually releases it when the muscle starts to work. Fibers that contain myoglobin are red because of the iron pigment. This is the red meat of a steak. Fibers that do not contain myoglobin are white, as in the meat of chicken.

HOW MUSCLES CONTRACT

SLIDING FILAMENT MECHANISM

Muscles can only pull, not push! To pull, muscles contract. When muscles contract, they shorten. Muscles shorten because the sarcomeres shorten, and the sarcomeres shorten because the thin and thick filaments slide past each other. Note how much shorter the contracted sarcomere appears compared with the relaxed sarcomere (see Figure 9-2, *C*). The following statements explain how the sarcomere shortens.

- When the contractile apparatus is stimulated, the myosin heads make contact with special sites on the actin, forming temporary connections called *cross-bridges*.
- Once the cross-bridges are formed, the myosin heads rotate, pulling the actin toward the center of the sarcomere. The rotation of the myosin heads causes the thin filaments to slide past the thick filaments. (The sarcomere shortens.)
- Muscle relaxation occurs when the cross-bridges are broken and the thin and thick filaments return to their original positions. (The sarcomere lengthens.)

Because of this sliding activity of the thin and thick filaments, muscle contraction is called the sliding filament mechanism of muscle contraction. *Repeat:* The sarcomeres shorten not because the thin and thick filaments shrink or shrivel up, but because they slide past one another. The sliding is like a trombone. The trombone shortens because the parts slide past one another, not because the metal shrinks. The thin and thick filaments do the same thing—they slide.

THE ROLE OF CALCIUM AND ADENOSINE TRIPHOSHATE

Adenosine triphosphate (ATP) and calcium play important roles in the contraction and relaxation of muscle. The ATP helps the myosin heads form and

Ramp It Up!

The Troponin-Tropomyosin Complex and Calcium

Muscle contraction occurs when the myosin heads bind to actin, thereby causing the thin and thick filaments to slide past one another. The sliding occurs only in the presence of calcium. What role does calcium play in muscle contraction and relaxation?

Panel A illustrates the components of the thin filament in the relaxed state. The thin filament is composed of two proteins: actin and the troponin-tropomyosin complex. (The cup-shaped troponin sits on the tropomyosin.) The actin protein contains sites to which myosin heads bind. In the relaxed state the myosin-binding sites on actin are blocked by the troponin-tropomyosin complex. Thus, cross-bridge formation and muscle contraction cannot occur.

Panel A: Thin Filament

Panel B illustrates the effects of calcium. When the calcium is released from the sarcoplasmic reticulum, it floods the troponin sites. The activation of the troponin with calcium causes the tropomyosin to move, thereby exposing the myosin-binding sites on actin. The myosin heads can now bind to the actin, forming cross-bridges. The swiveling of the cross-bridges causes the sliding movements of the thin and thick filaments and muscle contraction. What causes the muscle to relax? Calcium is pumped back into the SR away from the troponin.

The troponin-tropomyosin complex then moves back to its original position (panel A) where it blocks the myosin-binding sites on actin. Thus, the removal of calcium causes muscle relaxation.

An interesting clinical point! When muscle tissue (skeletal and cardiac) is injured, the contents of the muscle cell leak into the blood. Thus, following a heart attack, enzymes such as creatine phosphokinase and troponin elevate in the blood and act as biological markers in the diagnosis of a heart attack.

Panel B: Effect of Calcium

break cross-bridges with the actin. The ATP, however, can perform its role only if calcium is present. When the muscle is relaxed, the calcium is stored in the sarcoplasmic reticulum (SR), away from the thin and thick filaments. When the muscle is stimulated, calcium is released from the SR and causes the actin, myosin, and ATP to interact and slide. Muscle contraction then occurs. When calcium is pumped back into the SR, away from the actin, myosin, and ATP, the cross-bridges are broken and the muscle relaxes. (See "Ramp It Up: The Troponin-Tropomyosin Complex and Calcium" for further details of calcium and the thin filament.)

 Re-Think

Why is calcium necessary for muscle contraction? (Use the words *actin*, *myosin*, *cross-bridges*, and *sliding filaments*.)

 Sum It Up!

The three types of muscle are skeletal, smooth, and cardiac. A whole muscle is composed of many muscle fibers (muscle cells) arranged in bundles. Each muscle fiber contains actin-containing thin filaments and myosin-containing thick filaments, arranged into a series of sarcomeres. In accordance with the sliding filament mechanism, the sliding interaction of the actin and the myosin heads causes muscle contraction.

SKELETAL MUSCLES AND NERVES

SOMATIC MOTOR NEURON

Skeletal muscle contraction can take place only when the muscle is first stimulated by a nerve. The type of nerve that supplies the skeletal muscle is a somatic motor nerve (Figure 9-3, *A*). A motor nerve, composed of many nerve cells called *motor neurons*, emerges from the spinal cord and travels to the skeletal muscle. The interaction of the motor neuron and the muscle is described in terms of the motor unit and neuromuscular junction.

 Do You Know...

What the "Stiffness of Death" Is?

Both the formation of cross-bridges (muscle contraction) and the detachment of cross-bridges (muscle relaxation) depend on ATP. When a person dies, calcium leaks out of the SR, causing the muscles to contract. In addition, the production of ATP ceases. The deficiency of ATP prevents the detachment of the cross-bridges, so muscles remain contracted and become stiff. This change is called *rigor mortis*, or "stiffness of death." An assessment of rigor mortis often helps determine the exact time of death. For example, rigor begins 2 hours after death, peaks in 12 hours, and subsides in 36 hours. By assessing the degree of rigor, one can therefore determine the time of death. This fact has been used successfully in murder mysteries. By altering the environmental temperature, the murderer can alter the time course of rigor mortis and therefore make it difficult to determine the time of death.

THE MOTOR UNIT

As a motor neuron approaches the skeletal muscle, it forms many branches. Each branch innervates a single muscle fiber. The **motor unit** (see Figure 9-3, *A*) consists of a single motor neuron and the muscle fibers that are supplied by the motor neuron. Each muscle is innervated by many motor neurons, thereby forming many motor units. The strength of muscle contraction can vary, depending on the number of motor units that are stimulated. A stronger force of muscle contraction develops if many motor units are stimulated at the same time; a weaker force of muscle contraction develops when fewer motor units are stimulated. The consequences of activation of additional motor units is called **recruitment** and is discussed later.

THE NEUROMUSCULAR JUNCTION

The area where the motor neuron meets the muscle is called the **neuromuscular junction (NMJ)**. The NMJ includes the membrane at the end of the neuron, the space between the neuron and the muscle, and the receptors on the muscle membrane. What happens at the NMJ? The stimulated neuron causes the release of a chemical substance that diffuses across the NMJ and stimulates the muscle membrane. Four steps are involved in the transfer of the information from neuron to muscle at the NMJ (see Figure 9-3, *B*).

- Step 1. Stimulation of the neuron causes an electrical signal, or nerve impulse, to move along the neuron toward the ending of the neuron. Stored within its ending are vesicles, or membranous pouches, filled with a chemical substance called a *neurotransmitter*. The neurotransmitter at the NMJ is **acetylcholine** (ass-ee-til-KOH-leen) **(ACh)**.
- Step 2. The nerve impulse causes the vesicles to move toward and fuse with the membrane at the end of the neuron. ACh is released from the vesicles into the space between the neuron and the muscle membrane.
- Step 3. ACh diffuses across the space and binds to the receptor sites on the muscle membrane.
- Step 4. The ACh stimulates the receptors and causes an electrical signal to develop along the muscle membrane. The ACh then unbinds the receptor site and is immediately destroyed by an enzyme that is found within the NMJ, near the muscle membrane. The name of the enzyme is acetylcholinesterase (ass-ee-til-koh-lin-ES-ter-ase) or cholinesterase. The free binding sites are then ready for additional ACh when the neuron is stimulated again.

THE STIMULATED MUSCLE MEMBRANE

What happens to the electrical signal that forms in the muscle membrane? It travels along the muscle membrane and triggers a series of events that result

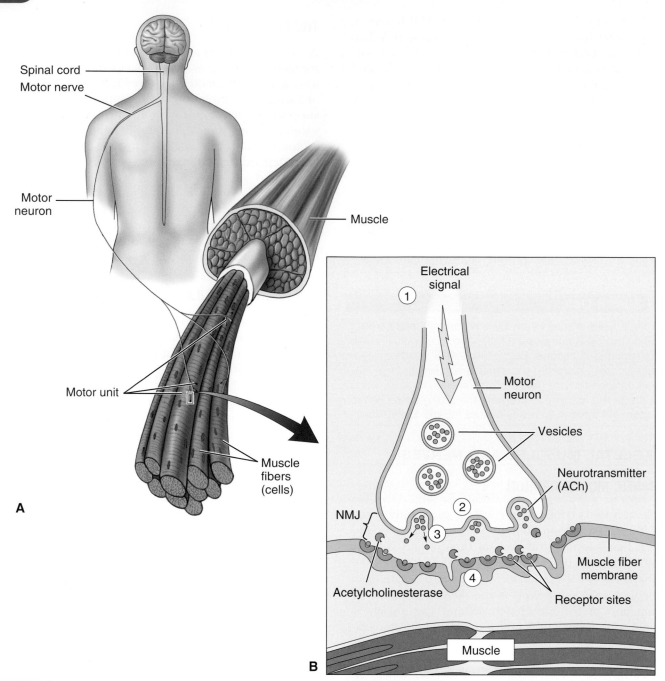

A

B

FIGURE 9-3 Innervation of a skeletal muscle. **A,** Motor unit. **B,** The four steps in the transmission of the signal at the neuromuscular junction (NMJ).

in muscle contraction (see Figure 9-2, *B* and *C*). Specifically, the electrical signal travels along the muscle cell membrane and penetrates into its interior through the T tubules. The electrical signal stimulates the SR to release calcium. The calcium floods the sarcomeres, thereby causing the thin and thick filaments to slide past one another, producing muscle contraction. Eventually, the calcium is pumped back into the SR, causing muscle relaxation.

DISORDERS OF THE NEUROMUSCULAR JUNCTION

Certain conditions affect events at the NMJ (Figure 9-4).

Myasthenia Gravis

Myasthenia gravis is a disease that affects the NMJ. The symptoms of the disease are caused by damaged receptor sites (N_M receptors) on the muscle membrane. The receptor sites are altered so that they cannot effectively bind ACh. Consequently, muscle contraction is impaired, and the person experiences extreme muscle weakness. (The word *myasthenia* means muscle weakness.) The muscle weakness first becomes noticeable as low tolerance to exercise. As the disease progresses, the person experiences difficulty in breathing because the breathing muscles are skeletal muscles.

🖊 Ramp It Up!

The Muscle Receptors (N$_M$) at the Neuromuscular Junction

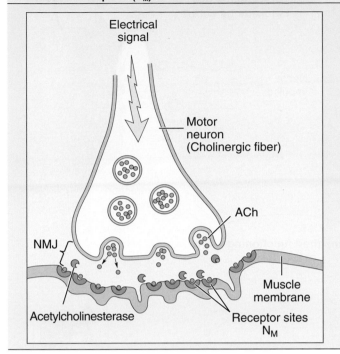

Follow the sequence of events within the neuromuscular junction (NMJ) as they are described. A nerve impulse travels along a somatic motor neuron causing the release of acetylcholine (ACh). The ACh diffuses across the NMJ and binds to the muscle membrane receptors. The receptor on the muscle membrane is a cholinergic receptor; it is called a *nicotinic receptor*. Because it is located on the muscle membrane, it is called a *nicotinic muscle (N$_M$) receptor*. Activation of the N$_M$ receptor causes a series of events that result in muscle contraction. A great deal of pharmacology involves the N$_M$ receptor. For example, curare is a skeletal muscle blocker because it blocks the N$_M$ receptors. Receptor blockade, in turn, prevents skeletal muscle contraction. What about a drug that activates the N$_M$ receptor? It stimulates muscle contraction. For example, neostigmine (Prostigmin) is a drug that inactivates acetylcholinesterase (the enzyme that destroys ACh), thereby increasing the amount of ACh that can bind to the N$_M$ receptors. (Because this drug inactivates acetylcholinesterase, it is called an *anticholinesterase agent*.) You can now understand why anticholinesterase agents improve the symptoms of myasthenia gravis and reverse postoperative sluggish intestinal activity. (Other nicotinic receptors are described in Chapter 12.)

Neuromuscular Blockade Caused by Curare

Curare is a drug classified as a skeletal muscle blocker. Skeletal muscle blockers are often used during surgery to promote muscle relaxation and paralysis. Curare works by blocking the receptor sites on the muscle membrane. Because the receptors are occupied by the drug, the ACh cannot bind with the receptor sites, and muscle contraction is prevented.

Because the respiratory muscles are also affected by curare, the patient must be mechanically ventilated until the effects of the drug disappear. Otherwise, the patient stops breathing and dies. Historically, curare was used as a paralyzing drug when hunting animals. The tip of an arrowhead was dipped in curare. When the arrow pierced the skin of the animal, the curare was absorbed and eventually caused skeletal muscle blockade and paralysis. Succinylcholine (Anectine) also blocks N$_M$ receptors and is used to induce muscle paralysis for short-term critical care situations such as intubation.

Effects of Neurotoxins on Muscle Function

Neurotoxins are chemical substances that in some way disrupt normal function of the nervous system. Neurotoxins are produced by certain bacteria. For example, *Clostridium tetani* (a bacterium) secretes a neurotoxin that causes excessive firing of the motor nerves. This, in turn, causes excessive release of ACh, overstimulation of the muscle membrane, and severe muscle spasm and tetanic contractions—hence the name *tetanus*. Because the muscles of the jaw are the first muscles affected, the disease is often called *lockjaw*.

A second neurotoxin is secreted by the bacterium *Clostridium botulinum*. This bacterium appears most often when food has been improperly processed and canned. Infection with this organism causes botulism, a very serious form of food poisoning. The neurotoxin works by preventing the release of ACh from the ends of the neurons within the NMJ. Without ACh, the muscle fibers cannot contract, and the muscles, including the breathing muscles, become paralyzed. On a more positive note, the injection of small amounts of this "poison" (Botox) has been used successfully to treat severe muscle spasm (torticollis, cerebral palsy) and migraine headaches, as well as, for cosmetic reasons, to erase muscle-induced wrinkles.

Note that muscle paralysis can occur if there is an excess or a deficiency of ACh activity. An excess of ACh causes spastic paralysis, a state of continuous muscle contraction. A deficiency of ACh activity causes flaccid paralysis, a state in which the muscles are limp and unable to contract.

❓ Re-Think

1. Explain how the signal is passed from the nerve to the muscle at the NMJ.
2. Explain the effects of curare at the NMJ.

FIGURE 9-4 Impaired functioning at the neuromuscular junction (NMJ).

 Do You Know...

What the Difference Is between Isometric Contraction and Isotonic Contraction?

An isotonic muscle contraction is a muscle contraction that causes movement, as in lifting a 20-lb object. An isometric muscle contraction is a muscle contraction that does not cause movement. For example, if you try to lift a 1000-lb object, your muscles contract but do not move the object (it is too heavy).

As you sit reading this text, you can do isometric exercises. Tighten the muscle in your thigh. Hold the tension for 30 seconds and then relax the muscle. Repetition of this type of exercise can provide you with a mini-workout without leaving your desk.

FORCE OF MUSCLE CONTRACTION

The sliding filament mechanism explains the contraction and relaxation of a single muscle fiber. A whole skeletal muscle, such as a large thigh muscle, is composed of thousands of muscle fibers. The contractile response of a whole muscle is much greater than that of a single muscle fiber. How does that happen?

CONTRACTILE FORCE OF A SINGLE MUSCLE FIBER

If a single electrical stimulus is delivered to a muscle fiber, the fiber contracts and then fully relaxes. This single muscle response is called a **twitch**. Twitches are not useful physiologically. However, if the muscle fiber is stimulated repeatedly, the muscle responds in two ways. First, repetitive stimulation increases the contractile force of the muscle fiber. Repetitive stimulation prolongs the presence of calcium within the sarcomere. Second, the muscle fiber has no time to relax and therefore remains contracted. Sustained muscle contraction is called **tetanus**. Thus, contractile force in the single muscle fiber develops in response to increasing the frequency of electrical stimulation.

MORE ABOUT TETANUS

In addition to increasing contractile force of a muscle, tetanus performs another important role; tetanic muscle contraction maintains posture. If the muscles that maintain our upright posture merely twitched, we would be unable to stand and would instead twitch and flop around on the ground (not a pretty sight). Because the muscle is able to tetanize, we are able to maintain an upright posture. (Do not confuse the "tetanus" described in this section with the disease called tetanus, or lockjaw.)

CONTRACTILE FORCE OF A WHOLE MUSCLE

A whole muscle increases its contractile force primarily by recruitment (see Figure 9-3). Recruitment of additional motor units increases contractile force because more muscle fibers are contracting. For example, the muscles in the arm contract when they lift a pencil; they contract more forcefully when lifting a 100-lb weight. Contraction and relaxation of the whole muscle is summarized in Figure 9-5.

MUSCLE TONE

Muscle tone, or **tonus**, refers to a normal continuous state of partial muscle contraction. Tone is caused by the contraction of different groups of muscle fibers within a whole muscle. To maintain muscle tone, one group of muscle fibers contracts first. As these fibers begin to relax, a second group contracts. This pattern of contraction and relaxation continues to maintain muscle tone. Muscle tone plays a number of important roles. For example, the tone of the skeletal muscles in the back of the neck prevents the head from falling forward.

 Re-Think

Why can a whole muscle develop a greater force of contraction than a single muscle fiber?

ENERGY SOURCE FOR MUSCLE CONTRACTION

Muscle contraction requires a rich supply of energy (ATP). As ATP is consumed by the contracting muscle, it is replaced in three ways:

The electrical signal (nerve impulse) travels down the nerve to the terminal and causes the release of the neurotransmitter ACh.

The ACh diffuses across the neuromuscular junction and binds to the receptor sites.

Stimulation of the receptor sites causes an electrical impulse to form in the muscle membrane. The electrical impulse travels along the muscle membrane and penetrates deep into the muscle through the T-tubular system.

The electrical impulse stimulates the sarcoplasmic reticulum to release calcium into the sarcomere area.

The calcium allows the actin, myosin, and ATP to interact, causing cross-bridge formation and muscle contraction. This process continues as long as calcium is available to the actin and myosin.

Muscle relaxation occurs when calcium is pumped back into the sarcoplasmic reticulum, away from the actin and myosin. When calcium moves in this way, the actin and myosin cannot interact, and the muscle relaxes.

FIGURE 9-5 Steps in the contraction and relaxation of skeletal muscle.

1. *Metabolism of creatine phosphate.* The resting muscle produces excess ATP and uses some of it to make creatine (KREE-ah-tin) phosphate. Creatine phosphate is a storage form of energy that can be used to replenish ATP quickly during muscle contraction. For example, a brief 15-second burst of intense muscle activity is sustained by ATP and creatine phosphate. When creatine phosphate supplies are depleted (15 seconds), the muscle switches to glycolysis for its supply of ATP.

2. *Glycolysis.* Glycolysis is a series of chemical reactions that break down glucose anaerobically (without oxygen), generating small amounts of ATP. The glucose is obtained from two sources: blood glucose and the glycogen that is stored in skeletal muscle. Glycolysis provides enough energy (ATP) for an additional 30 to 40 seconds of intense muscle

activity. In addition to ATP production, glycolysis also produces lactic acid. Some of the lactic acid is picked up by the blood and transported to the liver, where it is used to make glucose.

3. *Aerobic (oxygen-requiring) metabolism.* After 30 to 40 seconds, the supply of ATP from glycolysis is depleted and continued muscle activity relies on ATP production by aerobic respiration. In the presence of oxygen, pyruvic acid (formed from glycolysis) enters the mitochondria and is broken down completely to CO_2, H_2O, and ATP. Aerobic metabolism generates large amounts of ATP compared with glycolysis. The mitochondria receive their supply of oxygen from two sources: the blood (oxyhemoglobin) and myoglobin. Myoglobin is an oxygen-carrying protein found in the muscle fibers. Note the time sequence—creatine phosphate and ATP, glycolysis, and finally aerobic metabolism.

Why are your muscles sore after a heavy workout? Following a heavy workout, muscles can develop an immediate and latent soreness. Why is this? Muscles generate ATP aerobically and anaerobically through glycolysis. Lactic acid is the end-product of glycolysis, and its brief accumulation in the muscle tissue is thought to be the cause of the immediate soreness (30 to 60 minutes). The lactic acid is rapidly removed from the muscle and metabolized. The latent soreness (1 to 3 days after the workout) is attributed not to lactic acid but to tears of the connective tissue in the muscles and muscle cell membranes.

Do You Know...

What the Good News Is about Oxygen Debt?

Credit card debt? Bad! Oxygen debt? Good! What's so great about oxygen debt? The payment of an oxygen debt means that you continue to expend energy and burn fat long after you have come off the treadmill and have taken to your couch. In other words, you continue to exercise metabolically while recovering from your workout. When a person exercises strenuously, he or she burns fuel (fat). To do this, the body uses up available oxygen and borrows on the additional stores of oxygen found in the hemoglobin in blood and the myoglobin in muscles. When the person stops exercising, the body requires an increased intake of oxygen to do some additional, exercise-induced metabolic work (to convert lactic acid to glucose), so 30 minutes of exercise is actually more than 30 minutes of exercise.

MUSCLE FATIGUE

Muscle fatigue occurs if the muscle is not allowed to rest and is defined as the inability of a muscle to contract forcefully following prolonged activity. Muscle fatigue is the result of a number of factors, such as a decrease in the release of calcium from the SR, a depletion of nutrients, oxygen, glycogen, and energy stores, such as creatine phosphate, and a buildup of waste, such as lactic acid.

? Re-Think

What are the three ways that muscle obtains its energy for muscle contraction?

MUSCLE TERMS

ORIGIN AND INSERTION

The terms *origin* and *insertion* refer to the sites of muscle attachment. Most muscles cross or span at least one joint. When muscle contracts, one bone remains relatively stationary or immovable. The **origin** of the muscle attaches to the stationary bone, whereas the **insertion** attaches to the more movable bone (Figure 9-6). For example, the origin of the biceps brachii is the scapula and the insertion is on the radius. On contraction of the biceps brachii, the radius (insertion) is pulled toward the scapula (origin). Be sure that you understand origin and insertion because these terms will be used to describe muscle actions.

PRIME MOVER, SYNERGIST, AND ANTAGONIST

Although most movement is accomplished through the cooperation of groups of muscles, a single muscle is generally responsible for most of the movement. The "chief muscle" is called the **prime mover**. Assisting the prime mover are "helper muscles" called **synergists** (SIN-er-jists). Synergists are said to work with other muscles. In contrast, **antagonists** are muscles that oppose the action of another muscle. For example, contraction of the biceps brachii pulls the forearm toward the shoulder. The triceps brachii (posterior arm) is the antagonist. It opposes the action of the biceps brachii (see Figure 9-6).

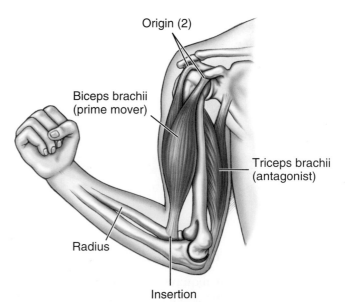

FIGURE 9-6 Origin and insertion: prime mover and antagonist.

MUSCLE OVERUSE AND UNDERUSE TERMS

HYPERTROPHY

Overused muscles increase in size. This response to overuse is called *hypertrophy*. Athletes intentionally cause their muscles to hypertrophy. Weight lifters, for example, develop larger muscles than couch potatoes.

Like skeletal muscle, cardiac muscle can also hypertrophy. Cardiac hypertrophy is undesirable and usually indicates an underlying disease, causing the heart to overwork. Hypertension, for example, causes the heart to push blood into blood vessels that are very resistant to the flow of blood. This extra work causes the heart muscle to enlarge.

ATROPHY

If muscles are not used, they will waste away, or decrease in size. A person with a broken leg in a cast, for example, is unable to exercise that leg for several months. This lack of exercise causes the muscles of the leg to atrophy, which is called *disuse atrophy*. When weight bearing and exercise are resumed, muscle size and strength can be restored. Muscle atrophy can also develop when the nerves to the muscle are severed, which is called *denervation atrophy*. Finally, muscle atrophy is part of the normal aging process; this is called *senile atrophy*. Senile atrophy can be delayed when the aging person carries out a regular exercise routine. Muscle motto: use it or lose it.

CONTRACTURE

If a muscle is immobilized for a prolonged period, it may develop a contracture, an abnormal formation of fibrous tissue within the muscle. It generally "freezes" the muscle in a flexed position and severely restricts joint mobility.

HOW SKELETAL MUSCLES ARE NAMED

The names of the various skeletal muscles are generally based on one or more of the following characteristics: size, shape, orientation of the fibers, location, number of origins, identification of origin and insertion, and muscle action.

SIZE

These terms indicate size: vastus (huge), maximus (large), longus (long), minimus (small), and brevis (short). Examples of skeletal muscles include the vastus lateralis and gluteus maximus.

SHAPE

Various shapes are included in muscle names, such as deltoid (triangular), latissimus (wide), trapezius (trapezoid), rhomboideus (rhomboid), and teres (round).

Examples include the trapezius muscle, latissimus dorsi, and teres major.

ORIENTATION OF FIBERS

Fibers are oriented, or lined up, in several directions: rectus (straight), oblique (diagonal), transverse (across), and circularis (circular). Examples include the rectus abdominis and the superior oblique.

LOCATION

The names of muscles often reflect their location in the body, such as pectoralis (chest), gluteus (buttock), brachii (arm), supra (above), infra (below), sub (underneath), and lateralis (lateral). Examples include the biceps brachii, pectoralis major, and vastus lateralis.

NUMBER OF ORIGINS

A muscle may be named according to the number of sites to which it is anchored: biceps (2), triceps (3), and quadriceps (4). Examples include the biceps brachii, triceps brachii, and quadriceps femoris.

ORIGIN AND INSERTION

Some muscles are named for sites of attachment both at their origin and insertion. The sternocleidomastoid, for example, has its origin on the sternum and clavicle and its insertion on the mastoid process of the temporal bone. This information allows you to determine the function of the muscle. The sternocleidomastoid flexes the neck and rotates the head. As noted here, many muscles have multiple points of origin and insertion.

MUSCLE ACTION

The action of the muscle may be included in the name. For example, an abductor muscle moves the limb away from the midline of the body, whereas an adductor moves the limb toward the midline. In the same way, a flexor muscle causes flexion, whereas an extensor muscle straightens the limb. A levator muscle elevates a structure, and a masseter muscle enables you to chew. Examples include the adductor magnus, flexor digitorum, and levator palpebrae superioris.

? Re-Think

What is the basis for the naming of the following muscles: quadriceps femoris, rectus abdominis, sternocleidomastoid, and vastus lateralis?

2+2 Sum It Up!

A skeletal muscle requires innervation by a somatic motor neuron. The electrical signal of the neuron causes the release of ACh into the NMJ, activation of the N_M receptors on the muscle membrane, and muscle contraction. A whole muscle contracts more forcefully than a single muscle fiber primarily because of recruitment of additional motor units. There are three energy sources for skeletal muscle contraction: aerobic metabolism, anaerobic metabolism, and metabolism involving creatine phosphate. Muscles are named according to their size, shape, orientation of fibers, location, number of origins, muscle action, and origin and insertion sites.

MUSCLES FROM HEAD TO TOE

Figure 9-7 shows the major skeletal muscles of the body. Details of muscle location and function are summarized in Table 9-1.

MUSCLES OF THE HEAD

The muscles of the head are grouped into two categories: the facial muscles and the chewing muscles (Figure 9-8).

FACIAL MUSCLES

Many of the facial muscles are inserted directly into the soft tissue of the skin and other muscles of the face. When the facial muscles contract, they pull on the soft tissue. This kind of muscular activity is responsible for our facial expressions like smiling and frowning.

- *Frontalis.* The frontalis (fron-TAL-is) is a flat muscle that covers the frontal bone. It extends from the cranial aponeurosis (origin) and inserts in the skin above the eyebrows. Contraction of the muscle raises the eyebrows, giving you a surprised look. It also wrinkles your forehead.
- *Orbicularis oculi.* The orbicularis (or-bik-yoo-LAR-is) oculi is a sphincter muscle that encircles the eyes. A sphincter (SFINGK-ter) is a ring-shaped muscle that controls the size of an opening. Contraction of the muscle closes the eye and assists in winking, blinking, and squinting.
- *Levator palpebrae superioris.* The levator palpebrae (leh-VAH-tor PAL-peh-bray) superioris muscle has its origin in the bony orbit of the eye and inserts on the upper eyelid. As its name implies, the muscle elevates the eyelid (opens the eye).
- *Orbicularis oris.* The orbicularis oris is a sphincter muscle that encircles the mouth. Contraction of this muscle assists in closing the mouth, forming words, and pursing the lips. It is sometimes called the kissing muscle.
- *Buccinator.* The buccinator (BUK-si-NAY-tor) is a muscle that has its origin on the maxilla and mandible and inserts into the orbicularis oris. The buccinator is used in actions requiring compression of

the cheeks, as in sucking, whistling, and playing the trumpet. The buccinator may also be considered a chewing muscle because, on contraction, it helps position the food between the teeth for chewing. The buccinator is particularly important for an infant because its contraction enables the infant to suck; it therefore plays an important role in the nourishment and comfort of a hungry infant.
- *Zygomaticus.* The zygomaticus (zye-goh-MAT-ik-us) is a smiling muscle; it extends from the corners of the mouth to the cheekbone (zygomatic bone).
- *Platysma.* Want to pout? The platysma (plah-TIZ-mah) is your muscle. It originates in the fascia of the shoulder and anterior chest and inserts on the mandible and tissue of the mouth and lower face. In addition to pouting, it allows you to open your mouth wide, per order of your dentist. Here's another platysmal downer—with aging, there is a loss of muscle tone of the platysma, creating loose skin in the throat area and the dreaded "turkey neck" look.

CHEWING MUSCLES

The chewing muscles are also called the muscles of mastication (chewing). All of them are inserted on the mandible, or lower jaw bone, and are considered some of the strongest muscles of the body (see Table 9-1).
- *Masseter.* The masseter (MAS-eh-ter) is a muscle that has its origin on the maxilla and zygomatic process of the temporal bone and its insertion on the mandible. Contraction of this muscle closes the jaw. It acts synergistically with the temporalis muscle to close the jaw.
- *Temporalis.* The temporalis (tem-poh-RAL-is) is a fan-shaped muscle that extends from the flat portion of the temporal bone (origin) to the mandible (insertion).

? Re-Think

1. Explain why the frontalis muscle can effect facial expression.
2. To which facial bone must the chewing muscles insert?

Do You Know...

About the "Droops and Drools" of Botox?

In the arsenal of anti-aging drugs, Botox is a star. It is the wrinkle-remover par excellence. Beware of Botox blunders, however. Misplaced Botox around the eyelids can cause droopy lids. Similarly, poor aim around the mouth region can cause drooling. Mercifully, the effects of Botox gradually wear off, although there may be many weeks during which you sport the droop-and-drool look. Botched batches of Botox have also caused severe, long-term paralysis.

Text continued on p. 160

A

Temporalis

Orbicularis oculi

Zygomaticus

Buccinator

Orbicularis oris

Trapezius

Deltoid

Biceps brachii

Brachialis

Rectus abdominis

Internal oblique

Abdominal muscles

External oblique

Transversus abdominis

Brachioradialis

Tensor fasciae latae

Iliopsoas

Adductor longus

Adductor magnus

Quadriceps femoris

Rectus femoris

Vastus lateralis

Vastus medialis

Vastus intermedius (not illustrated)

Tibialis anterior

Peroneus longus

Frontalis

Masseter

Sternocleidomastoid

Pectoralis major

Serratus anterior

Linea alba

Pectineus

Sartorius

Quadriceps tendon

Quadriceps ligament

Anterior view

FIGURE 9-7 Major muscles of the body. **A,** Anterior view. **B,** Posterior view.

Continued

B

Trapezius

Deltoid

Infraspinatus

Teres minor

Teres major

Triceps brachii

Latissimus dorsi

Gluteus medius

Gluteus maximus

Adductor magnus

Gracilis

Biceps femoris

Semitendinosus

Semimembranosus

Hamstring group

Gastrocnemius

Soleus

Achilles tendon (calcaneal tendon)

Posterior view

FIGURE 9-7, cont'd

Table 9-1	Muscles of the Body	
MUSCLE	**LOCATION, DESCRIPTION**	**FUNCTION**
Head		
Muscles of Facial Expression		
Frontalis	Flat muscle covering forehead; origin on cranial aponeurosis; inserts on skin above eyebrows	Raises eyebrows; surprised look; wrinkles forehead
Orbicularis oculi	Circular muscle around eye	Closes eyes; winking, blinking, and squinting
Levator palpebrae superioris	Origin on bony orbit of eye; inserts on upper eyelid	Elevates eyelid (opens eye)
Orbicularis oris	Encircles mouth	Closes, purses lips; kissing muscle
Buccinator	Horizontal cheek muscle; origin on maxilla and mandible; inserts on orbicularis oris	Flattens cheek; trumpeter's muscle; whistling muscle; helps with chewing by positioning food between teeth
Zygomaticus	Origin on cheekbone (zygomatic bone); inserts on corner of mouth	Elevates corner of mouth; smiling muscle
Platysma	Origin in fascia of shoulder and anterior chest; inserts on mandible, angle of lower mouth, soft tissue of lower face	Pouting muscle; "open your mouth wide" muscle
Chewing Muscles		
Temporalis	Flat fan-shaped muscle over temporal bone (origin); inserts on mandible	Closes jaw; retracts jaw
Masseter	Covers lateral part of lower jaw; origin on maxilla, zygomatic process of the temporal bone; inserts on mandible	Closes jaw; retracts jaw
Neck		
Sternocleidomastoid	Extends along each side of neck; strong narrow muscles that extend obliquely from sternum and clavicle (origin) upward to mastoid process of temporal bone (insertion)	Contraction of both muscles flexes the head at the neck; contraction of one rotates head toward opposite side
Trapezius	Large, flat, trapezoid-shaped muscle on back of neck and upper back; origin on occipital bone, C7, and all thoracic vertebrae; inserts on clavicle and scapula	Hyperextends head so as to look at sky; lateral flexion of head (see actions on shoulder)
Scalenes (3)	Origin on cervical vertebrae (C1–C7); insert on ribs 1 and 2	Act synergistically with sternocleidomastoid to flex neck
Muscles of the Trunk		
Muscles Involved in Breathing		
External intercostals	Located between ribs (intercostal space); both origin and insertion on ribs	Breathing (enlarges thoracic cavity during inhalation)
Internal intercostals	Located between ribs (intercostal space); both origin and insertion on ribs	Breathing (decreases thoracic cavity in forced exhalation)
Diaphragm	Dome-shaped muscle that separates thoracic and abdominal cavities	Breathing—chief muscle of inhalation (enlarges thoracic cavity)
Muscles of Abdominal Wall		
External oblique Internal oblique Transverse abdominis Rectus abdominis	As a group, muscles are arranged vertically, horizontally, and obliquely to strengthen abdominal wall	As a group, abdominal wall muscles compress the abdomen, thereby aiding in urination, defecation, childbirth, and forced expiration (breathing); also flex and rotate vertebral column

Continued

Table 9-1 Muscles of the Body—cont'd

MUSCLE	LOCATION, DESCRIPTION	FUNCTION
Muscles of Vertebral Column		
Trapezius	See trapezius above (Neck)	Helps to maintain spine in extension
Erector spinae	Extends length of vertebral column from cranium to sacrum	Extends and laterally flexes vertebral column; rotates head; assists in maintenance of erect posture
Sternocleidomastoid	See above (Neck)	Flexes and rotates cervical vertebral column
Abdominal muscles	See above (Muscles of Abdominal Wall)	Flexes and rotates vertebral column
Iliopsoas	Origin on ilium and lumbar vertebrae; inserts on femur	Flexes vertebral column
Muscles of Pelvic Floor		
	Flat muscle sheets	Support pelvic viscera; aid in urination and defecation
Muscles of Shoulder (Pectoral) Girdle and Arm		
Trapezius	See description above (Neck)	Causes shrugging and medial rotation of shoulders (by pulling shoulder blades and scapulae together)
Serratus anterior	Forms upper sides of chest wall; origin on upper ribs; inserts on scapula	Lowers shoulder and moves the arm forward as in pushing a cart
Pectoralis major	Large muscle that covers upper anterior chest; origin on clavicle, sternum, and cartilages of upper ribs; inserts on anterior humerus	Adducts and medially rotates arm across chest; flexes and extends arm at shoulder
Latissimus dorsi	Large, broad, flat muscle on mid and lower back; origin on lower vertebral column and lower ribs; inserts on posterior humerus	Adducts and rotates arm medially, behind the back; "swimmer's muscle"
Deltoid	Thick muscle that covers shoulder joint; origin on clavicle and scapula; inserts on humerus	Abducts arm as in "scarecrow" position; flexes, extends, and rotates arm at shoulder
Rotator cuff muscles Supraspinatus Subscapularis Infraspinatus Teres minor	Group of four muscles that attaches humerus (insertion) to scapula (origin); tendons form cuff over proximal humerus	Adduct, extend, and rotate arm at shoulder; the "cuff" stabilizes shoulder joint
Teres major	Origin on scapula; inserts on humerus	Extends and adducts arm at shoulder; medially rotates arm at shoulder
Muscles That Move Forearm		
Biceps brachii	Major muscle on anterior surface of arm; origin on scapula; inserts on radius	Flexes and supinates forearm at elbow and flexes arm at shoulder; muscle used to "make a muscle"; acts synergistically with brachialis and brachioradialis
Triceps brachii	Origin on posterior surface of arm (scapula and humerus); inserts on ulna	Extends forearm at elbow, extends arm at shoulder; "boxer's muscle"
Brachialis	Origin on humerus; inserts on ulna	Flexes forearm at elbow
Brachioradialis	Origin on humerus; inserts on radius	Flexes forearm at elbow
Supinator	Origin on humerus and ulna; inserts on radius	Supinates forearm (palm turns upward or faces forward, as in anatomical position)
Pronator teres	Origin on humerus and ulna; inserts on radius	Pronates forearm so that palm faces downward or backward

Table **9-1**   Muscles of the Body—cont'd

MUSCLE	LOCATION, DESCRIPTION	FUNCTION
Muscles That Move Wrist, Hand, and Fingers		
Flexor and extensor carpi group	Origin on humerus and ulna; inserts on tendon in wrist	Flex and extend hand at wrist; adduct and abduct hand at wrist
Flexor and extensor digitorum group	Origin on humerus, ulna, and radius; inserts on phalanges (fingers)	Flex and extend fingers; flex hand at wrist
Muscles That Move Thigh and Leg		
Gluteus maximus	Largest and most superficial of gluteal muscles; located on posterior surface of buttocks; origin on ilium of coxal bone, sacrum, coccyx, and local aponeurosis; inserts on femur	Forms buttocks; extends and rotates thigh laterally at hip; muscle for sitting and climbing stairs; produces backswing of leg while walking
Gluteus medius	Thick muscle partly behind and superior to gluteus maximus; origin on ilium; inserts on femur	Abducts and rotates thigh medially at hip; common site of intramuscular injections
Gluteus minimus	Smallest and deepest of gluteal muscles; origin on ilium; inserts on femur	Abducts and rotates thigh medially at hip
Iliopsoas	Located on anterior surface of groin; origin on ilium and lumbar vertebrae; inserts on femur	Flexes and rotates thigh laterally; antagonist to gluteus maximus
Tensor fasciae latae	Located on lateral thigh; origin on ilium; inserts on tibia	Flexes and abducts thigh at hip
Adductor group Adductor longus Adductor brevis Adductor magnus	As a group, located on anteromedial surface of thigh	Adducts and medially rotates thigh; muscles used by horseback riders to stay on horse
Gracilis	Located along medial thigh; origin on symphysis pubis; inserts on proximal tibia	Adducts and medially rotates thigh at hip; flexes leg at knee
Pectineus	Located on medial thigh; origin on pubis; inserts on femur	Adducts and flexes thigh at hip
Quadriceps femoris Rectus femoris Vastus lateralis Vastus medialis Vastus intermedius	Located on anterior thigh; all insert on tibia; rectus femoris originates on ilium (coxal bone); other "quads" originate on femur	Group used to extend leg at the knee (e.g., kicking a football); rectus femoris can flex thigh at hip; vastus lateralis is common site for intramuscular injections in children
Sartorius	Long muscle that crosses obliquely over anterior thigh; origin on ilium; inserts on tibia	Allows you to sit in crossed leg position; flexes, abducts, laterally rotates thigh at hip; flexes leg at knee
Hamstrings Biceps femoris Semitendinosus Semimembranosus	Located on posterior surface of thigh; as a group, attaches to ischium (origin) to their points of insertion on tibia. Biceps femoris also originates on femur and inserts on both tibia and fibula.	As a group, they flex leg at knee, extend thigh at hip; antagonistic to quadriceps femoris
Muscles That Move Ankle and Foot		
Tibialis anterior	Located on anterior leg; origin on tibia; inserts on tarsal and metatarsal bones	Dorsiflexes and inverts foot
Peroneus longus	Lateral surface of leg; origin on fibula and tibia; inserts on metatarsal and tarsal bones	Plantar flexion and eversion of foot; supports arch
Gastrocnemius	Posterior surface of leg; large two-headed muscle that forms calf; origin on femur; inserts on calcaneus (heel bone) by way of Achilles tendon	Plantar flexion of foot; toe dancer muscle; flexes leg at knee
Soleus	Posterior surface of leg; origin on fibula and tibia; inserts on calcaneus	Plantar flexion of foot

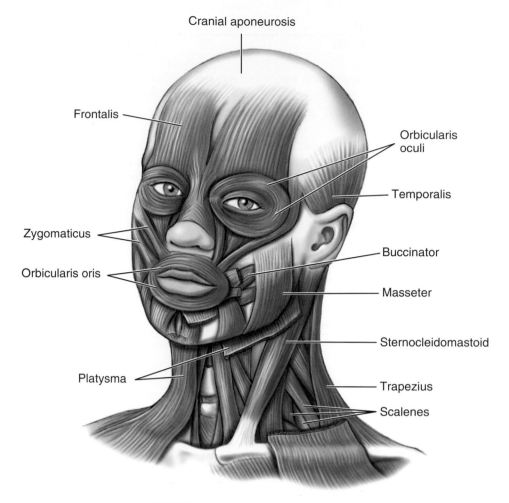

FIGURE 9-8 Muscles of the head and neck.

MUSCLES OF THE NECK

Many muscles are involved in the movement of the head and shoulders and participate in throat movements.

STERNOCLEIDOMASTOID

As the name implies, the sternocleidomastoid (STERN-oh-KLYE-doh-MAS-toyd) muscle extends from the sternum and clavicle to the mastoid process of the temporal bone in the skull. Contraction of both muscles on either side of the neck causes flexion of the head. Because the head bows as if in prayer, the muscle is called the *praying muscle*. Contraction of only one of the sternocleidomastoid muscles causes the head to flex and to rotate toward the opposite direction. A spasm of this muscle can cause torticollis, or wryneck. This condition is characterized by twisting of the neck and rotation of the head to one side. Botox has been used successfully in the treatment of torticollis. Although the sternocleidomastoid muscle is the prime mover of neck flexion, three scalene (SKAY-leen) muscles act synergistically to flex the neck. The scalenes have their origin on the cervical vertebrae (C1–C7) and insert on ribs 1 and 2.

TRAPEZIUS

The trapezius (trah-PEE-zee-us) has its origins at the base of the occipital bone of the cranium and on the spines of C7 to T4 of the upper vertebral column (see Figure 9-7). The trapezius inserts on both the scapula and clavicle. Contraction of the trapezius allows the head to tilt back (hyperextension) so that the face looks at the sky. The trapezius works antagonistically with the sternocleidomastoid muscle, which flexes and bows the head. The trapezius also causes lateral flexion of the head and shrugs the shoulder.

MUSCLES OF THE TRUNK

The muscles of the trunk are involved in breathing, form the abdominal wall, move the vertebral column, and form the pelvic region.

MUSCLES INVOLVED IN BREATHING

The muscles of the chest include the intercostal muscles and the diaphragm. These muscles are primarily responsible for breathing (Figure 9-9). The intercostal muscles are located between the ribs. They have their origin and insertion on the ribs and are responsible for raising and lowering the rib cage during breathing.

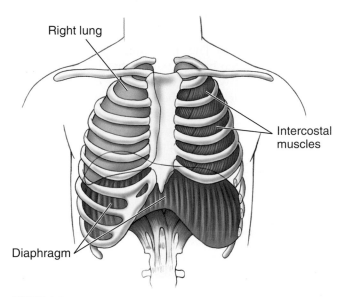

FIGURE 9-9 Breathing muscles: the intercostal muscles and the diaphragm.

The ribs that you barbecue are the intercostals (bone appétit!).

The diaphragm is a dome-shaped muscle that separates the thoracic cavity from the abdominal cavity. The diaphragm is the chief muscle of inhalation, or the breathing-in phase of respiration. Without the contraction and relaxation of the intercostal muscles and diaphragm, breathing cannot occur. The breathing muscles are more fully described in Chapter 22.

MUSCLES THAT FORM THE ABDOMINAL WALL

The abdominal wall consists of four muscles (see Figure 9-7, *A*) in an arrangement that provides considerable strength. The muscles are layered so that the fibers of each of the four muscles run in four different directions. This arrangement enables the muscles to contain, support, and protect the abdominal organs. Contraction of the abdominal muscles performs other functions. It causes flexion and rotation of the vertebral column and compression of the abdominal organs during urination, defecation, and childbirth.

The four abdominal muscles include the following:
- *Rectus abdominis.* As the name implies, the fibers of the rectus abdominis run in an up and down, or longitudinal, direction. They extend from the sternum to the pubic bone. Contraction of this muscle flexes the vertebral column.
- *External oblique.* Abdominal muscles called the external obliques make up the lateral walls of the abdomen. The fibers run obliquely (slanted).
- *Internal oblique.* The internal oblique muscles are part of the lateral walls of the abdomen. They add to the strength provided by the external oblique muscles; the fibers of the internal and external oblique muscles form a crisscross pattern.
- *Transversus abdominis.* The transversus abdominis muscles form the innermost layer of the abdominal

muscles. The fibers run horizontally across the abdomen.

To remember the abdominal muscles, think of that spare **TIRE**:

T	**t**ransversus abdominis
I	**i**nternal oblique
R	**r**ectus abdominis
E	**e**xternal oblique

The abdominal muscles are attached to fascia that forms a large aponeurosis along the midline of the abdominal wall. The aponeuroses of the abdominal muscles on opposite sides of the midline of the abdomen form a white line called the *linea alba*. The linea alba extends from the sternum to the pubic bone.

? Re-Think

1. Describe the movement of the head in response to contraction of the right sternocleidomastoid muscle.
2. Explain why the arrangement of the abdominal muscles conveys added strength to the abdominal wall.

MUSCLES THAT MOVE THE VERTEBRAL COLUMN

A number of muscles attach to the vertebrae and assist in the movement of the vertebral column; the movements include flexion, extension, hyperextension, lateral flexion, and rotation of the vertebral column. Muscles that move the vertebral column include the erector spinae, sternocleidomastoid, trapezius, abdominal muscles, and iliopsoas. Deep to the trapezius and the latissimus dorsi is the erector spinae (eh-REK-tor SPIN-ay); it extends the length of the vertebral column, from the sacrum to the cranium. As the erector spinae muscle ascends, it forms three columns of muscles. The erector spinae muscle causes extension and lateral flexion of the vertebral column and rotation of the head. This muscle assists in the maintenance of an erect posture. With aging, this muscle loses contractile strength and accounts in part for the stooped posture of an older person. Hungry? The erector spinae are best known by laypersons as pork chops and T-bone steaks.

Contraction of both sternocleidomastoid muscles causes flexion of the head at the neck, whereas contraction of one muscle rotates the head in the opposite direction (causes rotation of the cervical vertebral column). The trapezius maintains the vertebral column in extension. The abdominal muscles cause flexion and rotation of the vertebral column, and the iliopsoas (see later) flexes the vertebral column at the hip.

MUSCLES THAT FORM THE PELVIC FLOOR

The pelvic floor consists primarily of two flat muscle sheets and the attached fascia. These structures support the pelvic viscera and play a role in expelling the contents of the urinary bladder and rectum.

Do You Know...

What Is Wrong with Bulking Up?

Nothing is wrong with bulking up if it is done through weight lifting, exercise, and a healthy diet. Bulking up with the use of steroids, however, is dangerous. Steroids are thought to cause liver cancer, atrophy of the testicles in males, stunting of growth, and severe psychotic mood swings, among other health-related effects.

Then there is "'roid rage"—uncontrollable aggressive behavior. 'Roid rage has been implicated in many instances of serious sports-related injuries and has sent many a steroid abuser to prison for fighting, scrapping, brawling, and mauling—not a pretty picture.

MUSCLES OF THE SHOULDER (PECTORAL) GIRDLE AND ARM

Many muscles move the shoulder and the arm. The most important are the trapezius, serratus anterior, pectoralis major, latissimus dorsi, and deltoid and a group of muscles called the *rotator cuff muscles* (see Figure 9-7, *A* and *B*).

- *Trapezius.* The trapezius has its origin at the base of the occipital bone and the spines of all thoracic vertebrae; it inserts on the clavicle and scapula (shoulder blade). When contracted, the trapezius moves the clavicle and scapula and allows for a shrugging and rotating movement of the pectoral girdles. The trapezius causes medial rotation by pulling the shoulder blades (scapulae) together. The muscle gets its name because the right and left trapezius form the shape of a trapezoid.
- *Serratus anterior.* The serratus (sehr-AH-tis) anterior is located on the sides of the chest and extends from the upper ribs (origin) to the scapula (insertion). The serratus muscle has a jagged shape, much like the jagged edge of a serrated knife blade. When the serratus anterior contracts, the shoulders are lowered and the arm moves forward as if pushing a cart. The

trapezius and serratus anterior attach the scapula to the axial skeleton.

- *Pectoralis major.* The pectoralis (pek-toh-RAL-is) major is a large broad muscle that helps form the anterior chest wall. It connects the humerus (arm) with the clavicle (collarbone) and structures of the axial skeleton (ribs and sternum). Contraction of this muscle moves the arm across the front of the chest, as if pointing to an object in front of the body. (A more precise description of the function of the pectoralis major: It adducts and rotates the arm medially at the shoulder joint as well as flexes and extends the arm at the shoulder joint.) Many gym exercises are designed to hypertrophy the "pecs."
- *Latissimus dorsi.* The latissimus (LAT-iss-im-ahs) dorsi is a large broad muscle located in the middle and lower back region. Its origin is on the lower thoracic vertebrae, lumbar vertebrae, sacrum, and lower ribs; it inserts on the posterior humerus. Contraction of this muscle lowers the shoulders and brings the arm back, as if pointing to an object behind you. This same backward movement occurs in swimming and rowing. (A more precise description: The latissimus dorsi extends, adducts, and rotates the arm medially at the shoulder.) The pectoralis major and latissimus dorsi attach the humerus to the axial skeleton.
- *Deltoid.* The deltoid forms the rounded portion of the shoulder and forms the shoulder pad. The deltoid extends from its origins on the clavicle and scapula to its insertion on the humerus. Contraction of the deltoid muscle abducts the arm, raising it to a horizontal position (the scarecrow position). It also flexes, extends, and rotates the arm at the shoulder joint. Because of its size, location, and good blood supply, the deltoid is a common site of an intramuscular injection.
- *Teres major.* The teres (TER-eez) major is a long, round muscle that has its origin on the scapula and inserts on the humerus. It extends the arm at the shoulder joint and assists with the medial rotation and adduction of the arm at the shoulder joint.
- *Rotator cuff muscles.* The rotator cuff muscles are a group of four muscles that attach the humerus (insertion) to the scapula (origin). They include the subscapularis, supraspinatus, infraspinatus, and teres minor. The tendons of these muscles form a cap, or a cuff, over the proximal humerus, thus stabilizing the joint capsule. The muscles help rotate the arm at the shoulder joint. What about tennis buffs and their rotator cuffs? One of the most common causes of shoulder pain in athletes is known as *impingement syndrome*, or rotator cuff injury. It is caused by repetitive overhead motions and is commonly experienced by tennis players, swimmers, and baseball pitchers. The tendons are pinched and become inflamed, resulting in pain. If this continues, the inflamed tendon can degenerate

and separate from the bone. The condition can be a career-ending sports injury.

Note how many different movements are possible at the shoulder joint. The ball-and-socket joint and the many muscles that attach to the arm and pectoral girdle permit this freedom of movement.

Re-Think

Identify the origins and insertions of the following muscles: trapezius, pectoralis major, deltoid, and latissimus dorsi. Citing the origins and insertions of each, describe the movements caused by the contraction of the muscles.

MUSCLES THAT MOVE THE FOREARM

Most of the muscles that move the forearm (ulna and radius) are located along the humerus and are classified as flexors, extensors, supinators, or pronators. The flexors, those that cause flexion at the elbow joint, include the biceps brachii, brachialis, and brachioradialis. Extension is due to contraction of the triceps brachii.

The triceps brachii (TRY-seps BRAYK-ee-eye) lies along the posterior surface of the humerus; it has its origins on the scapula and humerus and its insertion on the ulna. Contraction causes extension of the forearm at the elbow joint; it also extends the arm at the shoulder joint. The triceps brachii is the muscle that supports the weight of the body when a person does push-ups or walks with crutches. It is also the muscle that packs the greatest punch for a boxer, hence the nickname "the boxer's muscle" (see Figure 9-7, *B*).

The biceps brachii is located along the anterior surface of the humerus; its two heads attach to the scapula (origin) and the distal end inserts on the radius of the forearm. The biceps brachii acts synergistically with the brachialis and brachioradialis to flex the forearm. The biceps brachii and brachialis are the prime movers for flexion of the forearm. When someone is asked to "make a muscle," the biceps brachii becomes most visible.

Pronation (palm down) is achieved by two pronator muscles located along the anterior forearm (origin on the humerus and ulna, insertion on the radius). The actions of the biceps brachii and a supinator muscle (origin on the humerus and ulna, insertion on the radius) located along the posterior forearm cause supination (palm up).

MUSCLES THAT MOVE THE WRIST, HAND, AND FINGERS

More than 20 muscles move the wrist, hand, and fingers. The muscles are numerous and small, making the wrist, hand, and fingers capable of delicate movements. The muscles are generally located along the forearm and consist of flexors and extensors. The flexors are located on the anterior surface of the forearm

and the extensors are located on the posterior surface. The tendons of these muscles pass through the wrist into the hand and fingers. The flexor carpi radialis and the flexor carpi ulnaris flex the hand at the wrist joint; they also adduct and abduct the hand at the wrist. Contraction of the flexor digitorum muscle (in the forearm) pulls on the tendons of the phalanges, thereby moving the fingers (like puppet strings). Imagine how fat your fingers would be if they were filled with muscle rather than tendons—your ring size would double or triple!

The puppet string setup, with the muscles in the forearm and tendons in the wrists and fingers, is responsible for another clinical mishap. If the tendons in the wrist are accidentally severed, the muscles in the forearm pull the tendons up into the forearm. The tendons "disappear" from the injured site. If the surgeon merely patches up the wrist injury and fails to retrieve and reattach the tendons, finger movement is lost.

The extensors of the wrist, hand, and fingers lie along the posterior forearm. The extensor carpi radialis longus extends and abducts the hand at the wrist. The extensor carpi ulnaris extends and adducts the hand at the wrist. The extensor digitorum extends the hand at the wrist and extends the fingers.

The flexors of the fingers are stronger than the extensors so that in a relaxed hand, the fingers are slightly flexed. If a person is unconscious for an extended period, the fingers remain in a flexed position. In response to inactivity, the tendons of the fingers shorten, thereby preventing extension of the fingers, which gives a clawlike appearance to the hand. This problem can be prevented by an exercise program that includes passive exercises of the hands and fingers.

THE CARPAL TUNNEL

Most of the tendons of the muscles that supply the hand pass through a narrow tunnel created by transversely oriented carpal ligaments and the carpal (wrist) bones (Figure 9-10). The flexor tendons in the carpal tunnel are encased in tendon sheaths and normally slide back and forth very easily. However, repetitive motion of the hand and fingers can cause the tissues within the carpal tunnel to become inflamed and swollen. The swelling puts pressure on the median nerve, which is also located in the carpal tunnel. The irritated nerve causes tingling, weakness, and pain in the hand and arm. The condition, carpal tunnel syndrome, is a major cause of disability in persons who must perform repetitive wrist motion (e.g., pianists, machinists, butchers, and keyboard operators).

Re-Think

Identify the origins and insertions of the following muscles: biceps brachii, brachialis, triceps brachii, and supinators. Citing the origins and insertions of each, describe the movements caused by the contraction of the muscles.

Carpal Tunnel Syndrome

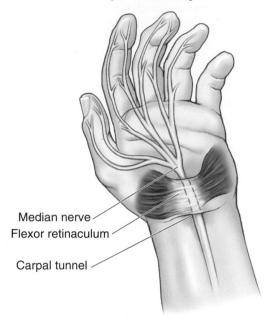

Median nerve
Flexor retinaculum
Carpal tunnel

FIGURE 9-10 Carpal tunnel syndrome.

MUSCLES THAT MOVE THE THIGH, LEG, AND FOOT

The muscles that move the thigh, leg, and foot are some of the largest and strongest muscles in the body. These muscles not only move the lower extremities, but also provide stability for the joints and help maintain posture.

MUSCLES THAT MOVE THE FEMUR (THIGH BONE)

The muscles that move the thigh at the hip all attach to some part of the pelvic girdle (coxal bones) and the femur (thigh bone). These include the gluteal muscles, the iliopsoas, the tensor fascia latae, and a group of adductor muscles. Contraction of these muscles causes movement at the hip joint (see Figure 9-7).

The gluteal muscles are located on the posterior surface and include the gluteus maximus, gluteus medius, and gluteus minimus. The gluteus maximus is the largest muscle in the body; it forms the area of the buttocks and is the muscle on which you sit.

The gluteus maximus has its origins on the ilium (coxal bone) and sacrum and inserts on the femur. It rotates the thigh laterally and extends the thigh at the hip, as in climbing stairs or walking. It produces the backswing of the leg while walking. The gluteus medius and gluteus minimus have their origins on the ilium (coxal bone) and insert on the femur. They abduct and rotate the thigh medially at the hip joint. Both the gluteus maximus and gluteus medius are commonly used sites for intramuscular injections.

The iliopsoas (il-ee-OHP-so-us) is located near the groin; it has its origins on the lower vertebrae and ilium (coxal bone) and its insertion on the femur. Contraction of this muscle flexes and rotates the thigh laterally.

The tensor fasciae latae (TEN-sor FASH-ee-ah LAT-ah) is on the lateral thigh; it has its origin on the ilium (coxal bone) and inserts on the tibia. Contraction of this muscle flexes and abducts the thigh at the hip joint.

The adductor muscles are located on the medial surface of the thigh; they have their origin on the lower coxal bones and insert on the medial and posterior surfaces of the femurs. This group of muscles adduct the thighs, pressing them together. These are the muscles that a horse rider uses to stay on the horse. The adductor muscles include the adductor longus, adductor brevis, adductor magnus, gracilis (GRAH-sil-is), and pectineus (pek-TIN-ee-us). In addition to adduction, most of the adductor muscles rotate the thigh. (See Table 9-1.)

The quadriceps femoris, sartorius, and hamstring muscles (described later) also move the thigh. The quadriceps femoris flexes the thigh at the hip, whereas the hamstrings extend the thigh at the hip. The sartorius allows you to sit cross-legged on the floor.

Note the many types of movement that occur at the hip, a ball-and-socket joint.

MUSCLES THAT MOVE THE LEG

The muscles that move the leg are located in the thigh. The extensor muscles lie along the anterior and lateral surfaces of the leg, whereas the flexors lie along the posterior and medial surfaces. Muscles that move the legs include the quadriceps femoris, sartorius, hamstring group, and the gastrocnemius.

The quadriceps femoris is located on the anterior thigh, is the most powerful muscle in the body, and has four heads as its origin. All four parts of the muscle insert on the tibia by the quadriceps ligament. (The quadriceps tendon extends distally to the tibial tuberosity as the quadriceps ligament.) The "quads" straighten, or extend, the leg at the knee, as in kicking a football. The four heads of the muscle give rise to four parts of the quadriceps femoris muscle, each of which has its own name: the vastus lateralis, vastus intermedius, vastus medialis, and rectus femoris. The vastus lateralis is frequently used as an injection site for children because it is more developed than the gluteal muscles.

The sartorius allows you to sit cross-legged on the floor. It assists in knee and hip flexion, abduction, and lateral rotation of the thigh. At one time tailors used to sit cross-legged as they worked. The Latin word for tailor is *sartor*, so this muscle was named the sartorius.

The hamstrings are a group of muscles located on the posterior surface of the thigh. All the muscles extend from the ischium (coxal bone) to the tibia. They flex the leg at the knee and are therefore antagonistic to the quadriceps femoris. Because these muscles also span the hip joint, they extend the thigh. The strong tendons of these muscles can be felt behind the knee. The tendons form the pit behind the knee called the *popliteal fossa*. These same tendons are found in hogs. In times past butchers used these tendons to hang the hams for smoking and curing—hence the name *hamstrings*. The hamstring muscles include the biceps femoris, semimembranosus, and semitendinosus. An athlete often pulls a hamstring or experiences a groin injury.

Because the gastrocnemius has its origin on the distal femur, it also flexes the leg at the knee. This large calf muscle is described later.

 Do You Know...

What a Wolf Knows about the Hamstrings?

Hungry wolves spot their prey—and the chase is on. The wolf will often attack the knee joint of its prey, severing the tendons of the hamstrings. Once the tendons are severed, the victim's legs are useless. Dinner is served!

MUSCLES THAT MOVE THE FOOT

The muscles that move the foot are located on the anterior, lateral, and posterior surfaces of the leg. See Figure 8-21 for movements of the foot. The tibialis anterior is located on the anterior surface. It has its origin on the tibia (shin bone) and inserts on the tarsal and metatarsal bones. It causes dorsiflexion and inversion of the foot. There are a number of muscles that cause plantar flexion. The peroneus (per-oh-NEE-us) longus muscle is on the lateral surface. It everts (turns outward) the foot, supports the arch of the foot, and assists in plantar flexion. The gastrocnemius (GAS-trok-NEE-mee-us) and soleus are the major muscles on the posterior surface of the leg and form the calf of the leg. They attach to the calcaneus (heel bone) by the calcaneal tendon, or Achilles tendon. Contraction of these muscles causes plantar flexion. The tibialis posterior also assists in plantar flexion and inverts the foot.

Plantar flexion aids in walking and allows a person to stand on tiptoes. For this reason the gastrocnemius is sometimes called the *toe dancer's muscle*. Runners, especially sprinters, occasionally tear or rupture the Achilles tendon. Because the heel then cannot be lifted, this injury severely impedes the ability of the runner to perform.

Finally, there are the toes. Like the fingers, some of the toes are tugged on by tendons whose muscles (flexors and extensors) lie in the leg. Other muscles have their origin in the tarsal and metatarsal bones.

Some muscles have acquired rather interesting names. Figure 9-11 shows the many interesting movements we are able to make.

 Re-Think

Identify the origins and insertions of the following muscles: gluteus maximus, quadriceps femoris, biceps femoris, tibialis anterior, soleus, and gastrocnemius. Citing the origins and insertions of each, describe the movements caused by the contraction of these muscles.

2+2 **Sum It Up!**

The skeleton is stabilized and covered with muscle. The ability of the muscles to contract and relax allows the skeleton to move about and engage in all the activities that make life so enjoyable. The location and function of the major muscles of the body are summarized in Table 9-1.

 As You Age

1. At about the age of 40, the number and diameter of muscle fibers decrease. Muscles become smaller, dehydrated, and weaker. Muscle fibers are gradually replaced by connective tissue, especially adipose or fat cells. By the age of 80, about 50% of the muscle mass has been lost.
2. Mitochondrial function in muscles decreases, especially in muscles that are not exercised regularly.
3. Motor neurons are gradually lost, resulting in muscle atrophy.
4. These changes lead to decreased muscle strength and slowing of muscle reflexes.

FIGURE 9-11 A medley of special muscles.

MEDICAL TERMINOLOGY AND DISORDERS   Disorders of the Musculoskeletal System

Medical Term	Word Parts	Word Part Meaning or Derivation	Description
Words			
adduction/ abduction	ad-	to, toward, or near	Adduction of the thigh indicates that the thigh is moving toward the midline of the body, whereas abduction means it is moving away from the midline of the body.
	ab-	away from	
	-duction	From the Latin word *ducere*, meaning "to lead"	
myalgia	my/o-	muscle	**Myalgia** means *muscle pain,* a characteristic of many musculoskeletal disorders.
	-algia	pain	
myopathy	my/o-	muscle	A **myopathy** is *a muscle disease where the primary defect is within the muscle itself and not in the neuromuscular junction or brain.*
	-path/o-	disease	
	-y	process or condition	
osteocyte	oste/o-	bone	**Osteocytes** are *bone cells.* Osteoblasts (-blast = immature) mature into osteocytes *(bone cells),* while osteoclasts (-clast = breakdown) break down osseous (bone) tissue.
	-cyte	cell	
periosteum	peri-	around	The **periosteum** is *the membrane around a bone.*
	-osteon	bone	
synergist	syn-	together	Refers to *muscles that work together to generate a movement.* Several muscles may work synergistically to flex the forearm.
	-erg-	From a Greek word meaning "to work"	
	-ist	one that specializes in	
Disorders			
arthralgia	arthr/o-	joint	**Arthralgia,** also called noninflammatory joint pain, has multiple causes: injury, infection, many diseases, or a reaction to medications.
	-algia	pain	
arthritis	arthr/o	joint	**Arthritis** is *inflammation of a joint.* There are over 25 types of arthritis; two common types are **osteoarthritis** and **rheumatoid arthritis.** **Osteoarthritis** is called *degenerative or "wear-and-tear" arthritis,* most frequently seen in older persons. It affects primarily the weight-bearing joints, but may also affect the hands. Bony nodules may develop in the interphalangeal joints. **Rheumatoid arthritis** (RA)—*the most debilitating type of arthritis*—is *an autoimmune disease characterized by inflammation of the joints and systemic symptoms such as fever, fatigue, and anemia.* Joint disease progresses from *thickening of joint tissue,* called **pannus formation,** to cartilage destruction and finally to deformity and fusion of the joints.
	-itis	inflammation	
bursitis	burs-	bursa	**Bursitis** is *the inflammation of one or more bursae, causing pain, swelling, and restriction of movement.* Common forms include subacromial bursitis (painful shoulder), olecranon bursitis (student's elbow, water on the elbow), and prepatellar bursitis (housemaid's knee, carpet layer's knee).
	-itis	inflammation	
luxation	lux-	From a Latin word meaning "to dislocate"	**Luxation** refers to *the displacement of a bone from its joint, with tearing of ligaments, tendons, and articular capsule.* The shoulder joint is a commonly dislocated joint. *A partial dislocation* is called a **subluxation**.
	-ation	condition or state	
fibromyalgia	fibr/o-	fiber	**Fibromyalgia** is *a syndrome characterized by pain in the muscles, tendons, and soft tissues.* Although the joints are not affected, the pain is experienced as originating in the joints. The musculoskeletal symptoms are accompanied by generalized feelings of fatigue, depression, headache, and anxiety.
	-my/o-	muscle	
	-algia	pain	

Continued

Medical Term	Word Parts	Word Part Meaning or Derivation	Description
fracture		From a Latin word meaning "to break"	**Fracture** refers to *a broken bone.* Most fractures are due to traumatic injuries; a small number are a result of another disease and are called **pathological fractures.** There are numerous ways to classify fractures: open/closed; stable/unstable; spiral, comminuted; transverse; stress.
multiple myeloma	myel/o-	bone marrow	Also called plasma cell myeloma, **multiple myeloma** refers to *malignant tumors of the bone marrow in which there are collections of abnormal plasma cells.* **CRAB** is a mnemonic that indicates the characteristic tetrad (four parts) of multiple myeloma: calcium (hypercalcemia), renal failure, anemia, and bone lesions.
	-oma	tumor	
muscular dystrophy	dys-	painful, difficulty, or faulty	**Muscular dystrophy** (MD) is *a group of inherited muscle disorders that cause progressive muscle weakness and degeneration of muscle tissue.* Numerous disorders are included in this category, with Duchenne MD being the most common.
	-troph/o-	nourishment or development	
	-y	condition or process of	
neoplasms (bone)	neo-	new	Osteogenic sarcoma or osteosarcoma is a highly malignant and rapidly metastasizing neoplasm. Osteoclastoma (tumor originating from osteoclasts) or giant cell tumor is most often nonmalignant, but highly destructive; it occurs in the long bones of the lower extremities. Ewing's sarcoma is a common malignancy of bone and soft tissue. Its rapid growth occurs within the pelvis and the medullary cavities of long bones of the extremities. Pathological fractures develop in response to the cancer-inducing osteonecrosis.
	plas/o-	formation	
osteomalacia	oste/o-	bone	**Osteomalacia** refers to *softening of the bones.* The loss of calcium and phosphorus is caused by vitamin D deficiency. The bone softening results in skeletal deformities and fractures. Osteomalacia in the growing bones of children is called *rickets.*
	-malacia	softening	
osteomyelitis	oste/o-	bone	**Osteomyelitis** is *a serious infection of the bone, bone marrow, and surrounding tissue.* It can be caused by many pathogens, the most common being *Staphylococcus aureus.* Infection can occur by direct (open wound) or indirect (hematogenous) entry.
	-myel/o-	bone marrow	
	-itis	inflammation	
osteoporosis	oste/o-	bone	A loss of bone mass that makes the bones so porous that they crumble under the ordinary stress of moving about. Osteoporosis is related to the loss of estrogen in older women, a dietary deficiency of calcium and vitamin D, and low levels of exercise. Osteopenia (-penia = abnormal reduction) is indicative of early osteoporosis.
	-por/os-	From a Greek word meaning "pore" or "passage"	
	-osis	condition of	
plantar fasciitis	fasci/o-	fascia	**Plantar fasciitis** is *inflammation of the plantar fascia on the bottom of the foot.* It is usually exercise-induced and painful.
	-itis	inflammation of	
rhabdomyolysis	rhabd/o-	rod-shaped or striated (skeletal)	**Rhabdomyolysis** is *the breakdown of muscle with the release of myoglobin into the blood.* It is a consequence of conditions in which muscle activity is excessive (seizures, drugs) or injurious (crush injuries).
	-my/o-	muscle	
	-lysis	breakdown	
strains and sprains			The two most common musculoskeletal injuries, usually as a result of twisting forces associated with physical activity. A **sprain** is *an injury or tearing of the ligaments of a joint.* A **strain** is *excess stretching of a muscle and its surrounding fascia.*
tendonitis	tend/o-	tendon	*Inflammation of a tendon causing pain and tenderness just outside the joint.* The joints most often affected are the elbows (tennis elbow, golfer's elbow), shoulders (pitcher's shoulder, swimmer's shoulder), wrists, and heels (Achilles tendonitis).
	-itis	inflammation	

Get Ready for Exams!

Summary Outline

The purpose of muscle is to contract and to cause movement.

I. Muscle Function: Overview
A. Types and functions of muscles
1. Skeletal muscle is striated and voluntary; its primary function is to produce movement.
2. Smooth (visceral) muscle is nonstriated and involuntary; it helps the organs perform their functions.
3. Cardiac muscle is striated and involuntary; it is found only in the heart and allows the heart to function as a pump.
B. Structure of the whole muscle
1. A large muscle consists of thousands of single muscle fibers (muscle cells).
2. Connective tissue binds the muscle fibers (cells) together, forming compartments in the limbs, and attaches muscle to bone and other tissue by tendons and aponeuroses.
C. Structure and function of a single muscle fiber
1. The muscle fiber (cell) is surrounded by a cell membrane (sarcolemma). The cell membrane penetrates to the interior of the muscle as the transverse tubule (T tubule).
2. An extensive sarcoplasmic reticulum (SR) stores calcium.
3. Each muscle fiber consists of a series of sarcomeres. Each sarcomere contains thin filaments (actin and troponin-tropomyosin complex) and thick filaments (myosin).
D. How muscles contract
1. Electrical signals run along the muscle membrane.
2. Electrical signal enters the T tubule system and stimulates the SR to release calcium.
3. Muscles shorten or contract as the actin and myosin (in the presence of calcium and ATP) interact through cross-bridge formation, according to the sliding filament mechanism.
4. Calcium is pumped back into the SR and the muscles relax.
E. Skeletal muscles and nerves: for a skeletal muscle to contract, it must be stimulated by a motor nerve.
1. Motor unit: formed by a motor neuron and the muscle fibers that it innervates (forms the basis of recruitment)
2. Neuromuscular junction (NMJ): the nerve terminal (ending) containing neurotransmitter (ACh), the space between the nerve terminal and muscle membrane, and the muscle membrane with its receptors
F. Force of muscle contraction
1. A single muscle fiber increases force of contraction through repetitive nerve stimulation.
2. A whole muscle increases its force of contraction in two ways: by repetitive nerve stimulation or recruitment of additional motor units.
G. Energy for muscle contraction can be obtained from three sources: burning fuel aerobically, burning fuel anaerobically, and metabolizing creatine phosphate.
H. Terms that describe muscle movement
1. Origin and insertion: the attachments of the muscles
2. Prime mover: the muscle most responsible for the movement achieved by the muscle group
3. Synergist or antagonist: works with or has an opposing action

II. Muscles from Head to Toe
A. Skeletal muscles are named according to size, shape, orientation of fibers, location, number of origins, place of origin and insertion, and muscle action.
B. See Table 9-1 for a list of the body's muscles.

Review Your Knowledge

Matching: Muscle Terms
Directions: Match the following words with their descriptions below. Some words may be used more than once, and others not at all.

a. origin
b. sarcoplasmic reticulum
c. smooth muscle
d. aponeurosis
e. actin
f. sarcomere
g. insertion
h. atrophy
i. synergist
j. skeletal muscle
k. myosin
l. tendon

1. ____ Cordlike structure that attaches muscle to bone
2. ____ Type of muscle classified as striated and voluntary
3. ____ Type of muscle that must be stimulated by a somatic motor nerve
4. ____ Flat, sheetlike fascia that attaches muscle to muscle or muscle to bone
5. ____ The head of this contractile protein binds to actin; forms a cross-bridge
6. ____ Calcium is stored within this muscle structure
7. ____ Series of contractile units that make up each myofibril: extends from Z line to Z line
8. ____ The muscle attachment to the movable bone
9. ____ Use it or lose it
10. ____ A helper muscle

Matching: Names of Muscles

Directions: Match the following words with their descriptions below. Some words may be used more than once, and others not at all.

a. quadriceps femoris
b. gastrocnemius
c. masseter
d. hamstrings
e. triceps brachii
f. deltoid
g. pectoralis major
h. latissimus dorsi
i. gluteus maximus
j. biceps brachii
k. diaphragm

1. ___ A muscle of mastication
2. ___ The major breathing muscle
3. ___ Major muscle of the anterior chest; attaches to the humerus
4. ___ The shoulder pad; pulls the arm into the scarecrow position
5. ___ A muscle that flexes the arm at the elbow
6. ___ A muscle that lies along the anterior thigh; flexes the thigh at the hip and extends the leg
7. ___ The muscle group that lies along the posterior thigh; flexes the leg at the knee
8. ___ The large muscle on which you sit
9. ___ Contraction of this muscle causes plantar flexion
10. ___ This muscle attaches to the calcaneus by the Achilles tendon

Multiple Choice

1. When the electrical signal travels along the T tubule and stimulates the sarcoplasmic reticulum (SR),
   a. calcium is released, causing cross-bridge formation between actin and myosin.
   b. acetylcholine (ACh) is released into the neuromuscular junction (NMJ).
   c. calcium is pumped into the SR from the sarcomere.
   d. ACh binds to the receptor on the muscle membrane.

2. Which of the following does not occur within the neuromuscular junction (NMJ)?
   a. ACh is released from the motor nerve terminal.
   b. ACh diffuses across the junction.
   c. Actin and myosin "slide."
   d. ACh is inactivated by an enzyme.

3. When skeletal muscle is stimulated quickly and repetitively,
   a. ACh within the NMJ is depleted.
   b. the muscle tetanizes and the force of contraction increases.
   c. the sarcoplasmic reticulum is depleted of calcium and the muscle becomes flaccid.
   d. the muscle merely twitches.

4. Which of the following slides?
   a. ACh and cholinesterase
   b. Calcium and ATP
   c. Troponin and tropomyosin
   d. Actin and myosin

5. Which of the following happens when calcium is pumped back into the sarcoplasmic reticulum?
   a. The muscle relaxes.
   b. ACh binds to the muscle membrane receptors in the NMJ.
   c. ACh is destroyed by cholinesterase.
   d. Actin and myosin slide.

6. Which of the following must occur to achieve flexion of the forearm?
   a. The triceps brachii contracts.
   b. The biceps brachii and brachialis contract.
   c. The brachioradialis relaxes.
   d. The deltoid and brachioradialis relax.

7. Which of the following does not characterize the quadriceps femoris?
   a. Has four heads, or points of attachment
   b. Is the prime mover for extension of the leg
   c. Inserts on the proximal tibia at the tibial tuberosity
   d. Causes plantar flexion as in toe dancing

8. Which of the following is true of the hamstrings?
   a. Located along the anterior thigh
   b. Is the prime mover for flexion of the leg
   c. Acts synergistically with the gastrocnemius to cause dorsiflexion
   d. Attaches to the Achilles tendon and inserts on the calcaneus

9. Which of the following is least descriptive of the masseter and temporalis muscles?
   a. Insert on the mandible
   b. Muscles of mastication
   c. Nonstriated and involuntary
   d. Innervated by somatic motor neurons

10. This muscle is best viewed on an anterior view of the body.
   a. Biceps femoris
   b. Pectoralis major
   c. Latissimus dorsi
   d. Gastrocnemius

Go Figure

1. According to Figure 9-1
   a. Visceral muscle is nonstriated and voluntary.
   b. The heart is primarily comprised of visceral or smooth muscle.
   c. Skeletal muscle is striated and voluntary.
   d. Cardiac muscle is smooth and involuntary.

2. According to Figure 9-2
   a. Panel C compares sarcomere length in the contracted and relaxed muscle.
   b. Panel C illustrates the location of the sarcoplasmic reticulum and T tubular system.
   c. Panel A indicates that we are using the biceps brachii to illustrate skeletal muscle function at the sarcomere level.
   d. Panel B illustrates the relationship of the thin and thick filaments within the sarcomere.

3. **According to Figure 9-3**
   a. The motor unit is another name for the neuromuscular junction (NMJ).
   b. Acetylcholine (ACh) is the neurotransmitter within the NMJ.
   c. Acetylcholinesterase is stored within the vesicles of the nerve terminal.
   d. The somatic motor neuron innervates only one muscle fiber (cell).

4. **According to Figure 9-4**
   a. Curare induces muscle paralysis because it blocks the release of acetylcholine (ACh) from the nerve terminal.
   b. *C. botulinum* induces paralysis because its toxin blocks muscle receptors.
   c. Myasthenia gravis is caused by the inability of the neuron to synthesize ACh.
   d. Curare induces paralysis because it blocks the muscle membrane receptors.

5. **According to Figure 9-5, which event occurs first?**
   a. Calcium is released from the sarcoplasmic reticulum.
   b. The electrical signal runs along the T tubule.
   c. ACh is released from the terminal of the somatic motor neuron.
   d. ACh binds to the receptors on the muscle membrane.

6. **According to Figure 9-6**
   a. The triceps brachii acts synergistically with the biceps brachii.
   b. Contraction of the biceps brachii causes extension of the arm at the elbow.
   c. The heads of the biceps brachii attach to the proximal humerus.
   d. The biceps brachii lies across the elbow joint.

7. **According to Figure 9-7 and Table 9-1, contraction of the pectoralis major causes**
   a. abduction of the arm at the shoulder.
   b. internal or medial rotation of the arm at the shoulder.
   c. flexion of the forearm at the elbow and external rotation of the arm, as if pointing behind you.
   d. movement of the arm into a "scarecrow" position.

8. **According to Figure 9-7 and Table 9-1, the sartorius**
   a. is visible only on the posterior view of the body.
   b. works synergistically with the muscles of the pectoral girdle.
   c. lies obliquely across the anterior thigh.
   d. inserts on the Achilles tendon.

9. **Which muscles are not illustrated in Figures 9-8 or 9-9?**
   a. Sternocleidomastoid, buccinator, and masseter
   b. Diaphragm, trapezius, and intercostals
   c. Latissimus dorsi, trapezius, and sartorius
   d. Frontalis, orbicularis oris, and platysma

Nervous System: Nervous Tissue and Brain

Key Terms

action potential (p. 175)
brain stem (p. 187)
cerebellum (p. 188)
cerebrospinal fluid (CSF) (p. 190)
cerebrum (p. 182)
depolarize (p. 176)
frontal lobe (p. 184)

hypothalamus (p. 187)
limbic system (p. 188)
medulla oblongata (p. 187)
meninges (p. 190)
myelin (p. 174)
neuroglia (p. 173)
neuron (p. 173)

neurotransmitters (p. 180)
occipital lobe (p. 186)
parietal lobe (p. 185)
repolarize (p. 176)
reticular formation (p. 188)
synapse (p. 179)
temporal lobe (p. 185)

Objectives

1. Define the two divisions of the nervous system.
2. List three general functions of the nervous system.
3. Discuss the cellular composition of the nervous system, including:
   - Compare the structure and functions of the neuroglia and neuron.
   - Explain the function of the myelin sheath.

- Explain how a neuron transmits information.
4. Describe the structure and function of a synapse.
5. Describe the functions of the four major areas of the brain and the four lobes of the cerebrum.
6. Describe how the skull, meninges, cerebrospinal fluid, and blood–brain barrier protect the central nervous system.

THE NERVOUS SYSTEM: STRUCTURE AND FUNCTION

If you have ever listened to an orchestra warming up before a performance, you know something about the need for its conductor. Without the conductor, the sound is more like noise than music. The conductor coordinates, interprets, and directs the sound into the beautiful strains of a symphony. So it is with the nervous system. The various organ systems of the body need an interpreter to coordinate and direct them. This role is performed magnificently by the nervous system. The music of the body is every bit as beautiful as the strains of a symphony!

DIVISIONS OF THE NERVOUS SYSTEM

The structures of the nervous system are divided into two parts: the central nervous system and the peripheral nervous system. The central nervous system (CNS) includes the brain and the spinal cord. The CNS is located in the dorsal cavity. The brain is located in the cranial cavity; the spinal cord is enclosed in the spinal cavity. The peripheral nervous system (PNS) is located outside the CNS and consists of the nerves that connect the CNS with the rest of the body (Figure 10-1).

FUNCTIONS OF THE NERVOUS SYSTEM

As the "conductor," the nervous system performs three general functions: a sensory function, an integrative function, and a motor function (Figure 10-2).

SENSORY FUNCTION

Sensory nerves gather information from inside the body and from the outside environment. The nerves then carry the information to the CNS. For example, information about a cat is picked up by special cells in the boy's eye.

INTEGRATIVE FUNCTION

Sensory information brought to the CNS is interpreted. The brain not only sees the cat, but also does much more. It recalls very quickly how a cat behaves. It may

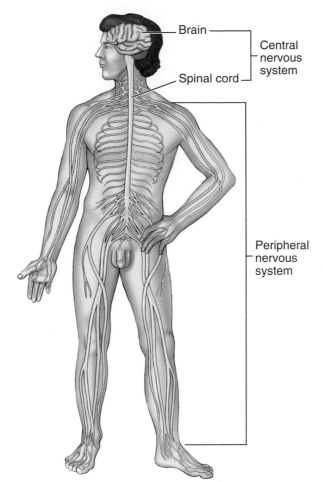

FIGURE 10-1 Nervous system: central nervous system and peripheral nervous system.

- Brain
- Central nervous system
- Spinal cord
- Peripheral nervous system

determine that the cat is acting hungry or is distressed and ready to attack. The brain integrates, or puts together, everything it knows about cats and then makes its plan.

MOTOR FUNCTION

Motor nerves convey information from the CNS toward the muscles and glands of the body. Motor nerves carry out the plans made by the CNS. For example, the person may decide to feed the hungry cat. Information must travel along the motor nerves from the CNS to all the skeletal muscles needed to feed the cat. The motor nerve converts the plan into action.

? Re-Think

Differentiate between sensory, integrative, and motor function; provide an example of each.

CELLS THAT MAKE UP THE NERVOUS SYSTEM

Nervous tissue is composed of two types of cells: the neuroglia and the neurons.

NEUROGLIA

Neuroglia (noo-ROHG-lee-ah), or glial cells, are the nerve glue. Neuroglia are the most abundant of the nerve cells; most glial cells are located in the CNS. Glial cells support, protect, insulate, nourish, and generally care for the delicate neurons. Some of the glial cells participate in phagocytosis; others assist in the secretion of cerebrospinal fluid. Glial cells, however, do not conduct nerve impulses.

Two of the more common glial cells are the astrocytes and the ependymal cells (Figure 10-3). The star-shaped astrocytes (ASS-troh-sytes) are the most abundant of the glial cells and have the most diverse functions; they support the neurons structurally, cover the entire surface of the brain, and help form a protective barrier, called the *blood–brain barrier*. This barrier helps prevent toxic substances in the blood from entering the nervous tissue of the brain and spinal cord. Astrocytes also secrete nerve growth factors that promote neuron growth and enhance synaptic development. A second glial cell is the ependymal (eh-PEN-di-mal) cell. These cells line the inside cavities of the brain and assist in the formation of cerebrospinal fluid. Other glial cells are listed in Table 10-1. Because glial cells undergo mitosis, most primary CNS tumors are composed of glial cells, such as astrocytomas.

NEURON

The second type of cell within the nervous system is the neuron. Of the two types of nerve cells, the neuron (NOO-ron) is the most important in the transmission of electrical signals. The neuron enables the nervous system to act as a vast communication network. Neurons have many shapes and sizes. Some neurons are extremely short; others are very long, with some measuring 4 feet in length. Unlike glial cells, neurons are nonmitotic and therefore do not replicate nor replace themselves when injured. Because they are nonmitotic, neurons generally do not give rise to primary malignant brain tumors.

PARTS OF A NEURON

Three Parts

The three parts of the neuron are the dendrites, cell body, and axon (Figure 10-4). Dendrites are treelike structures that receive signals from other neurons and then transmit the signals toward the cell body. One neuron may have thousands of dendrites, whereas other neurons have fewer dendrites. The neuron with the greater number of dendrites can receive signals from many other neurons. The cell body contains the nucleus and is essential for the life of the cell. The cell body usually receives thousands of signals from the dendrites and "decides" on the signal it wants to send to the axon. The axon is a long extension that transmits signals away from the cell body. The end of the axon

FIGURE 10-2 Three functions of the nervous system. **A,** Sensory function. **B,** Integrative function. **C,** Motor function.

undergoes extensive branching to form many axon terminals; it is within the axon terminals that the chemical neurotransmitters are stored. The arrow in Figure 10-4 indicates the direction in which signal travels over the neuron: from dendrites to cell body to axon.

The Axon: A Special Structure

What is so special about the axon? An enlarged view of the axon shows several unique structures: the myelin sheath, the neurilemma, and the nodes of Ranvier (see Figure 10-4). Most long nerve fibers of both the peripheral and central nervous systems are encased by a layer of white fatty material called the *myelin sheath*. **Myelin** (MY-eh-lin) protects and insulates the axon. Nerve fibers covered by myelin are said to be myelinated. Some neurons are not encased in myelin and are called *unmyelinated neurons*. Myelination begins during the fourth month of fetal life and continues into the teenage years. Because some axons of immature motor neurons lack myelination, the movements of an infant are slower and less coordinated than those of an older child. Severely restricting the fat intake of an infant or young child is unwise, because the child is still laying down myelin.

The formation of myelin sheath differs in the peripheral and central nervous systems. Surrounding the axon of a neuron in the peripheral nervous system is a layer of special cells called *Schwann* (shwon) *cells*. The Schwann cells form the myelin sheath that surrounds the axon. The nuclei and cytoplasm of the Schwann cells lie outside the myelin sheath and are

called the *neurilemma*. The neurilemma is important in the regeneration of a severed nerve.

In the CNS, the myelin sheath is formed not by Schwann cells but by oligodendrocytes (ohl-i-go-DEN-droh-sytes), a type of glial cell (see Table 10-1). Because there are no Schwann cells, there is no neurilemma. The lack of the neurilemma surrounding the axons accounts, in part, for the inability of the CNS neurons to regenerate. Failure of the neurons of the CNS to regenerate, however, is not fully explained by the lack of neurilemma; other factors include the formation of scar tissue and the lack of critical nerve growth factors.

Nodes of Ranvier, axonal areas not covered by myelin, appear at regular intervals along the myelinated axon.

 Re-Think

1. What is the biggest functional difference between glial cells and the neuron?
2. List the three main parts of a neuron.

TYPES OF NEURONS

The three types of neurons are the sensory neuron, the motor neuron, and the interneuron. A sensory neuron carries information from the periphery toward the CNS. Sensory neurons are also called *afferent neurons*.

A motor neuron carries information from the CNS toward the periphery. Motor neurons are also called *efferent neurons*.

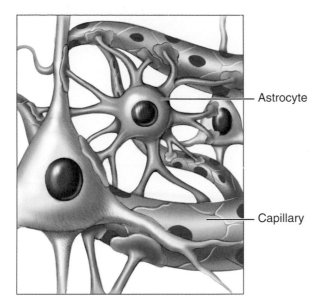

Astrocyte

Capillary

Table **10-1**	Types of Neuroglia
CELL NAME	**FUNCTION**
Astrocytes	Star-shaped cells present in blood–brain barrier; also anchor or bind blood vessels to nerves for support, act as phagocytes, and secrete nerve growth factors
Ependymal cells	Line the ventricles as part of the choroid plexus; involved in the formation of cerebrospinal fluid
Microglia	Protective role; phagocytosis of pathogens and damaged tissue
Schwann cells	Produce myelin sheath for neurons in the peripheral nervous system; assist in regeneration of damaged fibers
Oligodendrocytes	Produce myelin sheath for neurons in the central nervous system

in the CNS are generally referred to as *nuclei*. Small clusters of cell bodies in the peripheral nervous system are called *ganglia* (sing., ganglion). For example, patches of gray called the *basal nuclei* are located in the brain. (Sometimes, these patches of gray are called *basal ganglia*, despite their location in the CNS.)

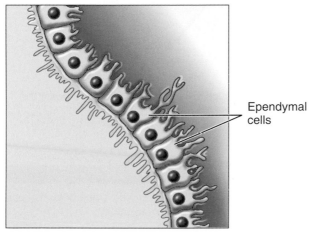

Ependymal cells

FIGURE 10-3 Neuroglia, or glia: astrocytes and ependymal cells.

Remember—what is the **SAME** about these fibers!

S	**s**ensory
A	**a**fferent
M	**m**otor
E	**e**fferent

The third type of neuron is the interneuron; it is found only in the CNS. Interneurons form connections between sensory and motor neurons. Interneurons also play a role in thinking, learning, and memory.

WHITE MATTER VERSUS GRAY MATTER

The tissue of the CNS is white or gray. White matter is white because of the myelinated axons, whereas gray matter is made up of unmyelinated axons, cell bodies, interneurons, and synapses.

Sometimes cell bodies appear in small clusters and are given special names. Clusters of cell bodies located

2+2 Sum It Up!

The nervous system plays a crucial role in allowing us to interact with our environment, both internal and external. The nervous system has two divisions: the central nervous system (CNS) and the peripheral nervous system. The nervous system performs three major functions: sensory, integrative, and motor. There are two types of cells in the nervous system: the neuroglia and the neurons. The neuron is responsible for the rapid communication of electrical signals. The three parts of the neuron are the dendrites, cell body, and axon.

THE NEURON CARRYING INFORMATION

Neurons allow the nervous system to convey information rapidly from one part of the body to the next. A stubbed toe makes itself known almost immediately. Think of how fast the information travels from your toe, where the injury occurred, to your brain, where the injury is interpreted as pain. Information is carried along the neuron in the form of a nerve impulse.

THE NERVE IMPULSE: WHAT IT IS

The nerve impulse is an electrical signal that conveys information along a neuron. A series of events cause the electrical charge inside the cell to move from its negative resting state (−) to its positive depolarized state (+) and back to its negative resting state (−). The nerve impulse is called the **action potential**. There

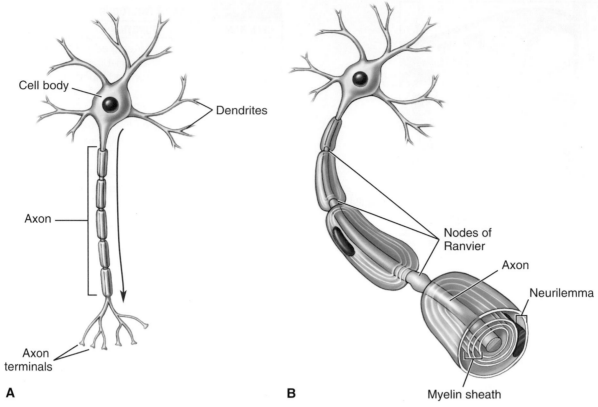

FIGURE 10-4 Structure of a neuron. **A,** Dendrites, cell body, axon, and axon terminals. **B,** Structure surrounding the axon, showing the myelin sheath, the nodes of Ranvier, and the neurilemma.

are two phases of an action potential: depolarization and repolarization. Follow Figure 10-5 through the events of the action potential, from its resting state (resting membrane potential) to depolarization to repolarization.

RESTING MEMBRANE POTENTIAL

The resting membrane potential refers to the electrical charge difference across the membrane of the resting neuron. The inside of a resting neuron is more negative (−) than the outside (+). The resting cell is said to be polarized. As long as the neuron is polarized, no nerve impulse is being transmitted. The cell is quiet, or resting.

DEPOLARIZATION

When the neuron is stimulated, a change occurs in the cell's electrical state. In the resting (polarized) state, the inside of the cell is negative. When the cell is stimulated, the inside becomes positive. As the inside of the cell changes from negative to positive, it is said to depolarize.

REPOLARIZATION

Very quickly, however, the inside of the cell again becomes negative; in other words, it returns to its resting state, or repolarizes. Unless the cell repolarizes, it cannot be stimulated again.

? Re-Think

What is the meaning of the resting membrane potential, polarization, depolarization, and repolarization?

THE NERVE IMPULSE: WHAT CAUSES IT

The changes associated with the action potential, or nerve impulse, are caused by the movement of specific ions across the cell membrane of the neuron. There is an ionic basis of the action potential. Follow the movement of the ions in Figure 10-6.

RESTING MEMBRANE POTENTIAL

What makes the inside of the cell negative in the resting state? The resting state is the result of the numbers and types of ions located inside the neuron. The chief intracellular ions include the positively charged potassium ions (K^+) and several anions (negatively charged ions). How do these ions get into the cell in such high concentrations? They are pumped in by ATP-driven pumps in the cell membrane. The chief intracellular cation is K^+. In the resting state, however, some of the K^+ ions leak out of the cell, taking with them the positive charge. The lost positive charge and the excess anions trapped in the cell make the inside of the cell negative. Remember: it is the outward leak of K^+ that is responsible for the resting membrane potential!

FIGURE 10-5 Nerve impulse (action potential). **A,** Polarization. **B,** Depolarization. **C,** Repolarization.

DEPOLARIZATION (STIMULATED STATE)

Why does the interior of the cell become positive when stimulated? When the neuron is stimulated, the permeability of the neuronal membrane changes in a way that allows sodium ions (Na^+) to diffuse rapidly across the membrane into the cell, carrying with it a positive (+) charge. Thus, it is the inward diffusion of Na^+ that causes depolarization. (Na^+ is the chief extracellular cation.)

REPOLARIZATION (RETURN TO RESTING)

Why does the inside of the cell quickly return to its resting negative state? Soon after the cell depolarizes, the neuronal membrane undergoes a second change. The change in the membrane permeability does two things: (1) it stops additional diffusion of Na^+ into the cell, and (2) it allows K^+ to rapidly diffuse out of the cell. The outward diffusion of K^+ decreases the positive charge from the inside of the cell, leaving behind the negatively charged anions. Thus, the outward movement of K^+ causes repolarization and a return to the resting state.

Eventually, membrane pumps restore intracellular ion concentrations; Na^+ is pumped out of the cell, while K^+ is pumped into the cell. Note that the repolarizing phase of the nerve impulse is not caused by the active transport pumps. Repolarization is caused by the rapid outward diffusion of K^+. In addition to their physiological roles, these active transport pumps are often the target of drugs. Digoxin, for example, poisons the Na^+/K^+ pumps, causing calcium to accumulate in cardiac muscle. This action accounts for the increased force of cardiac muscle contraction, a desired effect in the treatment of heart failure.

 Re-Think

What is the ionic basis of the resting membrane potential (polarization), depolarization, and repolarization?

THE NERVE IMPULSE: WHAT CAUSES IT TO MOVE

To convey information, a nerve impulse (action potential) must move the length of the neuron, from the cell

FIGURE 10-6 The cause of the nerve impulse. **A,** Polarization. **B,** Depolarization. **C,** Repolarization.

body to the axon terminal. Figure 10-7 shows that when nerve impulse one (NI-1) forms at point A, it also depolarizes the next segment of the membrane (point B), causing nerve impulse two (NI-2) to form. Nerve impulse 2 then depolarizes the next segment of membrane at point C, causing the formation of nerve impulse three (NI-3).

Because of the ability of each nerve impulse to depolarize the adjacent membrane, the nerve impulse moves toward the axon terminal much like a wave. In addition to showing the movement of the nerve impulse, Figure 10-7 also shows that each nerve impulse fires in an all-or-nothing manner. The all-or-nothing firing means that the height of each nerve impulse is the same. This is important because it ensures that the nerve impulse does not weaken as it travels the length of a long axon.

THE NERVE IMPULSE: WHAT CAUSES IT TO MOVE QUICKLY

We understand why the nerve impulse moves, but why does it move so quickly? Myelination increases the movement of the nerve impulse along the axonal membrane. Recall that the axons of most nerve fibers are wrapped in myelin, a fatty material. At the nodes of Ranvier, the axonal membrane is bare or unmyelinated.

The nerve impulse arrives at the axon but cannot develop on any part of the membrane covered with myelin. The nerve impulse can, however, develop at the nodes of Ranvier, the bare axonal membrane. Thus in a myelinated fiber, the nerve impulse jumps from node to node, much like a kangaroo, to the end of the axon (Figure 10-8). This "jumping" from node to

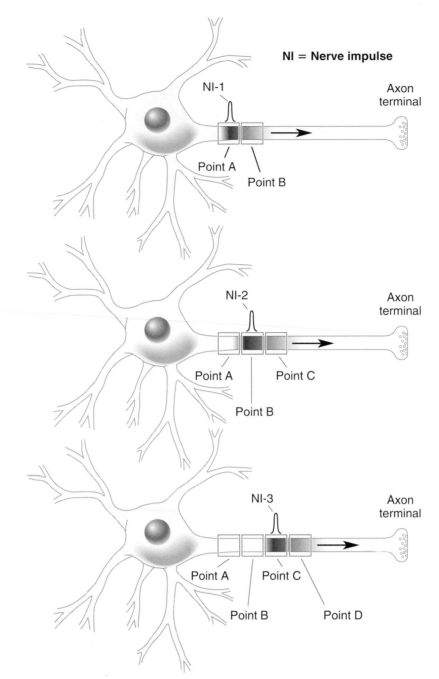

NI = Nerve impulse

FIGURE 10-7 What causes the nerve impulse to move from the cell body to the axon terminals?

node is called *saltatory conduction* (from the Latin word *saltare*, meaning "to leap"). Saltatory conduction increases the speed with which the nerve impulse travels along the nerve fiber. For this reason, myelinated fibers are considered fast-conducting nerve fibers.

❓ Re-Think

Explain how myelination affects the rate of nerve impulse (action potential) conduction.

SYNAPSE ACROSS NEURONS

The nerve impulse travels the length of the axon. However, the signal is unable to jump from one neuron to the next. A **synapse** helps information move from one neuron to the next. The big question is how.

PARTS OF A SYNAPSE

SYNAPTIC CLEFT

The synaptic (si-NAP-tik) cleft is a space (much like the neuromuscular junction in Chapter 9). The space

FIGURE 10-8 Jumping from node to node. **A,** A myelinated axon and the nodes of Ranvier. **B,** The nerve impulse jumps from node to node toward the axon terminal. **C,** The jumping of the nerve impulse resembles the jumping of a kangaroo.

exists because the axon terminal of neuron A (presynaptic neuron) does not physically touch the dendrite of neuron B (postsynaptic neuron). Follow Figure 10-9 as the synaptic structures listed below are described.

Receptors

The dendrite of neuron B contains receptor sites. Receptor sites are places on the membrane to which the neurotransmitters bind. For example, acetylcholine (ACh) binds to the receptors on dendrite B. Each receptor site has a specific shape and accepts only those neurotransmitters that "fit" its shape.

Neurotransmitters

The axon terminal of neuron A contains thousands of tiny vesicles that store chemical substances called neurotransmitters (noo-roh-TRANS-mit-ters). The most common neurotransmitters are ACh and norepinephrine (NE). Other CNS transmitters include epinephrine, serotonin, glutamate, dopamine, gamma-aminobutyric acid (GABA), and endorphins.

Inactivators

Inactivators are substances that terminate the activity of the neurotransmitters when they have completed their task. For example, the neurotransmitter ACh is terminated by acetylcholinesterase. Acetylcholinesterase is an enzyme located in the same area as the receptor sites on neuron B. Once ACh has completed its task, it is inactivated by acetylcholinesterase.

EVENTS AT THE SYNAPSE

The following details the events at the synapse (see Figure 10-9).
1. The nerve impulse travels along neuron A to its axon terminal.
2. The nerve impulse causes the vesicles to fuse with the membrane of the axon terminal. The vesicles open and release the neurotransmitter into the synaptic cleft.
3. The neurotransmitter diffuses across the synaptic cleft and binds to the receptor site. The binding of

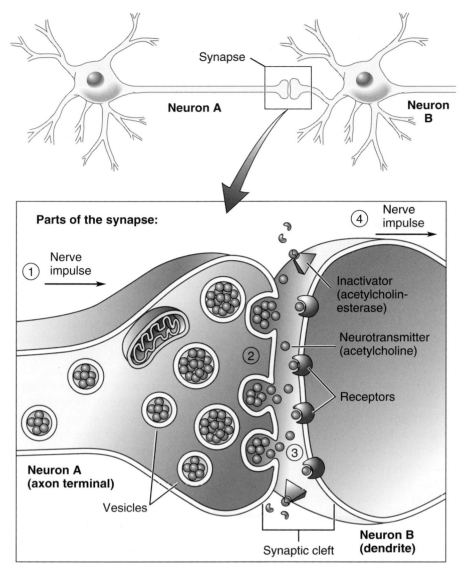

FIGURE 10-9 The synapse. The steps in the transfer of information across the synapse are shown.

the neurotransmitter to the receptor site causes a change in the membrane potential of the dendrite of neuron B, thereby developing a nerve impulse. The neurotransmitter vacates the receptor and is degraded.

4. Electrical information travels toward the cell body and axon of neuron B. What has happened at the synapse? Information from neuron A has been transmitted chemically to neuron B.

Re-Think

How does the nerve impulse (action potential) of the first neuron stimulate the dendrites of a second neuron?

2+2 Sum It Up!

The electrical signal that travels along the neuron is called the *nerve impulse* or *action potential*. The nerve impulse has two phases: depolarization and repolarization. The resting membrane potential and the phases of the nerve impulse are caused by the movement of ions, particularly Na^+ and K^+. The resting membrane potential is due to the outward leak of K^+. Depolarization is due to the influx of Na^+. Repolarization is due to the efflux of K^+. The nerve impulse travels along the neuron from the cell body to the end of the axon. Many of the axons are myelinated to increase the speed of the nerve impulse. During saltatory conduction, the nerve impulse jumps from node to node. The nerve impulse stimulates the release of neurotransmitters into the synaptic cleft; the transmitter diffuses across the synaptic cleft, binds to the postsynaptic receptor, and stimulates the dendrites of the second neuron. This is how information is transmitted from one neuron to the next.

BRAIN: STRUCTURE AND FUNCTION

You read a book, listen to music, sing a song, laugh, rage, remember, learn, feel, move, sleep, awaken, and so much more. All these are functions of the brain.

The brain is located in the cranial cavity. It is a pinkish-gray, delicate structure with a soft consistency. The surface of the brain appears bumpy, much like a walnut. The "boss of it all" weighs only 3 lb!

The blood supply to the brain is unique and is described in Chapter 18. Despite the fact that the brain weighs only 2% of the total body weight, it requires 20% of the body's oxygen supply. The primary source of energy for the brain is glucose. When blood glucose levels get very low (hypoglycemia), the person experiences mental confusion, dizziness, seizures, loss of consciousness, and death. No wonder that many of the body's hormones are concerned with making glucose available to the brain.

The brain is divided into four major areas: the cerebrum, the diencephalon, the brain stem, and the cerebellum (Figure 10-10).

CEREBRUM

The **cerebrum** (seh-REE-brum) is the largest part of the brain. It is divided into the right and left cerebral hemispheres. The cerebral hemispheres are joined together by bands of white matter that form a large fiber tract called the *corpus callosum*. The corpus callosum allows the right and left sides of the brain to communicate with each other. Each cerebral hemisphere has four major lobes: frontal, parietal, temporal, and occipital (Figure 10-11). These four lobes are named for the overlying cranial bones.

GRAY ON THE OUTSIDE, WHITE ON THE INSIDE

The cerebrum contains both gray and white matter. A thin layer of gray matter, called the *cerebral cortex*, forms the outermost portion of the cerebrum. The cerebral cortex is composed primarily of cell bodies and interneurons. The gray matter of the cerebral cortex allows us to perform higher mental tasks such as learning, reasoning, language, and memory.

The bulk of the cerebrum is composed of white matter located directly below the cortex. The white matter is composed primarily of myelinated axons that form connections between the parts of the brain and spinal cord. Scattered throughout the white matter are patches of gray matter called *nuclei*.

MARKINGS OF THE CEREBRUM

The lumpy, bumpy surface of the cerebrum has numerous markings with special names. The surface of the cerebrum is folded into elevations that resemble speed bumps on a road. The elevations are called *convolutions*, or *gyri* (sing., gyrus).

This extensive folding arrangement increases the amount of cerebral cortex, or thinking tissue. It is thought that intelligence is related to the amount of cerebral cortex and therefore to the numbers of convolutions or gyri. The greater the numbers of convolutions in the brain, the more intelligent the species. For example, the cerebral cortex of the human brain has many more convolutions than the brain of an elephant (except in the memory part of the brain). (Big bumps, big thoughts.)

Gyri are separated by grooves called *sulci* (sing., sulcus). A deep sulcus is called a *fissure*. Sulci and

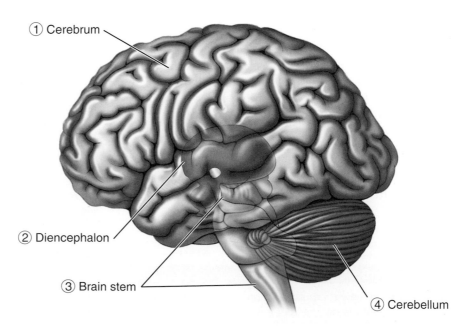

① Cerebrum
② Diencephalon
③ Brain stem
④ Cerebellum

FIGURE 10-10 Four major areas of the brain: cerebrum, diencephalon, brain stem, and cerebellum.

fissures separate the cerebrum into lobes. Figure 10-11 illustrates two of the numerous sulci and fissures: the central sulcus and the lateral sulcus. (Identify each structure on the diagram as it is described in the text.)

The central sulcus separates the frontal lobe from the parietal lobe. The central sulcus is an important landmark, separating the precentral and postcentral gyri. The precentral gyrus is located in the frontal lobe,

Do You Know...

If You Are a Left-Brain or a Right-Brain Person?

Some years ago, a surgeon severed the corpus callosum in the brain of a patient with severe epilepsy. This surgical procedure eliminated all communication between the left and right cerebral hemispheres. From these and other experiments, neuroscientists learned that there is a left brain and a right brain, and that these two brains have different abilities. The differences in function between the two cerebral hemispheres is called *cerebral lateralization*. The left brain is more concerned with language and mathematical abilities; it is the reasoning and analytical side of the brain. The right side of the brain is far superior with regard to spatial relationships, art, music, and the expression of emotions. The right brain is intuitive; it is the poet and the artist. Many of us are predominantly left-brain or right-brain persons. How much richer our lives are when we use both sides of our brains!

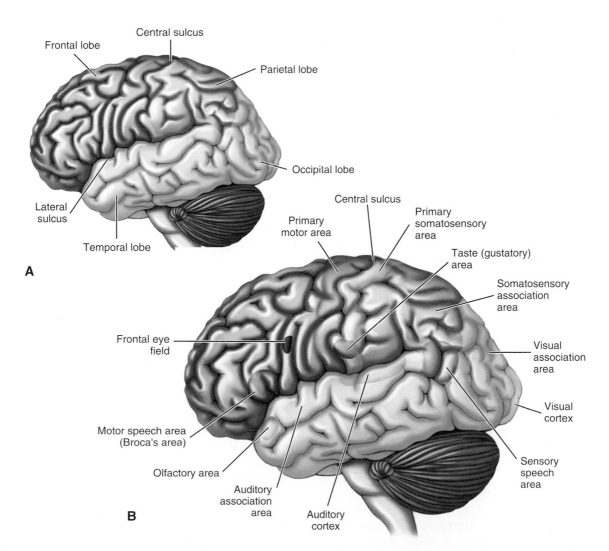

FIGURE 10-11 A, Lobes of the cerebrum: frontal lobe, parietal lobe, temporal lobe, and occipital lobe. **B,** Functional areas of the cerebrum.

Table 10-2	Brain Structure and Function
STRUCTURE	**FUNCTIONS**
Cerebrum	
Frontal lobe	Motor area, personality, behavior, emotional expression, intellectual functions ("executive" functions), memory storage
Parietal lobe	Somatosensory area (especially from skin and muscle; taste; speech; reading)
Occipital lobe	Vision, vision-related reflexes and functions (reading, judging distances, seeing in three dimensions)
Temporal lobe	Hearing (auditory area), smell (olfactory area), taste, memory storage, part of speech area
Diencephalon	
Thalamus	Relay structure and processing center for most sensory information going to the cerebrum
Hypothalamus	Integrating system for the autonomic nervous system; regulation of temperature, water balance, sex, thirst, appetite, and some emotions (pleasure and fear); regulates the pituitary gland and controls endocrine function
Brain Stem	
Midbrain	Relays information (sensory and motor); associated with visual and auditory reflexes
Pons	Relays information (sensory and motor); plays a role in respiration
Medulla oblongata	Vital function (regulation of heart rate, blood flow, blood pressure, respiratory centers); reflex center for coughing, sneezing, swallowing, and vomiting
Cerebellum	Smoothes out and coordinates voluntary muscle activity; helps in the maintenance of balance and muscle tone
Other Structures	
Limbic system	Experience of emotion and behavior (emotional brain)
Reticular formation	Mediates wakefulness and sleep; includes the reticular activating system (RAS)
Basal nuclei	Smoothes out and coordinates skeletal muscle activity

directly in front of the central sulcus, and the postcentral gyrus is located in the parietal lobe, directly behind the central sulcus. The lateral fissure separates the temporal lobe from the frontal and the parietal lobes. The longitudinal fissure separates the left and right cerebral hemispheres (not shown).

? Re-Think

1. What are the four major divisions of the brain?
2. What is the role of the corpus callosum?
3. In what cerebral lobe is the precentral gyrus? The postcentral gyrus?

LOBES OF THE CEREBRUM

What does each cerebral lobe do? (See Table 10-2.)

Frontal Lobe

The frontal lobe is located in the front of the cranium under the frontal bone (see Figure 10-11). The frontal lobe plays a key role in voluntary motor activity, personality development, emotional and behavioral expression, and performance of high-level tasks such as learning, thinking, and making plans; these are sometimes called *executive functions*. The frontal lobe contains the primary motor area. Nerve impulses that originate in the motor area control voluntary muscle

movement. When you decide to move your leg, the nerve impulse originates in the precentral gyrus, or primary motor cortex, of the frontal lobe. The axons of these motor neurons form the voluntary motor tracts that descend down the spinal cord.

The function of the precentral gyrus of the frontal lobe is illustrated by a homunculus, meaning "little man" (Figure 10-12). The homunculus represents the amount of brain tissue that corresponds to a function of a particular body part. The homunculus shows two important points; each part of the body is controlled by a specific area of the cerebral cortex of the precentral gyrus, and the complicated nature of certain movements requires large amounts of brain tissue. (Locate the specific points for the toe, foot, leg, trunk, hand, and face.)

For example, the movements of the hand are much more delicate and complicated than the movements of the foot. Therefore, the amount of brain tissue devoted to hand and finger movement is much greater than the amount devoted to foot and toe movement. Consequently, the homunculus has huge hands and small feet. Note also the amount of brain tissue required to run your mouth.

In addition to its role in voluntary motor activity, the frontal lobe plays a key role in motor speech. Motor speech refers to the movements of the mouth and tongue necessary for the formation of words.

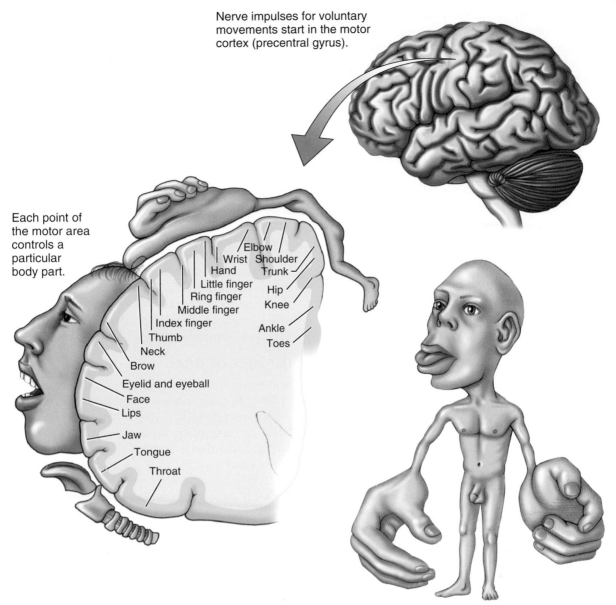

Nerve impulses for voluntary movements start in the motor cortex (precentral gyrus).

Each point of the motor area controls a particular body part.

Elbow
Wrist Shoulder
Hand Trunk
Little finger Hip
Ring finger Knee
Middle finger
Index finger Ankle
Thumb Toes
Neck
Brow
Eyelid and eyeball
Face
Lips
Jaw
Tongue
Throat

FIGURE 10-12 Motor area of the frontal lobe, illustrated with a homunculus.

The part of the frontal lobe concerned with motor speech is called *Broca's area*. In most persons, Broca's area is in the left hemisphere (see Figure 10-11). What happens when Broca's area is broken? If damaged, as happens with a stroke, the person develops a type of aphasia. The person knows what he or she wants to say but cannot say it. Just above Broca's area is an area called the *frontal eye field*. It controls voluntary movements of the eyes and the eyelids. Your ability to scan this paragraph is a function of this area.

Parietal Lobe

The parietal lobe is located posterior to the central sulcus (see Figure 10-11). The parietal lobe, particularly the postcentral gyrus, is primarily concerned with receiving general sensory information from the body. Because it receives sensations from the body, the parietal lobe is called the *primary somatosensory area*. This area receives information primarily from the skin and muscles and allows you to experience the sensations of temperature, pain, light touch, and proprioception (a sense of where your body is). The parietal lobe is also concerned with reading, speech, and taste. Like the motor homunculus in the precentral gyrus, a sensory homunculus can be drawn along the postcentral gyrus (not shown).

Temporal Lobe

The temporal lobe is located inferior to the lateral fissure in an area just above the ear. The temporal lobe contains the primary auditory cortex, the area that allows you to hear. It receives sensory information from the ears. Damage to the temporal lobe causes cortical deafness. The temporal lobe also receives sensory information from the nose; this area is called the *olfactory area*, the area that senses smell. Sensory information from the taste buds in the tongue is interpreted in both the temporal and parietal lobes. Wernicke's area is a broad region that is located in the parietal and temporal lobes; it is concerned with the translation of thought into words. Damage to this area, as occurs with chronic alcohol abuse, can result in severe deficits in language comprehension.

Occipital Lobe

The occipital (ok-SIP-it-al) **lobe** is located in the back of the head, underlying the occipital bone. The occipital lobe contains the visual cortex. Sensory fibers from the eye send information to the primary visual cortex of the occipital lobe, where it is interpreted as sight. The occipital lobe is also concerned with many visual reflexes and vision-related functions such as reading (through the visual association area). Damage to the primary visual cortex of the occipital lobe causes cortical blindness.

FUNCTIONS INVOLVING MANY CEREBRAL LOBES

Speech Area

Although specific functions can be attributed to each cerebral lobe, most functions depend on more than one area of the brain. The speech area, for example, is located in an area that includes the temporal, parietal, and occipital lobes. In most people, the speech area is located in the left hemisphere. The speech area allows you to understand words, whether written or spoken. When you have gathered your thoughts, Broca's area in the frontal lobe directs the muscles of the larynx, tongue, cheeks, and lips to speak.

 Do You Know...

Why a Person Might "Neglect" Half of his Face?

A person with a lesion in the parietal lobe may become unaware of the opposite side of his body. For example, he may not recognize his left leg as his own. When shaving, he may shave only one side of his face. When dressing, he may dress only one side of his body. When eating, he may eat only foods on one side of his plate. This neurological condition is called *contralateral neglect syndrome*.

Other functions require input from more than one brain structure. The ability to read, for example, requires interpretation of the visual information by the occipital lobe. It also requires understanding of the words and the coordination of the eyes as they scan the page. A vast amount of brain tissue beyond the occipital lobe is involved in vision and vision-related functions such as reading.

 Re-Think

1. Identify the cerebral lobes concerned with these functions: vision, hearing, taste, smell, and speech.
2. Identify one consequence of damage to Wernicke's area.

ASSOCIATION AREAS

Large areas of the cerebral cortex are called *association areas* (see Figure 10-11). These areas are concerned primarily with analyzing, interpreting, and integrating information. For example, a small area of the temporal lobe, called the *primary auditory cortex,* receives sensory information from the ear. The surrounding area, called the *auditory association area,* uses a large store of knowledge and experience to identify and give meaning to the sound. In other words, the auditory cortex hears the noise, and the auditory association area interprets the noise. The brain contains receiving and association areas for other sensations as well (e.g., visual association area, somatosensory association area).

PATCHES OF GRAY

Scattered throughout the cerebral white matter are patches of gray matter called *basal nuclei* (sometimes called *basal ganglia*). The basal nuclei help regulate body movement and facial expression. The neurotransmitter dopamine is largely responsible for the activity of the basal nuclei.

A deficiency of dopamine within the basal nuclei is called *Parkinson's disease*. It is a movement disorder or dyskinesia (dis-kin-EE-see-ah). Because of the characteristic shaking (tremors), Parkinson's disease is sometimes called *shaking palsy*. Dopamine-producing drugs are usually prescribed to treat this condition.

DIENCEPHALON

The diencephalon (dye-en-SEF-ah-lon) is the second main area of the brain. It is located beneath the cerebrum and above the brain stem. The diencephalon includes the thalamus and the hypothalamus (Figure 10-13).

The thalamus serves as a relay station for most of the sensory fibers traveling from the lower brain and spinal cord region to the sensory areas of the cerebrum. The thalamus sorts out the sensory information, gives us a hint of the sensation we are to experience, and then directs the information to the specific cerebral areas for more precise interpretation. For example, pain fibers coming from the body to the brain pass through the thalamus. At the level of the thalamus, we become aware of pain, but we are not yet aware of the type of pain or the exact location of the pain. Fibers that transmit pain information from the thalamus to the cerebral cortex provide us with that additional information.

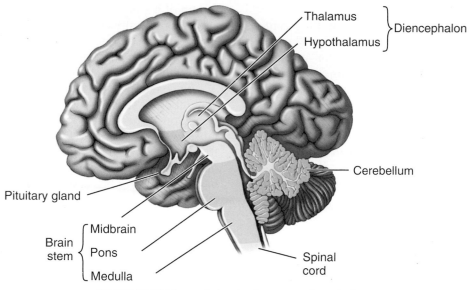

FIGURE 10-13 Diencephalon, brain stem, and cerebellum.

The **hypothalamus** is the second structure in the diencephalon. It is situated directly below the thalamus and helps regulate many body processes, including body temperature (thermostat), water balance, and metabolism. Because the hypothalamus helps regulate the function of the autonomic (involuntary) nerves, it exerts an effect on heart rate, blood pressure, and respiration.

Located under the hypothalamus is the pituitary gland. The pituitary gland directly or indirectly affects almost every hormone in the body. Because the hypothalamus controls pituitary function, the widespread effects of the hypothalamus are obvious. (The relationship of the hypothalamus to endocrine function is described in Chapter 14.)

 Re-Think

1. What role do association areas play? The basal nuclei?
2. What functions are influenced by the hypothalamus?

BRAIN STEM

The **brain stem** connects the spinal cord with higher brain structures. It is composed of the midbrain, pons, and medulla oblongata (see Figure 10-13). The white matter of the brain stem includes tracts that relay both sensory and motor information to and from the cerebrum. Scattered throughout the white matter of the brain stem are patches of gray matter called *nuclei*. These nuclei exert profound effects on functions such as blood pressure and respiration.

MIDBRAIN

The midbrain extends from the lower diencephalon to the pons. Like the rest of the brain stem structures, the midbrain relays sensory and motor information. The midbrain also contains nuclei that function as reflex centers for vision and hearing.

PONS

The pons (bridge) extends from the midbrain to the medulla oblongata. It is composed primarily of tracts that act as a bridge for information traveling to and from several brain structures. The pons also plays an important role in the regulation of breathing rate and rhythm.

MEDULLA OBLONGATA

The **medulla oblongata** (meh-DUL-ah oh-blohn-GAHT-ah) connects the spinal cord with the pons. The medulla acts as a relay for sensory and motor information. Several important nuclei within the medulla control heart rate, blood pressure, and respiration. Because of its importance with regard to vital functions, the medulla oblongata is called the *vital center*. Because these functions are vital to the body, you can understand the seriousness of a fracture at the base of the skull.

The medulla oblongata is also extremely sensitive to certain drugs, especially opioids such as morphine. An overdose of an opioid causes depression of the medulla oblongata and death because the person stops breathing. This danger is the reason for counting the respiratory rate before giving a patient an opioid. If the respiratory rate is less than 10 respirations per minute, the drug cannot be safely administered.

 Do You Know...

How the Brain Tranquilizes Itself?

The brain produces natural morphine-like substances called *endorphins* (endogenous morphine) and *enkephalins* (meaning "in the head"). Like morphine, these substances bind to opiate receptors in the CNS, moderating pain, relieving anxiety, and producing a sense of well-being. The "high" experienced by joggers may be caused by endorphins and enkephalins.

Vomiting Center

The medulla oblongata contains the vomiting center, or emetic center (emesis refers to vomiting). The vomiting center can be activated directly or indirectly. Direct activation includes stimuli from the cerebral cortex (fear), stimuli from sensory organs (distressing sights, bad odors, pain), and signals from the equilibrium apparatus of the inner ear (spinning). Indirect stimulation of the vomiting center comes from the chemoreceptor trigger zone (CTZ) located in the floor of the fourth ventricle. The CTZ can be stimulated by emetogenic compounds, such as anticancer drugs and opioids. Signals from the digestive tract, especially the stomach, travel via the vagus nerve to the CTZ. The CTZ, in turn, activates the vomiting center. Antiemetic agents can work on both the CTZ and medullary vomiting center to relieve nausea and vomiting. The pharmacological management of vomiting is a common clinical problem. Another interesting point is that nausea, which usually precedes vomiting, is derived from the Greek word for "ship," as in seasickness.

 Re-Think

1. List the three parts of the brain stem.
2. Why is the medulla oblongata called the "vital center"?
3. Differentiate between the vomiting center and the CTZ.

CEREBELLUM

The cerebellum (sair-eh-BELL-um), the fourth major area, is the structure that protrudes from under the occipital lobe at the base of the skull (see Figure 10-13). The cerebellum is connected to the brain stem by three pair of cerebellar peduncles (sair-eh-BELL-ahr peh-DUN-kuls); these stalks or connections allow the cerebellum to receive, integrate, and deliver information to many parts of the brain and spinal cord. The cerebellum is concerned with the coordination of voluntary muscle activity. Information is sent to the cerebellum from many areas throughout the body, including the eyes, ears, and skeletal muscles. The cerebellum integrates all the incoming information to produce a smooth, coordinated muscle response. Damage to the cerebellum produces jerky muscle movements, staggering gait, and difficulty maintaining balance or equilibrium. The person with cerebellar dysfunction may appear intoxicated. To help diagnose cerebellar dysfunction, the physician may ask the person to touch the tip of his or her nose with a finger. Why? The cerebellum normally coordinates skeletal muscle activity. In attempting to touch the nose, a patient with cerebellar dysfunction may overshoot, first to one side and then to the other.

The cerebellum also plays an important role in the evaluation of sensory input. For example, the cerebellum allows a person to evaluate the texture of different fabrics without seeing the fabric. It also "times" events, thereby allowing the person to predict where a moving object will be in the next few seconds. For example, a basketball player has a keen sense of where the ball is and should be in the next dribble or two. And, most of us can rhythmically drum our fingers on a desk—a task that is impaired in someone with cerebellar dysfunction.

 Do You Know...

Where and Why There Is a Tent in Your Brain?

At several areas in the brain, the dura mater forms rigid membranes that separate and support parts of the brain. One such membrane is the tentorium cerebelli; it forms a tentlike membrane over the cerebellum, separating it from the upper cerebral structures. The tentorium also functions as a common landmark in the brain. Brain tumors are classified according to their locations; those that occur in structures located above the tentorium are called *supratentorial brain tumors*, and those occurring below the tentorium are called *infratentorial brain tumors*. An increase in intracranial pressure can force the brain downward past the tentorium, causing life-threatening symptoms. The displacement is called *tentorial herniation*.

Re-Think

Locate and list two functions of the cerebellum.

STRUCTURES ACROSS DIVISIONS OF THE BRAIN

Three important structures are not confined to any of the four divisions of the brain because they "overlap" several areas. These structures are the limbic system, the reticular system, and the memory areas.

LIMBIC SYSTEM: THE EMOTIONAL BRAIN

Parts of the cerebrum and the diencephalon form a wishbone-shaped group of structures called the *limbic system*. The limbic system functions in emotional states and behavior. For example, when the limbic system is stimulated by electrodes, states of extreme pleasure or rage can be induced. Because of these responses, the limbic system is called the *emotional brain*.

RETICULAR FORMATION: WAKE UP!

What keeps us awake? Why don't we slip into a coma when we go to sleep? Extending through the entire brain stem, with numerous connections to the cerebral cortex, is a special mass of gray matter called the reticular formation. The reticular formation is concerned with the sleep–wake cycle and consciousness. Signals passing up to the cerebral cortex from the reticular formation stimulate us, keeping us awake and tuned in.

Other nuclei within the reticular formation include the gaze centers (allow the eyes to track an object) and special groups of cells that rhythmically send signals to the muscles that control breathing and swallowing. The reticular formation is also concerned with habituation, the process whereby the brain learns to ignore repetitive background information. For example, a parent may ignore the background noise of children playing and horns honking, but responds immediately to a crying child. Similarly, while driving a car, you ignore much of the background visual information, but are aware of traffic signals, nearby cars and, hopefully, any oncoming vehicles.

The reticular formation is very sensitive to the effects of certain drugs and alcohol. For example, the dangerous combination of benzodiazepines (tranquilizers) and alcohol can damage the reticular formation, causing permanent unconsciousness.

Consciousness, Sleep, and Coma

Consciousness is a state of wakefulness and is dependent on the reticular activating system (RAS). The RAS continuously samples sensory information from all over the body and then selects and presents essential, unusual, and threatening information to the higher structures in the cerebral cortex. The different levels of consciousness include attentiveness, alertness, relaxation, and inattentiveness. Sleep occurs when the RAS is inhibited or slowed. What causes sleep? In the sixth century BC, it was believed that sleep was caused by a temporary retreat of blood from the brain. Death was attributed to the permanent retreat of blood from the brain. As to the cause of sleep? We still do not know. What we do know is that neurotransmitters are replenished during sleep. We also know that most Americans do not get enough sleep (most adults require 7 to 8 hours of sleep) and that sleep deprivation is linked to numerous health problems, such as obesity, diabetes mellitus, and hypertension.

Coma is a hyporesponsive state with several stages, ranging from light to deep coma. In the lightest stages of coma, some reflexes are intact; the patient may respond to light, sound, touch, and painful stimuli. As the coma deepens, however, these reflexes are gradually lost, and the patient eventually becomes unresponsive to all stimuli. Damage to the reticular formation is associated with a state of deep coma, which can be permanent.

Many clinical conditions affect level of consciousness (LOC), often leading to coma. These include brain tumors, brain injury, drugs, toxins, hypoxia, hyperglycemia, acid-base imbalance, and electrolyte imbalance. As a clinician, you must be able to assess the patient's LOC.

? Re-Think

1. Locate the limbic system and explain why it is called the "emotional brain."
2. State a major role of the reticular activating system.
3. Why is LOC evaluated?

Stages of Sleep

The two types of sleep are non–rapid eye movement (NREM) sleep and rapid eye movement (REM) sleep. The four stages of NREM sleep progress from light to deep. In a typical 8-hour sleep period, a person regularly cycles through the various stages of sleep, descending from light to deep sleep and then ascending from deeper sleep to lighter sleep.

REM sleep is characterized by fluctuating blood pressure, respiratory rate and rhythm, and pulse rate. The most obvious characteristic of REM sleep is rapid eye movements, for which the sleep segment is named. REM sleep totals 90 to 120 minutes per night; most dreaming occurs during REM sleep. For unknown reasons, REM sleep deprivation is associated with mental and physical distress. Most sedatives and CNS depressants adversely affect REM sleep, perhaps accounting for that "hangover" feeling that often follows their use.

Do You Know...

About Chemo Fog?

We all know that many drugs exert profound effects on the brain. There is the euphoria of opioids, the hallucinogenic effects of LSD, the "buzz" of methamphetamines, the sedation of antihistamines, and the list goes on. For many years, breast cancer survivors have complained of (while being ignored) the lingering effects of their cancer chemotherapy. Many noted difficulty with memory, attention span, retrieving words, multitasking, and clarity of thought. (One woman filled the water glasses with turkey gravy at a Thanksgiving Day dinner.) They complained of "living in a fog"—hence, the term *chemo fog* or *chemobrain*. Chemo fog is real and lingers for many months, even years, after the chemo has ended! Today it has a new respectable name: *postchemotherapy cognitive impairment*, or *postchemotherapy cognitive dysfunction*.

MEMORY AREAS

Memory is the ability to recall thoughts and images. Many areas of the brain are concerned with memory. There are three categories of memory: immediate memory, short-term memory, and long-term memory. Immediate memory lasts for a few seconds. An example of your immediate memory is your ability to remember the words in the first part of the sentence so that you can get the thought of the entire sentence. Short-term memory lasts for a short period (seconds to a few hours). It allows you to recall bits of information, such as the price of those new jeans or a phone number that you looked up. Unfortunately, cramming for exams falls into this category—short-term memorization, 5-second retention, and then—BLANK. Long-term memory lasts much longer—years, decades, or lifetime. If you continuously use the new address or phone number, you will enter that information into your long-term memory. The same effect is achieved when you study over a longer period. Another interesting point: although memory is important, forgetting is also important. Imagine all the trivial information that you take in every second. Think of the many stones, trees, birds, street signs, and other things that you pass on your way to work. Persons who have difficulty in forgetting trivia have a great deal of difficulty in comprehension and in remembering things that need to be remembered.

 Re-Think

1. What is REM sleep?
2. List the three categories of memory. Explain why "cramming" for an exam is an ineffectual learning process.

Do You Know...

Why People in Ancient Times Bored Holes in the Skull?

Trephination refers to the drilling of holes into the skull for the purpose of reducing intracranial pressure. Today, it is performed in the operating room under sterile conditions; the surgically drilled holes are called *burr holes*. People in ancient times also performed trephination procedures. The patient sat on a log while the priest chipped a hole in the skull using a sharp stone. Ouch! It was thought that trephination could relieve headaches and release the devils of madness.

PROTECTING THE CENTRAL NERVOUS SYSTEM

The tissue of the CNS (brain and spinal cord) is very delicate. Injury to CNS neuronal tissue cannot be repaired. Thus, the CNS has an elaborate protective system that consists of four structures: bone, meninges, cerebrospinal fluid, and the blood–brain barrier.

BONE: FIRST LAYER OF PROTECTION

The CNS is protected by bone. The brain is encased in the cranium, and the spinal cord is encased in the vertebral column.

MENINGES: SECOND LAYER OF PROTECTION

Three layers of connective tissue surround the brain and spinal cord (Figure 10-14). These tissues are called the **meninges** (meh-NIN-jeez). The outermost layer is a thick, tough, connective tissue called the *dura mater,* literally meaning "hard mother." Inside the skull, the dural membrane splits to form the dural sinuses. These sinuses are filled with blood. Beneath the dura mater is a small space called the *subdural space.* The middle layer is the arachnoid (ah-RAK-noyd) mater (meaning "spider-like"), so-named because the membrane looks like a spider web.

The pia mater is the innermost layer and literally means soft, or gentle, mother. The pia mater is a very thin membrane that contains many blood vessels and lies delicately over the brain and spinal cord. These blood vessels supply the brain with much of its blood. Between the arachnoid layer and the pia mater is a space called the *subarachnoid space.* A fluid called the **cerebrospinal fluid (CSF)** circulates within this space and forms a cushion around the brain and spinal cord. If the head is jarred suddenly, the brain first bumps into this soft cushion of fluid. Specialized projections of the arachnoid membrane, called the *arachnoid villi* (sing., villus), protrude up into the blood-filled dural sinuses and are involved in the drainage of the CSF (described in the next section).

Remember—the meninges form a brain **PAD** (noting that the brain is closer to pia, the softer mother):

P	**p**ia mater
A	**a**rachnoid mater
D	**d**ura mater

The meninges can become inflamed or infected, causing meningitis. Meningitis is serious because the infection can spread to the brain, sometimes causing serious, irreversible brain damage. The bacterial or viral organism causing the meningitis can often be found in a sample of CSF obtained by lumbar puncture.

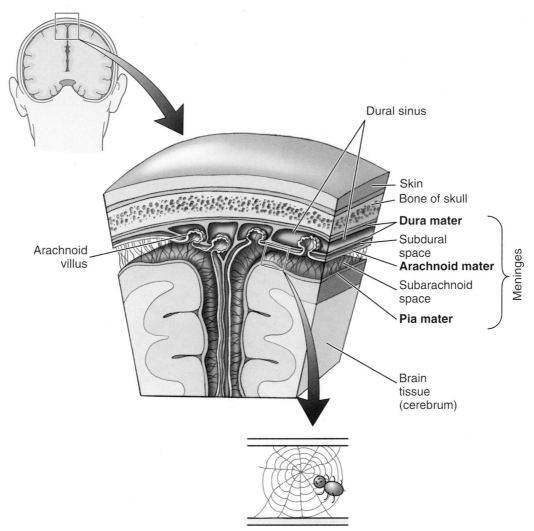

FIGURE 10-14 Three layers of meninges: the dura mater, arachnoid mater, and pia mater.

CEREBROSPINAL FLUID: THIRD LAYER OF PROTECTION

The CSF forms a third protective layer of the CNS. CSF is formed from the blood within the brain. It is a clear fluid that looks like clear soda and is similar in composition to plasma. The CSF is composed of water, glucose, protein, and several ions, especially Na$^+$ and Cl$^-$. An adult circulates about 130 mL of CSF; 500 mL is formed every 24 hours, so that CSF is replaced every 8 hours. In addition to its protective function, CSF also delivers nutrients to the CNS and removes waste.

Where is CSF formed? CSF is formed within the ventricles of the brain by a structure called the *choroid plexus* (Figure 10-15). The four ventricles are two lateral ventricles and a third and fourth ventricle. The choroid plexus, a grapelike collection of blood vessels and ependymal cells (see Table 10-1), is suspended from the roof of each ventricle. Water and dissolved substances are transported from the blood across the walls of the choroid plexus into the ventricles (see Figure 10-15).

Where does the CSF flow? As CSF leaves the ventricles, it follows two paths. Some of the CSF flows through a hole in the center of the spinal cord called the *central canal*. The central canal eventually drains into the subarachnoid space at the base of the spinal cord. The rest of the CSF flows from the fourth ventricle laterally through tiny holes, or foramina, into the subarachnoid space that encircles the brain.

How does the CSF leave the subarachnoid space? Eventually, CSF flows into the arachnoid villi; water and waste diffuse from CSF in the arachnoid villi into the blood of the dural sinuses. Blood then flows from the dural sinuses into the cerebral veins and back to the heart. Remember that the CSF is formed across the walls of the choroid plexus within the ventricles, circulates throughout the subarachnoid space around the brain and spinal cord, and then drains into the dural sinuses. The rate at which CSF is formed must equal the rate at which it is drained. If excess CSF is formed or drainage is impaired, CSF will accumulate in the ventricles of the brain, increasing the pressure within the skull. The resulting increase in intracranial pressure can cause brain damage and death.

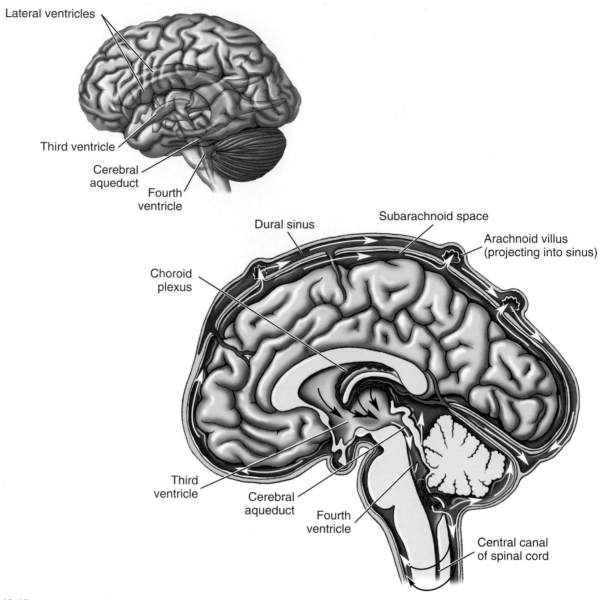

FIGURE 10-15 Cerebrospinal fluid: formation (choroid plexus in ventricles), circulation within the subarachnoid space, and drainage (arachnoid villus and dural sinus).

Do You Know...

Why an Infant May Develop Water on the Brain?

Occasionally, a newborn infant is born with an obstruction (e.g., tumor) in the ventricular system of the brain. Cerebrospinal fluid (CSF) is formed at a normal rate but cannot be drained because of the obstruction. The fluid accumulates within the ventricles, thereby increasing intracranial pressure and causing the skull to enlarge. This condition is called *hydrocephalus* (water on the brain). Head expansion in the infant is possible because the suture lines of the skull bones have not yet fused. If an obstruction were to occur in an older child or adult, the intracranial pressure would increase. The skull, however, could not expand because of the fused sutures. Without surgical intervention or the use of a shunt that bypasses the obstruction, the increased pressure would result in death.

Do You Know...

What a Little Red Worm's Doing in Your Brain?

In the 1300s, an anatomist claimed that mental function was controlled by a red worm. The worm referred to the fleshy choroid plexus of the ventricles of the brain. The plexi allegedly controlled brain functions by wiggling back and forth and modifying the flow of cerebrospinal fluid, which was supposed to contain the animal spirit. Several things have since been cleared up; mental function is the result of neuronal activity and not the flow of animal spirit, and the choroid plexus secretes cerebrospinal fluid and does not wiggle and shake. There is, however, a little red worm—the choroid plexus—and it is located in the ventricles of your brain where it secretes CSF.

? Re-Think

1. Trace the formation, flow, and drainage of cerebrospinal fluid.
2. What is the consequence of obstructed drainage of CSF?

BLOOD–BRAIN BARRIER: FOURTH LAYER OF PROTECTION

The blood–brain barrier is an arrangement of cells, particularly the glial astrocytes and the selectively permeable capillary cells; they act as a barrier to the movement of potentially harmful chemicals into the CNS. The astrocytes and the capillary cells select the substances allowed to enter the CNS from the blood. For example, oxygen, glucose, and certain ions readily cross the membrane. However, if a potentially harmful substance is present in the blood, the cells of the blood–brain barrier prevent that substance from entering the brain and the spinal cord.

Although the blood–brain barrier is successful in screening many harmful substances, not all toxic substances are blocked. Alcohol, for example, crosses the blood–brain barrier and affects brain tissue.

The blood–brain barrier may present a problem in the pharmacological treatment of infections within the CNS. Most antibiotics, for example, cannot cross the blood–brain barrier and therefore cannot reach the site of infection. Given this problem, how is an infection of the CNS treated? The two options are to select an antibiotic that does cross the blood–brain barrier or inject the antibiotic directly into the subarachnoid space; this mode of drug delivery is called an *intrathecal injection*.

2+2 Sum It Up!

The CNS, especially the brain, performs eloquently as a conductor. It coordinates the various organ systems of the body efficiently, with fine precision. The brain makes us humans—that is, thinking, caring, feeling, remembering persons. The brain is divided into four regions: the cerebrum, diencephalon, brain stem, and cerebellum. The cerebrum is the largest part of the brain and has four lobes: frontal, parietal, temporal, and occipital. The diencephalon is composed of the thalamus and the hypothalamus. The brain stem is composed of the midbrain, pons, and medulla oblongata. The medulla oblongata is considered the vital structure in that it affects basic functions such as respiration, cardiac function, and blood vessel tone. Three other areas are the reticular formation, which keeps us awake; the limbic system (emotional brain); and the memory areas. Because of the crucial role played by the CNS, it is afforded excellent protection—that is, bone, three layers of meninges, a soft cushion of fluid, and a blood–brain barrier.

? Re-Think

What effect may the blood–brain barrier have on drug distribution?

As You Age

1. Beginning at the age of 30, the number of neurons decreases. The number lost, however, is only a small percentage of the total number of brain cells and does not cause mental impairment. Although a decrease in short-term memory may cause some forgetfulness, most memory, alertness, intellectual functioning, and creativity remain intact. Severe alteration of mental functioning is generally caused by age-related diseases such as arteriosclerosis.
2. Impulse conduction speed decreases along an axon, amounts of neurotransmitters are reduced, and the number of receptor sites decreases at the synapses. These changes result in progressive slowing of responses and reflexes.

MEDICAL TERMINOLOGY AND DISORDERS   Disorders of the Brain

Medical Term	Word Parts	Word Part Meaning or Derivation	Description
Words			
meninges		From a Latin word meaning "membrane"	The **meninges** are *the three membranes that form the outer lining of the brain and spinal cord.* The Arabians referred to these membranes as *mater* (mother) because they believed these membranes were the "mother" of all membranes.
neurology	neur/o-	nerve	**Neurology** is *the study of the structure, function, and organic disorders of the nervous system.*
	-logy	study of	
polarize		From a French word meaning a "division within a group"	*Refers to a separation of electrical charge.* A **polarized** nerve cell has a negative charge on the inside of the cell membrane and a positive charge on the outside of the cell membrane. The electric charge of a **depolarized** (*de* = away from) cell becomes positive. A **repolarized** (*re* = again) cell has returned to an internal negative charge.
synapse	syn-	together	A **synapse** is *a junction or meeting place for two neurons.* The axon of one neuron interacts chemically at a **synapse** with the dendrite of a second neuron.
	-apse	From a Greek word, *haptein,* meaning "to clasp"	
Disorders			
cephalgia	cephal/o-	head	*Pain in the head or headache.* An example is the **migraine headache,** a severe, recurring headache that usually affects only one side of the head. (Migraine comes from the Latin *hemicranium,* meaning "one side of the head.") A simple **tension headache** may develop when a person is anxious or tense. Headaches may also develop secondarily in response to increased intracranial pressure (e.g., brain tumor), irritation of the meninges, or spasm of the cerebral blood vessels. **Cluster headaches** occur in cyclical patterns and are called "alarm clock headaches" because they often awaken the person with intense and sharp pain in and around one eye.
	-algia	pain	
cerebrovascular accident (CVA)			Called a **CVA, stroke,** or **brain attack.** A CVA is caused by a sudden lack of blood, causing oxygen deprivation and brain damage. Depending on the location and severity of the brain damage, a CVA can result in loss of sensory and motor function and speech impairment. The patient often experiences **hemiparalysis** (hemi- = half) and **hemiparesis.** In addition to loss of motor function, the patient experiences various types of **aphasia** (a- = without; phas/o = speech), *an impairment of language.* Prior to suffering a stroke, many persons will have experienced a **transient ischemic attack** (TIA), or *mini stroke.* During a TIA, blood flow to the brain is temporarily stopped or diminished.
dementia	de-	without	Originally from the Latin meaning "madness." **Dementia** is not a single disease, but *a group of symptoms affecting intellectual and social abilities to the extent that daily living is impaired.* There is a serious loss of cognitive ability, with impairment of language, problem solving, memory, attention, and judgment. Behavior may be disorganized, restless, and inappropriate. **Static dementia** is commonly caused by traumatic brain injury. **Progressive dementia** refers to a long-term decline and is caused by chronic conditions such as Alzheimer's disease, multiple sclerosis, and small or mini strokes **(vascular dementia).**
	-ment/o-	mind	
	-ia	condition of	

MEDICAL TERMINOLOGY AND DISORDERS | Disorders of the Brain—cont'd

Medical Term	Word Parts	Word Part Meaning or Derivation	Description
dyskinesias	dys-	difficulty	*Any medical disorder that is characterized by diminished voluntary muscle control (a movement disorder).* This broad term includes Parkinson's disease, Tourette's syndrome (muscle tics, verbal outbursts, sometimes profanity), chorea ("dance-like" muscle contractions that begin in one part of the body [toe] and work their way to another part [leg]), athetosis (graceful but purposeless movements primarily of the extremities), and asterixis ("flapping tremor" of the wrists). The term **dyskinesia** also includes many dystonias (impaired muscle tone), sustained muscle contractions that twist or contort the body. Some types of dyskinesias are localized, as in torticollis (lateral flexion of the neck caused by muscle spasm), whereas others are generalized, as in epileptic seizures. Tardive dyskinesias (TDs), often a result of antipsychotic drug therapy and dopaminergic antagonists, are characterized by involuntary movement of the lips (lip smacking), tongue (tongue rolling, protrusions), face, trunk, and extremities. Drug-induced TDs are usually irreversible.
	-kinesi/o-	movement	
	-ia	condition of	
encephalopathy	en-	within	*A broad term that refers to disease, damage, or dysfunction of the brain.* There are more than 150 types. The term **encephalopathy** is often described by its cause. **Anoxic encephalopathy** is due to a lack of oxygen, whereas **hepatic encephalopathy** is a response to liver disease. Chronic and excessive ingestion of alcohol causes irreversible injury to the nervous system. The result is mental deterioration, loss of memory, inability to concentrate, irritability, and uncoordinated movement. **Wernicke-Korsakoff syndrome** is an alcohol-related type of encephalopathy.
	-cephal/o-	head	
	-path/o-	disease	
	-y	condition or process	
epilepsy	epi-	upon	Historically referred to as the "sacred disease" by the ancients because they believed that epilepsy was a punishment for offending the gods. Epilepsy is a group of neurological disorders that all present with spontaneous seizure activity. Neurons in the brain fire suddenly, unpredictably, and repetitively, creating "electrical storms" in the brain. Although most cases of epilepsy are idiopathic (arising spontaneously; unknown) in origin, many underlying conditions cause seizure activity: brain tumors, toxins, trauma, fever **(febrile seizures),** and emotional stress. Epileptic seizures are classified as primarily generalized seizures (widespread electrical storm including both sides of the brain) and partial seizures (more limited brain involvement and localized responses). There are many types of seizures, two of which are **tonic-clonic seizures** (grand mal) and **absence seizures** (petit mal). **Grand mal** (big bad) seizures are described as tonic-clonic. The tonic phase of a grand mal seizure occurs when the motor areas fire repetitively, causing muscle stiffening, and loss of consciousness. The clonic phase is characterized by jerking activity. **Status epilepticus,** a medical emergency, refers to the failure of the seizures to resolve or to the rapid succession of seizure activity. **Petit mal** (small bad) seizures occur when sensory areas are affected, causing a brief period (5-15 sec) of altered consciousness. Petit mal seizures are not accompanied by generalized stiffening or prolonged unconsciousness and are often unnoticed. Epileptic seizures are described by the term **ictus.**
		From a Latin word meaning "seized upon" (by the gods)	
glioma	gli/o-	glue	**Glioma** is *the most common type of primary brain tumors in adults.* They arise from glial tissue, most commonly astrocytic (star-shaped) tissue (astrocytoma). The second most common brain tumor is a **meningioma,** arising from the meninges. Brain tumors can be malignant or benign.
	-oma	tumor	

Continued

MEDICAL TERMINOLOGY AND DISORDERS   Disorders of the Brain—cont'd

Medical Term	Word Parts	Word Part Meaning or Derivation	Description
head injury			*Due to trauma of the head, and may or may not involve the brain.* A **traumatic brain injury** (TBI) occurs when an external force traumatically injures the brain. TBI is a major cause of death and disability worldwide. Initially, brain injury is due to direct impact or by acceleration/deceleration alone; additional injury is sustained secondarily by injury-induced diminishment of blood flood and increases in intracranial pressure. A mechanism-related classification system divides TBIs into closed and penetrating head injuries. A **closed head injury** occurs when the brain is not exposed, as in blunt trauma. A **penetrating (open) head injury** occurs when the penetrating object pierces the dura mater. Depending on its severity and location, TBI causes numerous deficits: physical, emotional, social, and cognitive. Trauma to the head can cause bleeding and the formation of a **hematoma,** *a swelling or tumor formed by a collection of blood.* An **epidural hematoma** forms between the dura mater and the skull. A **subdural hematoma** forms under the dura mater.
hydrocephalus	hydro- -cephal/o-	water head	Called "water on the brain." There is an abnormal accumulation of cerebrospinal fluid (CSF) within the cerebral ventricles that can cause enlargement of the cranium. The clinical presentation is dependent on chronicity and age. There is also a **normal pressure hydrocephalus** (NPH), which develops more gradually in the elderly and is characterized by intermittent episodes of increased intracranial pressure.
infection		From the Latin word *inficere,* meaning transmission of disease by agency of air or water	The brain can be infected by a large number of microorganisms, most commonly bacteria and viruses. The pathogens cause inflammation of the surrounding tissue. **Encephalitis** is *inflammation of the brain itself.* **Meningitis** is *inflammation of the meninges.* A **brain abscess** is *a collection of infectious material within the brain.* Globally, bacterial meningitis is a major health concern in children. African children living in the "meningitis belt" are particularly vulnerable.
neurotoxin	neur/o- -tox/o-	nerve poison	*Any natural or artificial toxic substance that is toxic or harmful to nervous tissue.* Commonly encountered neurotoxins include chemotherapeutic drugs, organic solvents, pesticides, cosmetics, heavy metals, alcohol ingestion, and exposure to radiation. There are some naturally occurring neurotoxins, including beta-amyloid and glutamate.
palsy			A generalized term that refers to a loss of motor function. Three types of palsy are cerebral palsy, Bell's palsy, and brachial palsy (Erb's palsy). **Cerebral palsy** (CP), also called **spastic paralysis,** is a consequence of brain injury most often occurring in response to anoxic conditions around birth. All persons with CP experience muscle tightness and spasm causing limitations in muscle movement. **Bell's palsy** is due to inflammation or injury to the facial nerve (CN VII). **Brachial palsy** is usually caused by damage to the brachial plexus during a traumatic birth experience.
Parkinson's disease		Named after J. Parkinson, an English professor who wrote extensively about the disease	Called "shaking palsy." **Parkinson's disease** (PD) is *a dyskinesia that is classified as a movement disorder; it is due to diminished dopaminergic cell activity in the basal ganglia.* PD is characterized by tremors (rest tremors) or shaking of the extremities, especially the hands and jaw; rigidity (muscle stiffness), **akinesia** (inability to initiate voluntary movement), **bradykinesia** (slow voluntary movement), stooped posture, shuffling or freezing gait, poor balance, slow speech, and drooling. Cognitive abilities are generally preserved. **Parkinsonism** is a broad term that refers to disorders that present with similar symptoms. For instance, prolonged use of antipsychotic drugs and brain injuries sustained by boxers cause symptoms similar to PD.

Get Ready for Exams!

Summary Outline

The purpose of the nervous system is to bring information to the central nervous system, interpret the information, and enable the body to respond to the information.

I. The Nervous System: Overview
  A. Divisions of the nervous system
   1. The central nervous system (CNS) includes the brain and the spinal cord.
   2. The peripheral nervous system includes the nerves that connect the CNS with the rest of the body.
  B. Cells that make up the nervous system
   1. Neuroglia (glia) support, protect, and nourish the neurons.
   2. Neurons conduct the nerve impulse.
   3. The three parts of a neuron are the dendrites, cell body, and axon.
  C. Types of neurons
   1. Sensory, or afferent, neurons carry information toward the CNS.
   2. Interneurons are located in the CNS (make connections).
   3. Motor, or efferent, neurons carry information away from the CNS toward the periphery.
  D. White matter and gray matter
   1. White matter is the result of myelinated fibers.
   2. Gray matter is composed primarily of cell bodies, interneurons, and unmyelinated fibers.
   3. Clusters of cell bodies (gray matter) are called *nuclei* and *ganglia*.

II. The Neuron Carrying Information
  A. Nerve impulse
   1. The electrical signal is called the *action potential* or *nerve impulse*.
   2. The nerve impulse is caused by the following changes in the neuron: polarization, depolarization, and repolarization.
   3. The nerve impulse results from the flow of ions: polarization (outward leak of K^+), depolarization (influx of Na^+), and repolarization (outward flux of K^+).
   4. The nerve impulse jumps from node to node as it travels along a myelinated fiber. Myelination increases the speed of the nerve impulse.
   5. The nerve impulse causes the release of the neurotransmitter at the synapse.
  B. Synapse
   1. The synapse is a space between two neurons.
   2. The nerve impulse of the first (presynaptic) neuron causes the release of neurotransmitter into the synaptic cleft. The neurotransmitter diffuses across the synaptic cleft and binds to the receptors on the second (postsynaptic) membrane. The activation of the receptors stimulates a nerve impulse in the second neuron.

III. Brain: Structure and Function
  A. Cerebrum
   1. The right and left hemispheres are joined by the corpus callosum.
   2. The four main cerebral lobes are the frontal, parietal, temporal, and occipital lobes. Functions of each lobe are summarized in Table 10-2.
   3. Large areas of the cerebrum, called *association areas,* are concerned with interpreting, integrating, and analyzing information.
  B. Diencephalon
   1. The thalamus is a relay station for most sensory tracts traveling to the cerebrum.
   2. The hypothalamus controls many body functions such as water balance, temperature, and the secretion of hormones from the pituitary gland. It exerts an effect on the autonomic nervous system.
  C. Brain stem
   1. Brain stem: midbrain, pons, and medulla oblongata
   2. The medulla oblongata is called the *vital center* because it controls the heart rate, blood pressure, and respirations (the vital functions).
   3. The vomiting center is located in the medulla oblongata; it receives input directly and indirectly from activation of the chemoreceptor trigger zone (CTZ).
  D. Cerebellum
   1. The cerebellum is sometimes called the *little brain*.
   2. The cerebellum is concerned primarily with the coordination of voluntary muscle activity.
  E. Structures involving more than one lobe
   1. The limbic system is sometimes called the *emotional brain*.
   2. The reticular formation is concerned with the sleep–wake cycle. It keeps us conscious and prevents us from slipping into a coma state.
   3. The memory areas handle immediate, short-term, and long-term memory.

IV. Protection of the CNS
  A. Bone: cranium and vertebral column
  B. Meninges: pia mater, arachnoid mater, and dura mater
  C. Cerebrospinal fluid (CSF): circulates within the subarachnoid space
  D. Blood–brain barrier

Review Your Knowledge

Matching: Nerve Cells

Directions: Match the following words with their descriptions below.

a. efferent
b. ganglia
c. CNS
d. neuroglia
e. afferent
f. axon
g. nodes of Ranvier
h. Schwann cell
i. dendrite
j. myelin

1. ___ Also described as sensory neurons
2. ___ Nerve glue—astrocytes and ependymal cells
3. ___ Part of the neuron that carries the action potential away from the cell body
4. ___ Also described as motor neurons
5. ___ Composed of the brain and the spinal cord
6. ___ Clusters of cell bodies located outside of the CNS
7. ___ White insulating material that surrounds the axon; increases the speed that the signal travels along the axon
8. ___ Short segments of an axon that are not covered with myelin; allow for saltatory conduction
9. ___ A glial cell that makes myelin
10. ___ Treelike structure of the neuron that receives information from another neuron and transmits that information to the cell body

Matching: Brain

Directions: Match the following words with their descriptions below.

a. medulla oblongata
b. frontal
c. occipital
d. hypothalamus
e. temporal

1. ___ Cerebral lobe that performs the "executive functions" and contains the primary motor cortex
2. ___ Part of the brain stem that is called the *vital center*
3. ___ Part of the diencephalon that controls body temperature (thermostat) and endocrine function by its influence on the pituitary gland
4. ___ Cerebral lobe that contains the primary visual cortex
5. ___ Cerebral lobe that contains the primary auditory cortex

Multiple Choice

1. The precentral gyrus is
   a. located in the parietal lobe.
   b. the primary motor cortex.
   c. the primary visual cortex.
   d. a brain stem structure.
2. Which of the following is not descriptive of Broca's area?
   a. Located in the frontal lobe
   b. Concerned with motor speech
   c. Most often located in the left cerebral hemisphere
   d. Is the name of the frontal eye field area

3. Which of the following "brain claims" is true?
   a. The medulla oblongata is a cerebral structure.
   b. The hypothalamus is a brain stem structure.
   c. The medulla oblongata descends as the spinal cord.
   d. The midbrain, pons, and medulla oblongata are supratentorial structures.
4. Which of the following is not descriptive of the medulla oblongata?
   a. It is a brain stem structure.
   b. It is called the *vital center*.
   c. It is sensitive to the effects of narcotics (opioids).
   d. It performs the "executive" functions.
5. The postcentral gyrus
   a. is located in the parietal lobe.
   b. controls all voluntary motor activity.
   c. is the home of Broca's area.
   d. contains the primary visual cortex.
6. Cerebrospinal fluid (CSF)
   a. drains out of the subarachnoid space into the choroid plexus.
   b. circulates within the subarachnoid space.
   c. looks like blood.
   d. flows up the central canal into the fourth, third, and lateral ventricles.
7. Which of the following relationships is accurate?
   a. Temporal lobe: vision
   b. Frontal lobe: somatosensory (touch, pressure, pain)
   c. Occipital lobe: vision
   d. Parietal lobe: hearing
8. Neuroglia
   a. are classified as sensory and motor.
   b. include astrocytes, oligodendrocytes, Schwann cells, and ependymal cells.
   c. fire action potentials when stimulated.
   d. contain dendrites and axons.
9. Depolarization and repolarization
   a. are both caused by the movement of Na^+ into the neuron.
   b. are phases of the action potential.
   c. occur only in the neuroglia.
   d. are both caused by the movement of K^+ out of the neuron.
10. Activation of the emetic center or CTZ
    a. elevates blood pressure.
    b. lowers body temperature.
    c. causes diaphoresis.
    d. induces vomiting.
11. The hypothalamus
    a. is part of the diencephalon.
    b. synthesizes antidiuretic hormone and oxytocin.
    c. controls pituitary gland activity.
    d. All of the above are true.

Go Figure

1. **According to Figure 10-4**
   a. All axon terminals are myelinated.
   b. The electrical signal runs from the cell body, along the axon, to the axon terminals.
   c. Nodes of Ranvier are myelinated axonal membrane.
   d. All dendrites are myelinated.

2. **According to Figure 10-6**
   a. Panel B illustrates the influx of Na^+ and depolarization.
   b. Panel B illustrates the influx of Na^+ and repolarization.
   c. Panel C illustrates the influx of K^+ and depolarization.
   d. Panel C illustrates the efflux of K^+ and depolarization.

3. **Figure 10-8 illustrates**
   a. The formation of a nerve impulse at each node.
   b. The effect of myelination on conduction velocity (the speed that the nerve impulse travels along the axon).
   c. Saltatory conduction.
   d. All of the above are true.

4. **According to Figure 10-9**
   a. Acetylcholine (ACh) is an enzyme that inactivates acetylcholinesterase.
   b. Acetylcholinesterase inactivates ACh immediately after its release from the axon terminal.
   c. The receptors on the membrane of neuron B are activated by ACh.
   d. Both acetylcholine and acetylcholinesterase are stored within the vesicles of the axon terminal.

5. **According to Figures 10-10 and 10-11**
   a. The brain stem is located superior to the diencephalon.
   b. The primary motor cortex and the primary somatosensory area are separated by the lateral sulcus.
   c. The primary visual cortex is located within the cerebrum.
   d. The cerebellum is located anterior to the brain stem and superior to the diencephalon.

6. **According to Figures 10-12 and 10-13**
   a. The homunculus in Figure 10-12 is a sensory homunculus.
   b. The homunculus in Figure 10-12 lies over the cerebellum.
   c. The brain stem refers to the midbrain, pons, and medulla oblongata.
   d. The diencephalon is superior to the thalamus.

7. **According to Figures 10-14 and 10-15**
   a. Cerebrospinal fluid is secreted by the arachnoid villi and drained by the choroid plexus.
   b. The arachnoid villi protrude into the lateral ventricles where they are bathed in cerebrospinal fluid.
   c. Cerebrospinal fluid is secreted by Broca's area into the dural sinuses.
   d. The cerebral aqueduct drains cerebrospinal fluid from the third ventricle.

Nervous System: Spinal Cord and Peripheral Nerves

*e*volve

http://evolve.elsevier.com/Herlihy

Key Terms

afferent neuron (p. 205)
cranial nerves (p. 207)
dermatome (p. 214)
efferent neuron (p. 205)
gray matter (p. 201)

mixed nerves (p. 206)
motor nerves (p. 206)
nerve tracts (p. 206)
peripheral nervous system (p. 206)
plexus (p. 210)

reflex arc (p. 205)
sensory nerves (p. 206)
spinal nerves (p. 203)
white matter (p. 201)

Objectives

1. Describe the anatomy of the spinal cord and list its three functions.
2. Discuss reflexes and list four components of the reflex arc.
3. List and describe the functions of the 12 pairs of cranial nerves.

4. Do the following regarding the peripheral nervous system:
   • Identify the classification of spinal nerves.
   • List the functions of the three major plexuses.
   • Describe a dermatome.
   • Provide the functional classification of the peripheral nervous system.

The brain, spinal cord, and peripheral nervous system work together as an intricate communication system. The spinal cord continuously carries information to and from the brain. In the absence of spinal cord function, no sensory activity is present and the person cannot feel. The person also lacks voluntary motor activity and cannot move. The spinal cord plays a crucial role in reflex activity, and many of our rapid and patterned responses are processed by the spinal cord.

WHAT THE SPINAL CORD IS

LOCATION AND SIZE

The spinal cord is a continuation of the brain stem. It is a tubelike structure located within the spinal cavity. The diameter of the spinal cord is similar to the thickness of your thumb. The spinal cord is about 17 inches (43 cm) long and extends from the foramen magnum of the occipital bone to the level of the first lumbar vertebra (L1), just below the bottom rib. Like the brain, the spinal cord is well protected by bone (vertebrae), meninges, cerebrospinal fluid (CSF), and the blood–brain barrier (Figure 11-1).

An infant's spinal cord extends the full length of the spinal cavity. As the infant grows, however, the vertebral column grows faster than the cord. Because of the different rates of growth, the spinal cavity eventually becomes longer than the spinal cord, with the cord extending only to L1 in the adult. The meningeal membranes, however, extend the length of the spinal cavity.

This anatomical arrangement forms the basis for the site of a *lumbar puncture* (see Figure 11-1, *B* and *C*). In this procedure, a hollow needle is inserted into the subarachnoid space, between L3 and L4, at about the level of the top of the hip bone. A sample of CSF is withdrawn from the subarachnoid space. The CSF is then examined for pathogens, blood, or other abnormal signs. Because the spinal cord ends at L1, there is no danger of injuring the cord with the needle.

? Re-Think

1. Describe the length and location of the adult spinal cord.
2. Why is a lumbar puncture performed between L3 and L4?

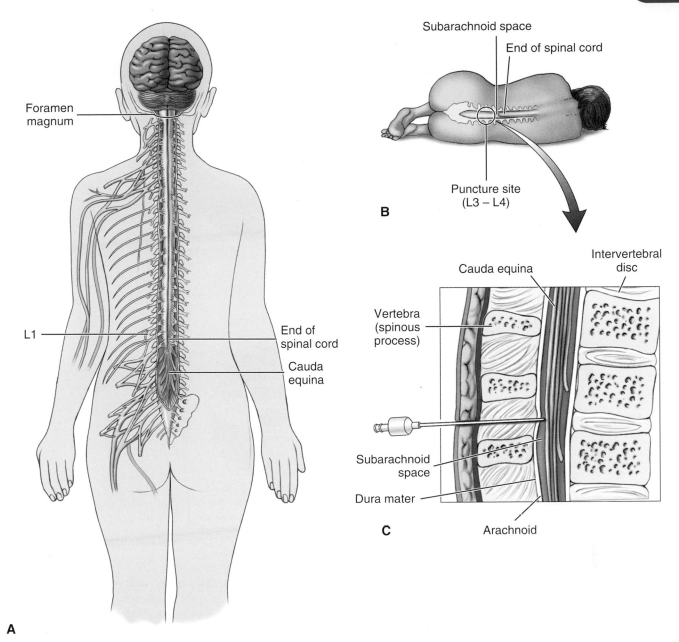

FIGURE 11-1 **A,** Location and length of the spinal cord. **B** and **C,** Lumbar puncture (spinal tap).

GRAY ON THE INSIDE, WHITE ON THE OUTSIDE

GRAY MATTER

A cross-section of the spinal cord shows an area of gray matter and an area of white matter (Figure 11-2). The **gray matter** is located in the center and is shaped like a butterfly. It is composed primarily of cell bodies, interneurons, and synapses. Two projections of the gray matter are the dorsal (posterior) horn and the ventral (anterior) horn. In the middle of the gray matter is the central canal. The central canal is an opening, or hole, that extends the entire length of the spinal cord. It is open to the ventricular system in the brain and to the subarachnoid space at the bottom of the spinal cord. CSF flows from the ventricles in the brain down through the central canal into the subarachnoid space

at the base of the spinal cord. The CSF then circulates throughout the subarachnoid space surrounding the spinal cord and brain.

WHITE MATTER

The **white matter** of the spinal cord is composed of myelinated and unmyelinated axons. These neuronal axons are grouped together into sensory and motor nerve tracts.

Sensory tracts carry information from the periphery, up the spinal cord, and toward the brain (see Figure 11-2). They are therefore called *ascending tracts*. The

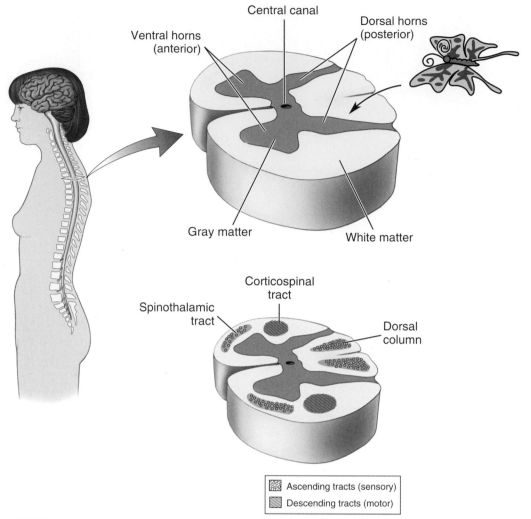

FIGURE 11-2 Cross-section of the spinal cord: inner gray matter ("butterfly") and outer white matter.

spinothalamic (spy-no-thah-LAM-ik) tract is an example of an ascending tract. It carries sensory information for touch, pressure, and pain from the spinal cord to the thalamus in the brain. Note that the name of the tract (spinothalamic) often indicates its origin (spinal cord) and destination (thalamus).

Motor tracts carry information from the brain, down the spinal cord, and toward the periphery. They are called *descending tracts*. The major descending tracts are the pyramidal and extrapyramidal tracts. The pyramidal tract, or corticospinal tract, is the major motor tract, originating in the precentral gyrus of the frontal lobe of the cerebrum. As its name (corticospinal) implies, motor information is carried from the cortex (origin) of the brain to the spinal cord (destination). Additional information concerning tracts and their functions is in Table 11-1.

Decussation

Most nerve tracts decussate (de-KUS-ate), or cross over, from one side to the other. For example, the corticospinal tract that originates in the left frontal lobe descends to the medulla oblongata, in the brain stem.

The fibers then decussate, descend down the right side of the spinal cord, and innervate the right side of the body. Stated in more clinical terms, the corticospinal tract decussates within the medulla oblongata and descends on the contralateral (opposite) side.

Table 11-1	Major Spinal Cord Tracts
TRACTS	**FUNCTIONS**
Ascending	
Spinothalamic	Temperature, pressure, pain, light touch
Dorsal column	Touch, deep pressure, vibration
Spinocerebellar	Proprioception
Descending	
Pyramidal (corticospinal)	Skeletal muscle tone, voluntary muscle movement
Extrapyramidal	Skeletal muscle activity (balance and posture)

Decussation accounts for the right-sided paralysis (hemiparalysis) in a person who has experienced a stroke on the left side of the brain. Some motor fibers do not decussate and therefore descend on the same (ipsilateral) side. Thus, a patient who has sustained a stroke in the left brain may experience both a right-sided paralysis and left-sided weakness. Whereas most motor tracts decussate at the level of the brain stem, most sensory tracts decussate in the spinal cord and travel contralaterally to the brain.

If injured, the neurons of the brain and spinal cord do not regenerate. If the neck is broken, the spinal cord might be severed. If the spinal cord is severed at the neck region, the trunk and all four extremities are paralyzed. This condition is called *quadriplegia*. This type of spinal cord injury is common in automobile, football, and diving accidents in which the neck is either compressed or bent excessively (Figure 11-3). If the spinal cord injury is lower, involving only the lumbar region of the spinal cord, the person has full use of the upper extremities but is paralyzed from the waist down. Paralysis of the lower extremities is called *paraplegia*.

2+2 Sum It Up!

The spinal cord and the peripheral nervous system allow the brain to communicate with the body and external environment. The spinal cord transmits information up and down the cord. Sensory information is brought to the brain from the lower cord region, whereas motor information is transmitted away from the brain, down the cord toward the periphery. Major spinal cord tracts are identified in Table 11-1. In addition to providing pathways for the flow of information, the spinal cord acts as a center of reflex activity.

? Re-Think

1. Differentiate between ascending and descending tracts.
2. What clue identifies the corticospinal tract as a motor tract?
3. What clue identifies the spinothalamic tract as a sensory tract?

SPINAL NERVES ATTACHED TO THE SPINAL CORD

Attached to the spinal cord are the spinal nerves. Each nerve is attached to the spinal cord by two roots: the dorsal root and the ventral root (Figure 11-4). Sensory nerve fibers from the periphery travel to the cord through the dorsal root. The cell bodies of the sensory fibers are gathered together in the dorsal root ganglia. The ventral root is composed of motor fibers. These motor fibers are distributed to muscles and glands. The dorsal and ventral roots are packaged together to form a spinal nerve.

WHAT THE SPINAL CORD DOES

The spinal cord serves three major functions: sensory pathway, motor pathway, and reflex center.

- *Sensory pathway.* The spinal cord provides pathways (ascending) for sensory information traveling from the periphery to the brain. For example, when you stick your finger with a sharp tack, sensory information travels from the finger toward the spinal cord. The information then ascends the spinal cord to the brain, where you experience the information as pain
- *Motor pathway.* The spinal cord provides pathways (descending tracts) for motor information coming

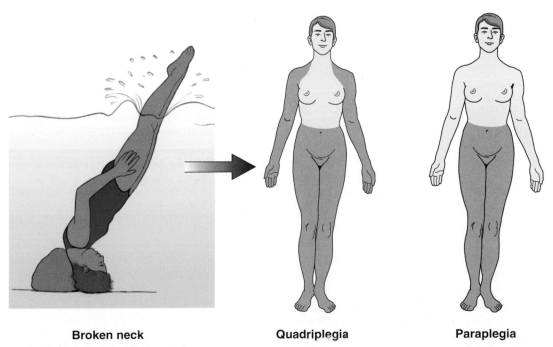

Broken neck   **Quadriplegia**   **Paraplegia**

FIGURE 11-3 Spinal cord injuries. Diving into a shallow pool can result in a damaged spinal cord (quadriplegia and paraplegia).

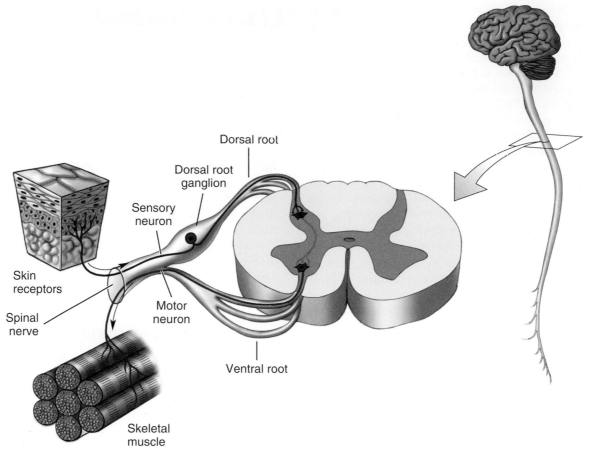

FIGURE 11-4 Attachment of the spinal nerves to the spinal cord.

from the brain and going to the periphery. For example, you decide to move your foot as in kicking a football. The information travels from the brain, down the spinal cord, and to the muscles of the leg and foot.

- *Reflex center.* The spinal cord acts as a major reflex center.

REFLEXES

WHAT REFLEXES ARE

What is a reflex? Many of the activities that we engage in every day occur very rapidly and without any conscious control. In other words, they happen reflexively. Many of the reflexes occur at the level of the spinal cord. A reflex is an involuntary response to a stimulus. If you touch a hot surface, for example, you very quickly remove your hand (withdrawal reflex). Your hand is safely away from the source of injury long before you consciously say, "This is hot. I must remove my hand!" Similarly, your ability to walk and maintain your balance requires hundreds of reflex movements. For example, you don't have to think about swinging your arms as you walk.

A typical reflex response is demonstrated by the patellar tendon, or knee-jerk, reflex (Figure 11-5). During a physical examination, the doctor taps the quadriceps ligament below your kneecap. In response to the tap, your leg quickly and involuntarily pops up. The physician has elicited the patellar tendon reflex. How does this reflex help you? If you are standing erect and your knee bends, even slightly, the patellar reflex is stimulated. In response to the bending, the quadriceps muscle in the thigh contracts, thereby straightening the leg and helping you maintain an upright position.

 Do You Know...

How Anesthesia Affects the Spinal Cord?

Anesthetic agents such as the "-caine" drugs may be injected into the subarachnoid space to achieve spinal anesthesia. When injected into the subarachnoid space, these drugs deaden, or anesthetize, the lumbar and sacral sensory nerves. Pain sensation from the areas innervated by these deadened nerves is temporarily lost.

How is epidural anesthesia used in childbirth? During the last, uncomfortable phase of childbirth, anesthetic agents may be continuously infused into the epidural space. The nerves that are deadened by the anesthesia supply the lower pelvic region of the body, thereby relieving the pain of childbirth.

Knee-jerk reflex arc

① When mallet taps
patellar ligament, receptors
in the muscle are stretched
(stimulated)

② The nerve impulse travels
along the sensory neuron
to the spinal cord

③ The nerve impulse
travels along the
motor neuron to
the muscle

④ The leg
moves up

FIGURE 11-5 Reflex arc. The knee-jerk reflex illustrates the components of the reflex arc.

THE REFLEX ARC

The knee-jerk reflex illustrates the four basic components of the reflex arc (see Figure 11-5). The reflex arc is the nerve pathway involved in a reflex. The four basic components of the reflex arc include the following:

1. *A sensory receptor.* By tapping the patellar ligament, the mallet stimulates sensory receptors in the anterior thigh muscles (quadriceps femoris).
2. *An* afferent, *or sensory,* neuron. The nerve impulse is carried from the receptors along a sensory neuron to the spinal cord. *An integrating center.* The gray matter of the spinal cord contains interneurons that determine the motor response to the sensory input. In the simplest reflex arc (knee jerk reflex), there is a single synapse with no interneuron. All other reflexes require two or more interneurons.
3. *An* efferent, *or motor,* neuron. The nerve impulse is carried by a motor nerve to the muscles of the thigh.
4. *An effector organ.* The muscles of the thigh, the quadriceps femoris, are effector organs for this reflex. In response to the motor nerve impulse, the muscles contract and move the leg in an upward movement (extension of the leg).

MANY, MANY REFLEXES

OUCH! THE WITHDRAWAL REFLEX

The withdrawal reflex (Figure 11-6, *A*) helps protect you from injury. For example, this reflex quickly moves your finger away from a hot iron, thereby preventing a severe burn. The "ouch" occurs after your finger is safely away from the hot iron.

Organ Reflexes

Reflexes also help regulate organ function. Figure 11-6 illustrates some of the reflexes that regulate body function. The pupillary reflex, for example, regulates the amount of light that enters the eye. When a bright light is directed at the eye, the muscles that control pupillary size constrict. The size of the pupil diminishes, thereby restricting the amount of additional light entering the eye. Blood pressure is also under reflex control. When blood pressure changes abruptly, the baroreceptor reflex causes the heart and blood vessels to respond in a way that restores blood pressure to normal.

In addition to performing important physiological functions, some reflexes are used diagnostically to assess nerve function. Abnormal findings may indicate central nervous system (CNS) lesions, tumors, and other neurological diseases such as multiple sclerosis. You may have observed a physician elicit the Babinski reflex (Figure 11-6, *D*) by stroking the lateral sole of the foot in the direction of heel to toe with a hard blunt object. In the adult, the Babinski reflex is normal, or negative, if the response to the stroking is plantar flexion, or a curling of the toes. An abnormal, or positive, Babinski reflex is dorsiflexion of the big toe, sometimes with fanning of the other toes. An infant normally dorsiflexes the big toe, an indicator of the immaturity of the infant's nervous system. Some clinically significant reflexes and their functions are listed in Table 11-2.

FIGURE 11-6 Many reflexes. **A,** Withdrawal reflex. **B,** Pupillary reflex. **C,** Blood pressure, or baroreceptor, reflex. **D,** Babinski reflex. **E,** Knee-jerk reflex.

2+2 Sum It Up!

The spinal cord and the peripheral nervous system allow the brain to communicate with the body and the external environment. The spinal cord transmits sensory and motor information to and from the brain. It also acts as a reflex center. A reflex is an involuntary response to a stimulus. A reflex arc has four components: sensory receptor, afferent neuron, efferent neuron, and effector organ. Clinically significant reflexes are identified in Table 11-2.

? Re-Think

Describe the steps of the withdrawal reflex in response to sticking your finger on a sharp tack.

PERIPHERAL NERVOUS SYSTEM

The **peripheral nervous system** consists of the nerves and ganglia located outside the CNS.

NERVES

Before classifying the nerves, you need to differentiate between a nerve and a neuron (see Chapter 10). A neuron is a single nerve cell. The nerve contains many neurons bundled together with blood vessels and then wrapped in connective tissue (Figure 11-7). Nerves are located outside the CNS. Within the CNS, bundles of nerve fibers are called **nerve tracts**. Nerves are classified as the following:

- **Sensory nerves**, composed only of sensory neurons
- **Motor nerves**, composed only of motor neurons
- **Mixed nerves**, containing both sensory and motor neurons. Most nerves are mixed and all spinal nerves are mixed.

CLASSIFYING THE PERIPHERAL NERVOUS SYSTEM

The peripheral nervous system can be classified in two ways: structurally (by the anatomy) or functionally (according to what they do).

STRUCTURAL CLASSIFICATION OF THE PERIPHERAL NERVOUS SYSTEM

The structural classification of the peripheral nervous system divides the nerves into cranial and spinal nerves. The classification is based on the origin of the fiber (where it originates).

Table 11-2	Clinically Significant Reflexes	
REFLEX	**DESCRIPTION**	**MEANING OF ABNORMAL RESPONSE**
Patellar tendon (knee-jerk reflex)	A stretch reflex. The mallet strikes the patellar ligament below the knee; in response, the leg kicks up.	Impaired in damage to nerves involved in the reflex Impaired in damage to lumbar region of spinal cord Impaired in patients with diseases that affect the nerves and spinal cord (e.g., diabetes mellitus, neurosyphilis, and chronic alcoholism)
Achilles tendon (ankle-jerk reflex)	A stretch reflex. The mallet strikes the Achilles tendon, causing plantar flexion.	Impaired in damage to nerves involved in the reflex Impaired in damage to lower spinal cord (L5–S2)
Abdominal	With stroking of the lateral abdominal wall, the abdominal wall contracts and moves the umbilicus toward the stimulus.	Impaired in lesions of peripheral nerves Impaired in lesions of spinal cord (thoracic) and in patients with multiple sclerosis
Babinski	With stroking of the lateral sole of the foot from heel to toe, the toes curl, with slight inversion of the foot (see text).	Impaired in lesions or damage of the spinal cord In children younger than 2 years old, the Babinski reflex appears positive.

Cranial Nerves

Names and Numbers of Cranial Nerves. Twelve pairs of **cranial nerves** are shown in Figure 11-8. Each cranial nerve has a specific number, always designated by a Roman numeral, and a name. The numbers indicate the order in which the nerves exit the brain from front to back. Ten of the twelve cranial nerves originate in the brain stem.

In general, the name of the nerve indicates the specific anatomical area served by the nerve. For example, the optic nerve serves the eye. The cranial nerves primarily serve the head, face, and neck region, but one pair—the vagus—branches extensively and extends throughout the thoracic and abdominal cavities.

A common mnemonic used to memorize the cranial nerves in proper order is shown in Table 11-3: On Old Olympus Towering Tops A Finn Viewed Germans Vaulting And Hopping. The first letter of each word is the same as the first letter of each cranial nerve. (My personal mnemonic is Oh! Oh! Oh! Tough, Tricky Anatomy Final … Very Grave Vibes … Aching Head.) Try to develop your own creative mnemonic, or search the Web for others. Unfortunately, you must know the name and Roman numeral of each cranial nerve. For instance, the vestibulocochlear nerve is CN VIII.

Functions of Cranial Nerves. Cranial nerves perform four general functions that carry different types of information:

- Sensory information for the special senses: smell, taste, vision, and hearing
- Sensory information for the general senses: touch, pressure, pain, temperature, and vibration
- Motor information that results in contraction of skeletal muscles
- Motor information that results in the secretion of glands and the contraction of cardiac and smooth muscle

Cranial nerve function is summarized in Table 11-3. Locate each cranial nerve on Figure 11-8 as it is described below.

CN I, olfactory nerve. A sensory nerve that carries information from the nose to the temporal lobe of the cerebrum. The olfactory nerve is concerned with the sense of smell. A person who damages the olfactory nerve may lose the sense of smell (anosmia). In addition, the person may complain of loss of taste

Neuron

Blood vessels

Nerve

FIGURE 11-7 Difference between a neuron and nerve.

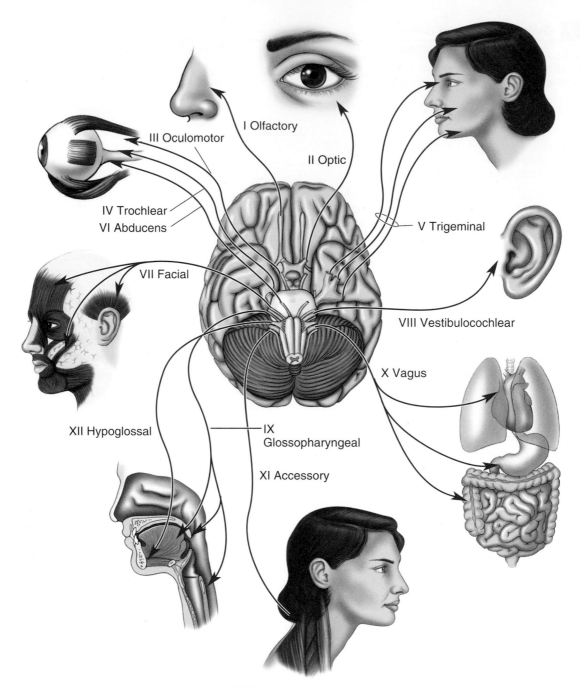

FIGURE 11-8 Cranial nerves.

because the appeal of food is determined by both taste and smell.

CN II, optic nerve. A sensory nerve that carries visual information from the eye to the primary visual cortex of the occipital lobe of the cerebrum. Damage to the optic nerve causes diminished vision or blindness in the affected eye.

CN III, oculomotor nerve. Primarily a motor nerve that causes contraction of most of the extrinsic eye muscles, thereby moving the eyeball in its socket. The oculomotor nerve also raises the eyelid and constricts the pupil of the eye.

Because the oculomotor nerve is located close to the hard tentorium within the cranium, it is easily compressed by brain tumors or by increased intracranial pressure. Compression of the nerve interferes with the ability of the pupil of the eye to respond to light (sluggish pupillary response). With more severe compression, the pupils may become dilated and fixed. Compression of CN III also interferes with raising the eyelid; the person experiences ptosis (TOH-sis) of the eyelid. Observation of the eyes provides excellent clinical clues to neurological status.

Table 11-3   Cranial Nerves

MNEMONIC	NUMBER/NERVE	TYPE	FUNCTION
On	I/Olfactory	Sensory	Sense of smell
Old	II/Optic	Sensory	Sense of sight
Olympus	III/Oculomotor	Mixed (mostly motor)	Movement of eyeball, raising of eyelid, change in pupil size
Towering	IV/Trochlear	Mixed (mostly motor)	Movement of eyeball
Tops	V/Trigeminal	Mixed	Chewing of food; sensations in face, scalp, cornea (eye), and teeth
A	VI/Abducens	Mixed (mostly motor)	Movement of eyeball
Finn	VII/Facial	Mixed	Facial expressions, secretion of saliva and tears, taste, blinking
Viewed	VIII/Vestibulocochlear	Sensory	Sense of hearing and balance
Germans	IX/Glossopharyngeal	Mixed	Swallowing, secretion of saliva, taste, sensory for the reflex regulation of blood pressure, part of the gag reflex
Vaulting	X/Vagus	Mixed	Visceral muscle movement and sensations, especially movement and secretion of the digestive system; sensory for reflex regulation of blood pressure
And	XI/Accessory	Mixed (mostly motor)	Swallowing, head and shoulder movement, speaking
Hopping	XII/Hypoglossal	Mixed (mostly motor)	Speech and swallowing

CN IV, trochlear nerve. Primarily a motor nerve that innervates one of the extrinsic muscles of the eyeball, thereby helping move the eyeball. Damage may cause double vision and an inability to rotate the eye properly.

CN V, trigeminal nerve. A mixed nerve with three branches supplying the facial region. The two sensory branches carry information regarding touch, pressure, and pain from the face, scalp, eye, and teeth to the brain. The ophthalmic branch of the trigeminal nerve detects sensory information from the cornea. For example, if you touch the surface of the cornea, the ophthalmic branch is stimulated and sends information to the brain. In response to the corneal irritation, motor fibers of the facial nerve (CN VII) respond by eliciting blinking and the secretion of tears. Thus, both the trigeminal and facial nerves help to relieve the irritation. The motor branch of the trigeminal nerve innervates the muscles of mastication (chewing). Nerve damage causes a loss of sensation and impaired movement of the mandible (lower jaw).

A person may experience an inflammation of the trigeminal nerve. This condition is called *trigeminal neuralgia,* or *tic douloureux.* It is characterized by bouts of severe facial pain. The pain may be triggered by events such as eating, shaving, and exposure to cold temperatures. In an effort to avoid these triggers, the patient often becomes a prisoner of the disease, refusing to eat, shave, or leave the house in cold weather.

CN VI, abducens nerve. Primarily a motor nerve that, like the trochlear, controls eye movement by innervating only one of the extrinsic eye muscles. Nerve damage prevents a lateral rotation of the eye; at rest, the eye drifts medially (toward the nose).

CN VII, facial nerve. A mixed nerve that performs mostly motor functions. It is called the nerve of facial expression and allows you to smile, frown, and "make other faces." It also stimulates the secretion of saliva and tears. The facial nerve innervates the orbicularis oculi, the muscle involved in blinking. Blinking not only protects the eye from foreign objects, such as dust, but also washes tears over the cornea, thereby keeping the cornea moist and preventing corneal ulceration. Its sensory function is taste.

If the facial nerve is damaged, facial expression is absent on the affected side of the face. This condition is called *Bell's palsy* (see next page). Cosmetically, this condition is very distressing because one side of the face may smile and look alive, but the other side of the face sags, drools, and is expressionless. Salivation and the secretion of tears are diminished, thereby requiring the use of eyedrops to protect the cornea. Fortunately, Bell's palsy often responds well to steroid therapy.

Bell's palsy

CN VIII, vestibulocochlear nerve. A sensory nerve that carries information for hearing and balance from the inner ear to the brain. The vestibular branch of this nerve is responsible for equilibrium, or balance, and the cochlear branch is responsible for hearing. Damage to this nerve may cause loss of hearing or balance or both (see Chapter 13).

CN IX, glossopharyngeal nerve. A mixed nerve that carries taste sensation from the posterior tongue to the brain. Motor fibers stimulate the secretion of salivary glands in the mouth. Other motor fibers innervate the throat and aid in swallowing. The glossopharyngeal nerve is also associated with the gag reflex. The gag reflex plays an important role in preventing food and water from entering the respiratory passages. Normally, when something goes down the wrong way, you gag and cough until the airway is cleared. Gagging is a good thing—and clinically important when depressed. Loss of the gag reflex places you at risk for choking. A second sensory function of this nerve involves the regulation of blood pressure via the baroreceptor reflex (see Chapter 19).

CN X, vagus nerve. A mixed nerve that innervates the tongue, pharynx (throat), larynx (voice box), and many organs in the thoracic and abdominal cavities (lungs, stomach, intestines). Nerve damage causes hoarseness or loss of voice, impaired swallowing, and diminished motility of the digestive tract. Damage to both vagus nerves can be fatal. The word *vagus* literally means wanderer; the name refers to the far-reaching distribution of this nerve. The sensory fibers of the vagus nerve also participate in the regulation of blood pressure via the baroreceptor reflex (see Chapter 19).

CN XI, accessory nerve. Primarily a motor nerve that supplies the sternocleidomastoid and the trapezius muscles, thereby controlling movement of the head and shoulder regions. Nerve damage impairs your ability to shrug your shoulders and rotate your head.

CN XII, hypoglossal nerve. Primarily a motor nerve that controls movement of the tongue, thereby affecting speaking and swallowing activities. Nerve damage causes the tongue to deviate toward the injured side.

A neurological assessment includes simple procedures that test the ability of each cranial nerve to perform these functions. Table 11-4 illustrates some methods used to test cranial nerve function. The table also includes common disorders and abnormal findings involving the cranial nerves.

 Do You Know...

About the "Wandering" Characteristics of the Tenth Cranial Nerve?

Check the local jail, and you will find a couple of unsavory characters locked up on charges of vagrancy—the habit of wandering around and generally getting into trouble. (The word *vagrant* means someone who wanders about.) The vagus nerve, the tenth cranial nerve (CN X), is also a wanderer. Unlike the other cranial nerves that are confined to the head and shoulder area, the vagus nerve leaves the head and wanders, or makes its way through, the thoracic and abdominal cavities. The vagus nerve is named for these vagrant or wandering characteristics.

 Re-Think

1. CNs II, III, IV, and VI all innervate eye structures. What is the difference in function of each?
2. List two effects of a damaged CN VIII.
3. Why is the vagus nerve called the "wanderer" nerve?

SPINAL NERVES

Names and Numbers of Spinal Nerves

Thirty-one pairs of spinal nerves emerge from the spinal cord (Figure 11-9). Each pair is numbered according to the level of the spinal cord from which it arises. The 31 pairs are grouped as follows: 8 pairs of cervical nerves, 12 pairs of thoracic nerves, 5 pairs of lumbar nerves, 5 pairs of sacral nerves, and 1 pair of coccygeal nerves. The lumbar and sacral nerves at the bottom of the cord extend the length of the spinal cavity before exiting from the vertebral column. These nerves are called the *cauda equina* because they look like a horse's tail. The nerves exit from the bony vertebral column through tiny holes in the vertebrae called *foramina*.

Spinal Nerve Plexuses

As the spinal nerves exit from the vertebral column, they divide into many fibers. At various points, most nerve fibers converge, or come together again, into nerve **plexuses** (PLEX-sus-ez), or networks. The three major nerve plexuses are the cervical plexus, the brachial plexus, and the lumbosacral plexus (see Figure 11-9). Each plexus sorts out the many fibers and sends them to a specific part of the body. The three plexuses and the major nerves that emerge from each plexus are

Table 11-4   Cranial Nerves: Assessment and Disorders

NERVE	ASSESSMENT	SOME DISORDERS
I Olfactory	Person is asked to sniff and identify various odors (e.g., vanilla).	Inability to smell (anosmia)
II Optic	Examination of the interior of the eye by ophthalmoscopic visualization. Use of eye charts and tests of peripheral vision.	Diminished or loss of vision
III Oculomotor	Observation of eyelids. Test the ability of the eyes to follow a moving object. Examination of pupils for size, shape, and size equality. Pupillary reflex is tested with a penlight (the pupils should constrict). Test the ability of the eyes to converge.	Drooping upper eyelids (ptosis) Difficulty in focusing eyes on an object Absence of pupillary reflex (e.g., dilated and fixed pupils that may indicate an increase in intracranial pressure)
IV Trochlear	Test ability of the eyes to follow a moving object.	Inability to move eyeball in a particular direction
V Trigeminal	Sensations (pain/touch/temperature) are tested with sharp pin and hot/cold objects. Corneal reflex (sensory) is tested with a cotton wisp. Motor function is tested by asking the person to open the mouth (against resistance) and to move the jaw from side to side.	Loss of sensation (pain/touch); paresthesias (tingling, itching, and numbness) Pain, tearing, and blinking Shift of jaw to side of lesion when opened Difficulty in chewing
VI Abducens	Test ability of the eyes to follow a moving object.	Inability to move eyes laterally
VII Facial	Person is asked to cause facial muscle movement (e.g., smile, close eyes, wrinkle forehead, whistle). Test anterior two thirds of tongue for sweet, salty, sour, and bitter taste. Ability to secrete tears is tested by asking person to sniff ammonia fumes.	Bell's palsy (expressionless face, drooping mouth and drooling, inability to close eyes and blink) Loss of taste on anterior two thirds of tongue on side of lesion
VIII Vestibulocochlear	Hearing is checked by air and bone conduction (use of tuning fork).	Loss of hearing, noises in ear (tinnitus) Loss of balance (vertigo)
IX Glossopharyngeal	Check gag and swallowing reflex. Test posterior two thirds of tongue for taste. Person is asked to speak and cough.	Loss of gag reflex Difficulty in swallowing (dysphagia) Loss of taste on posterior two thirds of tongue Decreased salivation Hoarseness of voice
X Vagus	Similar to testing for CN IX (because they both innervate throat).	Sagging of soft palate Hoarseness of voice resulting from paralysis of vocal fold
XI Accessory	Ask person to rotate head from side to side and to shrug shoulders (against resistance).	Drooping shoulders Inability or difficulty in rotating head (wryneck)
XII Hypoglossal	Person is asked to stick out tongue—note any deviation in position of the protruded tongue.	Some difficulty in speaking (dysarthria), chewing, and swallowing (dysphagia)

listed in Table 11-5 and described as follows. The results of damage to major peripheral nerves are listed in Table 11-6.

Cervical plexus (C1 to C4). Fibers from the cervical plexus supply the muscles and skin of the neck. Motor fibers from this plexus also pass into the phrenic nerve. The phrenic nerve stimulates the contraction of the diaphragm, the major breathing muscle (Figure 11-10; see Figure 11-9).

If the spinal cord is severed below the C5 level, the person is paralyzed but can breathe without ventilator assistance. If the level of injury is higher, at C2, the phrenic nerve is injured, motor impulses to the diaphragm are interrupted, and the person cannot breathe normally. To breathe, the injured person generally needs the assistance of a ventilator.

Brachial plexus (C5 to C8, T1). The nerves that emerge from the brachial plexus supply the muscles and

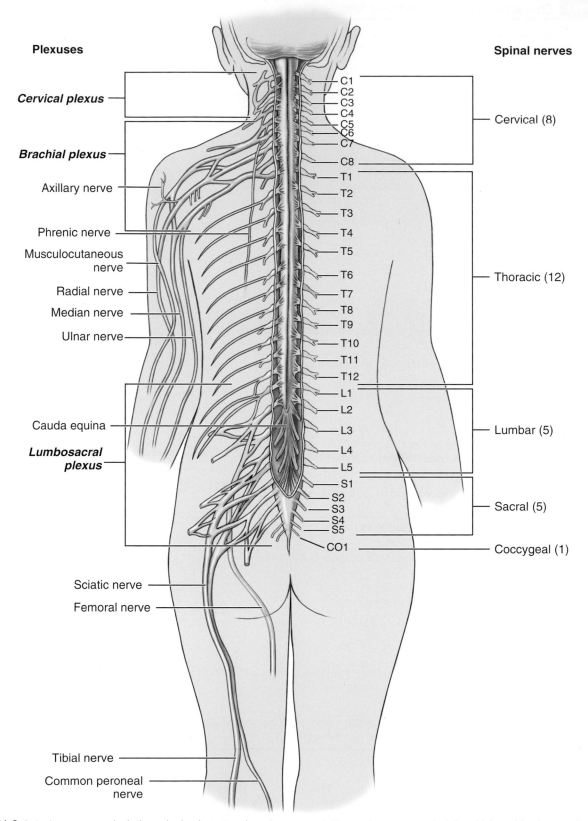

Plexuses

Cervical plexus

Brachial plexus

Axillary nerve

Phrenic nerve

Musculocutaneous nerve

Radial nerve

Median nerve

Ulnar nerve

Cauda equina

Lumbosacral plexus

Sciatic nerve

Femoral nerve

Tibial nerve

Common peroneal nerve

Spinal nerves

C1
C2
C3
C4
C5
C6
C7
C8

Cervical (8)

T1
T2
T3
T4
T5
T6
T7
T8
T9
T10
T11
T12

Thoracic (12)

L1
L2
L3
L4
L5

Lumbar (5)

S1
S2
S3
S4
S5

Sacral (5)

CO1

Coccygeal (1)

FIGURE 11-9 Spinal nerves: cervical, thoracic, lumbar, sacral, and coccygeal. Nerve plexuses: cervical, brachial, and lumbosacral plexuses.

Table 11-5   Spinal Nerve Plexuses

PLEXUS	SPINAL NERVE ORIGIN	REGION INNERVATED	MAJOR NERVES EMERGING FROM PLEXUS
Cervical	C1 to C4	Skin and muscles of the neck and shoulder, diaphragm	Phrenic
Brachial	C5 to C8, T1	Skin and muscles of the upper extremities	Axillary Radial Median Musculocutaneous Ulnar
Lumbosacral	T12, L1 to L5, S1 to S4	Skin and muscle of lower torso and lower extremities	Femoral Obturator Sciatic Pudendal

Table 11-6   Major Peripheral Nerves: Results of Damage

NERVE	BODY AREA SERVED	RESULTS OF NERVE DAMAGE
Phrenic	Diaphragm	Impaired breathing
Axillary	Muscles of shoulder	Crutch palsy
Radial	Posterior arm, forearm, hand; thumbs and first two fingers	Wristdrop (inability to lift or extend hand at wrist)
Median	Forearm and some muscles of the hand	Inability to pick up small objects
Ulnar	Wrist and many muscles in hand	Clawhand—inability to spread fingers apart
Intercostal	Rib cage	Impaired breathing
Femoral	Lower abdomen, anterior thigh, medial leg, foot	Inability to extend leg and flex hip
Sciatic	Lower trunk; posterior thigh and leg	Inability to extend hip and flex knee
Common peroneal	Lateral area of leg and foot	Footdrop—inability to dorsiflex foot
Tibial	Posterior area of leg and foot	Shuffling gait caused by inability to invert and dorsiflex foot

CERVICAL PLEXUS

Phrenic nerves

"Breathing muscles"

Damage to phrenic nerve

BRACHIAL PLEXUS

Damage to axillary nerve

Damage to median nerve

LUMBOSACRAL PLEXUS

Irritation of sciatic nerve

FIGURE 11-10 Examples of nerve damage.

skin of the shoulder, arm, forearm, wrist, and hand. The axillary nerve emerges from this plexus and travels through the shoulder into the arm.

The axillary nerve in the shoulder region is susceptible to damage. For example, a person using crutches should be taught to bear the weight of the body on the hands and not on the armpit, or axillary region. The weight of the body can damage the axillary nerve, causing crutch palsy.

The radial and ulnar nerves, which serve the forearm, wrist, and hand, also emerge from the brachial plexus. Damage to the radial nerve can cause a wristdrop, and injury to the ulnar nerve causes the hand to appear clawlike; the person is unable to spread the fingers apart.

Lumbosacral plexus (T12, L1 to L5, S1 to S4). The lumbosacral plexus gives rise to nerves that supply the muscles and skin of the lower abdominal wall, external genitalia, buttocks, and lower extremities. The sciatic nerve, the longest nerve in the body, arises from this plexus. The sciatic nerve supplies musculature of the thigh, leg, and foot. The sciatic nerve can become inflamed and cause intense pain in the buttock and posterior thigh region. A common cause of sciatica is a ruptured or herniated vertebral disc (see Figure 11-10).

What a Dermatome Is

A dermatome is a sensory thing. Each dorsal root of a spinal nerve innervates a particular area of the skin; this distribution of nerves is called a **dermatome** (DER-mah-tohm). Figure 11-11 illustrates the dermatomes for the entire body. Each dermatome is named for the particular nerve that serves it. For example, the C4 dermatome is innervated by the C4 spinal nerve. Dermatomes are useful clinically; for example, if the skin of the shoulder region is stimulated with the tip of a pin and the person cannot feel it, the clinician has reason to believe that the C4 nerve is impaired.

 Do You Know...

About Tingling Thigh Syndrome?

Although tight, low-slung jeans are "in," your thigh nerves are on edge about this fashion craze. The snug jeans are compressing nerves in your thighs, causing a tingling sensation. The "tingling thigh syndrome" is easily cured, but the jeans have to go—or go higher.

 Re-Think

1. Explain the difference between a cranial and spinal nerve.
2. What happens at a nerve plexus?
3. Explain why a quadriplegic with a C2 injury is ventilator-dependent, whereas a quadriplegic with a C5 injury is not ventilator-dependent.

 Do You Know...

What Was on Dr. Herby Zoster's Shingle?

The doctor's shingle indicates that he specializes in chickenpox, shingles, and postherpetic neuralgia; all three are caused by the herpes zoster virus. Following a chickenpox infection, the herpes virus "hides out" in nerves and often reactivates in later life, causing shingles. Clusters of vesicles develop along cranial or spinal dermatomes. The painful lesions eventually crust over. For months after the "crusting over period," a significant number of patients with shingles develop a persistent and painful neuralgia, called *postherpetic neuralgia*. The term *shingles* comes from a word meaning "girdle," a reference to the usual appearance of lesions around the waist.

Any pharmacological help for shingles? Yes! Analgesics are prescribed for pain. Antiviral drugs may be used if the shingles is diagnosed quickly. On a preventive note, a shingles vaccine is now available.

Are shingles contagious? No! However, a person with shingles can transmit chickenpox to a person with no immunity to the disease. Also, a child with chickenpox can activate the dormant herpes virus in a person who has had chickenpox in the past.

FIGURE 11-11 Dermatomes.

FUNCTIONAL CLASSIFICATION OF THE PERIPHERAL NERVOUS SYSTEM

The functional classification explains where the nerves go and what they do. The functional classification for the peripheral nervous system includes the following:

- The somatic afferent nerves, which bring sensory information from the different parts of the body, particularly the skin and muscles, to the CNS (see Chapter 13).
- The somatic efferent nerves, which bring motor information from the CNS to the skeletal muscles throughout the body (see Chapter 9).
- The autonomic nervous system (ANS) is composed of nerves that supply the organs (viscera), smooth muscle, and glands. The ANS is the topic of Chapter 12.

2+2 Sum It Up!

The peripheral nervous system consists of the nerves and ganglia located outside the CNS. Nerves are sensory, motor, or mixed. Mixed nerves carry both sensory and motor neurons. The peripheral nervous system can be classified structurally and functionally. The structural classification divides the nerves into cranial and spinal nerves. The 12 pairs of cranial nerves contain fibers that originate in the brain (see Figure 11-8 and Table 11-3). There are 31 pairs of spinal nerves; their fibers originate in the spinal cord (see Figure 11-9 and Tables 11-5 and 11-6). Most spinal nerve fibers converge into nerve plexuses, or networks. The three major nerve plexuses are the cervical plexus, brachial plexus, and lumbosacral plexus. The functional classification of nerves include: somatic afferent nerves, somatic efferent nerves, and autonomic nerves.

Note: The As You Age box and the Medical Terminology and Disorders table appear in Chapter 12.

Get Ready for Exams!

Summary Outline

The brain, spinal cord, and peripheral nerves act as a vast communication system. The spinal cord transmits information to and from the brain. The peripheral nervous system brings information to the CNS (its sensory role) and delivers information from the CNS to the periphery (its motor role).

I. What the Spinal Cord Is
 A. The spinal cord is a tubelike structure located in the spinal cavity, extending from the foramen magnum (occipital bone) to L1.
 B. Arrangement of nervous tissue
  1. The gray matter is a butterfly-shaped area located centrally; it is composed primarily of cell bodies, interneurons, and synapses.
  2. The white matter is composed of myelinated and unmyelinated fibers arranged in tracts. Ascending tracts are sensory tracts; descending tracts are motor tracts.
  3. Spinal nerves are attached to the spinal cord. All spinal nerves are mixed (they contain sensory and motor fibers).
  4. Sensory nerve fibers travel to the cord through the dorsal root. Motor nerve fibers travel in the ventral root.

II. What the Spinal Cord Does: Functions
 A. The spinal cord relays sensory information (ascending tracts).
 B. The spinal cord relays motor information (descending tracts).
 C. The spinal cord acts as a major reflex center.

III. Reflexes
 A. A reflex is an involuntary response to a stimulus.
 B. The four components of a reflex are a sensory receptor, an afferent neuron, an efferent neuron, and an effector organ.

IV. Peripheral Nervous System
 A. Nerve
  1. A nerve is a group of neurons, blood vessels, and connective tissue.
  2. There are sensory nerves, motor nerves, and mixed nerves.
 B. Structural classification of nerves
  1. A classification of nerves on the basis of structure (anatomy) divides nerves into cranial nerves and spinal nerves. There are 12 pairs of cranial nerves (see Table 11-3) and 31 pairs of spinal nerves (see Figure 11-9).
  2. Spinal nerves are sorted out at nerve plexuses. The three major plexuses are the cervical plexus, the brachial plexus, and the lumbosacral plexus.
  3. A dermatome is the area of skin innervated by each spinal nerve; a dermatome is purely sensory.
 C. Functional classification of nerves
  1. Somatic afferent nerves carry sensory information to the CNS.
  2. Somatic efferent nerves carry motor information to skeletal muscles.
  3. Autonomic nerves carry motor information to the organs (viscera).

Review Your Knowledge

Matching: Reflexes
Directions: Match the following words with their descriptions below.

a. gag reflex
b. baroreceptor reflex
c. withdrawal reflex
d. Achilles tendon reflex
e. pupillary reflex
f. patellar tendon reflex

1. ___ Helps you maintain balance; also called the *knee-jerk reflex*
2. ___ Regulates blood pressure
3. ___ Controls the amount of light that enters the eye
4. ___ When you pull your finger away from a sharp object
5. ___ Helps prevent food and water from entering the respiratory passages
6. ___ Tapping of the calcaneal tendon; causes plantar flexion

Matching: Nerves
Directions: Match the following words with their descriptions below. Some words may be used more than once.

a. oculomotor
b. optic
c. vagus
d. facial
e. sciatic
f. olfactory
g. phrenic
h. vestibulocochlear

1. ___ Innervates the skeletal muscles that move the eyeball
2. ___ Carries sensory information to the primary visual cortex of the occipital lobe
3. ___ Carries sensory information for hearing and balance
4. ___ Innervates the diaphragm, causing it to contract
5. ___ Innervates muscles of the thigh
6. ___ "Wanderer" nerve that is distributed throughout the thoracic and abdominopelvic cavities
7. ___ The "smell" nerve
8. ___ The nerve of facial expression
9. ___ Ototoxicity refers to this damaged nerve
10. ___ "Fixed and dilated" describes this injured nerve

Multiple Choice

1. Which of the following does not describe the oculomotor nerve?
   a. It is also CN III.
   b. It innervates the skeletal muscles that move the eyeball.
   c. It is the carrier of information to the primary visual cortex in the occipital lobe.
   d. It innervates skeletal muscle that raises the eyelids.
2. The trigeminal nerve
   a. is CN V.
   b. has both sensory and motor fibers.
   c. affects chewing.
   d. All of the above are true.
3. The sciatic nerve
   a. is a motor nerve that innervates thigh muscles.
   b. is a cranial nerve.
   c. enters the cervical plexus for distribution to the periphery.
   d. travels within the spinothalamic tract.
4. Which of the following is descriptive of the spinothalamic tract?
   a. It carries sensory information regarding touch, pressure, and pain.
   b. It is the major motor tract.
   c. It is also called the *pyramidal tract*.
   d. It is a descending tract.
5. Which of the following is least descriptive of the corticospinal tract?
   a. Descending tract
   b. Major motor tract
   c. Pyramidal tract
   d. Carries information from the spinal cord to the thalamus
6. What is the final step in the reflex arc?
   a. Response of the effector organ(s)
   b. Activation of the sensory receptor
   c. Communication of the sensory neuron with an interneuron within the spinal cord
   d. Traveling of the nerve impulse along the motor neuron
7. Which of the following is not true of the gag reflex?
   a. It is impaired in a paraplegic person.
   b. It is associated with CN IX.
   c. It is associated with the glossopharyngeal nerve.
   d. It prevents food and water from entering the respiratory passages.
8. Damage to the phrenic nerve
   a. interferes with the pupillary response to light.
   b. impairs breathing.
   c. eliminates the gag reflex.
   d. causes dysphagia.
9. CN IX, CN X, and the baroreceptor reflex are concerned with the regulation of
   a. the amount of light that enters the eye.
   b. facial expression.
   c. the movement of the eyeballs and elevation of the eyelids.
   d. blood pressure.
10. Which of the following cranial nerves is not classified as sensory?
   a. Olfactory
   b. CN II
   c. Vestibulocochlear
   d. Vagus

Go Figure

1. **According to Figure 11-1**
   a. The spinal cord fills the entire spinal cavity.
   b. The usual lumbar puncture site is between L6 to L7.
   c. The cauda equina exits from the distal end of the spinal cord.
   d. The subarachnoid space ends at L1.

2. **According to Figure 11-2**
   a. The corticospinal tract, spinothalamic tract, and dorsal columns ascend and descend in the gray matter.
   b. The corticospinal tract runs only in the left side of the spinal cord.
   c. The ventral and posterior horns are composed of white matter.
   d. All tracts ascend and descend in white matter.

3. **According to Figure 11-5**
   a. The effector organ of the patellar tendon reflex is the patellar tendon.
   b. A sensory neuron carries information to the gray matter in the spinal cord.
   c. The response to the patellar tendon reflex is flexion of the leg at the knee.
   d. A motor neuron carries information from the patellar tendon to the spinal cord.

4. **According to Figure 11-8**
   a. The facial nerve only innervates the lower jaw.
   b. The vagus (CN X) is restricted to the thoracic cavity.
   c. CN V has two branches: vestibular and cochlear.
   d. CN VIII is the vestibulocochlear nerve.

5. **According to Figure 11-9**
   a. The sciatic and femoral nerves innervate the thoracic cavity.
   b. The phrenic nerve exits the spinal cord at the level of T6.
   c. The radial, median, and ulnar nerves exit from the lumbosacral plexus.
   d. Transection of the spinal cord at C2 causes quadriplegia.

Autonomic Nervous System

Key Terms

adrenergic fiber (p. 223)
alpha-adrenergic receptor (p. 225)
autonomic nervous system
    (ANS) (p. 218)
beta-adrenergic receptor (p. 225)
cholinergic fiber (p. 223)

craniosacral outflow (p. 222)
muscarinic receptors (p. 224)
nicotinic receptors (p. 224)
norepinephrine (NE) (p. 223)
parasympathetic
    nervous system (p. 220)

preganglionic fiber (p. 221)
postganglionic fiber (p. 221)
sympathetic nervous system
    (p. 219)
thoracolumbar outflow (p. 221)

Objectives

1. Describe the function and pathway of autonomic (visceral) reflexes.
2. Do the following regarding the autonomic nervous system:
   • Describe the function of the autonomic nervous system.
   • Identify the two divisions of the autonomic nervous system.
   • State the anatomical and functional differences between the sympathetic and parasympathetic nervous systems.
   • Define autonomic terminology used in pharmacology.

   • Differentiate between autonomic tone and vasomotor tone.
3. Discuss autonomic nervous system neurons, including:
   • Define *cholinergic* and *adrenergic* fibers.
   • Name the major neurotransmitters of the autonomic nervous system.
   • Name and locate the cholinergic and adrenergic receptors.
4. Explain the terms used to describe the effects of neurotransmitters and drugs on autonomic receptors.

Throughout the day, you are busy doing various things. You walk across a room, run up the stairs, write, tie your shoes, and chew your food. You perform all these activities voluntarily and consciously. Your body, however, performs many more activities automatically. For example, when you eat, you don't think, "I am eating. Therefore, I should increase the flow of my digestive enzymes and then increase the rate of contraction of my intestinal muscles in order to enhance the digestive process." Instead, your body automatically makes these decisions and carries them out for you. This automatic response is the function of the **autonomic nervous system (ANS)**. Autonomic = automatic!

AUTONOMIC (VISCERAL) REFLEXES

WHAT THEY DO

Mention the word *reflex* and what comes to mind is the knee-jerk reflex. Tap the patellar ligament and up pops the leg. The knee-jerk reflex is mediated by somatic nerves. There are also visceral reflexes. These reflexes are mediated by the ANS. As the name implies, visceral reflexes regulate organ function. Visceral reflexes control such things as heart rate, blood pressure, body temperature, digestion, air flow through respiratory passages, elimination, and pupillary (eye) responses. Note the wide variety of functions controlled by autonomic activity. It takes a load off your mind!

PATHWAY

A visceral reflex is mediated in a manner similar to the knee-jerk reflex: activation of a receptor, transmission of sensory information to the central nervous system (CNS), the processing of the information by the CNS, and the motor response sent to the effector organ(s). For example, a sudden decrease in blood pressure activates pressure receptors (baroreceptors). The information about the low blood pressure is carried to the medulla oblongata in the brain stem by sensory nerves. The medulla oblongata determines that the blood pressure is low and sends motor signals to the visceral effector organs (heart and blood vessels). The motor response results in changes in the heart and blood vessels that elevate blood pressure. What has been accomplished? A sudden decrease in blood pressure stimulates a visceral reflex that restores blood pressure to normal. All this has been accomplished without conscious input.

 Do You Know...

What Pinocchio and Your Autonomic Nervous System Have in Common?

Although Pinocchio's nose was a dead giveaway to his lying ways, most of us do not do "the nose thing" in response to fibbing. But fibbers beware! Your ANS can act like the puppet's nose. Lying, even those little white lies, activates the sympathetic nervous system and causes physiological responses that are readily found by a polygraph machine. A modern-day Gepetto knew that we are generally unable to control the ANS and so invented the lie detector.

Why does 007 wear shades? The ANS is constantly adjusting our innards to environmental stresses. The adjustments are noticeable in our eye responses, particularly in the changes in pupil size. Bored, you say? Pupils constrict. Got your eye on a "person of interest"? Pupils dilate. James Bond certainly doesn't want to give away any of his autonomic cues and therefore wears his shades—as do poker players.

ORGANIZATION AND FUNCTION OF THE AUTONOMIC NERVOUS SYSTEM

DIVISION OF THE AUTONOMIC NERVOUS SYSTEM

The ANS is the part of the peripheral nervous system that supplies motor activity to the visceral effector organs: glands, smooth muscles within organs and tubes, and the heart.

The two divisions of the ANS are the sympathetic (sim-pah-THET-ik) and parasympathetic (pair-ah-sim-pah-THET-ik) nervous systems. The distribution of sympathetic and parasympathetic nerves to the viscera varies. A single organ most often receives fibers from both divisions of the ANS; this is called *dual innervation*. In most instances, stimulation of one division of the ANS causes a specific effect, whereas stimulation by the other division causes an opposing effect. For example, the cells of the heart that determine heart rate receive both sympathetic and parasympathetic fibers. Stimulation of the sympathetic fibers increases heart rate, whereas stimulation of the parasympathetic fibers decreases heart rate. There are exceptions to this arrangement. In a few organs that receive dual innervation, the effects of sympathetic and parasympathetic activity are complementary rather than opposite. For example, in the male, erectile activity is regulated by the parasympathetics, whereas ejaculation is regulated by the sympathetics. The sympathetics and parasympathetics work in a complementary way to achieve the desired effect: penetration of the female and ejection of the sperm. Finally, not all organs have dual innervation. For example, the blood vessels are innervated only by the sympathetic nervous system. Regulation of blood vessel diameter is achieved through an adjustment of sympathetic activity. Increased sympathetic activity causes constriction of the blood vessels, and decreased sympathetic activity causes the blood vessels to dilate.

Table 12-1 indicates the effects of sympathetic and parasympathetic stimulation on some major organs of the body.

SYMPATHETIC NERVOUS SYSTEM: FIGHT OR FLIGHT

In general, the sympathetic nervous system is activated during periods of stress or times when a person feels threatened in some way (Figure 12-1). For this reason, the sympathetic nervous system is called the *fight-or-flight* division of the ANS. In other words, the

Table 12-1 Autonomic Nervous System: Organ Responses

ORGAN	SYMPATHETIC RESPONSE	PARASYMPATHETIC RESPONSE
Heart	Increases rate and strength of contraction	Decreases rate: no direct effect on strength
Bronchial tubes	Dilates (↑ air flow)	Constricts (↓ air flow)
Iris of eye	Dilates (pupil enlarges)	Constricts (pupil becomes smaller)
Blood vessels	Constricts	No innervation
Sweat glands	Stimulates	No innervation
Intestine	Inhibits motility and secretion	Stimulates motility and secretion
Uterus	Relaxes muscle	No effect
Adrenal medulla	Stimulates secretion of epinephrine and norepinephrine	No effect
Salivary glands	Stimulates thick secretion	Stimulates watery secretion

Urinary system
  Bladder wall
  Internal sphincter
	
	Relaxes muscle
	Closes sphincter
		
		Contracts muscle
		Opens sphincter

Parasympathetic nervous system

CNS

Sympathetic nervous system

Feed and breed

Fight or flight

FIGURE 12-1 Autonomic nervous system: parasympathetic nervous system and sympathetic nervous system.

sympathetic nervous system causes you to be prepared either to confront (fight) or to remove yourself from the threatening situation (flight). Recall a time when you were frightened. Your heart raced and pounded in your chest. The pupils of your eyes opened wide. You breathed more quickly and more deeply. The palms of your hands became wet with perspiration, and your mouth became so dry you could hardly speak. The easiest way to remember the sympathetic responses is to recall your personal response to your own worst nightmare. You can check Table 12-1 to see if your responses matched the sympathetic column.

Although the sympathetic nervous system is activated during periods of stress, these periods are normally short-lived. If you keep yourself stressed out, however, the sympathetic nervous system keeps the body in a state of high alert. Over time, this state takes its toll on the body through stress-induced illnesses. Laughter, play, rest, and relaxation diminish sympathetic outflow and are good buffers against stress. So relax and be happy!

 Do You Know...

About the Sympathetic Nervous System Gone Wild?

Several clinical conditions are caused by out-of-control sympathetic activity. One condition is called *autonomic dysreflexia*. Autonomic dysreflexia is experienced by a person who has sustained a high cervical spinal cord injury (e.g., C4 transection and quadriplegia). With this condition, the quadriplegic patient develops a distended urinary bladder, usually from a kinked urinary catheter. The distended bladder sends signals to the spinal cord, setting off massive thoracolumbar (sympathetic) discharge. The intense sympathetic activity severely elevates blood pressure, sometimes to the point of causing a cerebral hemorrhage (stroke). The sympathetic stimulation continues as long as the bladder remains distended. The ANS cannot counteract the sympathetic firing because of the spinal cord injury. Immediate treatment is to remove the stimulus (distended bladder), which then lowers the blood pressure. Out-of-control sympathetic activity is life threatening and is always taken seriously.

PARASYMPATHETIC NERVOUS SYSTEM: FEED AND BREED

The **parasympathetic nervous system** is most active during quiet, nonstressful conditions. It has a calming effect on the body. The parasympathetic nervous system plays an important role in the regulation of digestion and in reproductive function. For this reason, it is sometimes referred to as the *feed-and-breed* division of the ANS. Another descriptive term for the parasympathetic nervous system is *resting and digesting*.

What is "paradoxical fear"? Although the sympathetics are usually associated with fear reactions, the parasympathetics can be activated in situations that are perceived as hopeless and where fight or flight seems futile. The massive parasympathetic discharge can result in uncontrolled urination and defecation. It can also cause the heart rate to decrease so severely that the person faints or experiences a potentially lethal electrical disturbance of the heart. Clinically, this type of cardiac stress reaction is described as "bradying down," a reference to severe bradycardia (dangerously slow heart rate). Yes, one can die of fright!

 Re-Think

1. Explain why sympathetic activity is called *fight or flight*.
2. Explain why parasympathetic activity is called *feed and breed*.

AUTONOMIC TERMINOLOGY AND PHARMACOLOGY

Many drugs work by altering autonomic activity. Thus, many pharmacology terms refer to the autonomic nervous system. In fact, you cannot understand pharmacology without knowing ANS terminology. So get ready for some challenging words.

If a drug causes effects similar to the activation of the sympathetic nervous system, it is called a *sympathomimetic* (sim-pah-thoh-mim-ET-ik) (as in mimicking) drug. A sympathomimetic agent increases heart rate, force of cardiac contraction, and blood pressure. If the drug causes effects that are similar to a situation where the sympathetic nervous system cannot be activated, the drug is called a *sympatholytic* (sim-pah-thoh-LIT-ik) drug (*-lytic* means "inhibiting"). The administration of a sympatholytic drug prevents an increase in cardiac activity when the sympathetic nerves are fired.

If a drug causes effects similar to the activation of the parasympathetic nervous system, it is called a *parasympathomimetic* (pair-ah-sim-pah-thoh-mim-ET-ik) drug. A parasympathomimetic agent decreases heart rate and increases digestive activity. The administration of a *parasympatholytic* (pair-ah-sim-pah-thoh-LIT-ik) agent prevents activation of the parasympathetic nervous system. As if this isn't confusing enough! Most parasympathetic fibers travel with the vagus nerve (CN X). If a drug causes effects similar to parasympathetic activity, it is also called *vagomimetic*. If a drug slows parasympathetic activity, it is called *vagolytic*. The vagomimetic and vagolytic terminology is more commonly used. If an organ, such as the heart, is being driven excessively by the parasympathetic nervous system, the heart rate becomes dangerously slow (bradycardia). The administration of a parasympatholytic or vagolytic drug, such as atropine, blocks the parasympathetic effect on the heart, thereby allowing the heart rate to increase.

AUTONOMIC TONE AND VASOMOTOR TONE

The sympathetics and parasympathetics are active at the same time, creating a background (continuous, low-level) firing of the ANS. This background autonomic activity is called *autonomic tone*. In the resting state, parasympathetic activity is generally stronger. For example, parasympathetic tone maintains the resting heart rate at around 72 beats per minute. When physical activity increases, however, the sympathetic nerves fire more intensely, whereas parasympathetic activity decreases. The shift to sympathetic discharge during exercise results in an increase in heart rate, thereby supplying more oxygen and energy to the exercising muscles. The balance between sympathetic and parasympathetic activity is maintained by the hypothalamus and parts of the brain stem.

A second example of autonomic tone involves the blood vessels. Blood vessels are innervated only by the sympathetic nerves; there is no parasympathetic innervation. Thus, the autonomic tone of the blood vessels is determined by the sympathetic nervous system. Background sympathetic firing keeps the blood vessels somewhat constricted. This sympathetically induced continuous state of blood vessel constriction is called *vasomotor tone* or *sympathetic tone*. Additional sympathetic firing causes blood vessels to constrict, thereby elevating blood pressure. A decrease in sympathetic firing causes blood vessels to dilate, thereby lowering blood pressure. A change in vasomotor tone is clinically very important. For example, loss of vasomotor tone can dangerously lower blood pressure, plunging a person into a lethal shock.

? Re-Think

1. What is a sympathomimetic effect? A parasympathomimetic effect?
2. What is the effect of a vagomimetic drug on heart rate? What is the effect of a vagolytic drug on heart rate?

AUTONOMIC NERVOUS SYSTEM NEURONS

NUMBERS AND GANGLIA

The numbers and arrangement of the neurons of the ANS are important. The pathways of the ANS use two neurons with a ganglion between each neuron (Figure 12-2, *A*). The cell body of neuron 1 is located in the CNS, in the brain or the spinal cord. The axon of neuron 1 leaves the CNS and extends to the ganglion where it synapses on neuron 2. The axon of neuron 1 is called the **preganglionic fiber** (because it comes before [*pre*] the ganglion). The axon of neuron 2 leaves the ganglion and extends to the effector or target organ. This axon is called the **postganglionic fiber** (because it comes after [*post*] the ganglion). Pay particular attention to the postganglionic fibers; they are key to understanding autonomic function. The postganglionic fibers of the sympathetic and parasympathetic nervous systems secrete different neurotransmitters. These different neurotransmitters account for the different effects caused by the sympathetic and parasympathetic nervous systems.

NEURONS OF THE SYMPATHETIC NERVOUS SYSTEM

The neurons of the sympathetic nervous system leave the spinal cord at the thoracic and lumbar levels (T1 to L2) (see Figure 12-2, *B*). The sympathetic nervous system is therefore called the **thoracolumbar outflow**. Most preganglionic sympathetic fibers travel a short distance and synapse within ganglia located close to the spinal cord. The sympathetic ganglia form a chain that runs parallel to the vertebral column. This chain is called the *paravertebral ganglia* or *sympathetic chain*

A

Sympathetic

Parasympathetic

B

C

FIGURE 12-2 **A,** Arrangement of autonomic fibers. **B,** Sympathetic nervous system. **C,** Parasympathetic nervous system.

ganglia. Postganglionic fibers leave the ganglia and extend to the various target organs.

The location of the paravertebral ganglia is important. The paravertebral ganglia provide a site where each preganglionic fiber synapses with multiple postganglionic fibers. Why is this important? The firing of a single sympathetic neuron is capable of providing a generalized, widespread sympathetic response; many organs respond to sympathetic firing. This makes sense—if you are confronted with an emergency situation, you want the entire body to respond immediately!

The adrenal gland (adrenal medulla) acts as a modified sympathetic ganglion. Preganglionic sympathetic fibers supply the adrenal medulla, causing it to secrete hormones (epinephrine and norepinephrine) that resemble the neurotransmitters of the sympathetic nervous system. These hormones circulate in the blood throughout the body. Thus, the sympathetic nervous system and the adrenal medulla function together to achieve a sustained response.

NEURONS OF THE PARASYMPATHETIC NERVOUS SYSTEM

The neurons of the parasympathetic nervous system leave the CNS at the level of the brain stem and sacrum (S2 to S4; see Figure 12-2, *C*). The parasympathetic nervous system is therefore called the **craniosacral outflow.**

Because the ganglia of the parasympathetic nervous system are located close to or within the target organs, the parasympathetic nerves do not have a chain of ganglia running parallel to the spinal cord. The preganglionic fibers are long because the ganglia of the parasympathetic nervous system are located near the target organ. Short postganglionic fibers run from the ganglia to the smooth muscle or glands within the organ. Because of the location of the ganglia close to the target organs, parasympathetic activity generates a more localized response (as opposed to the generalized sympathetic response). Table 12-2

Table 12-2	Autonomic Nervous System: Comparison	
CHARACTERISTIC	**SYMPATHETIC**	**PARASYMPATHETIC**
Origin of fibers	Thoracolumbar	Craniosacral
Functions	Fight or flight	Feed and breed
Ganglia	Paravertebral ganglia	Located near or in target organ
Effects	Generalized, widespread	Localized
Neurotransmitter	Norepinephrine (postganglionic)	Acetylcholine

compares the anatomical arrangement of the sympathetic and parasympathetic nervous systems.

? Re-Think

1. Why is the preganglionic fiber of the sympathetic nervous system shorter than that of the parasympathetic nervous system?
2. Why are the sympathetic nerves referred to as *thoracolumbar outflow*?
3. Why are the parasympathetic nerves referred to as the *craniosacral outflow*?

RUNNING WITH CRANIAL NERVES

Parasympathetic fibers travel from the brain stem with four cranial nerves (CNs): oculomotor (CN III), facial (CN VII), glossopharyngeal (CN IX), and vagus (CN X).

Oculomotor Nerve (CN III)

The oculomotor nerve innervates most of the extrinsic eye muscles (skeletal muscles) that move the eyeball. The oculomotor nerve also carries parasympathetic fibers to two intrinsic eye muscles: the constrictor muscle of the eye, which causes pupillary constriction, and the ciliary muscle, which controls the shape of the lens of the eye. Observation of pupillary reflexes is used clinically to observe for signs of increasing intracranial pressure and other neurological disorders. In addition, many drugs alter parasympathetic activity of the intrinsic eye muscles, and you will need to assess their clinical effects. You will have to do "eye checks"; pay close attention to the eye muscles and nerves of the eye (described in Chapter 13).

Facial Nerve (CN VII)

The facial nerve carries parasympathetic fibers to the tear glands (eyes), salivary glands (mouth), and nasal glands (nose).

Glossopharyngeal Nerve (CN IX)

The glossopharyngeal nerve (with the assistance of the trigeminal nerve) carries parasympathetic fibers to the salivary glands in the mouth.

Vagus Nerve (CN X)

The vagus nerve (the "wanderer" nerve) carries over 80% of the parasympathetic fibers. It travels from the brain stem to organs within the thoracic and abdominal cavities.

2+2 Sum It Up!

The sympathetic nervous system is called the *thoracolumbar outflow*; the parasympathetic nervous system is called the *craniosacral outflow*. Each system has preganglionic and postganglionic fibers. The ganglia of the sympathetic nerves are located in the paravertebral ganglia, and the ganglia of the parasympathetics are located near the target organ. Parasympathetic fibers travel from the brain stem with four cranial nerves: oculomotor, facial, glossopharyngeal, and vagus nerves.

NAMING FIBERS AND NEUROTRANSMITTERS

The key to understanding autonomic function and autonomic pharmacology is based on knowledge of the autonomic neurotransmitters and their receptors. The two major neurotransmitters of the ANS are acetylcholine (ACh) and **norepinephrine** (nor-ep-i-NEF-rin) **(NE)**.

The neurotransmitter is used to name the fibers of the ANS. For example, a fiber that secretes NE as its neurotransmitter is called an **adrenergic fiber** (NE is also called nor*adrenaline*). A fiber that secretes ACh (acetyl*choline*) as its neurotransmitter is called a **cholinergic fiber**.

Now, here's the challenging part. Remember, we are concerned with four fibers (two preganglionic and two postganglionic fibers, sympathetic and parasympathetic). All preganglionic fibers secrete ACh and are therefore cholinergic fibers. The postganglionic fibers of the parasympathetic nervous system secrete ACh and are also cholinergic. The postganglionic sympathetic nervous system fibers, however, secrete NE and are called *adrenergic fibers*. Refer to Figure 12-2, *B* and *C*, and note the color coding that differentiates the adrenergic from the cholinergic fibers. The cholinergic fibers are colored green, whereas the adrenergic fibers are colored red. You absolutely need this fiber-neurotransmitter information to learn autonomic pharmacology.

NEUROTRANSMITTERS: TERMINATION OF ACTIVITY

ACh is secreted by cholinergic fibers and diffuses to its receptor. After ACh exerts its effect on its receptor, it is quickly degraded by acetylcholinesterase (AChE), an enzyme found in the synapse.

NE is secreted by adrenergic fibers. The effects of NE are more prolonged because of the manner in which NE is terminated. Most of the NE is reabsorbed by the adrenergic nerve terminals themselves. The termination of NE is called *reuptake*. Note that its termination differs from that of ACh. The NE taken up by the nerve terminal is processed in two ways. Most of the NE is simply reused. Excess NE can be degraded by an enzyme located within the adrenergic nerve terminal and is called *monoamine oxidase* (MAO). Some of the NE is merely "washed away" from the synapse and is degraded by another enzyme found in surrounding tissue. The name of this enzyme is *catechol-O-methyltransferase* (COMT).

 Do You Know...

Why You Might Have to "Hold the Beer and Sausage" If You Are Taking an MAO Inhibitor?

Monoamine oxidase (MAO) is an enzyme that breaks down norepinephrine in the CNS. An MAO-inhibitor drug prevents the breakdown of NE and is used in the treatment of depression. Although the drug relieves the depression by increasing NE in the CNS, it can also cause serious adverse effects such as a dangerously elevated blood pressure. Certain foods (e.g., beer, cheese, sausage) contain an amino acid that is used in the synthesis of NE. The combination of the drugs and food increases NE and blood pressure and the possibility of a stroke. Some herbals such as St. John's wort have MAO inhibitor activity and may also dangerously elevate blood pressure. Taking an MAO inhibitor? Hold the beer and sausage!

2+2 Sum It Up!

The two major neurotransmitters of the ANS are acetylcholine (ACh) and norepinephrine (NE). ACh is secreted by cholinergic fibers. The effects of ACh are short lived; the ACh is degraded by acetylcholinesterase located in the synapse. NE is secreted by adrenergic fibers. The effects of the sympathetic nervous system are primarily caused by NE. The effects of NE are more prolonged because of how NE is terminated (through reuptake). Excess NE is degraded by monoamine oxidase (MAO). Some NE is simply washed away and degraded at distal sites by another enzyme.

? Re-Think

1. What is the difference between a cholinergic and adrenergic fiber?
2. Explain how neurotransmitter activity is ended.

RECEPTORS OF THE AUTONOMIC NERVOUS SYSTEM

The neurotransmitters of the ANS—ACh and NE—bind to receptors on target cells (cardiac muscle, smooth muscle, and glands). A receptor is any site on the cell to which a neurotransmitter binds, causing an alteration in cellular function. For example, ACh binds to a receptor on a heart cell and causes the heart rate to decrease. NE binds to a different receptor on the heart cell and causes the heart rate to increase. The ANS has two receptor types: cholinergic and adrenergic receptors.

CHOLINERGIC RECEPTORS

Cholinergic receptors are activated by ACh. There are two types of cholinergic receptors: **muscarinic** (mus-kar-IN-ik) **receptors** and **nicotinic receptors**. The different types of cholinergic receptors explain the variety of effects of cholinergic receptor activation by ACh.

Where are these receptors located? Muscarinic receptors are located on the effector or target organs (cardiac muscle, smooth muscle, and glands) of the parasympathetic nerves (Figure 12-3, *A*). Thus, activation of the parasympathetic nervous system releases ACh and stimulates muscarinic receptors. Refer to Table 12-3 and note several of the effects of muscarinic activation. For example, activation of the muscarinic receptors on the constrictor muscle of the iris causes pupil size to decrease. Activation of the muscarinic receptors in the heart (sinoatrial node) causes the heart rate to decrease. Muscarinic activation of the urinary bladder causes the bladder muscle to contract and the outlet sphincter muscle of the urinary bladder to relax; these coordinated muscarinic responses of the bladder promote urination.

There are two types of nicotinic receptors in the peripheral nervous system. The nicotinic neural (N_N) receptors are located within the ganglia of the ANS (see Figure 12-3, *A* and *B*). Because these nicotinic receptors are located in both the sympathetic nervous system and parasympathetic nervous system, the responses to N_N activation are difficult to predict. Nicotinic receptors are also located outside the ANS. For example, the receptors located on skeletal muscles in the neuromuscular junction are nicotinic muscle

Table 12-3 Cholinergic Receptors and Responses*

ORGAN	RECEPTOR	ACTIVATION RESPONSE
Heart	Muscarinic	Decreases heart rate
Bronchial tubes	Muscarinic	Constricts (↓ air flow)
Iris of eye	Muscarinic	Constricts (pupil becomes smaller)
Urinary system		
Bladder wall	Muscarinic	Contracts
Internal sphincter	Muscarinic	Relaxes and opens sphincter

*Muscarinic receptors that are commonly targeted by pharmacological agents are listed in this table.

FIGURE 12-3 Receptors: adrenergic and cholinergic.

receptors (N_M; see Figure 12-3, C). Activation of the N_M receptors in the neuromuscular junction causes skeletal muscle contraction. Remember, the N_N receptors are part of the ANS; the N_M receptors are part of the somatic motor nervous system and skeletal muscle. The cholinergic receptor subtypes are important in pharmacology and are worthwhile learning. However, in this chapter we will refer only to the muscarinic receptors.

ADRENERGIC RECEPTORS

There are two main types of adrenergic receptors: **alpha- (α) adrenergic** and **beta- (β) adrenergic receptors** (see Figure 12-3, B). There are subtypes of the adrenergic receptors: alpha$_1$-, alpha$_2$-, beta$_1$-, and beta$_2$-adrenergic receptors. Adrenergic receptors are located on the target organs of the sympathetic nerves, so that stimulation of the sympathetic nervous system causes activation of adrenergic receptors. See Table 12-4 for the effects of adrenergic receptor activation. Note that activation of the alpha$_1$ receptors of the blood vessels of the mucous membrane causes constriction, thereby decreasing blood flow and shrinking swollen membranes to relieve the discomfort of a stuffy nose. Activation of the alpha$_1$ receptors on blood vessels causes vasoconstriction, thereby elevating blood pressure. These drugs are used in the treatment of conditions that involve low blood pressure, such as shock. Activation of the beta$_1$ receptors in the heart increases heart rate and the strength of cardiac muscle contraction. Activation of the beta$_2$ receptors dilates the breathing tubes, thereby increasing air flow; this action is the

basis of the bronchodilators used in the treatment of asthma. Activation of the alpha$_1$ receptors in the iris (eye) causes the radial muscle to contract and the pupil to dilate. Finally, activation of the beta$_2$ receptors in the pregnant uterus causes the uterine muscles to relax, thereby preventing the premature delivery of the fetus. The adrenergic receptors are activated by NE and other natural catecholamines, such as epinephrine and dopamine.

There are a small number of dopamine receptors (also classified as adrenergic receptors) located in the blood vessels of the kidney. Activation of the dopamine receptors causes the blood vessels in the kidney to dilate, thereby increasing blood flow to the kidneys. Dopamine is often administered clinically to maintain blood flow to the kidneys during shocklike episodes that would normally diminish blood flow to the kidneys.

Table **12-4**	Adrenergic Receptors and Responses*	
ORGAN	**RECEPTOR**[†]	**ACTIVATION RESPONSE**
Heart	β_1	Increases heart rate and strength of contraction
Bronchial tubes	β_2	Dilates ($\uparrow$ air flow)
Iris of eye	α_1	Dilates (pupil enlarges)
Blood vessels	α_1	Constricts
Uterus	β_2	Relaxes

*Adrenergic receptors commonly targeted by pharmacological agents are listed in this table.
[†]α, Alpha; β, beta.

1. Name and locate the cholinergic receptors. Name the neurotransmitter that activates cholinergic receptors.
2. Name and locate the adrenergic receptors. Name a neurotransmitter that activates adrenergic receptors.

AUTONOMIC TERMINOLOGY: "DOING" AUTONOMIC PHARMACOLOGY

Autonomic pharmacology classifies drugs according to their receptors. For example, a beta$_1$-adrenergic agonist is a drug that activates the beta$_1$-adrenergic receptors. (An agonist is a drug that activates a receptor.) A beta$_1$-adrenergic antagonist is a drug that blocks the effect of beta$_1$-adrenergic activation. (An antagonist or blocker is a drug that prevents receptor activation.) A muscarinic agonist activates the muscarinic receptor, whereas a muscarinic antagonist blocks muscarinic receptor activation. The same terminology (agonist/antagonist) is applied to drugs that interact with cholinergic and adrenergic receptors.

Let's see if you can figure out some autonomic physiology and pharmacology.

- *Question 1.* Mr. T was admitted to the ER experiencing respiratory distress caused by asthma. Why was he given a beta$_2$-adrenergic agonist (albuterol)? Check Table 12-4 for the respiratory effects of beta$_2$-adrenergic activation. *Answer.* Activation of the beta$_2$-adrenergic receptors on the bronchioles (airways) causes the airways to dilate (open up), thereby improving the flow of air and relieving the respiratory distress of asthma.

- *Question 2.* A very anxious Mr. Q was admitted with a rapid heart rate. Why was he given a beta$_1$-adrenergic blocker (propranolol)? Check Table 12-4 for the cardiac (heart) effects of beta$_1$-adrenergic response. *Answer.* Mr. Q's heart rate was elevated because of excess sympathetic stimulation (an anxiety effect). A beta$_1$-adrenergic blocker prevents activation of the beta$_1$-adrenergic receptors on the heart, thereby reducing heart rate.

- *Question 3.* A patient has had a heart attack and is experiencing a very slow heart rate caused by excessive parasympathetic (vagal) activity. Why was he given a muscarinic antagonist (atropine)? Check Table 12-3 for the effects of muscarinic activation on heart rate. *Answer.* Muscarinic activation (caused by excess parasympathetic activity) slows heart rate. By blocking muscarinic receptors with atropine, heart rate increases.

- *Question 4.* Ms. S is diagnosed with hypertension (high blood pressure). Why did her physician prescribe an alpha$_1$-adrenergic blocker? Check Table 12-4 for the effect of an alpha$_1$-adrenergic response on blood vessels. *Answer.* The alpha$_1$-adrenergic antagonist blocks the alpha$_1$ receptors in the blood vessels, causing them to dilate. Blood vessel dilation decreases blood pressure.

- *Question 5.* A postoperative patient is unable to urinate because of the anticholinergic drugs used during the perioperative period. Why was she given a muscarinic agonist such as bethanechol? *Answer.* Activation of the muscarinic receptors stimulates contraction of the urinary bladder and relaxation of the bladder sphincter. Both actions facilitate urination.

- *Question 6.* A patient goes to his eye doctor for an eye exam. Why did the physician put anticholinergic eyedrops in his eyes (see Table 12-3)? *Answer.* Activation of the muscarinic receptor on the pupillary muscles causes pupillary constriction. By using anticholinergic (antimuscarinic) eyedrops, the muscarinic receptors are blocked, and the pupil dilates. The dilated pupils facilitate the eye exam.

- *Question 7.* A canine friend (Dillon) routinely "bradys down" in response to general anesthesia and is therefore premedicated with atropine. What happens to Dillon without and with the atropine? *Answer.* The general anesthesia causes sustained vagal discharge to the heart and a significant decrease in heart rate (bradycardia). By premedicating with a vagolytic or antimuscarinic drug (see Table 12-3), atropine, the decline in heart rate is prevented.

This is how to analyze autonomic function and "do" autonomic pharmacology. Learn the receptors and the consequences of receptor activation (agonist) and blockade (antagonist).

Do You Know...

About the Parasympathetics, Nitric Oxide, Erections ... and, By the Way, Viagra?

In response to sexual stimulation, parasympathetic fibers stimulate the endothelial cells of the blood vessels of the penis to secrete nitric oxide, a gas that triggers a series of reactions that produce cyclic guanosine monophosphate (cGMP). cGMP relaxes the smooth muscle of the blood vessels, thereby increasing blood flow to the penis. Hence, the erection. Having done its job, the cGMP is degraded by an enzyme called *phosphodiesterase*. Most men with erectile dysfunction have difficulty in sustaining their erections. Enter Viagra (sildenafil)! Viagra inhibits the activity of phosphodiesterase, thereby prolonging the life of cGMP and sustaining the erection.

Sum It Up!

The neurotransmitters, ACh and NE, bind to receptors. There are two types of autonomic receptors: cholinergic and adrenergic. Cholinergic receptors are activated by ACh. There are two types of cholinergic receptors: muscarinic and nicotinic. The muscarinic receptors are located on the target organs of the parasympathetic nerves. The adrenergic receptors are activated by NE. There are two types of adrenergic receptors: alpha- and beta-adrenergic receptors. The adrenergic receptors are located on the target organs of the sympathetic nervous system.

🍂 As You Age

1. Aging causes an increase in synaptic delay and a 5% to 10% decrease in the speed of nerve conduction. Consequently, nerve reflexes become slower.
2. Aging causes a loss of the sense of vibration at the ankle after the age of 65. This change is accompanied by a decrease of the ankle-jerk reflex and may affect balance, increasing the chance of falling.
3. An aging ANS causes many changes. For example, a less-efficient sympathetic nervous system may cause transient hypotension and fainting. A decreased responsiveness of the baroreceptor reflex contributes to the fainting episodes.
4. Decreased autonomic nerve activity supplying the eyes causes changes in pupil size and pupillary reactivity. There is some decline in function of the cranial nerves mediating taste and smell.

👤 MEDICAL TERMINOLOGY AND DISORDERS — Disorders of the Somatic Efferent and Autonomic Nervous Systems

Medical Term	Word Parts	Word Part Meaning or Derivation	Description
Words			
autonomic	auto-	self	**Autonomic** means *automatic*. In response to changing body needs the autonomic nervous system (ANS) automatically helps regulate organ function, such as heart rate. The sympathetic division increases heart rate, whereas the parasympathetic division lowers heart rate.
	-nom(os)-	law	
	-ic	pertaining to	
contralateral	contra-	opposite	*A reference to the opposite side of the body.* For example, a patient suffered a brain attack on the left side of her brain and experienced hemiparalysis on the contralateral side (right) of her body.
	-later/o-	side	
	-al	pertaining to	
decussate		From a Latin word meaning "to mark with a cross"	Means *to cross over.* For example, the pyramidal tract decussates at the medulla oblongata and descends on the contralateral side of the spinal cord.
ipsilateral	ipse-	same	*A reference to the same side of the body.* For example, a patient suffered a brain attack (left brain) and suffered right-sided hemiparalysis and ipsilateral paresis (left side of the body).
	-lateral	side	
Disorders			
amyotrophic lateral sclerosis	a-	without	Also called **ALS** or **Lou Gehrig disease**. ALS refers to *progressive deterioration of motor nerve cells resulting in a progressive loss of muscle control.* Muscle atrophy is caused by hardening of nerve tissue on the lateral columns of the spinal cord. Disability increases from muscle weakness in the extremities, muscles of speech and swallowing, and muscles of respiration to total paralysis and death.
	-myo-	muscle	
	-throph/o-	nourishment	
	later/o	side	
	scler/o-	hardening	
	-osis	condition of	
autonomic dysreflexia	dys-	difficult or faulty	See the "Do You Know" feature on p. 220.
	-reflexia	reflex	
meningocele	mening/o-	meninges	*Protrusion of the meninges through a defect in the skull or vertebra (spina bifida).* A **myelomeningocele** is *a protrusion of the spinal cord and meninges through a defect in the vertebrae.* Disability is related to the location and size of the protruding spinal cord and nervous tissue.
	-cele	protrusion, hernia	
multiple sclerosis	scler/o-	hardening	**Multiple sclerosis** (MS) is *a progressive demyelination of the neurons, especially the oligodendrocytes; the demyelination produces sclerotic lesions along the neurons, thereby interfering with nerve conduction.* The most common form of MS is called *relapsing-remitting MS,* in which the symptoms appear and disappear (exacerbations and remissions). Degenerative changes affect cognitive, sensory, and motor activity. Fatigue, weakness, paresthesias, ataxia (a- = without; -tax/o- = coordination), and optic neuritis are common. Optic neuritis causes a variety of visual disturbances: diplopia, nystagmus, diminished vision, and blindness.
	-osis	condition of	

Continued

MEDICAL TERMINOLOGY AND DISORDERS — Disorders of the Somatic Efferent and Autonomic Nervous Systems—cont'd

Medical Term	Word Parts	Word Part Meaning or Derivation	Description
neuralgia	neur/o-	nerve	**Neuralgia** is *pain that involves a nerve.* Sciatica is a form of neuralgia; pain moves along the sciatic nerve and its branches through the buttocks and into the thigh and leg. Shingles or herpes zoster sometimes causes postherpetic neuralgia, a severe pain that persists long after the lesions have healed. Pain and a vesicular rash progress along the course of one or more spinal nerves, usually the intercostal nerves and sometimes the trigeminal nerve. Trigeminal neuralgia is due to inflammation of the trigeminal nerve (CN V); it causes excruciating pain in the facial area.
	-algia	pain	
paralysis	para-	alongside of or abnormal	**Paralysis** refers to *the complete loss of muscle function in one or more muscle groups.* Paralysis (-plegia) may be accompanied by loss of sensation. Most episodes of paralysis in adults are due to CVA and spinal cord injury. Paralysis may be described as being flaccid or spastic. Flaccid paralysis is described as flabby or lack of muscle control and is caused by damaged nerves. With spastic paralysis there is stiff and poorly coordinated muscle control. It is due to CNS disorders such as cerebral palsy. Infantile paralysis or polio is a contagious viral infection that destroys the motor neurons in the grey matter (polio means "grey") of the brain stem and the spinal cord. Bell's palsy is a weakness or paralysis of one side of the face in response to inflammation of the facial nerve (CN VII). The word part paresis means "slight paralysis," as in hemiparesis (slight paralysis or weakness of the right or left half of the body). Gastroparesis causes weak stomach (gastr/o- = stomach) muscle contractions and delayed gastric emptying. Vocal cord paresis causes diminishment in voice quality and volume.
	-lysis	breakdown	
paresthesia	para-	alongside of or abnormal	*Refers to abnormal sensation such as burning, numbness, prickling, or tingling.* Paresthesias can be caused by lesions of both the central and peripheral nervous system and often are symptomatic of other disorders such as multiple sclerosis and diabetes mellitus. **Anesthesia** is *a lack of sensation* and hyperesthesia is *an increased sensitivity to a sensory stimulus (skin/touch).*
	-esthesia	sensation or feeling	
peripheral neuropathy	neur/o-	nerve	*A loss of normal sensation caused by peripheral nerve damage.* There are many causes of neuropathies. The pain has different intensities (severe to mild), multiple distribution patterns (hands, foot, pain), and a variety of descriptions (numbness, burning, tingling, prickly, akin to electric shock).
	-path/o-	disease	
	-y	condition of	
spinal cord injury			*Any condition or event that damages the spinal cord.* Complete transection of the cord produces quadriplegia or paraplegia, depending on the level of injury. Immediately after the injury, the person experiences spinal shock that may last from several hours to several weeks.

Get Ready for Exams!

Summary Outline

I. Autonomic or Visceral Reflexes
A. What they do: autonomic nerves reflexively regulate organ function.
B. Pathway: the sequence is receptor activation, sensory input (→ CNS), motor neuron response, and effector response.

II. Organization and Function of the Autonomic Nervous System
A. Divisions of the ANS: two divisions
   1. Sympathetic nervous system, called *fight or flight*
   2. Parasympathetic nervous system, called *feed and breed*

B. Autonomic terminology and autonomic pharmacology
   1. Drugs that affect the sympathetic nervous system are called *sympathomimetic* and *sympatholytic*.
   2. Drugs that affect the parasympathetic nervous system are called *parasympathomimetic* (vagomimetic) and *parasympatholytic* (vagolytic).

C. Autonomic tone and vasomotor tone
   1. Background firing of the ANS causes autonomic tone.

2. Background sympathetic stimulation of the blood vessels causes vasomotor or sympathetic tone.

III. **Autonomic Nervous System: Neurons**
  A. Numbers and ganglia
    1. Preganglionic fibers are fibers that extend from the CNS to the ganglia.
    2. Postganglionic fibers are fibers that extend from the ganglia to the effector or target organ.
  B. Neurons of the sympathetic nervous system
    1. The sympathetic nervous system is called the *thoracolumbar outflow*.
    2. The sympathetic ganglia are located in a chain close to the spinal cord; the chain is called *paravertebral ganglia*.
    3. The adrenal medulla secretes hormones that mimic the sympathetic nervous system.
  C. Neurons of the parasympathetic nervous system
    1. The parasympathetic nervous system is called the *craniosacral outflow*.
    2. Some parasympathetic fibers travel with cranial nerves; most parasympathetics run with the vagus nerve (CN X).
  D. Naming fibers and neurotransmitters
    1. Cholinergic fibers secrete acetylcholine (ACh).
    2. Adrenergic fibers secrete norepinephrine (NE).
  E. Neurotransmitters: termination of activity
    1. ACh is degraded immediately by acetylcholinesterase.
    2. NE activity is ended primarily by reuptake of the NE into the nerve terminal and by MAO activity in the nerve terminal. Distally, NE is degraded by COMT.

IV. **Receptors of the Autonomic Nervous System**
  A. Cholinergic receptors
    1. Activated by ACh
    2. Two types: muscarinic and nicotinic (and subtypes)
  B. Adrenergic receptors
    1. Activated by NE
    2. Two types: alpha and beta (and subtypes)
  C. Receptor activation and blockade can be determined by examining Tables 12-1, 12-3, and 12-4.
  D. Autonomic receptors—doing autonomic pharmacology
    1. Clinical examples where drugs target autonomic receptors

Review Your Knowledge

Matching: Sympathetic or Parasympathetic
Directions: Indicate if the following statements describe the sympathetic nervous system (S) or the parasympathetic nervous system (P).
  1. ___ Paravertebral ganglia
  2. ___ Feed-and-breed function
  3. ___ Thoracolumbar outflow
  4. ___ Postganglionic fiber is adrenergic.
  5. ___ The target organs are stimulated by norepinephrine (NE).
  6. ___ Fight-or-flight function
  7. ___ The postganglionic fiber is cholinergic.

  8. ___ The target organs are stimulated by acetylcholine (ACh).
  9. ___ Craniosacral outflow
  10. ___ The effects of this system are more widespread and prolonged.

Matching: Norepinephrine or Acetylcholine
Directions: Indicate if the statements are descriptive of norepinephrine (NE) or acetylcholine (ACh).
  1. ___ Secreted by adrenergic fibers
  2. ___ Causes activation of alpha-adrenergic receptors
  3. ___ Secreted by the postganglionic fibers of the parasympathetic nervous system
  4. ___ Causes activation of muscarinic receptors
  5. ___ Action terminated by acetylcholinesterase, an enzyme located within the synapse
  6. ___ Action terminated by reuptake of the neurotransmitter and MAO
  7. ___ Causes activation of beta-adrenergic receptors
  8. ___ Causes activation of nicotinic receptors, including the N_M receptors in the neuromuscular junction of skeletal muscle
  9. ___ Mediates fight or flight (postganglionic)
  10. ___ Mediates feed and breed

Multiple Choice
  1. Which of the following is least related to the sympathetic nervous system?
     a. Includes the paravertebral ganglia
     b. Is also called the *fight-or-flight* response
     c. Is also called *craniosacral outflow*
     d. Uses norepinephrine as a transmitter
  2. Which of the following is most related to the parasympathetic nervous system?
     a. Uses norepinephrine as a postganglionic transmitter
     b. Mediates feed-and-breed activities
     c. Is also called the *fight-or-flight* response
     d. Postganglionic fiber is adrenergic
  3. What is the role of monoamine oxidase (MAO)?
     a. Destroys norepinephrine
     b. Activates the muscarinic receptors
     c. Activates the beta$_1$-adrenergic receptors
     d. Inactivates acetylcholine
  4. Activation of the beta$_2$-adrenergic receptors
     a. is a response to the binding of ACh.
     b. causes wheezing.
     c. dilates the breathing passages.
     d. slows the heart rate.
  5. Activation of the muscarinic receptors
     a. dilates the breathing passages.
     b. slows the heart rate.
     c. dilates the pupil.
     d. is a response to norepinephrine.
  6. Blockade of the alpha$_1$-adrenergic receptors is the basis for what group of drugs?
     a. Hypoglycemic agents
     b. Antihypertensive drugs
     c. Cardiac stimulants
     d. Bronchodilators

7. Pupillary dilation, an increase in heart rate, and an inability to urinate are effects of
   a. alpha$_1$-adrenergic activation.
   b. beta$_2$-adrenergic activation.
   c. muscarinic blockade.
   d. vagomimetic activity.

8. A vagolytic drug exerts the same effects as
   a. a sympathomimetic agent.
   b. a beta$_1$-adrenergic agonist.
   c. a muscarinic agonist.
   d. an antimuscarinic agent.

9. Fight or flight, paravertebral ganglia, and norepinephrine are most related to
   a. cholinergic fibers.
   b. sympathetic nervous system.
   c. nicotinic and muscarinic receptors.
   d. craniosacral outflow.

10. Feed and breed, craniosacral outflow, and ACh are most related to the
    a. sympathetic nervous system.
    b. adrenergic fibers.
    c. nicotinic and muscarinic receptors.
    d. paravertebral ganglia.

Go Figure

1. **According to Figure 12-1**
   a. The sympathetic nervous system is called the *craniosacral outflow*.
   b. The parasympathetic nervous system is called the *thoracolumbar outflow*.
   c. Activation of the craniosacral outflow mediates a calming effect.
   d. Fight-or-flight best describes craniosacral outflow.

2. **According to Figure 12-2**
   a. All preganglionic fibers secrete ACh.
   b. All postganglionic fibers secrete ACh.
   c. Cholinergic fibers are restricted to the parasympathetic nervous system.
   d. Adrenergic fibers are restricted to the parasympathetic nervous system.

3. **According to Figure 12-2**
   a. The postganglionic fibers of the sympathetic nervous system are longer than those of the parasympathetic nervous system.
   b. All fibers of the sympathetic nervous system secrete norepinephrine.
   c. Paravertebral ganglia are found only within the parasympathetic nervous system.
   d. The ganglia of sympathetic fibers are found near or in the organ of innervation.

4. **According to Figure 12-3**
   a. ACh activates muscarinic receptors.
   b. Parasympathetic nervous system discharge activates muscarinic receptors.
   c. Sympathetic nervous system discharge activates alpha- and beta-adrenergic receptors.
   d. All of the above are true.

5. **According to Tables 12-3 and 12-4**
   a. Activation of the muscarinic receptors decreases heart rate.
   b. Activation of the nicotinic receptors on skeletal muscle is an autonomic effect.
   c. Activation of the adrenergic receptors decreases heart rate and dilates all blood vessels.
   d. All of the above are true.

Sensory System

Key Terms

chemoreceptors (p. 231)
cochlea (p. 250)
cornea (p. 241)
equilibrium (p. 236)
eustachian tube (p. 249)
mechanoreceptors (p. 231)

olfactory receptors (p. 236)
optic chiasm (p. 247)
ossicles (p. 248)
pain receptors (p. 231)
photoreceptors (p. 231)
proprioception (p. 236)

referred pain (p. 234)
refraction (p. 245)
retina (p. 241)
sclera (p. 241)
thermoreceptors (p. 231)
vestibule (p. 251)

Objectives

1. State the functions of the sensory system.
2. Define the five types of sensory receptors.
3. Describe the four components involved in the perception of a sensation and two important characteristics of sensation.
4. Describe the five general senses.
5. Describe the special senses of smell and taste.
6. Describe the sense of sight, including:
   • Describe the structure of the eye.
   • Explain the movement of the eyes.
   • Describe how the size of the pupils changes.

7. Describe the sense of hearing, including:
   • Describe the three divisions of the ear.
   • Describe the functions of the parts of the ear involved in hearing.
   • Explain the role of the ear in maintaining the body's equilibrium.

The sensory system allows us to experience the world. Senses let you see the trees, hear the voices of your friends and family, feel the heat of the sun, and taste your favorite foods. When the external environment becomes threatening, the sensory system also acts as a warning system. For example, if you place your hand on a hot surface, the sensory system experiences the episode as pain. The pain is a danger signal indicating that the body must make an adjustment to remove the harmful stimulus.

In addition to sensing outside information, the sensory system also allows us to keep track of what is happening within our bodies. For example, when the stomach fills with food, sensory information is carried to the central nervous system (CNS). In response to this information, the stomach is told to digest the food.

RECEPTORS AND SENSATION

CELLS THAT DETECT STIMULI

Sensory neurons transmit information to the CNS (Table 13-1). A receptor is a specialized area of a sensory neuron that detects a specific stimulus. For example, the receptors in the eye respond to light, whereas the

receptors on the tongue respond to chemicals in food. The five types of sensory receptors are as follows:

• **Chemoreceptors** (kee-moh-ree-SEP-tors): Receptors stimulated by changes in the chemicals such as hydrogen ion (H^+), calcium, and food
• **Pain receptors**, or nociceptors (noh-see-SEP-tors): Receptors stimulated by tissue damage or distention
• **Thermoreceptors**: Receptors stimulated by changes in temperature
• **Mechanoreceptors**: Receptors stimulated by changes in pressure or movements of body fluids
• **Photoreceptors**: Receptors stimulated by light

WHAT SENSATION IS

A sensation is the conscious awareness of incoming sensory information. Yelling "Ouch," for example, indicates that you have become aware of a painful stimulus.

EXPERIENCING A SENSATION

FOUR COMPONENTS

Four components are involved in the perception of a sensation. Using the sense of sight as an example, these

Table 13-1 Types of Sensory Receptors

RECEPTOR	STIMULUS	EXAMPLE
Chemoreceptors	Changes in chemical concentrations of substances	Taste and smell
Pain receptors (nociceptors)	Tissue damage	Pain
Thermoreceptors	Changes in temperature	Heat and cold
Mechanoreceptors	Changes in pressure or movement of fluids	Hearing and equilibrium
Photoreceptors	Light energy	Sight

four components are illustrated in Figure 13-1 and described as follows:

- *Stimulus:* Light is the stimulus for the sense of sight. In the absence of light, you cannot see.
- *Receptor:* Light waves stimulate the photoreceptors in the eye, producing a nerve impulse.
- *Sensory nerve:* The nerve impulse is conducted by a sensory nerve (optic nerve) to the occipital lobe of the brain.
- *Special area of the brain:* The sensory information is interpreted as sight in the occipital lobe of the brain. This is an important point; the sensation is experienced by the brain and not by the sensory receptor. For example, you see an object, hear a voice, or feel pain because the sensory information has stimulated a part of the brain.

As you study each sensation, identify the stimulus, type of receptor, name of the sensory nerve, and specific area of the brain that interprets the sensation.

TWO CHARACTERISTICS OF SENSATION

Two important characteristics of sensation are projection and adaptation. Projection describes the process whereby the brain, after receiving a sensation, refers that sensation back to its source. You see with your eyes, hear with your ears, and feel pain in your injured finger because the cortex of your brain receives the sensation and projects it back to its source. Projection answers the question, "If pain is experienced by the brain, why does my injured finger hurt?" (Figure 13-2, *A*).

The experience of "phantom limb pain" is another example of projection. If a leg is amputated, the person may still feel pain in the amputated leg (see Figure 13-2, *B*). The missing leg often throbs with pain. What is the cause of phantom limb sensation? The severed nerve endings of the amputated leg continue to send sensory information to the parietal lobe of the brain. The brain interprets the information as pain and

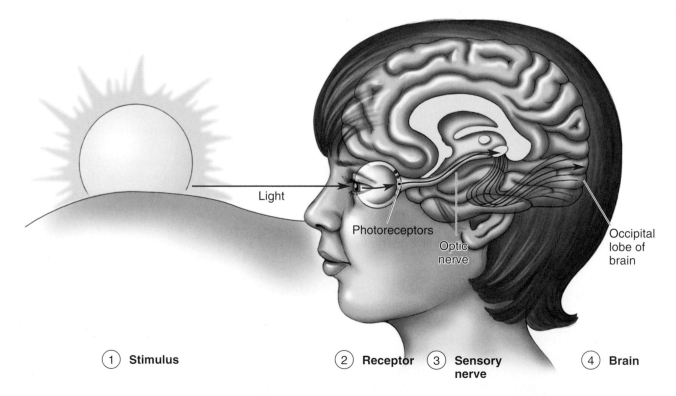

Light

Photoreceptors

Optic nerve

Occipital lobe of brain

① **Stimulus**　　② **Receptor**　③ **Sensory nerve**　　④ **Brain**

FIGURE 13-1 Four components of sensation.

A   **B**

FIGURE 13-2 **A,** Projection . . . ouch! **B,** Phantom limb. The *dashed line* represents the amputated part.

projects the feeling back to the leg area. For most amputees, the phantom limb pain diminishes as the severed nerves heal, but the person often experiences a phantom limb presence. The amputated leg still feels as though it is attached. There is some good news about phantom limb sensation—the sensation often "locates" the amputated limb and helps a patient learn to use an artificial limb.

Sensory adaptation is another characteristic of sensation; it is illustrated by the sense of smell. When you enter a room with a strong odor, the odor at first seems overwhelming. After a short time, however, the odor becomes less noticeable. The sensory receptors in the nose have adapted. When continuously stimulated, these receptors send fewer signals to the area of the brain that interprets sensory information as smell.

Receptors vary in their ability to adapt. Pain receptors do not adapt, whereas the receptors for the smell adapt rapidly. Generally, receptors that regulate homeostatic mechanisms adapt very slowly or not at all.

There are two groups of senses: general and special senses. General senses are called *general*, or *somatic*, because their receptors are widely distributed throughout the body. The special senses are localized within a particular organ in the head. The special senses include taste, smell, sight, hearing, and balance.

? Re-Think

1. Predict what would happen to the sense of sight if the optic nerve were severed (cut)?
2. Define *projection* and *adaptation*.

THE GENERAL SENSES

General senses include pain, touch, pressure, temperature, and proprioception (Figure 13-3). Receptors for the general senses are widely distributed and are found in the skin, muscles, joints, and viscera.

PAIN

The receptors for pain, called *nociceptors,* consist of free nerve endings that are stimulated by tissue damage. Pain receptors do not adapt and may continue to send signals after the stimulus is removed. Pain receptors are widely distributed throughout the skin, the visceral organs, and other internal tissues. Oddly enough, the nervous tissue of the brain lacks pain receptors; there is no pain in the brain. Tissues surrounding the brain, like the meninges and the blood vessels, however, do contain pain receptors. You can feel a headache.

Pain serves a protective function. Being unpleasant, pain motivates the person to remove its cause. The failure of the pain receptors to adapt is also protective. For example, if a person complains of right lower quadrant (RLQ) abdominal pain, the pain is used as a valuable clue about what is wrong. In this example, the pain is indicative of acute appendicitis, requiring an appendectomy (surgical removal of the appendix). Once the diagnosis is made, the pain is treated. If the physician merely relieved the pain, surgical intervention might have been delayed, resulting in a ruptured appendix and life-threatening peritonitis. Although unpleasant and undesirable, pain serves the body well.

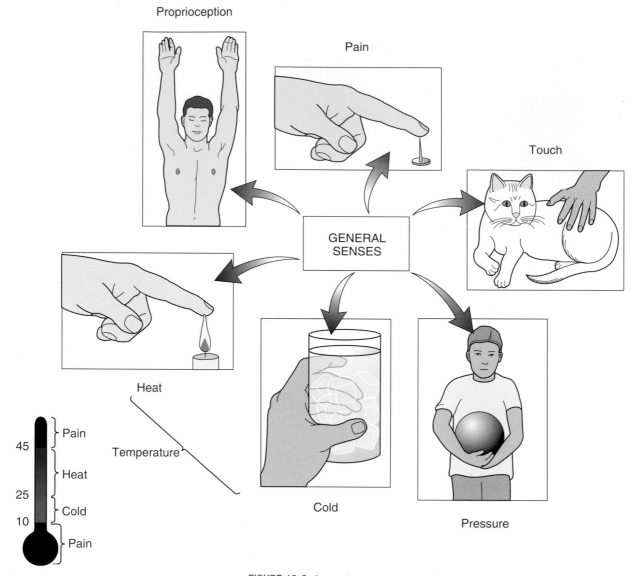

Proprioception

Pain

Touch

GENERAL SENSES

Heat

Pain

45

Temperature

Heat

25

Cold

10

Pain

Cold

Pressure

FIGURE 13-3 General senses.

Some patients are at risk because of a diminishment or alteration in the sensation of pain. Patients with diabetes mellitus, for example, often develop nerve damage in their legs and feet; the nerve damage is called *diabetic neuropathy*. Because they cannot feel the pain, persons with neuropathy may develop blisters on their feet because of poorly fitting shoes. The blistered site continues to expand and eventually becomes infected and gangrenous, requiring amputation. This is a common experience among diabetic persons and is the reason for meticulous attention to their foot care.

What stimulates nociceptors? The specific signals that stimulate pain are not well understood. Three pain triggers have been identified. First, tissue injury promotes the release of chemicals that stimulate pain receptors. Second, a deficiency of oxygen stimulates pain receptors. For example, if the blood supply to an internal organ is diminished, a condition called *ischemia*, the tissue is deprived of oxygen and the person experiences pain. The pain of a heart attack is caused

in part by the oxygen deprivation experienced by the cardiac muscle. The administration of oxygen helps relieve pain. Third, pain may be experienced when tissues are stretched or deformed. The stimulus is mechanical (distention, distortion) rather than chemical. For example, if the intestine becomes distended, the person will often experience a severe cramping pain.

Why is pain originating in the heart often experienced in the shoulder and left arm? When pain feels as if it is coming from an area other than the site where it originates, it is called **referred pain** (Figure 13-4). Patients with heart disease often complain of pain or an aching sensation that starts in the shoulder region and moves down the left arm into the fourth and fifth fingers. In other words, stimulation of pain receptors in the heart causes pain that is experienced as being away from the heart.

What is the explanation for referred pain? The occurrence of referred pain is the result of shared sensory nerve pathways. The nerve pathways that

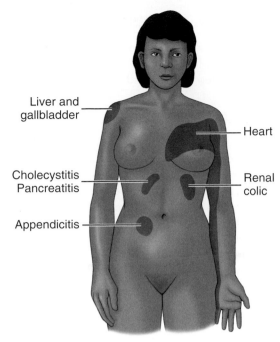

Liver and gallbladder

Heart

Cholecystitis
Pancreatitis

Renal
colic

Appendicitis

FIGURE 13-4 Sites of referred pain.

carry information from the heart are the same pathways that carry information from the shoulder and left arm. As a result, the brain interprets heart pain as shoulder and arm pain.

Once the pain receptors are stimulated, where does the information go? Pain impulses for most of the body travel up the spinal cord in a sensory nerve tract called the *spinothalamic tract*. The information is then transmitted to the thalamus, where the person first becomes aware of the pain, and then to the parietal lobe. The parietal lobe can identify the source of the pain and judge its intensity and other characteristics.

You will spend much time assessing pain. You will determine the location of the pain, its duration, and what the pain "feels like"—sharp, dull, deep, superficial, burning, throbbing, cramping, aching, gnawing, stabbing, and a host of other descriptive terms. You will also use a pain scale that will help you evaluate the intensity of pain. For example, you may ask your patient to rate his or her pain from 1 (pain-free) to 5 (horrible pain). Create your own pain scale (1 to 5) using the following "smiley face" approach.

No pain

Horrible
pain

◯ ◯ ◯ ◯ ◯

Relief of pain is achieved in many ways, such as rest, change of position, meditation techniques, surgical intervention, the administration of oxygen, and the use of drugs. Drugs called *analgesics,* including aspirin, acetaminophen, ibuprofen, and opioids (morphine),

relieve pain. Pain management is a huge clinical problem!

 Re-Think

1. List five words used to describe pain.
2. Provide an example of referred pain.

TOUCH AND PRESSURE

The receptors for touch and pressure are mechanoreceptors; they respond to forces that press, move, or deform tissue. Touch receptors are also called *tactile receptors* and are found mostly in the skin; they allow us to feel a cat's soft fur (see Figure 13-3). They are particularly numerous in the lips and tips of the fingers, toes, tongue, penis, and clitoris. Fingers have the highest concentration of touch receptors. Receptors for heavy pressure are located in the skin, subcutaneous tissue, and the deep tissue. Pressure receptors are stimulated by the heavy ball in the boy's arms in Figure 13-3.

Touch is the first sensory system to develop in the fetus and is essential to its growth and development. The importance of touch extends throughout the lifespan. If an infant is not touched, it does not thrive and will likely die (failure-to-thrive syndrome). An appreciation of touch in the health of a preterm infant forms the basis of "kangaroo care"; the tiny, diaper-clad infant is placed in the blouse or shirt of its parent. The warmth and physical contact with the parent causes many neurobiological changes that calm the infant, stabilize its temperature, and improve feeding. Sadly, you will often encounter infants or "warehoused" older persons who have been diagnosed with failure to thrive. They are generally the untouched and ignored. Touch is life-sustaining!

TEMPERATURE

The receptors for temperature are called *thermoreceptors*. The two types of thermoreceptors are heat and cold receptors. Thermoreceptors are found in free nerve endings, as well as in other specialized sensory cells beneath the skin, and are scattered widely throughout the body. Note the temperature scale in Figure 13-3. The cold receptors are stimulated at between 50° and 76°F (10° and 25°C). Heat receptors are stimulated between 76° and 112°F (25° and 45°C). At both ends (extremes) of the temperature scale, pain receptors are stimulated, producing a freezing or burning sensation. Both heat and cold thermoreceptors display adaptation so that the sensation of heat or cold fades rapidly. Immerse your hand in warm water and note how quickly the feeling of warmth disappears, even though the temperature of the water has not decreased. Your heat receptors have adapted.

Remember that pain receptors do not adapt. If you place your hand in boiling water, you will feel intense continuous pain. Sensory information regarding temperature is sent to the parietal lobe. What about the cooling effects of menthol? Menthol anesthetizes the heat receptors. Thus, the only thermoreceptors that can be activated are the cold receptors.

PROPRIOCEPTION

Proprioception (proh-pree-oh-SEP-shun) is the sense of orientation, or position. This sense allows you to locate a body part without looking at it. In other words, if you close your eyes, you can still locate your arm in space; you do not have to see your arm to know that it is raised over your head (see Figure 13-3). Proprioception plays an important role in maintaining posture and coordinating body movements.

The receptors for proprioception, called *proprioceptors,* are located in muscles, tendons, and joints. Proprioceptors are also found in the inner ear, where they function in **equilibrium**. The cerebellum, which plays a major role in coordinating skeletal muscle activity, receives sensory information from these receptors. Sensory information regarding movement and position is also sent to the parietal lobe of the cerebrum. Think how busy the proprioceptors are in the midst of a basketball game!

[?] Re-Think

1. What receptors are stimulated when you immerse your hand in boiling water?
2. Name three triggers that activate nociceptors.

[2+2] Sum It Up!

The sensory system is designed to detect information from within and outside the body and to convey that information to the CNS for interpretation. Receptors located on sensory neurons respond to specific stimuli. There are five types of receptors: chemoreceptors, nociceptors, thermoreceptors, mechanoreceptors, and photoreceptors. There are four components necessary for experiencing a sensation: stimulus, receptor, sensory nerve, and special area of the brain. Two characteristics of a sensation are adaptation and projection. Senses are classified as general or special. The general senses include pain, touch, pressure, temperature, and proprioception.

THE SPECIAL SENSES

The five special senses are smell, taste, sight, hearing, and balance (Table 13-2). The receptors for the special senses are located in the head.

SENSE OF SMELL: THE NOSE

The sense of smell, olfaction, is associated with sensory structures located in the upper nose (Figure 13-5). These **olfactory** (ol-FAK-tor-ee) **receptors** are very sensitive and classified as chemoreceptors, meaning that they are stimulated by chemicals that dissolve in the moisture of the nasal tissue. Once the olfactory receptors have been stimulated, the sensory impulses travel along the olfactory nerve (CN I). The sensory information is eventually interpreted as smell within the olfactory area of the temporal lobe. Faint odor? Sniff harder, because the olfactory receptors are located high in the nose where the air circulation is poor.

WHAT A SMELL CAN TELL

Think of the many pleasant "smell experiences" you have each day: food, flowers, home, fragrant candles, your child, a pet—the list goes on, as do the functions served by the sense of smell. Food odors can stimulate the digestive tract secretions, literally causing you to drool and ingest necessary nutrients. The sense of smell can function as a protective warning, telling you of spoiled food and threatening environments, such as a room filled with leaking gas. Other familiar odors pack an emotional punch, often eliciting memories (pleasant and not-so pleasant). Aromatherapy uses the sense of smell for its healing and calming effects on the body. And, of course, Mr. and Ms. Rover, in the heat of the moment, illustrate well the role of pheromones (sex odors) in mating and reproduction. By the way, each person has a unique odor as distinctive as fingerprints.

Some odors are harsh and unpleasant. For example, ammonia fumes activate both the olfactory receptors and the trigeminal nociceptors. Thus, "smelling salts" quickly and uncomfortably revive a semiconscious person. Unpleasant odors can trigger distressing

Table **13-2**   Special Senses

TYPE OF SENSE	ORGAN	SPECIFIC RECEPTOR	STIMULUS	RECEPTOR
Smell	Nose	Olfactory cell	Changes in chemical concentrations of substances	Chemoreceptor
Taste	Tongue	Gustatory cell	Changes in chemical concentrations of substances	Chemoreceptor
Sight	Eye	Rods and cones	Light energy	Photoreceptor
Hearing	Inner ear: cochlea	Organ of Corti (hair cells)	Movement of fluids	Mechanoreceptor
Balance	Inner ear, vestibular apparatus	Hair cells	Movement of fluids	Mechanoreceptor

FIGURE 13-5 Sense of smell: olfactory receptors, olfactory nerve, and the olfactory cortex (temporal lobe).

visceral responses. For example, putrid odors can stimulate the emetic center, causing the person to vomit in response to the noxious stimulus.

Some persons experience an olfactory aura, meaning that they smell an odor that is not present. Olfactory auras most often occur prior to seizure activity or before the onset of a migraine headache. The person may "smell" chicken soup, bleach, rotting flesh, or worse. Sometimes, the aura is a distortion of an odor. For example, a person may experience body odor as a smell of beer. These strange smell events are called *olfactory hallucinations*.

Your sense of smell is also a valuable diagnostic tool. You can smell the acetone breath of a person in diabetic ketoacidosis, the putrid odor of an infected wound, and the odor of alcohol on the breath of an intoxicated person. Think that's good? Rover can smell the presence of melanoma and his ears perk right up when he smells the breath of a person with pulmonary tuberculosis. Cranial nerve (CN I) assessment? Have the person identify various odors such as vanilla; an intact olfactory nerve identifies the vanilla odor. Clearly, the olfactory receptors that hang out in the nose are very busy and do much more than just smell perfume.

SENSE OF TASTE: THE TONGUE

The sense of taste is often called the social sense, as in "let's do lunch"; it is also called the *gustatory* (GUS-tah-tor-ee) *sense* or *gustation*. Taste buds are the special organs of taste. The taste receptors are located primarily on the tongue and are classified as chemoreceptors, meaning that they are activated by the chemicals in our food. A small number of taste buds are also located on the palate, tonsils, and throat. Rover, of course, has many taste buds in his throat. So not to worry when he gulps his treat; he is tasting and thoroughly enjoying it despite its rapid disappearance. The four basic taste sensations are salty, sweet, sour, and bitter. Each sensation is concentrated on a particular area of the tongue, as illustrated in Figure 13-6. The tip of the tongue is most sensitive to sweet and salty substances. Sour sensations are found primarily on the sides of the tongue, and bitter substances are most strongly tasted on the back part of the tongue.

When the taste receptors are stimulated, the taste impulses travel along three cranial nerves (facial, glossopharyngeal, and vagus nerves) to various parts of the brain, eventually arriving in the parietal and temporal lobes of the cerebral cortex. Note that because the taste sensation is carried by three cranial nerves, when assessing cranial nerve function, you will be asking the patient to detect specific tastes and stimulating only parts of the tongue. For example, a person with damage to the facial nerve may experience loss of taste only on the anterior two thirds of the left side of the tongue.

SOME TASTEFUL COMMENTS

- The salty receptors can trigger a "salt craving." For example, as her blood volume expands during pregnancy, the woman's taste buds may sense a decrease

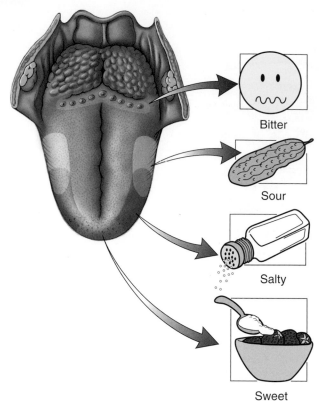

FIGURE 13-6 Sense of taste. The four taste sensations are bitter, sour, salty, and sweet.

Bitter

Sour

Salty

Sweet

? Re-Think

1. Locate and classify olfactory receptors.
2. Why does food taste different when you have a cold?

2+2 Sum It Up!

The special senses include smell, taste, sight, hearing, and balance. The nose houses the receptors for smell, the olfactory receptors. CN I (olfactory nerve) carries information from the nose to the temporal lobe of the cerebrum. Distortions in the sense of smell are common and include anosmia and olfactory auras/hallucinations. The sense of taste is called the *gustatory sense*. Sensory information from the taste buds is carried by three cranial nerves (CN VII, IX, and X) to the temporal and parietal lobes of the cerebrum.

SENSE OF SIGHT: THE EYE

The sense of sight (vision) is one of our most cherished senses. Think of all that you see that brings so much joy to your life—the smiles of children, the faces of your friends and pets, and the beautiful colors of the trees and flowers. The eyes are the organs of vision; they contain the visual receptors. Assisting the eyes in their function and protecting them from injury are the visual accessory organs. The study of the eye is called *ophthalmology*.

VISUAL ACCESSORY ORGANS

The visual accessory organs include the eyebrows, eyelids, conjunctiva, eyelashes, lacrimal apparatus, and extrinsic eye muscles (Figure 13-7).

Eyebrows

The eyebrows, patches of hair located above the eyes, perform a protective role. They keep perspiration out of the eyes and shade the eyes from glaring sunlight. Eyebrows also participate in your facial expression, as in the "raised eyebrow" look.

Eyelids

The eyelids, or palpebrae, protect the eyes. They prevent the entrance of foreign objects and wash tears over the surface of the eye. The upper and lower eyelids meet at the corners of the eyes. The corners are called the *medial (inner) canthus* and *lateral (outer) canthus*. The eyelids are composed of four layers: skin, skeletal muscle (orbicularis oculi), connective tissue, and an inner lining called the *conjunctiva*. The margin of the eyelids contains tarsal or meibomian glands, special types of sebaceous glands that secrete an oil that coats the surface of the eye and reduces evaporation of the tears. Skeletal muscles open and close the eyelids. The levator palpebrae superioris muscle (*levator* means "to raise," like an elevator) is attached to the eyelid and the upper bony orbit; contraction of this muscle opens the eye. Contraction of the orbicularis oculi muscle closes it.

of salt in her blood, causing her to increase her intake of salt. Because salt plays a crucial role in blood volume regulation, the salt craving has an important survival role. Ever notice the gathering of deer around a salt lick?

- Taste receptors seem especially sensitive to bitter-tasting substances. This sensitivity serves a protective role because the poisonous substances in plants are often bitter.
- Food often tastes differently when you have a cold. The senses of taste and smell are closely related. When interpreted in the cerebral cortex, information from both senses may combine to produce a different taste sensation. Therefore, food often tastes different when you have a cold or stuffy nose.
- The sense of taste can be lost or altered. Drugs and radiation used in the treatment of cancer often change or destroy the sensation of taste. Obviously, the loss of taste affects appetite and nutrition.
- Two other tastes have been suggested. A metallic taste has been attributed to the effects of certain drugs. A second taste has been described by a Japanese word, *umami,* which means yummy or delicious and refers to a meaty flavor.
- There is also some evidence that the tongue can taste the texture and shape of food.

FIGURE 13-7 Visual accessory organs and lacrimal apparatus.

Look in the mirror. Lid levels matter. Your eyelid normally covers a small part of the upper iris (colored part of your eye); it should not cover the pupil (hole). Sometimes, a patient cannot lift the eyelid completely and the person has a sleepy look. This condition is called *ptosis of the eyelid*. The upper eyelid of a person with an overactive thyroid may appear to be pulled up too high, thereby exposing the white sclera above the iris. This is called "lid lag." Thus, the eyelids often provide diagnostic clues about underlying diseases or disorders. While you are looking in the mirror, pull down your lower lid and note its inner lining; it forms a sac (the conjunctival sac). Eyedrops are temporarily held in this sac until the blinking eyelids wash the medication over the surface of the eye.

Occasionally, a hair follicle at the edge of the lid becomes infected, usually by *Staphylococcus*. This infection is called a *stye*, or *hordeolum*; it is red, swollen, and painful.

Conjunctiva

The conjunctiva (kon-junk-TIE-vah) is a thin mucous membrane that lines the inner surface of the eyelids. The conjunctiva also folds back to cover a portion of the sclera on the anterior surface of the eyeball; this part of the sclera is called *the white of the eye*. The conjunctiva does not cover the cornea; it secretes a thin mucous film that moistens the surface of the eye. The anterior surface of the eye must be kept moist; otherwise, it will ulcerate and scar. Figure 13-7 identifies the limbus, the meeting place of the white of the eye with the cornea that overlies the colored iris.

The conjunctiva is very vascular, meaning that it has many blood vessels. Evidence of its rich vascularity is

its bloodshot appearance when the blood vessels are dilated. Eyedrops that claim to "get the red out" cause the blood vessels of the conjunctiva to constrict, thereby decreasing the amount of blood. Pink eye, also associated with dilated blood vessels, is a highly contagious bacterial or viral conjunctivitis. It is commonly seen in groups of children in whom it is difficult to maintain good hygienic conditions. Conjunctivitis can also be caused by irritation and allergies.

Eyelashes

Eyelashes line the edges of the eyelid and help trap dust. Touching the eyelashes stimulates blinking—a mascara challenge! Interestingly, the camel has three eyelids and two layers of eyelashes to deal with its sandy environment. Imagine how long it would take to get out of the house with so many lids and lashes to paint!

Lacrimal Apparatus: It's Tearing Me Up!

The lacrimal (LAK-ri-mal) apparatus is concerned with the secretion, distribution, and drainage of tears. It is composed of the lacrimal gland and a series of ducts called *tear ducts* (see Figure 13-7). The lacrimal gland is located in the upper lateral part of the orbit. The lacrimal gland secretes tears, which flow across the surface of the eye toward the nose. The tears drain through small openings called *lacrimal puncta* and then into the lacrimal sac and nasolacrimal ducts. The nasolacrimal ducts eventually empty into the nasal cavity. Normally, tears flow to the back of the throat and are swallowed. If the secretion of tears increases, as in crying, the nose begins to run. The excess tears may overwhelm the drainage system and spill onto the cheeks. Similarly, the nasolacrimal ducts can become swollen and close when a person has a cold. The tears cannot drain and thus spill out onto the cheeks.

Tears perform several important functions. They moisten, lubricate, and cleanse the surface of the eye. Tears also contain an enzyme called *lysozyme*, which helps destroy pathogens and prevents infection. Blinking stimulates lacrimation and helps spread the tears over the surface of the eye. Routine use of eyewashes may do more harm than good by washing away natural antibacterial secretions.

Extrinsic Eye Muscles

Extrinsic eye muscles also function as visual accessory organs (see "Muscles of the Eye" later in this chapter).

 Re-Think

1. List the visual accessory organs.
2. Trace the flow of tears from their origin to their destination.

THE EYEBALL

The eyeball has a spherical shape and is approximately $\frac{3}{4}$ to 1 inch (2 to 3 cm) in diameter (Figure 13-8, *A*). Most of the eyeball sits within the bony orbital cavity

A

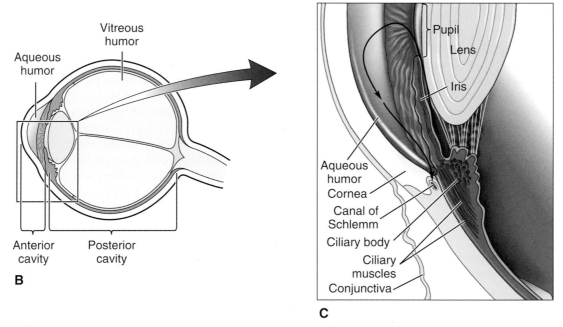

B

C

FIGURE 13-8 **A,** Structure of the eyeball. **B,** Cavities and fluids. **C,** Flow of aqueous humor from the ciliary body to the canal of Schlemm *(arrow).*

of the skull, partially surrounded by a layer of orbital fat. Thus, the eyeball is recessed and well protected. Interestingly, our eyes are the same size from infancy to adulthood. Think about it: the large eyeballs in young animals are what make them so stinkin' cute!

The eyeball is composed of three layers: the sclera, the choroid, and the retina. Identify the structures in Figure 13-8 as they are described in the following text.

Layers of the Eyeball

Sclera. The outermost layer is called the **sclera** (SKLEH-rah). The sclera is a tough fibrous connective tissue that covers most of the eyeball. The sclera helps contain the contents of the eye; it also shapes the eye and is the site of attachment for the extrinsic eye muscles. The sclera extends toward the front of the eye. The anterior sclera is covered by conjunctiva and, as indicated earlier, is called *the white of the eye*. A transparent extension of the sclera is called the **cornea** (KOR-nee-ah). The cornea covers the area over the iris (the colored portion of the eye).

The cornea is avascular (contains no blood vessels) and transparent, meaning that light rays can go through this structure. Because light enters the eye first through the cornea, it is called *the window of the eye*. The cornea has a rich supply of sensory nerve fibers and is therefore sensitive to touch. If the surface of the cornea is touched lightly, the eye tears and blinks to remove the source of irritation. This response is called the *corneal reflex* and serves a protective function. The corneal reflex involves two cranial nerves. A branch of the trigeminal nerve (CN V) provides sensory fibers to the surface of the cornea; the facial nerve (CN VII) provides motor fibers that result in tearing and blinking. Think of how your eye responds to a piece of dust—through pain, tearing, and blinking.

Choroid. The middle layer of the eye is the choroid (KOH-royd). The choroid layer is highly vascular and is attached to the innermost layer, the retina. The choroid performs two functions: (1) it provides the retina with a rich supply of blood, and (2) dark pigments located in the choroid absorb any excess light to prevent glare.

The choroid extends toward the front of the eyeball to form the ciliary body and the iris. Collectively, the middle layer (choroid, ciliary muscle, and iris) is called the *uvea*. The ciliary body secretes a fluid called *aqueous humor* and gives rise to a set of intrinsic eye muscles called the *ciliary muscles*. The most anterior portion of the choroid is the iris, the colored portion of the anterior eye. The song "Beautiful Brown Eyes" is a serenade to the iris.

The opening, or hole, in the middle of the iris is called the *pupil*. The size of the pupil is determined by two sets of intrinsic eye muscles located in the iris. The iris regulates the amount of light entering the eye.

Do You Know...

Why the "Beautiful Lady" Can't See?

A group of drugs, including atropine and scopolamine (muscarinic receptor antagonists), belongs to a drug classification called *belladonna*, or "beautiful lady." Why beautiful? When belladonna is placed in the eyes of the young lady, the pupils dilate, becoming wide, dark, and very seductive. Dilated pupils may indeed be beautiful, but they do not promote acute vision. "Beautiful lady" may be beautiful, but she needs an escort because she certainly cannot see.

Today, belladonna drugs are still used, primarily for their mydriatic and cycloplegic effects in eye examinations and surgical procedures. Interestingly, atropine is still used by photographers to create pictures of "beautiful ladies."

Retina. The innermost layer of the eyeball is the **retina** (RET-i-nah). It lines the posterior two thirds of the eyeball. The retina is the nervous layer containing the visual receptors, which are sensitive to light and are therefore called *photoreceptors*. The two types of photoreceptors are rods and cones. The rods are scattered throughout the retina but are more abundant along its periphery. The rods are sensitive to dim light and provide us with black-and-white vision. The cones are most abundant in the central portion of the retina and provide us with color vision. The area of the retina that contains the highest concentration of cones is called the *fovea centralis,* an area in the center of a yellow spot called *macula lutea* (see Figure 13-8, *A*). Because the fovea centralis contains so many cones, it is considered the area of most acute vision.

A second small circular area of the retina is in the back of the eye. The neurons of the retina converge there to form the optic nerve; it contains no rods or cones. This area is called the *optic disc*. Because there are no photoreceptors on the optic disc, images that focus on this area are not seen. The optic disc is therefore called the *blind spot*. You can locate your own blind spot. Draw a rectangle with a small X on the left side and a dot on the right. Using only one eye (cover the second eye), look at the X as you move it closer to your eye. At some point, you will not be able to see the dot on the right when it focuses on your blind spot.

Here's another interesting fact about the optic disc. A head-injured person may develop increased intracranial pressure. This increased pressure pushes the optic disc forward. The bulging optic disc seen on ophthalmic examination is described as a choked disc or papilledema. The eyes can provide a wealth of information about a patient with a head injury.

? Re-Think

1. List the three layers of the eyeball.
2. Name the anterior extensions of the choroid and the sclera.
3. Why might a detached retina cause retinal death and blindness?

Cavities and Fluids

There are two cavities in the eyeball: the posterior and anterior cavities (see Figure 13-8, *B*). The posterior cavity is larger and is located between the lens and the retina. The posterior cavity is filled with a gel-like substance called the *vitreous humor*. The vitreous humor gently pushes the retina against the choroid layer, thereby ensuring that the retina receives a good supply of oxygenated blood. For the forensic sleuths: Immediately after death, the concentration of potassium ion (K$^+$) in the vitreous humor increases slowly and consistently. Thus, its measurement is used to determine time of death and is considered more accurate than the onset of rigor mortis.

 Do You Know...

Why We Sometimes See Spots in Front of Our Eyes?

The spots are called *floaters* or *muscae volitantes*, meaning "flying flies." They are either particles or red blood cells that have escaped from the capillaries in the eye. These substances float through the vitreous humor, occasionally getting in our line of vision. The presence of these substances is usually considered normal and harmless. However, the sudden appearance of floaters or an increase in the number of floaters may indicate that a hole has formed in the retina. The development of a retinal tear often precedes retinal detachment and demands immediate professional attention.

The anterior cavity is located between the lens and the cornea. The anterior cavity is filled with a watery fluid called *aqueous humor*. Aqueous humor is produced by the ciliary body and circulates through the pupil into the space behind the cornea (see Figure 13-8, *B*). The aqueous humor performs two functions: (1) it maintains the shape of the anterior portion of the eye, and (2) it provides nourishment for the cornea. The aqueous humor leaves the anterior cavity by way of tiny canals located at the junction of the sclera and the cornea. These outlet canals are called *venous sinuses* or the *canals of Schlemm* (see Figure 13-8, *C*).

Drainage of aqueous humor through the canals of Schlemm may become impaired. Consequently, aqueous humor accumulates in the eye and elevates the pressure in the eye. An elevated intraocular pressure is called *glaucoma*. Glaucoma is serious because the elevated pressure compresses the choroid, chokes off the blood supply to the retina, and damages the optic nerve. Glaucoma is a leading cause of retinal damage and blindness. Treatment of glaucoma is aimed at decreasing the formation of aqueous humor and improving the drainage of aqueous humor through the canal of Schlemm.

 Re-Think

Trace the origin, path, and drainage of aqueous humor.

2+2 **Sum It Up!**

The eyeball has three layers: sclera, choroid, and retina. The sclera extends anteriorly as the cornea. The choroid extends anteriorly as the ciliary body and iris. (The middle layer and its extensions are called the *uvea*.) The inner retinal layer contains the photoreceptors, the rods and cones. There are two cavities: the posterior cavity that contains vitreous humor, and the anterior cavity that contains aqueous humor. Aqueous humor is secreted by the ciliary body, flows anteriorly through the pupil, and is drained through the canal of Schlemm. Impaired drainage of aqueous humor increases intraocular pressure (glaucoma), leading to blindness.

MUSCLES OF THE EYE

The two groups of muscles associated with the eye are the extrinsic and intrinsic eye muscles. The extrinsic eye muscles move the eyeball in its bony orbit. The intrinsic eye muscles move structures within the eyeball.

Extrinsic Eye Muscles

How do you move your eyes? The extrinsic eye muscles are skeletal muscles located outside the eye (Figure 13-9, *A*). Six extrinsic eye muscles attach to the bone of the eye orbit and the sclera, the tough outer connective tissue layer of the eyeball. There are four rectus muscles and two oblique muscles:

- Superior rectus
- Inferior rectus
- Medial rectus
- Lateral rectus
- Superior oblique
- Inferior oblique

The extrinsic eye muscles move the eyeball in various directions. You can move your eyes up, down, and sideways because of the rectus muscles. You can also roll your eyes because of the oblique muscles. The extrinsic eye muscles are innervated by three cranial nerves, with the most important being the oculomotor nerve (CN III). Then there is LR$_6$SO$_4$, which sounds like a nasty chemical formula. However, it helps you remember that the lateral rectus (LR) muscle is innervated by the abducens nerve (CN VI) whereas the superior oblique (SO) muscle is innervated by the trochlear nerve (CN IV). Cranial nerve assessment of CN III, IV, and VI: observe movement of the eyeballs up, down, medial, lateral, and around.

Back to the mirror. Note that both eyes move together in a coordinated way; when one eye moves, the other eye moves. Both eyes focus on the same object. In the event of a traumatic injury to an eye, you may need to immobilize the injured eye, usually by applying a loose covering over it. However, because both eyes move in a coordinated way, if you want to immobilize the injured eye, you must cover both eyes. Then it is off to the ophthalmologist for treatment.

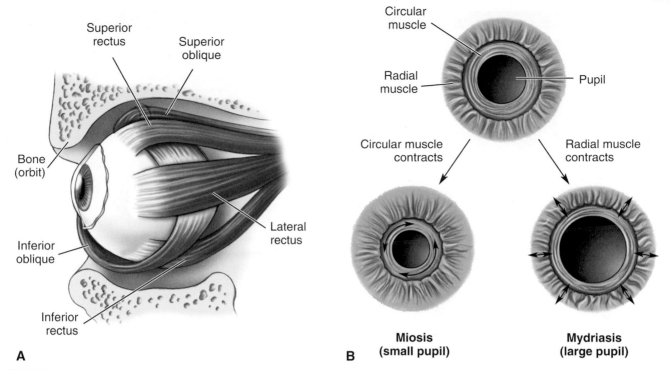

FIGURE 13-9 A, Extrinsic muscles: four rectus muscles and two oblique muscles (only five are shown). **B,** Intrinsic eye muscles: iris (circular and radial muscles).

Occasionally, the eyeballs are not aligned and do not focus on a desired point. This condition is called *strabismus* (Figure 13-10). If the eye deviates medially toward the nasal side, the eyes look crossed; hence, the term *cross-eyed*. If uncorrected, strabismus not only presents a serious cosmetic problem, but can also lead to loss of vision.

 Do You Know...

About Lazy Eye?

Normally, both eyes work together and focus on one object; in response, the brain forms a single image. Sometimes, both eyes do not focus on the same object, usually because the muscles of one eye are weak (lazy) and therefore unable to move the affected eye into position. The occipital lobe is then presented with different information from each eye. The occipital lobe, however, can't process both signals; it receives information from one eye and suppresses information from the lazy eye. If uncorrected, the "lazy" eye will become nonfunctional (blind). Loss of vision resulting from lazy eye is called *suppression amblyopia*. It is common and preventable; treatment, however, must begin early.

Intrinsic Eye Muscles

The intrinsic muscles are smooth muscles located in the eyeball, specifically in the iris and the ciliary body. There are three intrinsic eye muscles, as described in the following text.

Muscles of the Iris. The iris is composed of two eye muscles: the radial muscle and the circular muscle (see Figure 13-9, *B*). These muscles control the size of the pupil and therefore regulate the amount of light that enters the eye. The muscle fibers of the radial muscle are arranged like the spokes of a wheel. Just as the spokes radiate from the center of the wheel, the radial muscle fibers radiate from the area of the pupil. Contraction of the radial muscle causes the pupil to dilate, thereby increasing the amount of light entering the eye. Sympathetic nerve fibers supply the radial muscles. Thus, sympathetic nerve stimulation causes pupillary dilation, or mydriasis (mi-DRY-ah-sys). Drugs that dilate the pupil are called *mydriatic agents*.

The second muscle located in the iris is the circular muscle. Contraction of the circular muscles causes the pupil to constrict, thereby decreasing the amount of light entering the eye. The circular muscle is supplied by parasympathetic nerve fibers in the oculomotor nerve (CN III). Parasympathetic nerve stimulation causes pupillary constriction, or miosis (see Figure 13-9, *B*). Drugs that constrict the pupils are called *miotic agents*. Some drugs, such as opioids (narcotics), constrict the pupils so intensely that the pupils are described as pinpoint. (An easy way to remember the difference between mydriasis and miosis is that the words *dilate* and *mydriasis* both contain the letter *d*.)

Ramp It Up!

Pupil Size and Drugs that Affect the Autonomic Receptors on the Iris

the alpha$_1$ receptor by norepinephrine (NE) causes pupillary dilation or mydriasis. The circular muscle of the iris is innervated by parasympathetic fibers and contains muscarinic receptors. Activation of the muscarinic receptors causes pupillary constriction or miosis. There are several clinical important implications.

1. An ophthalmologist may want to examine the interior of the eye; dilation of the pupils and paralysis of the muscles of accommodation (ciliary muscles) facilitates the exam. Eyedrops containing an antimuscarinic drug (e.g., atropine, other drugs included in the belladonna drug class) achieve mydriasis and cycloplegia (paralysis of the muscles of accommodation). Remember that muscarinic activation causes pupillary constriction, so muscarinic blockade causes pupillary dilation, or mydriasis.

2. Patients with glaucoma (increased intraocular pressure) are advised to avoid taking drugs that cause mydriasis because mydriasis diminishes the drainage of aqueous humor and further elevates intraocular pressure. Patients often take a number of drugs. Many commonly used drugs, such as antidepressants, have antimuscarinic effects. Therefore, while treating the primary problem of depression, you must also consider other secondary clinical conditions, such as glaucoma. Otherwise, the depression may improve in response to the antidepressant drug, but the glaucoma may worsen because of its antimuscarinic effect on the eye.

3. A neurological assessment includes the response of the photopupillary reflex. Drugs that activate or block the receptors on the iris affect the pupillary response and interfere with the neurological assessment.

Pupillary size is also affected by drugs that do not affect the autonomic receptors. For example, opioids, such as morphine, cause miosis; the pupils may be described as pinpoint pupils. The eyes reveal much about the patient.

Many drugs affect pupillary size, and you must understand these effects so that you can make sound clinical judgments. The effects of drugs on pupil size are described in terms of autonomic receptor terminology. (You may need to review cholinergic and adrenergic receptors in Chapter 12.)

The radial muscle of the iris is innervated by sympathetic fibers and contains alpha$_1$-adrenergic receptors. Activation of

HERE'S LOOKING AT YOU!

Ptosis

Hordeolum (stye)

Conjunctivitis ("pink eye")

Strabismus

FIGURE 13-10 Conditions of the eye.

Photopupillary Reflex. When one eye is exposed to light, the pupil immediately constricts, thereby restricting the amount of light entering the eye. This response is called the *photopupillary reflex.* The pupil of the other eye also constricts even if no light is directed at it. The second eye is said to constrict consensually; it consents to constrict when the photopupillary reflex is stimulated in the opposite eye. Both of these effects are assessed when an eye exam is performed.

Who is PERRLA? Pupillary function is evaluated by noting the size, shape, and reactivity to light. PERRLA is an assessment term for pupillary function: *P*upils *E*qual, *R*ound, *R*eact to *L*ight, and *A*ccommodation.

Ciliary Muscle. The third intrinsic eye muscle is the ciliary muscle. Locate the ciliary muscles in Figure 13-8, *C.* The ciliary muscles arise from the ciliary body. The ciliary muscles attach to the suspensory ligaments, which, in turn, tug on the lens, causing the lens to change its shape. Why tug? Read on.

> **? Re-Think**
>
> 1. List the extrinsic eye muscles and state their function.
> 2. List the intrinsic eye muscles and state their functions.
> 3. Describe the effect of the photopupillary reflex on pupillary size.

REFRACTION AND ACCOMMODATION

For us to see, the light waves must enter the eye and bend to focus on the retina. The bending of light waves is called **refraction**. Let's see how this happens. Although the cornea and aqueous humor are all capable of refracting light, the lens can change its shape and its refracting power. The need for refraction by the lens is illustrated in Figure 13-11, *A.* The light waves are shown traveling in a straight line toward the retina. Unless light waves 1 and 3 are bent, they will not focus on point X.

How does the lens bend light waves (see Figure 13-11, *B*)? The bottom part of light wave 1 hits the lens first and is slowed before penetrating it. The top of the light wave continues to travel until it hits the lens. For a split second, the top of the light wave travels faster than the bottom. The light wave therefore bends. This illustrates how the lens bends several light waves. For sharp vision, light waves must be refracted to focus on one particular area of the retina.

Why and how does the lens change its shape? The lens can change its shape, becoming fatter or thinner. The lens is an elastic structure held in place by the suspensory ligaments attached to ciliary muscles (see Figure 13-8, *A*). When the ciliary muscles contract and relax, the tension on the lens causes the changes in the shape of the lens. The lens either thins out or becomes fatter. The change in shape affects how much the light is bent. For example, if the lens becomes fatter, the light wave is bent at a sharper angle. If the lens thins, the degree of refraction lessens and the light wave is not bent as much.

FIGURE 13-11 Refraction. **A,** Path that the light waves travel (without lens). **B,** Refraction of the first and third light waves (with lens).

The ability of the lens to change its shape allows the eye to focus objects close up or at a distance. For example, if you hold a pencil 6 inches in front of your eyes, you will be able to see it clearly. The focusing of the close-up object (pencil) on the retina is caused primarily by the lens. The lens becomes fatter and bends the light waves more acutely so as to focus them on the retina. This ability of the lens to change its shape to focus on a close object is called *accommodation.* A professional who assesses the ability of the eyes to refract light is called an *optometrist.* Optometrists prescribe lenses to correct the errors of refraction. (Do not confuse ophthalmologist with optometrist.)

Accommodation is accompanied by pupillary constriction and by convergence, the movement of the eyes medially toward the nose. Accommodation, pupillary constriction, and convergence all work together to focus both eyes on one object.

Emmetropia (em-eh-TROHP-ee-ah) refers to the ability of the eye to refract light without the assistance of a corrective lens. With advancing age, the lens loses some of its ability to change shape, thereby diminishing the ability to accommodate for close objects. This condition, which is often evident after age 40, is called *presbyopia* (pres-bee-OH-pee-ah) (*presbyter* means "an old man"). Persons with presbyopia have difficulty adjusting to close objects. Presbyopia accounts for the tendency of older persons to hold the newspaper at arm's length. You may have heard older persons comment good naturedly on how their arms have gotten shorter as they have gotten older!

 Do You Know...

What Is Meant by 20/20 Vision?

The ability of the eye to focus an image on the retina is assessed by use of the Snellen chart. This chart is composed of lines of letters arranged in decreasing size. The person is placed at a distance 20 feet away from the chart and is asked to cover one eye and read a line of letters. A score of 20/20 means that the person can see at 20 feet what a person with normal eye function can see. Thus, 20/20 vision is considered normal. A score of 20/40 means that a person can see at 20 feet what a person with normal vision can see at 40 feet. Thus, 20/40 vision is less perfect than 20/20 vision. A score of 20/200 indicates severely impaired vision, and the person is considered legally blind.

? **Re-Think**

1. Define refraction and explain how the lens refracts light.
2. With regard to refraction, why does a person with presbyopia move his or her arms to see a newspaper more clearly?

2+2 **Sum It Up!**

There are two groups of muscles associated with the eyeball: extrinsic eye muscles and intrinsic eye muscles. The extrinsic eye muscles move the eyeball and are innervated by CN III, IV, and VI. The intrinsic eye muscles control pupillary size and the shape of the lens. By changing pupillary size, the iris regulates the amount of light that enters the posterior cavity. By changing the curvature of the lens, the muscles enable the lens to refract light.

STIMULATION OF THE PHOTORECEPTORS

Once the light penetrates the various eye structures, it must stimulate the photoreceptors (rods and cones). Why do you see black and white at night and color during daylight?

Night Vision

The rods are widely scattered throughout the retina but are more abundant in the periphery. In low light conditions the pupil dilates, thereby allowing more light to enter the eye. The dilated pupil allows the light rays to scatter along the periphery of the retina, thereby stimulating the rods. Rods provide us with black-and-white vision. The image produced by the stimulation of rods is somewhat fuzzy. Because rods respond to dim light, stimulation of rods is often called *night vision*.

 Do You Know...

What Night Blindness Is?

Stimulation of the rods (night vision photoreceptors) by light waves causes the breakdown of a chemical substance called *rhodopsin*. This breakdown, in turn, stimulates nerve impulses. As nerve impulses are formed, the amount of rhodopsin is used up and must be replaced. The synthesis of additional rhodopsin requires vitamin A. Because night vision depends on an adequate supply of rhodopsin, a deficiency of vitamin A can cause night blindness.

Color Vision

Cones are the photoreceptors for color vision. Cones are most abundant in the central portion of the retina, especially in the macula lutea. When in a well-lit environment the pupil is constricted and directs the light toward the central cone-rich part of the retina. The image produced by the stimulation of cones is colored and sharp. Why colored? There are three types of cones, each with a different visual pigment (a light-sensitive chemical). One type of cone produces a green color, another produces blue, and a third produces red. Stimulation of combinations of these cones produces the many different colors and shades of colors that we enjoy.

INFORMING THE BRAIN: THE VISUAL PATHWAY

Nerve impulses that arise from the photoreceptors leave the eye (retina) by way of the optic nerve (CN II). The nerve impulses travel along the fibers of the optic nerve to the occipital lobe of the brain. This pathway from the retina to the brain is called the *visual pathway*.

Figure 13-12 illustrates the pathways of the optic nerves as each leaves the eye. Note that half of the fibers from the left eye cross over and travel to the right side of the brain, and half of the fibers from the right eye cross over and travel to the left side of the brain. The crossing over of the fibers allows the occipital lobe

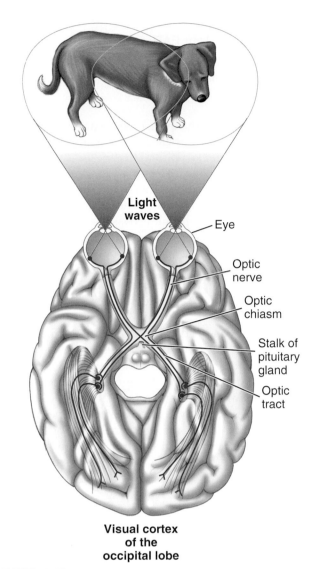

Light waves

Eye

Optic nerve

Optic chiasm

Stalk of pituitary gland

Optic tract

Visual cortex of the occipital lobe

FIGURE 13-12 Visual pathway. Note the optic chiasm and the pituitary gland (behind the optic chiasm).

to integrate the information from both eyes and produce only one image. The point at which the fibers from the left and right eyes crisscross is called the **optic chiasm** (KYE-ass-im). The optic chiasm is located directly in front of the pituitary gland. An enlargement of the pituitary gland can therefore cause visual disturbances as the tumor presses on the optic chiasm and interferes with the transmission of the nerve impulse to the occipital lobe.

SEEING HAPPENS WHEN...

When all the parts of the eye, visual pathway, and brain are working correctly, you can see. Light waves enter your eye, are refracted, and are focused on the photoreceptors of the retina. The photoreceptors translate the light signal to a nerve impulse, which is then transmitted from the retina, along the optic nerve, and finally to the occipital lobe of the brain, where you experience vision.

SEEING DOESN'T HAPPEN WHEN...

When the parts of the eye and visual pathway do not work normally, a person may experience diminished vision or blindness. Any defect along this pathway from the cornea to the brain can interfere with vision. Certain conditions may prevent the entrance of light into the eye. For example, a scarred cornea or a cloudy lens (cataract) may block the entrance of light, thereby preventing the stimulation of the rods and cones. Errors of refraction such as nearsightedness and farsightedness can adversely affect the focusing of light on the retina (Figure 13-13). Light waves are focused either in front of the retina (nearsightedness) or beyond the retina (farsightedness). Although these conditions can diminish vision, they are generally treatable. The more serious and often untreatable conditions affect the retina in the following ways:

- Increased intraocular pressure (glaucoma) may squeeze the blood vessels of the choroid, depriving the retina of an adequate blood supply. The cells of the retina then die and blindness results.
- The photoreceptors of the macula lutea can degenerate, causing macular degeneration and a loss of vision.
- A person with diabetes often experiences severe damage of the retinal blood vessels. The blood vessels develop microaneurysms. The aneurysms rupture, causing bleeding and scar formation throughout the retina. Retinal photoreceptor cells are replaced with scar tissue. This is called *diabetic retinopathy*.
- Another type of retinal damage includes a detached retina (the retina falls away from the choroid, its blood supply). Activities that cause jarring movements of the head, such as boxing and basketball, increase the risk of retinal detachment.
- Certain conditions or injuries can destroy the optic nerve. For example, a tumor on the optic nerve or at the optic chiasm can interfere with the transmission of the nerve impulse along the nerve to the brain.
- Finally, tumors, blood clots, or trauma can damage the primary visual cortex of the occipital lobe of the brain, causing cortical blindness.

 Do You Know...

About High Concentrations of Oxygen and Blindness?

The administration of oxygen is generally beneficial and often lifesaving. Oxygen (O_2) therapy, however, must be delivered with care, particularly in preterm infants. In "preemies" younger than 32 weeks' gestation, the administration of very high concentrations of oxygen can cause blindness. The oxygen is usually administered to a severely hypoxemic infant. While relieving the hypoxemia, the high concentration of O_2 also causes constriction of the developing blood vessels of the retina. Deprived of its blood supply, the retina dies and is replaced by a retrolental membrane of fibrous tissue. The O_2-induced blindness is called *retrolental fibroplasia* or the *retinopathy of prematurity*.

Myopia (nearsightedness)

Hyperopia (farsightedness)

FIGURE 13-13 Errors of refraction: myopia and hyperopia.

? Re-Think

1. Describe the pathway of light to the retina.
2. Describe the path of the nerve impulses (action potentials) generated in the photoreceptors to the primary visual cortex in the occipital lobe.

2+2 Sum It Up!

Light stimulates the photoreceptors, rods (black and white) and cones (color), generating nerve impulses or electrical signals (action potentials) that are carried by the optic nerve (CN II) and visual pathway to the primary visual cortex of the occipital lobe. By tracing these pathways of light and action potentials, you can understand the sequence of events in seeing.

SENSE OF HEARING: THE EAR

Listen to the sounds around you. Perhaps some of it is background noise that you mostly ignore. Other sounds provide you with information. Most importantly, you can hear sounds that you enjoy, such as the voices of friends and sounds of music. The ear is the organ of the sense of hearing.

Refer to Figure 13-14 to identify the structures described as follows.

STRUCTURE OF THE EAR

The ear is divided into three parts: the external ear, the middle ear, and the inner ear.

External Ear

The external ear is the part of the ear you can see. It is composed of the auricle and the external auditory canal. The auricle, or pinna (Latin for "wing"), is composed of cartilage covered by a layer of loose-fitting skin. The auricle functions like a satellite dish gathering sound waves. The auricle opens into the external auditory canal, a passageway for sound waves to enter the ear. The external auditory canal is hollowed out of the temporal bone. It is about 1 inch long (2.5 cm) and ½ inch (1.25 cm) wide and extends to the tympanic membrane, or eardrum. The tympanic membrane separates the external ear from the middle ear.

The external auditory canal is lined with tiny hairs and glands that secrete cerumen, a yellowish waxy substance also known as earwax. The hairs and cerumen help prevent dust and other foreign objects from entering the external ear. Cerumen tends to be a victim of our cleanliness fetish; we insert hairpins, toothpicks, and other sharp objects into the canal in an attempt to dig out the wax. These objects may damage the tympanic membrane. Cotton-tipped applicators, although appearing safer, actually remove very little wax and can push any accumulated wax up against the eardrum and impair hearing. It is best not to insert *any* objects into the ear canal. This practice is more common than you think. A young child may insert an object such as a bean into the external canal; over time, the bean accumulates moisture and swells, making it difficult to remove. Off to the ear doctor for bean removal!

Middle Ear

The middle ear is a small, air-filled chamber located between the tympanic membrane at one end and a bony wall at the other end. The middle ear contains several structures: the tympanic membrane, three tiny bones, several small muscles, and the eustachian tube (also called the *pharyngotympanic tube*).

The tympanic membrane is composed primarily of connective tissue and has a rich supply of nerves and blood vessels. The tympanic membrane vibrates in response to sound waves entering the ear through the external auditory canal. The vibration of the tympanic membrane is passed on to the tiny bones in the middle ear.

The middle ear contains three tiny bones, or **ossicles**, which are the tiniest bones in the body—the malleus (hammer), incus (anvil), and stapes (stirrup). The ossicles transmit vibration from the tympanic membrane to the oval window, a membranous structure that separates the middle ear from the inner ear.

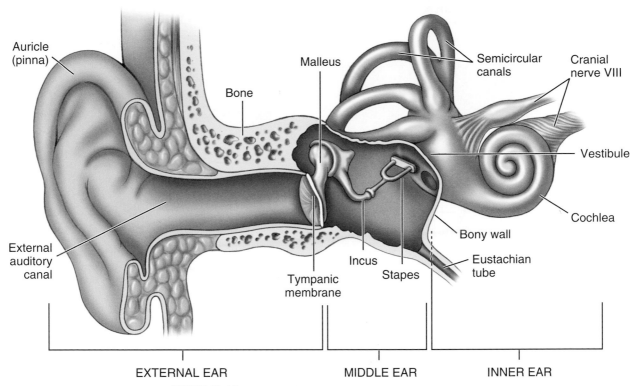

FIGURE 13-14 Three divisions as well as structures of the ear.

The middle ear has a passageway connecting it to the pharynx, or throat. This passageway is called the *auditory tube,* or the **eustachian tube.** The purpose of the eustachian tube is to equalize the pressure on both sides of the tympanic membrane by permitting air to pass from the pharynx into the middle ear. If the pressures across the membrane become unequal, the tympanic membrane bulges. As the tympanic membrane is stretched, pain receptors are stimulated. Pain caused by stretched tympanic membranes is why your ears sometimes hurt when you take off and land in an airplane. Hints to prevent a pressure difference across the tympanic membrane include chewing gum, drinking water through a straw, yawning, and swallowing. Babies can suck on a nipple or pacifier.

Inner Ear

The inner ear consists of an intricate system of tubes, or passageways, hollowed out of the temporal bone. This coiled network of tubes is called a *bony labyrinth* (Figure 13-15). Inside the bony labyrinth is a similarly shaped *membranous labyrinth.* The bony labyrinth is filled with a fluid called *perilymph.* The membranous labyrinth is surrounded by perilymph and is itself filled with a thick fluid called *endolymph.* (For our purposes, the endolymph is the more important fluid.) The inner ear has three parts: the vestibule, the semicircular canals, and the cochlea. The cochlea is concerned with hearing. The vestibule and semicircular canals are concerned with balance.

Do You Know...

Why Children Tend to Outgrow Ear Infections?

The size and position of the eustachian tube in a child are different than in an adult. The eustachian tube of a child is shorter and lies in a more horizontal position than the adult eustachian tube. The child who develops a cold will often sniffle, thereby forcing the nasal drainage from the throat region into the eustachian tubes and middle ear. This drainage results in a middle ear infection called *otitis media.*

As the child grows, the eustachian tube grows longer and becomes more vertical. There is less chance for bacteria to enter the middle ear from the throat. In this sense, children are said to outgrow ear infections.

Child   **Adult**

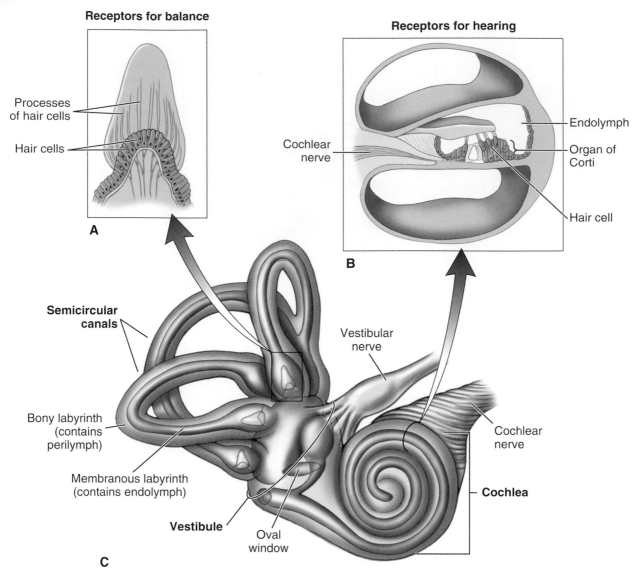

Receptors for balance

Processes of hair cells

Hair cells

A

Receptors for hearing

Cochlear nerve

Endolymph

Organ of Corti

Hair cell

B

Semicircular canals

Vestibular nerve

Bony labyrinth (contains perilymph)

Membranous labyrinth (contains endolymph)

Vestibule

Oval window

Cochlear nerve

Cochlea

C

FIGURE 13-15 Inner ear. **A,** The receptors for balance. **B,** The receptors for hearing (organ of Corti). **C,** Structures of the inner ear.

The cochlea is a snail-shaped part of the bony labyrinth. Sitting on a membrane within the cochlea and immersed in endolymph are the receptors for hearing (see Figure 13-15, *B*). The receptors are cells that contain tiny hairs; these are called the *organ of Corti*. When the hairs on the receptor cells are bent, a nerve impulse is sent by the cochlear branch of the vestibulocochlear nerve (CN VIII) to the primary auditory cortex of the temporal lobe of the brain, where the sensation is interpreted as hearing. Note that the receptors are stimulated by the bending of the hairs; hence, the receptors are classified as mechanoreceptors.

HEARING HAPPENS WHEN…

How do we hear the sounds of music? As Figure 13-16 illustrates, the vibrating guitar strings disturb the air, causing sound waves. The sound waves are gathered by the auricle, travel through the external auditory canal, and hit the tympanic membrane, causing the tympanic membrane to vibrate. This vibration, in turn, causes the middle ear bones (malleus, incus, and stapes) to vibrate. The stapes, sitting within the oval window, then causes the fluid in the inner ear to move. Because the hairs (organ of Corti) are sitting within the endolymph, movement of the fluid causes the hairs to bend. The bending of the hairs triggers a nerve impulse carried by the cochlear branch of the vestibulocochlear nerve (CN VIII) to the primary auditory cortex of the temporal lobe, where it is interpreted as sound.

HEARING DOESN'T HAPPEN WHEN…

What happens when the parts do not work? Following the steps listed in Figure 13-16, consider the number

FIGURE 13-16 Steps in hearing.

of ways our hearing may become impaired. For example, the vibration of the tympanic membrane may become blunted if a plug of cerumen (earwax) becomes lodged against the tympanic membrane. The sound waves may then be unable to vibrate the eardrum. The tiny ossicles may also become fused to one another. This condition diminishes the ability of the bones to transmit vibration from the tympanic membrane to the oval window. This problem often develops in children who have experienced repeated middle ear infections.

Another problem is that the stapes may become glued, or fixed, to the oval window. This condition diminishes the transmission of vibration to the inner ear. Deafness resulting from impaired function of the ossicles is called *bone conduction deafness*. The cochlear branch of CN VIII in the inner ear may also be damaged. The damaged nerve cannot conduct nerve impulses from the ear to the brain. This condition develops in persons exposed to prolonged periods of loud noise. For example, "rock and roll deafness" is hearing loss associated with loud music. Nerve damage also occurs in response to certain drugs, especially antibiotics. Drugs that cause damage to the vestibulocochlear nerve are called *ototoxic agents*. Nerve conduction deafness is commonly experienced by older persons. Finally, the primary auditory cortex of the temporal lobe may be damaged. The person will then experience a cortical deafness.

? Re-Think

1. List the three parts of the ear.
2. Describe the pathway of hearing from the collection of sound waves in the external ear to the primary auditory cortex in the temporal lobe of the cerebrum.

SENSE OF BALANCE: THE EAR

We all appreciate our ears as organs of hearing, but we may not realize that our ears play an important role in equilibrium or balance. Damage to the inner ear, for example, may make it impossible for us to stand without losing balance.

The receptors for balance are mechanoreceptors. These cells contain hairlike projections immersed in a gel-like fluid within the vestibule and semicircular canals of the inner ear (see Figure 13-15). The **vestibule** contains the receptors that provide information about the position of the head at rest. The receptors in the semicircular canals provide information about the position of the body as it moves about. These receptors sense the changing positions of the head. When the positions change, the hairs are bent, and the receptor cells send nerve impulses through the vestibular branch of the vestibulocochlear nerve (CN VIII) to several parts of the brain, including the cerebellum, midbrain, and temporal lobe. The brain dispatches signals to the various muscles to restore balance.

Because the vestibulocochlear nerve carries sensory information concerning both hearing and balance, someone with an ear infection may complain of feeling dizzy. The person should be assured that as the ear infection resolves, the dizzy feeling will also disappear.

 Do You Know...

Why Rocks in Your Head Keep You Balanced?

Tiny hairs on the inner ear cells concerned with balance (vestibule and the semicircular canals) bend in response to movement of the head. The tiny hair receptors contain little stones called *otoliths*. The stones make the hairs much more sensitive to a change in head position. So otoliths, the rocks in your head, keep you balanced. Notably, sharks have elaborate otoliths. Ask any Great White about his otoliths and he will quickly tell you that the rocks in his head keep him balanced, coordinated, and fine-tuned for Xtreme fishing. He would quickly starve without his array of otoliths.

 Sum It Up!

The ear is the organ of hearing. There are three parts of the ear: external, middle, and inner ear. Sound waves enter the external ear, vibrate the tympanic membrane, which, in turn vibrates the middle ear ossicles (malleus, incus, stapes). The stapes, sitting in the oval window, vibrates the endolymph in the inner ear. Movement of the endolymph activates the hearing mechanoreceptors, the organ of Corti, forming nerve impulses. The nerve impulses travel along the cochlear branch of CN VIII to the primary auditory cortex in the temporal lobe. The ear is also the organ that contains the sense receptors for balance. The mechanoreceptors are located within the inner ear and specifically within the semicircular canals and vestibule. Activation of the receptors causes nerve impulses that are carried by the vestibular branch of CN VIII to various parts of the brain (cerebellum, midbrain, and temporal lobe).

 As You Age

1. The general senses diminish with age. A decrease in the number and sensitivity of sensory receptors, dermatomes, and neurons results in dulling of pain, touch, and tactile sensation.
2. A gradual loss in taste and smell begins around the age of 50 years.
3. Cumulative damage to hair cells in the organ of Corti occurs after the age of 60. Older adults can lose the ability to hear high-pitched sounds and the consonants *ch, f, g, s, sh, t, th,* and *z.* Also, 25% of older adults are hearing impaired.
4. Vision diminishes by the age of 70, primarily because of a decrease in the amount of light that reaches the retina and impaired focusing of the light on the retina.
5. The muscles of the iris become less efficient, so the pupils usually remain somewhat constricted.
6. The lacrimal glands become less active, and the eyes become dry and more susceptible to bacterial infection and irritation.

MEDICAL TERMINOLOGY AND DISORDERS   Disorders of the Senses: Eyes and Ears

Medical Term	Word Parts	Word Part Meaning or Derivation	Description
Eye			
aphakia	a-	without	**Aphakia** refers to *the absence of the lens when the cataract is extracted.* **Pseudoaphakia (pseudo = false or fake)** refers to *an eye that has an artificial lens.*
	-phak/o-	lens	
	-ia	condition of	
blepharitis	blephar/o-	eyelid	**Blepharitis** is *an inflammation of the eyelid.*
	-itis	inflammation	
cataracts		From a Latin word meaning "waterfall or broken water"	*Clouding of the lens, thereby diminishing the amount of light that enters the posterior eye.*
lacrimal	lacrim/o-	tear	The **lacrimal** gland secretes tears that wash over the cornea and drain through the lacrimal ducts.
	-al	pertaining to	
ocular	ocul/o-	eye	**Ocular** is a word that *refers to the eye,* as in an ocular disease such as glaucoma.
	-ar	pertaining to	

	MEDICAL TERMINOLOGY AND DISORDERS	Disorders of the Senses: Eyes and Ears—cont'd	

Medical Term	Word Parts	Word Part Meaning or Derivation	Description
ophthalmoscope	ophthalm/o-	eye	An **ophthalmoscope** is *an instrument used to examine the eye.*
	-scope	instrument used for examination	
photophobia	phot/o-	light	A patient with a corneal abrasion may be described as being **photophobic,** or having *a fear of pain-inducing exposure to light.*
	-phob/o-	fear of	
	-ia	pertaining to	
Disorders			
conjunctivitis	conjunctiv/o-	conjunctiva	Refers to *inflammation or infection of the conjunctiva; it is usually viral, bacterial, or allergenic in origin.*
	-itis	inflammation	
errors of refraction	*refringere*	From a Latin word meaning "to break up" (referring to light)	Refers to *distorted vision resulting from improper refraction of light as it enters the eye.* **Emmetropia** (emmetros = well-proportioned/relaxed; -opia = condition of vision) refers to *normal refractive condition of the eye.* Errors of refraction are described in the text.
glaucoma	From the Greek word *glaukos*	Name given to any condition in which gray or green replaces the black color of the pupil	Also called the "silent thief of sight," glaucoma is the second most common cause of blindness in the United States. **Glaucoma** is *a group of eye conditions that cause damage to the optic nerve (CN II) and blindness.* The damage is due to increased intraocular pressure (IOP). There are four major types of glaucoma: open-angle glaucoma, angle-closure glaucoma, congenital glaucoma, and secondary glaucoma. Secondary glaucoma is due to drugs (corticosteroids), eye infections/trauma, or systemic diseases such as diabetes mellitus.
keratitis	kerat/o-	cornea	*Refers to inflammation of the cornea.* **Keratitis** is most often caused by pathogens associated with the use of contact lenses. **Exposure keratitis** is caused by drying and ulceration of the cornea in response to incomplete closure of the eyelids (as occurs with **exophthalmos,** protrusion of the eyeball). **Photokeratitis** is due to excess UV radiation (snow blindness or welder's arc eye). Healing may cause scarring and necessitate a corneal transplant, or keratoplasty (-plasty = surgical repair of).
	-itis	inflammation	
macular degeneration		From a Latin word *macula* meaning "spot"	Called **age-related macular degeneration (AMD)** and *results from damage of the macular cells of the retina with loss of vision in the center of the visual field (like a hole punched in the center of a picture).* **Dry AMD** is due is atrophy of the retina and loss of photoreceptors. **Wet AMD,** or **exudative AMD,** is due to neovascularization (new blood vessel growth), which causes blood or fluid to leak below the macula.
nystagmus		From a Latin word meaning "a nodding" or drowsiness	*Involuntary and rapid oscillating movements of the eyeball.* The movement may be side-to side **(horizontal nystagmus),** up and down **(vertical nystagmus),** or rotary **(rotary or torsional nystagmus).**

Continued

MEDICAL TERMINOLOGY AND DISORDERS   Disorders of the Senses: Eyes and Ears—cont'd

Medical Term	Word Parts	Word Part Meaning or Derivation	Description
retinopathy	retin/o-	retina	*Refers to permanent damage of the retina.* Retinopathy is often characterized by microvascular retinal changes and angiogenesis (formation of new blood vessels). The new blood vessels are fragile and leak fluid or blood into the eye; this causes retinal scarring and severe loss of vision or blindness. There are many causes of retinopathy, the most common being **diabetic retinopathy**.
	-pathy	disease	
strabismus		From a Greek word *strabismos* meaning "to squint"	Also called "crossed eyes." *A disorder in which two eyes do not align in the same direction and therefore do not focus on the same point.* There is **convergent strabismus**, whereby the eye(s) deviates medially, and **divergent strabismus**, whereby the eye(s) deviates laterally.
uveitis	uvea-	From a Latin word meaning "grape"	*Inflammation of the uvea, the middle layer of the eye.* **Anterior uveitis** affects the front part of the eye, usually the iris, causing **iritis. Posterior uveitis** affects the choroid, the layer that supplies most of the blood to the retina. Posterior uveitis is most apt to cause loss of vision.
	-itis	inflammation	
Ear			
myringotomy	myring/o-	eardrum	A **myringotomy** is *an incision into the eardrum usually in an attempt to insert a plastic tube for the purpose of preventing the accumulation of fluid within the middle ear* as occurs in **otitis media.** Also called a *tympanoplasty* (tympan/o- = eardrum).
	-otomy	incision into	
otoscope	ot/o-	ear	An **otoscope** is *an instrument used to visualize the external auditory canal and the tympanic membrane (eardrum).*
	-scope	instrument for examination	
otosclerosis	ot/o-	ear	*Refers to an abnormal bone growth in the middle ear causing a gradual loss of hearing; causes bone conduction deafness.*
	-scler/o-	hard	
	-osis	condition of	
ototoxic	ot/o-	ear	Many drugs are considered to be ototoxic, harmful to the ear and causing a loss of hearing.
	-toxo-	poison	
	-ic	pertaining to	
presbycusis	presby/o-	old age	**Presbycusis** refers to *impaired hearing that develops with advancing age.*
	-acous/os	hearing condition	
Disorders			
Ménière's disease		Named after the French physician Ménière, who first described the disorder	*A disorder of the inner ear thought to be caused by a buildup of inner ear fluid (endolymph).* There are four main symptoms: hearing loss, a feeling of pressure in the ear, tinnitus or a roaring sound, and vertigo. The vertigo is most distressing, causing the person to experience a spinning sensation that, in turn, causes severe nausea, vomiting, and sweating.
kinetosis	kinesi/o-	From a Greek word *kinein,* meaning "to put in motion"	Also called **motion sickness** and **travel sickness** (car, plane, boat). Motion sickness occurs in response to excessive stimulation of the equilibrium receptors in the inner ear. The Greek word for *nausea* means "ship," a reference to seasickness.
	-osis	condition of	

MEDICAL TERMINOLOGY AND DISORDERS   Disorders of the Senses: Eyes and Ears—cont'd

Medical Term	Word Parts	Word Part Meaning or Derivation	Description
otitis	ot/o-	ear	*A general term for inflammation or infection of the ear and causes* otalgia *or* otodynia, *an earache.* It is classified as otitis externa, otitis media, and otitis interna. **Otitis externa** is *an outer ear infection, most commonly "swimmer's ear."* **Otitis media** is *a middle ear infection with fluid or pus accumulation behind the tympanic membrane (eardrum). The drum may burst, causing scarring of the tympanic membrane. Offending pathogens enter the middle ear from the pharynx (throat) via the eustachian tube.* **Aerotitis media** is *inflammation of the middle ear caused by changes in atmospheric pressure, as in air travel.* **Otitis interna** *(inner ear inflammation/ infection) affects the sensory cells for both hearing and balance; vertigo is a common symptom.*
	-itis	inflammation	

Get Ready for Exams!

Summary Outline

The sensory system allows us to experience the world through a variety of sensations: touch, pressure, pain, proprioception, temperature, taste, smell, vision, hearing, and equilibrium.

I. Receptors and Sensation
  A. Receptor
    1. A receptor is a specialized area of a sensory neuron that detects a specific stimulus.
    2. The five types of receptors are chemoreceptors, pain receptors (nociceptors), thermoreceptors, mechanoreceptors, and photoreceptors.
  B. Sensation
    1. A sensation is a conscious awareness of incoming sensory information.
    2. There are four components of a sensation.
    3. Two characteristics of sensation are projection and adaptation.

II. General Senses
  A. Pain
    1. Pain receptors (nociceptors) are free nerve endings.
    2. The stimuli for pain are tissue damage, lack of oxygen, and stretching or distortion of tissue.
  B. Touch and pressure
    1. Receptors are mechanoreceptors that respond to forces that press, move, or deform tissue.
    2. The receptors for pressure are located in the skin, subcutaneous tissue, and deep tissue.
  C. Temperature
    1. There are thermoreceptors for heat and cold.

  2. Thermoreceptors are found in free nerve endings and in other specialized sensory cells beneath the skin.
  D. Proprioception
    1. Proprioceptors are located primarily in the muscles, tendons, and joints.
    2. Proprioceptors sense orientation or position.

III. Special Senses
  A. Sense of smell: The nose
    1. Olfactory receptors are chemoreceptors.
    2. Sensory information travels along the olfactory nerve to the temporal lobe.
  B. Sense of taste: The tongue
    1. Taste buds contain chemoreceptors for taste.
    2. There are four basic taste sensations: sweet, salty, sour, and bitter.
    3. Sensory information travels along the facial, glossopharyngeal, and vagus nerves to the gustatory cortex in the parietal lobe.
  C. Sense of sight: The eye
    1. The visual accessory organs include the eyebrows, eyelids, eyelashes, lacrimal apparatus, and extrinsic eye muscles.
    2. The eyeball has three layers: the sclera, choroid, and retina (contains the photoreceptors, rods, and cones).
    3. The eyeball has two cavities. One is a posterior cavity filled with vitreous humor; the other is an anterior cavity filled with aqueous humor.
    4. There are two sets of eye muscles: extrinsic and intrinsic eye muscles.
    5. The extrinsic eye muscles move the eyeball.
    6. The intrinsic eye muscles control the size of the pupil and shape of the lens for refraction.

7. Light stimulates the photoreceptors.
8. The electrical signal is carried to the occipital lobe via the optic nerve and visual pathway.
D. Sense of hearing: The ear
  1. There are three parts of the ear: the external ear, middle ear, and inner ear.
  2. The middle ear contains the ossicles.
  3. The inner ear structure concerned with hearing is the cochlea. It contains the hearing receptors, or the organ of Corti (mechanoreceptors).
  4. Hearing information is carried by the cochlear (CN VIII) to the temporal lobe.
  5. Steps in hearing are summarized in Figure 13-16.
E. Sense of balance: The ear
  1. The receptors are mechanoreceptors located in the vestibule and semicircular canals of the inner ear.
  2. The receptors are activated when the head changes position.
  3. Balance information travels along the vestibular nerve (CN VIII) to many areas of the brain (cerebellum, midbrain, and temporal lobe).

Review Your Knowledge

Matching: Senses
Directions: Match the following words with their descriptions below. Some words may be used more than once.
a. sight
b. taste
c. smell
d. hearing
e. balance

1. ___ Involves rods and cones, the retina, and CN II
2. ___ Involves the organ of Corti and CN VIII
3. ___ Is the olfactory sense; uses chemoreceptors
4. ___ Uses mechanoreceptors; sensory information transmitted by the vestibular branch of CN VIII
5. ___ Gustatory sensation
6. ___ From photoreceptors to the occipital lobe
7. ___ From receptors to the auditory cortex

Matching: Structures of the Eye
Directions: Match the following words with their descriptions below. Some words may be used more than once.
a. choroid
b. vitreous humor
c. lens
d. cornea
e. iris
f. aqueous humor
g. conjunctiva
h. retina

1. ___ The layer of the eyeball that contains the photoreceptors
2. ___ The colored muscle portion of the eye that determines the size of the pupil
3. ___ The shape of this structure determined by the ciliary muscles; refracts light

4. ___ Layer of the eyeball that provides the blood supply for the retina
5. ___ Secreted by the ciliary body and drained by the canal of Schlemm
6. ___ Gel-like substance in the posterior cavity; maintains the shape of the eye and helps hold the retina in place
7. ___ Contains the radial and circular muscles; mydriasis and miosis
8. ___ The window of the eye; an avascular structure
9. ___ Includes the macula lutea
10. ___ Inner lining of the lids; "pink eye"

Matching: Structures of the Ear
Directions: Match the following words with their descriptions below. Some words may be used more than once.
a. external ear
b. middle ear
c. inner ear

1. ___ Contains the malleus, incus, and stapes
2. ___ Connected to the pharynx by the eustachian tube
3. ___ Home of cerumen
4. ___ Location of the organ of Corti and CN VIII
5. ___ Cochlea, semicircular canals, and vestibule
6. ___ Endolymph and perilymph; mechanoreceptors
7. ___ Separated from the middle ear by the tympanic membrane
8. ___ Separated from the inner ear by the oval window
9. ___ Bone conduction deafness
10. ___ Nerve conduction deafness

Multiple Choice
1. The retina
  a. refracts light.
  b. contains rods and cones.
  c. covers the optic disc, the area of most acute vision.
  d. secretes vitreous humor.
2. What is the consequence of diminished blood flow to the choroid?
  a. Aqueous humor cannot be formed and the intraocular pressure increases.
  b. Light cannot be refracted.
  c. The retina dies.
  d. The pupil constricts.
3. A drug or effect that is described as mydriatic
  a. decreases intraocular pressure.
  b. dilates the pupil.
  c. increases the secretion of aqueous humor.
  d. increases the numbers of cones.
4. Which of the following does not describe the middle ear?
  a. It contains the malleus, incus, and stapes.
  b. It connects with the pharynx by the eustachian tube.
  c. It is the location of the organ of Corti.
  d. It is concerned with bone conduction.
5. The organ of Corti
  a. is the receptor for hearing.
  b. refers to the ossicles within the middle ear.
  c. leans up against the tympanic membrane and "feels" its vibration.
  d. activates CN II.

6. Touch, pressure, pain, and temperature are
   a. mediated through mechanoreceptors.
   b. classified as general senses.
   c. interpreted in the precentral gyrus.
   d. general senses that are interpreted in the occipital lobe.
7. Cranial nerves III, IV, and VI
   a. carry sensory information from the retina to the occipital lobe.
   b. carry sensory information from the organ of Corti to the primary auditory cortex.
   c. innervate the extrinsic eye muscles.
   d. are the motor nerves involved in the corneal reflex.
8. Which of the following is not a sense?
   a. Gustation
   b. Lacrimation
   c. Olfaction
   d. Proprioception
9. Which of the following best describes these structures: superior oblique, inferior oblique, superior rectus, inferior rectus, medial rectus, and lateral rectus?
   a. Cranial nerves that stimulate the extrinsic eye muscles
   b. Muscles that form the iris
   c. Middle ear structures
   d. Extrinsic eye muscles
10. Which of the following is least related to the eyelids?
   a. Levator palpebrae superioris
   b. CN III
   c. Ptosis, causing a "sleepy" appearance
   d. Optic nerve

Go Figure

1. **According to Figures 13-1 and 13-3 and Table 13-1**
   a. The general senses include touch, pressure, smell, temperature, and proprioception.
   b. Pain receptors are stimulated on either extreme of the thermoreceptors.
   c. Figure 13-3 identifies the four components of a sensation that are specific to the special senses.
   d. All the receptors in Table 13-1 are represented in Figure 13-3.

2. **According to Figures 13-5 and 13-6, and Table 13-1**
   a. Olfactory receptors are mechanoreceptors.
   b. Activation of chemoreceptors in the nasal membrane elicits the sensation of smell in the olfactory cortex of the temporal lobe.
   c. The tip of the tongue is responsible for differentiating among bitter, sour, salty, and sweet tastes.
   d. The gustatory sense (taste) is mediated by a nociceptor.

3. **According to Figure 13-7**
   a. The lacrimal gland is located medially and secretes aqueous humor.
   b. Tears are drained through openings in both the medial and lateral canthi.
   c. The lacrimal sac is located laterally and inferior to the lacrimal gland.
   d. The lacrimal puncta are part of the drainage system for tears.

4. **According to Figure 13-8**
   a. Vitreous humor fills the anterior cavity and gives shape to the cornea.
   b. Aqueous humor fills the posterior cavity and gently presses the retina against the choroid.
   c. The retina lies against the choroid in the posterior portion of the eyeball.
   d. The optic nerve receives sensory information from all structures within the eye, particularly the lens.

5. **According to Figure 13-8**
   a. Aqueous humor drains from the anterior cavity by way of the canal of Schlemm.
   b. Vitreous humor drains from the posterior cavity by way of the optic disc.
   c. The macula lutea and fovea centralis are areas of the choroid.
   d. All of the above are true.

6. **According to Figure 13-8**
   a. The retina, choroid, and sclera are layers of the posterior eyeball.
   b. Suspensory ligaments attach the lens to the cornea.
   c. The macula lutea and fovea centralis are intrinsic eye muscles.
   d. The iris is located posterior to the lens.

7. **According to Figures 13-8 and 13-9**
   a. The ciliary muscles are extrinsic eye muscles.
   b. The iris is composed of circular and radial muscles.
   c. The intrinsic eye muscles include the ciliary muscles and the superior and inferior oblique muscles.
   d. Mydriasis occurs in response to the constriction of the circular muscles of the iris.

8. **According to Figures 13-11 and 13-13**
   a. Refraction is accomplished by the contractile activity of the extrinsic eye muscles.
   b. Hyperopia and myopia are called *errors of refraction*.
   c. Refraction is accomplished by the contraction and relaxation of the iris.
   d. The lens focuses the light rays on the optic disc.

9. **According to Figure 13-12**
   a. The optic chiasm is located in the primary visual cortex.
   b. All fibers from the right eye cross at the optic chiasm and travel to the left side of the brain.
   c. All fibers from the left eye cross at the optic chiasm and travel to the right side of the brain.
   d. Some fibers from both the left and right eyes cross at the optic chiasm and travel to opposite sides of the brain.

10. **According to Figures 13-14 and 13-15**
    a. Bone conduction is an inner ear event.
    b. Nerve conduction is a middle ear event.
    c. The external ear is separated from the middle ear by the oval window.
    d. CN VIII receives input from receptors for both hearing and balance.

11. **According to Figures 13-14, 13-15, and 13-16**
    a. Vibration of the tympanic membrane is caused by fluid movement in the inner ear.
    b. The eustachian tube connects the middle ear with the semicircular canals.
    c. The semicircular canals and vestibule house the organ of Corti.
    d. The cochlear branch of CN VIII carries information to the temporal lobe.

Endocrine System

Key Terms

adenohypophysis (p. 263)
adrenal glands (p. 271)
catecholamines (p. 271)
endocrine glands (p. 259)

hormone (p. 259)
neurohypophysis (p. 266)
pancreas (p. 274)
parathyroid glands (p. 269)

pineal gland (p. 277)
steroids (p. 261)
thymus gland (p. 277)
thyroid gland (p. 267)

Objectives

1. List the functions of the endocrine system.
2. Discuss the role and function of hormones in the body, including:
   - Define *hormone*.
   - Explain the process by which hormones bind to the receptor sites of specific tissues (targets).
   - Explain the three mechanisms that control the secretion of hormones.

3. Discuss the pituitary gland, including:
   - Describe the relationship of the hypothalamus to the pituitary gland.
   - Describe the location, regulation, and hormones of the pituitary gland.
4. Identify the other major endocrine glands and their hormones, and explain the effects of hyposecretion and hypersecretion.

While performing his mating ritual, Rooster is dancing out the meaning of the word *hormone*, the main focus of the endocrine system. It is a Greek term meaning "to arouse or to set into motion." Rooster's testosterone has truly set him in motion. It has him prancing and dancing his mating ritual and has both him and Hen aroused.

The nervous system and the endocrine system are the two chief communicating and coordinating systems in the body. They regulate almost all organ systems. Although the nervous and endocrine systems work together closely, they have several differences. The nervous system communicates through electrical signals called *nerve impulses*. Nerve impulses communicate information rapidly and generally achieve short-term effects. The endocrine system, in contrast, communicates through chemical signals called *hormones*. The endocrine system responds more slowly and generally exerts longer-lasting effects.

ENDOCRINE GLANDS

The endocrine system is composed of endocrine glands that are widely distributed throughout the body (Figure 14-1). **Endocrine glands** secrete the chemical substances called *hormones*. Endocrine glands are ductless glands—that is, they secrete the hormones directly into the blood and not into ducts. For example, the pancreas secretes the hormone insulin into the blood, which then delivers the insulin to cells throughout the body. Many hormones are also secreted by organs, such as the stomach, kidney, and heart: these hormones will be described in later chapters.

HORMONES

A **hormone** is a chemical messenger that influences or controls the activities of other tissues or organs. In general, the endocrine system and its hormones help regulate metabolic processes involving carbohydrates, proteins, and fats. Hormones also play an important role in growth and reproduction and help regulate water and electrolyte balance. When you become hungry, thirsty, hot, or cold, your body's response includes the secretion of hormones. Finally, hormones help your body meet the demands of infection, trauma, and stress. The study of the endocrine system is called *endocrinology*.

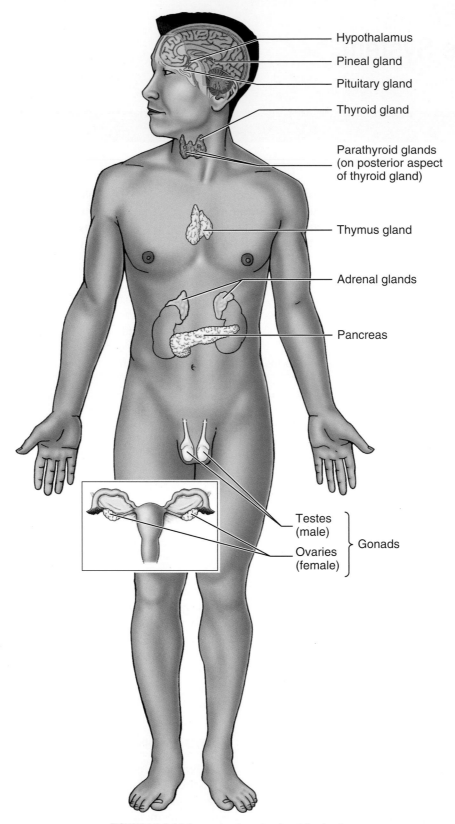

FIGURE 14-1 Major endocrine glands of the body.

Hypothalamus

Pineal gland

Pituitary gland

Thyroid gland

Parathyroid glands
(on posterior aspect
of thyroid gland)

Thymus gland

Adrenal glands

Pancreas

Testes
(male)

Ovaries
(female)

Gonads

CLASSIFICATION OF HORMONES

Chemically, hormones are classified as either proteins (and protein-related substances) or **steroids**. With the exception of secretions from the adrenal cortex and the sex glands, all hormones are protein or protein related. The adrenal cortex and the sex glands secrete steroids.

TARGETS

Each hormone binds to a specific tissue, called its *target tissue* or *organ* (Figure 14-2, *A*). The target tissue may be located close to or at a distance from the endocrine gland. Some hormones, such as thyroid hormone and insulin, have many target tissues and therefore exert more widespread, or generalized, effects. Other hormones, such as parathyroid hormone (PTH), have fewer target tissues and therefore exert fewer effects.

HORMONE RECEPTORS

Hormones bind to the receptor sites of the cells of their target tissues. The two types of receptors are those located on the outer surface of the cell membrane (membrane receptors) and those located within the cell (intracellular receptors).

How do hormones recognize their target tissues? The hormone and its receptor can be compared to a lock and key. The key must fit the lock. The same is true for the hormone and receptor; a part of the hormone (key) "fits into" its receptor (lock) on the target. Unless the match is perfect, the hormone cannot lock into and stimulate the receptor. For example, the hormone insulin circulates throughout the body in the blood and is therefore delivered to every cell in the body. Insulin, however, can only stimulate the cells that have insulin receptors. Insulin does not affect cells that lack insulin receptors. The lock-and-key theory guarantees that a particular hormone affects only certain cells. The hormone-receptor relationship ensures specificity, meaning that there is a specific hormone for each receptor.

Protein hormones generally bind to receptor sites located on the cell membrane (see Figure 14-2, *B*). The interaction of the hormone with its receptor stimulates the production of a second messenger such as cyclic adenosine monophosphate (cAMP). The cAMP, in turn, helps activate the enzymes in the cell. For

A

B   C

FIGURE 14-2 What hormones do. **A,** Hormones: aim at target tissues or target organs. **B,** Protein hormones and membrane receptors. **C,** Steroid hormones and intracellular receptors.

example, when epinephrine stimulates its receptors on the heart, cAMP is formed and then stimulates the heart itself.

The second type of receptor is located intracellularly (see Figure 14-2, C). Steroid hormones, which are lipid soluble, pass through the plasma membrane of the target cell and bind to receptors in the nucleus. The steroid-receptor complex then stimulates protein synthesis. The newly synthesized protein alters cellular function.

? Re-Think

1. What is a target organ?
2. How does a hormone recognize its target cell?

CONTROL OF HORMONE SECRETION

Three mechanisms control the secretion of hormones: feedback control loops, biorhythms, and control by the central nervous system (CNS).

NEGATIVE FEEDBACK LOOP, OR "ENOUGH IS ENOUGH"

Normal endocrine function depends on the normal plasma levels of hormones. Life-threatening complications develop when the glands hypersecrete or hyposecrete hormones. For example, if too much or too little steroid is secreted by the adrenal cortex, the person develops signs and symptoms that are potentially life threatening. So how does the adrenal cortex, a steroid-secreting gland, know when it has secreted enough steroid?

The pattern of adrenocorticotropic hormone (ACTH) and cortisol secretion is one example of a negative feedback loop (Figure 14-3). ACTH, secreted by the anterior pituitary gland, stimulates its target organ (adrenal cortex) to secrete cortisol. As blood levels of cortisol increase, the cortisol in the blood chemically "tells" the anterior pituitary gland to slow further secretion of ACTH. The diminished ACTH, in turn, decreases the secretion of cortisol by the adrenal cortex.

What information was fed back to the anterior pituitary gland? It was the increasing level of cortisol in the blood. What was the response of the anterior

pituitary gland? The gland decreased its secretion of ACTH. Because the cortisol diminished the secretion of the anterior pituitary gland, the response is referred to as *negative feedback control*. Why doesn't the adrenal cortex completely stop its secretion of cortisol? Over time, the plasma level of cortisol declines as the hormone is degraded and eliminated from the body; the negative inhibition by cortisol is relieved and ACTH is again secreted. (ACTH regulation is described more completely later in the chapter.)

POSITIVE FEEDBACK LOOP, OR "GIVE ME MORE"

Unlike the inhibition of a negative feedback loop, a positive feedback loop causes an enhanced response, a self-amplification cycle in which a change is the stimulus for an even greater change in the same direction—the "give me more" effect. For example, during early labor, the head of the baby stretches the cervix, the neck of the uterus. The stretch causes nerve impulses to travel from the cervix to the brain, which in turn causes the secretion of a hormone called *oxytocin*. The oxytocin is carried by the blood to the uterus, where it stimulates the contraction of the uterus. In response to uterine contraction, the cervix is stretched further by the baby's head, causing the release of additional oxytocin. This positive feedback cycle continues until the baby is born. Positive feedback loops are often designed to produce a rapid response.

BIORHYTHMS

Blood levels of most hormones are also controlled by biorhythms. A biorhythm is a rhythmic alteration in a hormone's rate of secretion. Some hormones, such as cortisol, are secreted in a circadian rhythm. A circadian rhythm (*circa-* means "around"; *-dian* means "day") is a 24-hour rhythm; its pattern repeats every 24 hours. Because of its circadian rhythm, cortisol secretion is highest in the morning hours (peak at 8 AM) and lowest in the evening hours (lowest at midnight). The female reproductive hormones represent another biorhythm. They are secreted in a monthly pattern—hence, the monthly menstrual cycle.

Unfortunately, biorhythms can be disturbed by travel and alterations in sleep patterns. For example, jet lag and the symptoms of fatigue experienced by persons who work the night shift are related to alterations of biorhythms. More recently alterations in biorhythms have also been linked to disturbances in cholesterol metabolism and diseases such as cancer. The problem has become so acute that some hospitals have developed staffing schedules based on biorhythms.

Sometimes drugs are administered on a schedule that mimics normal biorhythms. For example, steroids are administered in the morning, when natural steroid levels are highest. Coordinating with the natural rhythms increases the effectiveness of the drug and

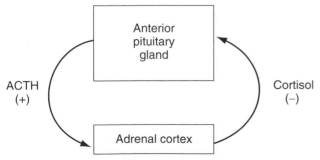

FIGURE 14-3 Negative feedback loop.

causes fewer side effects. The effect of biorhythms on drug effects is so important that a branch of pharmacology addresses this issue: chronopharmacology.

CONTROL BY THE CENTRAL NERVOUS SYSTEM

The CNS helps control the secretion of hormones in two ways: activation of the hypothalamus and stimulation of the sympathetic nervous system. Think about this. The CNS exerts a powerful influence over the endocrine system. Because the CNS is also the center for our emotional life, it is not surprising that our emotions, in turn, affect the endocrine system.

For example, when we are stressed out, the CNS causes several of the endocrine glands to secrete stress hormones, thereby alerting every cell in the body to the threat. Many women have experienced the effect of stress on the menstrual cycle. Stress can cause the menstrual period to occur early or late; it may even cause the cycle to skip a month. These effects illustrate the power of emotions on our body. In fact, the functions of the nervous system and the endocrine system are so closely related that the word *psychoneuroendocrinology* is used.

 Re-Think

Referring to Figure 14-3, explain the concept of negative feedback control.

 Sum It Up!

The endocrine system is composed of endocrine glands widely distributed throughout the body. The endocrine glands secrete hormones. Hormones stimulate target tissues by binding to cell receptors. The receptors are located either on the cell membrane or within the cell. Three control mechanisms regulate the secretion of hormones: negative and positive feedback loops, biorhythms, and CNS activity.

PITUITARY GLAND

PITUITARY GLAND AND HYPOTHALAMUS

The pituitary gland, also called the *hypophysis* (hye-POF-is-sis), is a pea-sized gland located in a depression of the sphenoid bone. It is attached to the undersurface of the hypothalamus by a short stalk called the *infundibulum*. The pituitary contains two main parts: the anterior pituitary gland and posterior pituitary gland. A tiny third lobe exists only in the fetus. The major hormones and their target glands are shown in Figure 14-4, *A*.

The secretion of the anterior pituitary gland is controlled by the hypothalamus. Although it is part of the brain, the hypothalamus secretes several hormones and is therefore considered to be an endocrine gland. These hormones are called *releasing hormones* and *release-inhibiting hormones*. They either stimulate or inhibit the secretion of anterior pituitary hormones.

For example, prolactin-releasing hormone, secreted by the hypothalamus, stimulates the pituitary gland to secrete prolactin. Prolactin-inhibiting hormone (PIH), secreted by the hypothalamus, inhibits the secretion of prolactin by the anterior pituitary gland.

How do the hypothalamic hormones reach the anterior pituitary gland? The hypothalamus secretes its hormones into a network of capillaries (tiny blood vessels) that connect the hypothalamus with the anterior pituitary gland (see Figure 14-4, *B*). These connecting capillaries are called the *hypothalamic-hypophyseal portal system*. Thus, hormones secreted by the hypothalamus flow through the portal capillaries to the anterior pituitary.

 Do You Know...

Why the Pituitary Gland Is "Uppity" but Not Snotty?

The pituitary gland is also known as the *master gland*, and a pretty important gland it is! When first discovered, however, the pituitary gland was relegated to the lowly role of mucus secretion (*pituita* is the Greek word for "mucus"). The gland was credited with secreting mucus as a cooling agent. After cooling the body, mucus was then eliminated through the nose. Obviously, this is not true. Mucus is secreted by the mucous membrane that lines the nasal passages and does not act as a coolant. Mucus merely does the nasal housework—it traps the dust and gets blown out of your nose. The pituitary gland, on the other hand, has more important things to do. It secretes many hormones and controls much of the endocrine function of the body. Unfortunately, this master gland is stuck with the name *pituitary* (mucus-making). Its other name, hypophysis, isn't much more flattering; it means "undergrowth" (referring to its location under the brain). Mucus and undergrowth—humbling for a master gland!

ANTERIOR PITUITARY GLAND

The anterior pituitary gland is composed of glandular epithelial tissue and is also called the **adenohypophysis** (ad-eh-no-hye-POF-i-sis). The anterior pituitary gland secretes six major hormones (Table 14-1; Figure 14-4, *A*). These hormones control other glands and affect many organ systems. In fact, the anterior pituitary affects so many other glands that it is often called the *master gland*.

The hormones of the anterior pituitary include thyroid-stimulating hormone (TSH), ACTH, growth hormone (GH), the gonadotropins, and prolactin (PRL).

Remember!	
PRO	Prolactin
ATHletes	ACTH
Got	Gonadotropins (FSH, LH)
To	TSH
GROW	Growth hormone

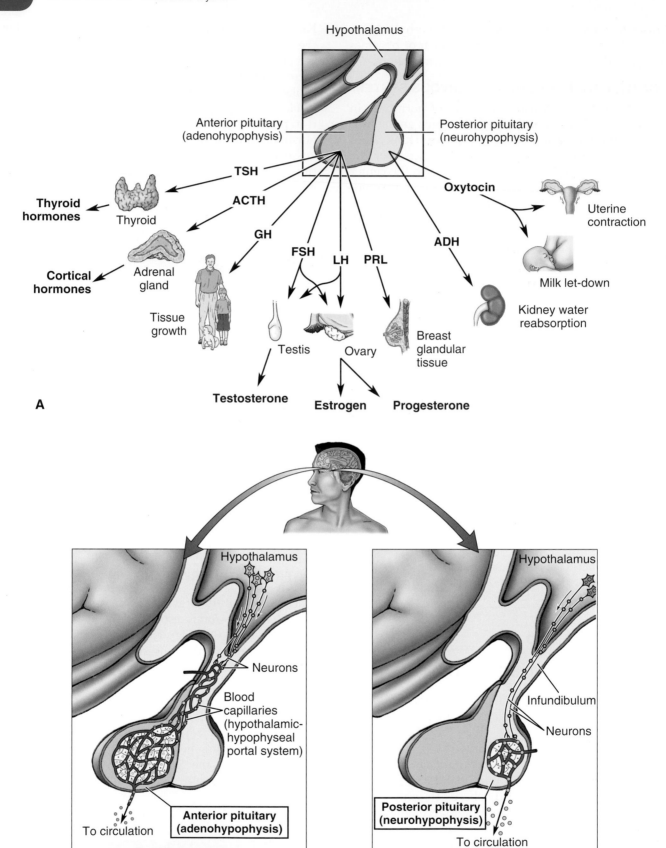

FIGURE 14-4 Pituitary gland. **A,** Hormones and target organs of the anterior and posterior pituitary glands. **B,** Relationship of the hypothalamus to the anterior pituitary gland. **C,** Relationship of the hypothalamus to the posterior pituitary gland.

Table 14-1   Hormones and Their Functions

HORMONE	FUNCTION
Anterior Pituitary Gland	
Growth hormone (GH)	Stimulates the growth of bone, cartilage, and skeletal muscle; stimulates the synthesis of glucose during periods of fasting
Prolactin	Stimulates the breast to develop and produce milk
Thyroid-stimulating hormone (TSH)	Stimulates the thyroid gland to produce thyroid hormones (T_3 and T_4)
Adrenocorticotropic hormone (ACTH)	Stimulates the adrenal cortex to secrete steroids, especially cortisol

Gonadotropic hormones
  Follicle-stimulating hormone (FSH)
  Luteinizing hormone (LH)
	
	Stimulates the development of ova and sperm
	Causes ovulation in women; stimulates secretion of progesterone in women and testosterone in men

Posterior Pituitary Gland	
Antidiuretic hormone (ADH)	Stimulates water reabsorption by the kidneys; also constricts blood vessels
Oxytocin	Contracts uterine muscle during labor; releases milk from the mammary glands (during breast-feeding)
Hormones of the Thyroid and Parathyroid Glands	
Thyroid hormones (T_3, T_4)	Triiodothyronine (T_3) and tetraiodothyronine (T_4, or thyroxine) secreted by the thyroid gland; control metabolic rate and regulate growth and development
Calcitonin	Secreted by the thyroid gland; decreases plasma levels of calcium
Parathyroid hormone (PTH)	Secreted by the parathyroid glands; increases plasma calcium
Hormones of the Adrenal Gland	

Catecholamines
  Epinephrine
  Norepinephrine
	Stimulate the "fight-or-flight" response

Steroids
  Cortisol
 	
  Aldosterone
 	
  Sex hormones
	
	Glucocorticoid that helps regulate glucose, fat, and protein metabolism; is part of the stress response
	Mineralocorticoid that causes the kidneys to reabsorb sodium and water and excrete potassium; helps regulate fluid and electrolyte balance
	The androgens (especially testosterone) help develop the secondary sex characteristics in the female and male

Hormones of the Pancreas	
Insulin	Secreted by beta cells of the islets of Langerhans; helps regulate the metabolism of carbohydrates, proteins, and fats; lowers blood glucose levels
Glucagon	Secreted by the alpha cells of the islets of Langerhans; raises blood glucose levels
Other Hormones	
Estrogens and progesterone	Secreted by the ovaries; stimulate the development of the ova (eggs) and development of secondary sex characteristics in the female
Testosterone	Secreted primarily by the testes; chief male androgen; stimulates development of sperm and secondary sex characteristics in the male
Thymosins	Stimulates maturation of the T lymphocytes
Melatonin	Secreted by the pineal gland; helps set the biorhythms

GROWTH HORMONE

Growth hormone (GH) is also called *somatotropin* or *somatotropic hormone*. Its primary effects are on the growth of bones, cartilage, and skeletal muscles, thereby determining a person's size and height. GH also exerts powerful metabolic effects. It causes amino acids to be built into proteins and fats to be broken down and used for energy. It also stimulates the conversion of protein to glucose (gluconeogenesis),

especially during periods of fasting between meals. GH thus causes blood glucose levels to rise. GH also affects electrolyte balance: it stimulates the kidneys to reabsorb sodium (Na^+), potassium (K^+), and chloride (Cl^-) and the digestive tract to absorb dietary calcium. These electrolytes then become available to growing tissue. In addition to the direct effects of GH on tissue growth, it also stimulates growth indirectly. GH stimulates the liver to produce growth stimulants called *insulin-like growth factors* (or somatomedins). GH is secreted during periods of exercise, sleep, and hypoglycemia. Like your mother said, "Plenty of rest and exercise makes you grow big and strong." (And you thought she didn't know her physiology!)

As its name implies, GH exerts a profound effect on growth. A person who hypersecretes GH as a child develops gigantism and will grow very tall, often achieving a height of 8 or 9 feet. If hypersecretion of GH occurs in an adult after the epiphyseal discs of the long bones have sealed, only the bones of the jaw (called "lantern jaw"), eyebrow ridges, nose, hands, and feet enlarge. This condition is called *acromegaly*. GH deficiency in childhood causes the opposite effect, a pituitary dwarfism. With this condition, body proportions are normal, but the person's height is very short.

PROLACTIN

Prolactin (PRL) is also called *lactogenic hormone*. As its name suggests (*pro-* means "for"; *-lact-* means "milk"), PRL promotes milk production in women. PRL stimulates the growth of the mammary glands and the production of milk after childbirth. As long as the lactating mother continues to breast-feed, PRL levels remain high and milk is produced. (PRL is discussed in more detail in Chapter 27.) The role of PRL in males is not fully understood but is known to increase the secretion of testosterone.

TROPIC HORMONES

The remaining hormones of the anterior pituitary gland are tropic hormones, which are aimed at and control other glands. The names of tropic hormones usually end in *-tropin*, or *-tropic*, as in thyrotropin or adrenocorticotropic hormone. The tropic hormones include the following:

- *Thyrotropin, or thyroid-stimulating hormone (TSH).* The target gland for TSH is the thyroid gland. TSH stimulates the thyroid gland to secrete two thyroid hormones.
- *Adrenocorticotropic hormone (ACTH).* The target gland for ACTH is the adrenal cortex. ACTH stimulates the adrenal cortex to secrete steroids.
- *Gonadotropic hormones.* The target glands for the gonadotropic hormones are the gonads, or sex glands (ovaries and testes). The two gonadotropins are follicle-stimulating hormone (FSH) and luteinizing hormone (LH). FSH stimulates the development of ova (eggs) in the female and sperm in the male. LH causes ovulation in the female and causes the secretion of sex hormones in both the male and the female. LH in the male is also called *interstitial cell–stimulating hormone* (ICSH) because it stimulates the interstitial cells in the testes to synthesize and secrete testosterone. (These hormones are described further in Chapter 26.)

POSTERIOR PITUITARY GLAND

The posterior pituitary gland is an extension of the hypothalamus (see Figure 14-4, *C*). The posterior pituitary is composed of nervous tissue and is therefore called the **neurohypophysis** (noo-roh-hye-POF-i-sis). The two hormones of the posterior pituitary gland are produced in the hypothalamus and transported to the gland, where they are stored until needed. The two hormones are antidiuretic hormone (ADH) and oxytocin. The secretion of the posterior pituitary gland is controlled by neuroendocrine reflexes. In other words, the hormones are released in response to signals from the nervous system.

ANTIDIURETIC HORMONE

Antidiuretic hormone (ADH) is released from the posterior pituitary gland in an attempt to conserve water. The primary target organ for ADH is the kidney. ADH causes the kidney to reabsorb water from the urine and return it to the blood. By so doing, the amount of urine that the kidney excretes decreases—hence, the term *antidiuretic hormone* (*anti-* means "against"; *diuresis* means "urine flow").

What is the signal for the release of ADH? ADH is released in response to a concentrated blood (increased osmolarity) and decreased blood volume; both occur in dehydration. Other triggers for the release of ADH are stress, trauma, and drugs such as morphine. Alcohol, in contrast, inhibits ADH secretion—hence, the excessive urination that accompanies beer drinking!

In the absence of ADH, a profound diuresis occurs, and the person may excrete up to 25 L/day of dilute urine. This ADH deficiency disease is called *diabetes insipidus* and should not be confused with the more common *diabetes mellitus,* which is an insulin deficiency. (The effect of ADH on the kidneys is described in Chapter 24.)

ADH also causes the blood vessels to constrict, thereby elevating blood pressure. Because of this blood pressure–elevating effect, ADH is also called *vasopressin* (vay-so-PREHS-in). (A vasopressor agent is one that elevates blood pressure.)

OXYTOCIN

The second posterior pituitary hormone is oxytocin. The target organs of oxytocin (ahk-see-TOH-sin) in the female are the uterus and the mammary glands (breasts). Oxytocin stimulates the muscles of the uterus to contract and plays a role in labor and the delivery of a baby. The word *oxytocin* literally means "swift birth," and an oxytocic drug is one that causes uterine contractions and hastens delivery. You have probably heard of the use of IV "pit" (or Pitocin, the trade name for oxytocin) to initiate labor.

Oxytocin also plays a role in breast-feeding. When the baby suckles at the breast, oxytocin is released and stimulates contraction of the smooth muscles around the mammary ducts within the breasts, thereby releasing breast milk. The release of milk in response to suckling is called the *milk let-down reflex* (discussed further in Chapter 27). The role of oxytocin in the male is not fully understood; it is thought to help move the semen along the male reproductive tract. Oxytocin has recently been dubbed the bonding or relationship hormone; it seems that a high blood level of oxytocin generates feelings of goodwill and an urge to be cooperative, protective, and friendly. It makes sense that breast-feeding (and the release of oxytocin) facilitates bonding between Mom and Baby.

A TINY THIRD LOBE ... A FETAL STRUCTURE

MELANOCYTE-STIMULATING HORMONE

Like the adult, the fetal pituitary gland is divided into two main parts: the anterior and posterior pituitary. The fetal pituitary gland, however, has a tiny third lobe (pars intermedia) that secretes melanocyte-stimulating hormone (MSH). MSH influences pigmentation of the skin. What eventually happens to the tiny third lobe? The cells are incorporated into the tissue of the anterior pituitary gland; hence, the adult pituitary has no tiny third lobe. These cells do not secrete MSH; instead, they produce a polypeptide called *pro-opiomelanocortin* (POMC). POMC is not secreted as a hormone; rather, it is degraded in the pituitary gland to ACTH and endorphins. Adrenal cortical insufficiency also causes a hypersecretion of ACTH derived from the POMC, causing the person to appear bronzed.

? Re-Think

1. Why is the pituitary gland sometimes called the *master gland*? Why do some call the hypothalamus the *master gland*?
2. What "happens" in the hypothalamic-hypophyseal portal system?
3. List the six hormones secreted by the anterior pituitary gland and two hormones secreted by the posterior pituitary gland.

2+2 Sum It Up!

The pituitary gland is called the *master gland* because it controls many other endocrine glands. The anterior pituitary gland (adenohypophysis) is controlled by hypothalamic hormones, called *releasing hormones* and *release-inhibiting hormones*. These hormones are secreted by the hypothalamus into the hypothalamic-hypophyseal portal system. The anterior pituitary gland secretes six major hormones, most of which are tropic hormones. The posterior pituitary gland is an extension of the hypothalamus and is called the *neurohypophysis*. The posterior pituitary gland secretes two hormones.

THYROID GLAND

The **thyroid gland** is located in the anterior neck; it is situated on the front and sides of the trachea

(Figure 14-5, *A*) and is easily palpated (i.e., you can feel thyroid nodules or enlargement). The thyroid gland is butterfly shaped and has two lobes connected by a band of tissue called the *isthmus* (ISS-muss). The thyroid gland contains two types of cells: the follicular cells, located within the thyroid follicle, and the parafollicular cells, located between the follicles. Each type of cell secretes a particular hormone (see Table 14-1).

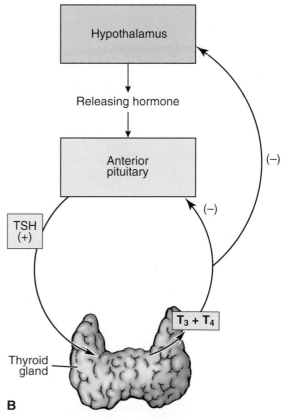

FIGURE 14-5 Thyroid gland. **A,** Location; the thyroid follicle. **B,** Control of the secretion of T_3 and T_4.

THYROID FOLLICLE

The thyroid gland is composed of many secretory units called *follicles*. The cavity in each follicle is filled with a clear, viscous substance called *colloid*. Follicular cells secrete two thyroid hormones: triiodothyronine (try-eye-oh-doh-THY-roh-neen) (T_3) and tetraiodothyronine (tet-rah-eye-oh-doh-THY-roh-neen) (T_4, or thyroxine). The term *thyroid hormones* refers to T_3 and T_4 collectively.

WHAT THYROID HORMONES (T_3 AND T_4) DO

The thyroid hormones T_3 and T_4 have similar functions, although T_3 is more potent. Thyroid hormones regulate all phases of metabolism and are necessary for the proper functioning of all other hormones. Thyroid hormones are necessary for the normal maturation of the nervous system and for normal growth and development. In addition to its many actions, thyroid hormones stimulate the secretion of GH by the anterior pituitary gland. If you were a tadpole, you would require adequate thyroid hormones before you could develop into a frog.

Perhaps the best way to describe the effects of thyroid hormones is to observe the signs and symptoms of thyroid hormone deficiency (hypothyroidism) and excess (hyperthyroidism).

HYPOTHYROIDISM

Hypothyroidism in an adult results in a condition called *myxedema*. Myxedema (mik-seh-DEE-mah) is a slowed-down metabolic state characterized by a slow heart rate, sluggish peristalsis resulting in constipation, a low body temperature, low energy, loss of hair, and weight gain. The skin becomes thick and puffy because of the accumulation of a thick fluid under the skin—hence, the name *myxedema* (*myx* means "mucus").

If an infant is born with no thyroid gland, a condition called *cretinism* develops. An infant with cretinism fails to develop both physically and mentally. The child will be short and stocky, with abnormal skeletal development and severe signs of developmental delay.

Early diagnosis and prompt treatment with thyroid hormone can prevent further developmental delay.

HYPERTHYROIDISM

An excess of thyroid hormones produces hyperthyroidism, a speeded-up metabolic state. A common type of hyperthyroidism is Graves' disease. It is characterized by an increase in heart rate, increase in peristalsis resulting in diarrhea, elevation in body temperature (heat intolerance), hyperactivity, weight loss, and wide emotional swings. The hyperthyroid person exhibits an increased sensitivity to the effects of catecholamines (epinephrine) and is at risk for the development of fast rhythm disorders of the heart. Graves' disease is also characterized by bulging eyes, a condition known as *exophthalmia* (ek-soff-THAL-mee-ah). In exophthalmia, the eyes are thought to bulge because the fat pads behind the eyeballs enlarge, pushing the eyeballs forward in the eye socket. Severe exophthalmia may make it difficult for the patient to close his or her eyelids over the cornea of the eye; the exposed cornea may then dry out, ulcerate, and scar, leading to a loss of vision.

REGULATION OF SECRETION

The regulation of thyroid gland activity is illustrated in Figure 14-5, *B*. The hypothalamus secretes a releasing hormone, which stimulates the anterior pituitary to secrete TSH. TSH stimulates the thyroid gland to secrete T_3 and T_4. When the plasma levels of the thyroid hormones increase sufficiently, negative feedback inhibition prevents further secretion of TSH.

 Do You Know...

Why an Overactive Thyroid Gland Is Hot Stuff?

An overactive thyroid gland secretes excess thyroid hormones. Thyroid hormones increase the utilization of oxygen by most cells of the body. As oxygen is used, excess heat is made by the working or metabolizing cells and body temperature rises. The heat-producing effect of the thyroid hormones is called its *calorigenic effect* and is responsible for the higher body temperature of someone who is hyperthyroid. Hot stuff, that thyroid disease!

THE NEED FOR IODINE

SYNTHESIS OF THYROID HORMONE

The synthesis of T_3 and T_4 requires iodine. The iodine in the body comes from dietary sources. Most of the iodine in the blood is actively pumped into the follicular cells of the thyroid gland, where it is used in the synthesis of the thyroid hormones. Tetraiodothyronine, or thyroxine, contains four (tetra-) iodine atoms and therefore is called T_4. Triiodothyronine (tri-) contains three iodine atoms and is called T_3.

IODINE DEFICIENCY

Why does an iodine-deficient diet cause the thyroid gland to enlarge? In an iodine-deficient state, the amount of T_3 and T_4 production decreases because iodine is necessary for the synthesis of the thyroid hormones. With insufficient iodine, thyroid hormones cannot be made in quantities great enough to shut off the secretion of TSH through negative feedback control. Persistent stimulation of the thyroid gland by TSH causes the thyroid gland to enlarge; an enlarged thyroid gland is called a *goiter* (GOYH-ter).

 Do You Know...

What a Goiter Is Doing on the Ceiling of the Sistine Chapel?

Like many artists of the Renaissance period, Michelangelo had a fascination with goiters (from the Latin *guttur*, meaning "throat"). One of his paintings, called the "Separation of Light from Darkness," shows the Creator with a very obvious nodular goiter. It is no accident that the artist equates the appearance of the goiter with the first day of creation. Why? Michelangelo was very familiar with goiters, having grown up in the iodine-poor region of Italy (before the days of iodized salt). Michelangelo was obsessed with anatomy, having spent many hours dissecting corpses and sketching innards. He shared the view of his contemporaries that goiters were a sign of beauty and privilege, so of course he gifted God a huge goiter. Other artists not only painted gnarly goiters, but they also illustrated rather hefty body types, thereby connecting the goiter with the weight gain of hypothyroidism.

Some medical historians offer a different "take" on Michelangelo's divine goiter. It has been suggested by some that Michelangelo himself had a goiter and actually painted God in his own goitrous image. This view is certainly consistent with Michelangelo's lofty opinion of himself. It has also been suggested that the "self-portrait" theory represents his petulant response to the demand of Pope Julius that he paint the ceiling, a task that Michelangelo did not enjoy.

Clinical assessment of thyroid function makes use of the iodine-pumping activity of the gland. For example, if a patient drinks radioactive iodine (^{131}I), the thyroid gland pumps the radioactive iodine from the blood into the gland. The rate of iodine uptake by the thyroid gland can be determined by a gamma ray scanner placed over the thyroid gland. Increased iodine uptake is observed in hyperthyroid and iodine-deficient patients, whereas a decrease in iodine uptake is noted with hypothyroid patients. Larger therapeutic doses of ^{131}I can be used to destroy thyroid tissue in the hyperthyroid state.

? Re-Think

1. Why does a hypothyroid person have an elevated plasma TSH level?
2. Why does an iodine-deficient diet cause goiter formation?
3. What is the calorigenic effect of thyroid hormones?

CALCITONIN

The parafollicular cells of the thyroid gland secrete a hormone called *calcitonin*. Although calcitonin is a thyroid hormone, its effects are very different from those of T_3 and T_4. Calcitonin helps regulate blood levels of calcium. Calcitonin is secreted in response to elevated blood levels of calcium. It decreases blood calcium primarily by stimulating osteoblastic (bone-making) activity in the bones, thereby moving calcium from the blood into the bone. Calcitonin also increases the excretion of calcium in the urine. In general, calcitonin acts as an antagonist to parathyroid hormone.

PARATHYROID GLANDS

Four tiny parathyroid glands lie along the posterior surface of the thyroid gland (Figure 14-6). The **parathyroid glands** secrete PTH. The stimulus for the release of PTH is a low blood level of calcium. PTH has three target organs: bone, digestive tract (intestine), and kidneys. The overall effect of PTH is to increase blood calcium levels, which it does in four ways:

1. PTH increases the release of calcium from bone tissue, called *resorption*. (Do not confuse the word *resorption* with *reabsorption*.) It does so by stimulating osteoclastic (bone breakdown) activity. In response, calcium moves from the bone to the blood.
2. PTH stimulates the kidneys to reabsorb calcium from the urine. At the same time, PTH causes the kidneys to excrete phosphate. The excretion of phosphate by the kidneys is called its *phosphaturic* (foss-foh-TOOR-ik) *effect*. The urinary excretion of phosphate is important because of the inverse relationship of phosphate and calcium in the blood. The inverse relationship means that as phosphate levels decrease, calcium levels increase; when phosphate levels increase, calcium levels decrease. Thus, to raise blood calcium levels, it is necessary to lower blood phosphate levels.
3. Working with vitamin D, PTH increases the absorption of dietary calcium by the digestive tract (intestine). Thus, a vitamin D deficiency can decrease the dietary absorption of calcium. Remember, from Chapter 7, that a daily but brief exposure to sunlight increases the production of vitamin D by the skin.
4. Blood calcium levels control the secretion of both calcitonin and PTH through negative feedback control. High blood calcium levels stimulate secretion of calcitonin, whereas low blood calcium levels inhibit secretion of calcitonin and stimulate secretion of PTH.

BLOOD CALCIUM REGULATION: IMBALANCES

HYPOCALCEMIA

What is the hand in Figure 14-7 doing? The hand and wrist muscles are contracted and cannot relax, thereby

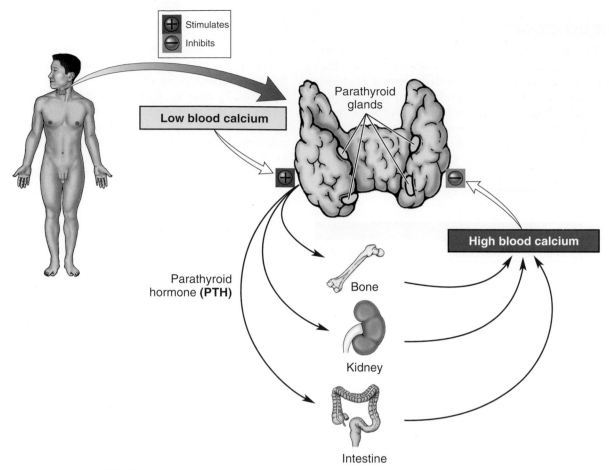

FIGURE 14-6 Parathyroid glands. Parathyroid hormone (PTH) and three target organs.

producing a carpal spasm. What causes the carpal spasm? Calcium normally stabilizes nerve and muscle membranes. With insufficient PTH, blood calcium declines, causing hypocalcemia. Consequently, the nerve and muscle membranes become unstable and continuously fire electrical signals, causing the muscles to remain contracted. Sustained skeletal muscle contraction is referred to as *tetany* (TET-ah-nee). Hypocalcemic tetany not only contorts the wrist; more seriously, it causes sustained contractions of the muscles of the larynx (laryngospasm) and the breathing muscles.

Inability of these muscles to relax causes asphyxiation and death. Hypocalcemia is life threatening!

HYPERCALCEMIA

The clinical effects of hypercalcemia are best summarized as "Bones, Stones, Moans, and Groans." The patient develops hyperparathyroidism in response to a tumor in the parathyroid gland. The PTH stimulates osteoclastic activity in the bones, thereby moving calcium from the bones to the blood and causing hypercalcemia. Bone pain results from persistent osteoclastic activity (bones and groans). Hypercalcemia causes excess calcium to be filtered into the urine, causing hypercalciuria (hye-per-kal-see-YOOR-ee-ah); the excess calcium in the urine precipitates out as kidney stones (bones, stones, and groans). Hypercalcemia also depresses the nervous, cardiac, and gastrointestinal systems causing a variety of symptoms, including depression (moans), fatigue, bradycardia, anorexia, and constipation. The Groan Zone, indeed!

FIGURE 14-7 Carpal spasm.

? Re-Think

1. List the target organs of PTH.
2. Why does a deficiency of PTH cause hypocalcemia?

Do You Know...

Why Mr. Graves's Face Is a-Twitching?

Mr. Graves just had a thyroidectomy. As part of his postsurgical care, his nurse periodically tapped the area over the facial nerve. "He is twitching," observed his nurse and immediately reported this observation as a positive Chvostek's sign. Hyperirritability of the facial nerve occurs when the blood levels of calcium decrease. Sometimes the parathyroid glands, which are embedded in the thyroid gland, are mistakenly removed or injured during thyroid surgery. If the parathyroid glands are removed, blood calcium levels decrease because there is no PTH. The nerves become so irritable that they fire continuously, causing continuous muscle contraction (tetany). Unless treated with intravenous calcium, the person may develop a fatal hypocalcemic tetany.

2+2 Sum It Up!

The thyroid gland and parathyroid glands are located in the anterior neck region. The thyroid gland secretes two iodine-containing hormones: T_3 and T_4. These hormones regulate the body's metabolic rate. Excess secretion of T_3 and T_4, called *hyperthyroidism*, increases the body's metabolic rate. Hypothyroidism causes a hypometabolic state. The thyroid gland also secretes calcitonin, which decreases blood levels of calcium. The parathyroid glands secrete PTH, which increases blood calcium levels through its effect on three target organs: bone, kidneys, and digestive tract.

ADRENAL GLANDS

The two small glands located above the kidneys are called **adrenal glands** (*ad* means "near"; *renal* means "kidney"; Figure 14-8, *A*). An adrenal gland consists of two regions: an inner medulla and an outer cortex. The medulla and the cortex secrete different hormones (see Table 14-1).

ADRENAL MEDULLA

The adrenal medulla is the inner region of the adrenal gland and is considered an extension of the sympathetic nervous system. Remember from Chapter 12 that the sympathetic nervous system is called the "fight-or-flight" system. Chromaffin cells in the adrenal medulla secrete two hormones: epinephrine (85%) and norepinephrine (15%).

Epinephrine (adrenaline) and norepinephrine, classified as **catecholamines** (kat-eh-KOHL-ah-meens), are secreted in emergency or stress situations. You may have heard the expression, "I can feel the adrenaline flowing." It is another way of saying, "I'm ready to meet the challenge." The catecholamines, like the sympathetic nervous system, help the body respond to stress by causing the following effects:

- Elevating blood pressure
- Increasing heart rate
- Converting glycogen to glucose in the liver, thereby making more glucose available to the cells

- Increasing metabolic rate of most cells, thereby providing more energy
- Causing bronchodilation (opening up of the breathing passages) to increase the flow of air into the lungs
- Changing blood flow patterns, causing dilation of the blood vessels to the heart and muscles and constriction of the blood vessels to the digestive tract

Some medullary cells extend into the inner cortical layer. When stress activates the sympathetic "fight-or-flight" response, the medullary cells stimulate the cortex to secrete steroids (also stress hormones).

Occasionally, a person develops a tumor of the adrenal medulla and displays signs and symptoms that resemble sympathetic nervous system excess. The tumor is called a *pheochromocytoma* (FEE-oh-kroh-moh-cye-TOH-mah); it causes life-threatening high blood pressure. Immediate treatment is directed at lowering the blood pressure. Long-term treatment involves surgical removal of the tumor.

ADRENAL CORTEX

The adrenal cortex, the outer region of the adrenal gland (see Figure 14-8, *A*), secretes hormones called *steroids*. Steroids are lipid-soluble hormones made from cholesterol. The adrenal cortex secretes three steroids: glucocorticoids, mineralocorticoids, and sex hormones. Adrenal cortical hormones are essential for life. If the adrenal cortex is removed or its function is lost, death will occur unless steroids are administered. An easy way to remember the functions of the adrenal cortical steroids is that they regulate sugar, salt, and sex.

Remember!

Glucocorticoids	Sugar
Mineralocorticoids	Salt
Sex hormones	Sex

GLUCOCORTICOIDS

As their name implies, the glucocorticoids affect carbohydrates. They convert amino acids into glucose (gluconeogenesis) and help maintain blood glucose levels between meals. This action ensures a steady supply of glucose for the brain and other cells. Glucocorticoids also affect protein and fat metabolism, burning both substances as fuel to increase energy production.

The chief glucocorticoid is cortisol. Cortisol is a hormone that is secreted in greater amounts during times of stress. Stress refers to physiological stress such as disease, physical injury, hemorrhage, infection, pregnancy, extreme temperature, and emotional stress, such as anger and worry. In fact, it is thought that the abdominal fat associated with heart disease is deposited in response to stress-induced chronic secretion of cortisol. Yet another reason to relax! Cortisol also has

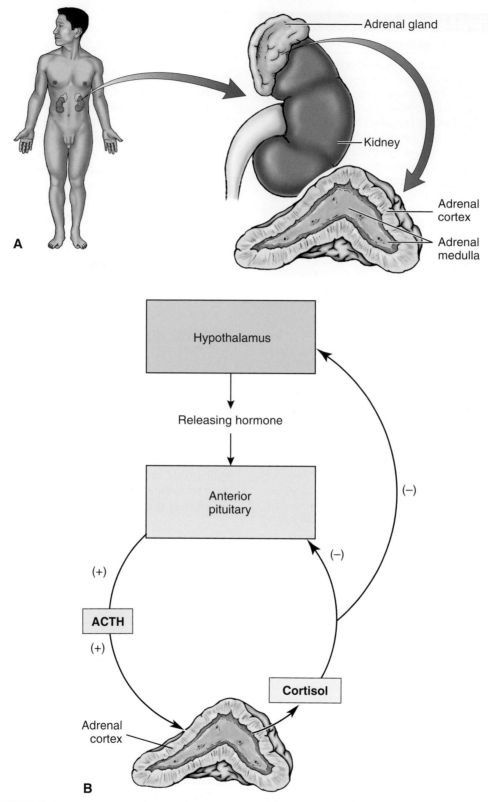

FIGURE 14-8 **A,** Adrenal glands: adrenal medulla and adrenal cortex. **B,** Control of the secretion of cortisol.

an anti-inflammatory effect. In other words, it prevents injured tissues from responding with the classic signs of inflammation: redness, heat, swelling, and pain. For this reason, cortisol is used as a drug to prevent inflammation in the treatment of arthritis and severe allergic responses.

Control of Cortisol Secretion

The secretion of cortisol involves the hypothalamus, anterior pituitary gland, and adrenal gland (see Figure 14-8, *B*). The hypothalamus secretes a releasing hormone, which then stimulates the anterior pituitary gland to secrete ACTH. ACTH, in turn, stimulates the adrenal cortex to secrete cortisol. Through negative feedback control, the cortisol inhibits the further secretion of ACTH and additional cortisol.

MINERALOCORTICOIDS

The chief mineralocorticoid is aldosterone (al-DOS-ter-own). Aldosterone plays an important role in the regulation of blood volume, blood pressure, and the concentration of electrolytes, especially Na^+ and K^+. Aldosterone is often called the salt-retaining (NaCl) hormone. The primary target organ of aldosterone is the kidney. Aldosterone reabsorbs sodium and water from the urine and eliminates potassium in the urine. The role and regulation of aldosterone are described in Chapter 24.

SEX HORMONES

The sex hormones—secreted in small amounts—include the female hormones, primarily estrogens, and male hormones, called *androgens* (primarily testosterone). The sex hormones of the ovaries usually mask the effects of the adrenal sex hormones. In females, the masculinizing effects of the adrenal androgens, such as increased body hair, may become evident after menopause, when levels of estrogen and progesterone from the ovaries decrease.

What's with the cat? His name is Steroid **CAT**. Steroid **CAT** secretes **C**ortisol, **A**ldosterone, and **T**estosterone.

```
STEROID  C  A  T
         O  L  E
         R  D  S
         T  O  T
         I  S  O
         S  T  S
         O  E  T
         L  R  E
            O  R
            N  O
            E  N
               E
```

HYPOSECRETION AND HYPERSECRETION

Hyposecretion

In some persons, the adrenal cortex fails to secrete adequate amounts of steroids. This condition is called *chronic adrenal cortical insufficiency*, or *Addison's disease*. It is characterized by generalized weakness, muscle atrophy, a bronzing of the skin, hyperkalemia (elevated K^+ in the blood), and severe loss of fluids and electrolytes, especially Na^+. Left untreated, adrenal insufficiency becomes acute and progresses to low blood volume, shock, and death. Adrenal insufficiency is life threatening and must be treated with steroids and replacement of fluids and electrolytes.

Hypersecretion

More commonly, some persons have an excess of adrenal cortical hormones. This condition may be caused by a hypersecretion of either ACTH by the anterior pituitary gland or cortisol by the adrenal cortex. Most often, however, elevated levels of cortisol are caused by the administration of steroids as drugs such as prednisone. Elevated blood levels of steroids cause a condition called *Cushing's syndrome*. It is characterized by truncal obesity, a rounded facial appearance (moon face), excess fat deposition between the shoulders (buffalo hump), masculinizing effects (virilization), facial hair (hirsutism), thin skin that bruises easily, bone loss, and muscle weakness. Salt and water retention cause blood volume and blood pressure to increase. Prolonged use of steroids causes many harmful effects, particularly in young athletes who take steroids to improve their athletic performance.

The Case of the Lazy Gland (Acute Adrenal Cortical Insufficiency)

The effects of steroid drugs on adrenal cortical function provide a dramatic example of negative feedback control. Consider this situation. A patient is given prednisone (cortisol-like) as a drug for the treatment of arthritis. As blood cortisol levels rise, the secretion of ACTH by the anterior pituitary gland is inhibited by negative feedback. In the absence of ACTH, the adrenal gland becomes "lazy" and stops its production of cortisol. As long as the person continues to take the prednisone, blood cortisol levels remain high. If, however, the person suddenly discontinues the drug, the lazy adrenal gland no longer produces cortisol, and the person eventually develops acute adrenal insufficiency and will die unless treated. (Remember: Steroids are essential for life.) Because of lazy adrenal function, steroid drugs are never discontinued abruptly; dosage is tapered off over an extended period. This gradual reduction in drug dose gives the lazy gland time to recover and regain its ability to respond to ACTH.

? Re-Think

1. List the three groups of steroids secreted by the adrenal cortex.
2. Explain the following: A person has been taking prednisone for 1 year. She suddenly stops taking the drug and develops a life-threatening acute adrenal insufficiency.

2+2 Sum It Up!

The adrenal glands are composed of the medulla and the cortex; both secrete stress hormones. The adrenal medulla is an extension of the sympathetic nervous system ("fight or flight") and secretes two catecholamines called *epinephrine* (adrenaline) and *norepinephrine*. The adrenal cortex secretes three steroids: the glucocorticoids (cortisol), the mineralocorticoids (aldosterone), and the sex hormones. The adrenal cortex is controlled by a hypothalamic-releasing hormone and ACTH from the anterior pituitary gland. The functions of the adrenal cortex are concerned with the regulation of sugar, salt, and sex.

PANCREAS

The **pancreas** (PAN-kree-ass) is a long slender organ that lies transversely across the upper abdomen, extending from the curve of the duodenum to the spleen (see Figure 14-1). The pancreas functions as both an exocrine gland and an endocrine gland. (Its exocrine function is concerned with the digestion of food and is discussed in Chapter 23.)

The pancreas secretes at least five hormones; we are concerned primarily with two hormones: insulin and glucagon. Consult Ms. PIG in Figure 14-9; she will help

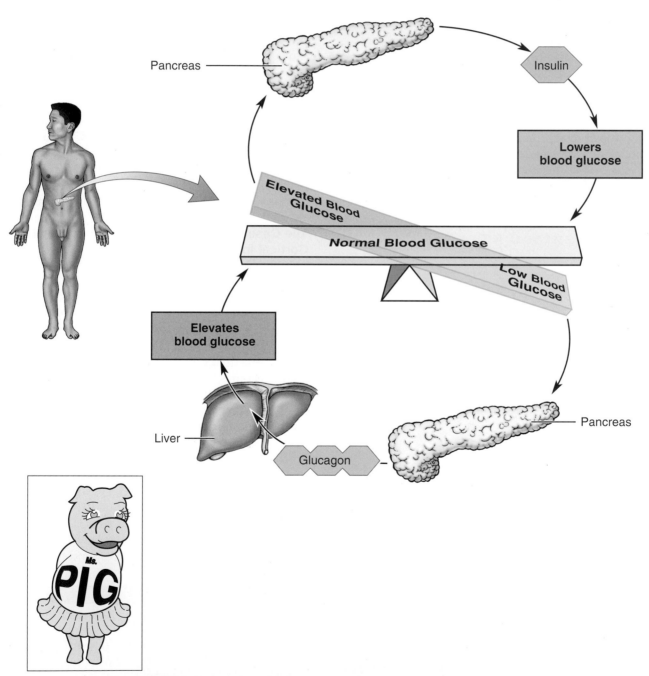

FIGURE 14-9 Pancreatic regulation of blood glucose: insulin and glucagon.

remind you that the *pancreas* secretes *insulin* and *glucagon* (**P**ancreas, **I**nsulin, **G**lucagon). The hormone-secreting cells of the pancreas are called the *islets of Langerhans*. The islets of Langerhans have several types of cells: the alpha cells, which secrete glucagon, and the beta cells, which secrete insulin. Both insulin and glucagon help regulate blood glucose levels.

INSULIN

SECRETION AND EFFECTS

Figure 14-9 illustrates the relationship of the blood glucose level to the pancreatic hormones. Insulin is released in response to increased blood levels of glucose, such as what occurs after a meal. The secretion of insulin decreases as blood levels of glucose decrease. Insulin has many target tissues and therefore exerts widespread effects:

- Insulin helps transport glucose into most cells. Without insulin, glucose remains outside the cells, thereby depriving the cell of its fuel. (The liver and brain require glucose for their metabolic needs but do not require insulin for the transport of glucose across the cell membrane.)
- Insulin helps control carbohydrate, protein, and fat metabolism in the cell. Insulin stimulates the breakdown of glucose (glycolysis) for energy and stimulates the liver and skeletal muscles to store excess glucose as glycogen (glycogenesis). Insulin also increases the transport of amino acids into cells and then stimulates the synthesis of protein from the amino acids. Finally, insulin promotes the making of fats from fatty acids.

 Do You Know...

Why Some Diabetic Persons Require an Injection of Insulin Whereas Others Can Take a Pill?

Some diabetic persons require insulin injections, and others control their diabetes with a pill. The difference is that the pancreas of a person with severe diabetes produces no insulin, so this person must receive insulin injections. Such people have insulin-dependent diabetes. In contrast, the pancreas of a person with another form of diabetes may still be able to produce some insulin. This person may not require insulin injections and may benefit from oral medication. Some diabetic pills work by stimulating the person's pancreas to produce more insulin. Others work by preventing the hepatic (liver) synthesis of glucose. A person with diabetes who does not require insulin injections is considered to have non–insulin-dependent diabetes.

INSULIN AND BLOOD GLUCOSE

Insulin decreases blood glucose levels for two reasons. First, insulin increases the transport of glucose from the blood into the cells. Second, insulin stimulates the cells to burn glucose as fuel. *Insulin is the only hormone that lowers blood glucose levels.* All other hormones increase blood glucose levels.

DIABETES MELLITUS: "A MELTING DOWN OF THE FLESH AND LIMBS INTO URINE"

Because insulin plays such an important role in the metabolism of all types of foods (carbohydrates, proteins, and fats), a deficiency of insulin causes severe metabolic disturbances. Insulin deficiency or insulin ineffectiveness is called *diabetes mellitus* (dye-ah-BEE-teez mell-EYE-tus). Before insulin therapy was discovered, diabetes mellitus was described as a "melting down of the flesh and the limbs into urine." This description attests to the devastating effects of untreated juvenile-onset diabetes mellitus. The child took one year literally to "melt away." Read on to understand the physiological effects of insulin deficiency; note specifically the three *"polys"* of diabetes mellitus: polyuria, polydipsia, and polyphagia.

 Do You Know...

How One Rebounds with Somogyi?

A diabetic person takes insulin to lower his or her blood glucose level. If too much insulin is taken, the blood glucose level becomes too low (hypoglycemia). The hypoglycemia, in turn, stimulates the secretion of glucose-elevating hormones such as glucagon, cortisol, growth hormone, and epinephrine; this causes hyperglycemia. The hyperglycemia requires additional insulin to lower blood glucose levels. The additional insulin again causes hypoglycemia; thus, a vicious cycle of hypoglycemia and hyperglycemia occurs. The Somogyi effect is a rebound phenomenon in which hypoglycemia is followed by hyperglycemia as a result of a hormonal overreaction to the low blood sugar level.

- *Hyperglycemia.* Excess glucose in the blood is called *hyperglycemia.* This condition is caused by two factors. The first is the inability of glucose to enter the cells, where it can be burned for energy. Failure to move the glucose into the cells causes it to accumulate in the blood. The second is the making of additional glucose. In the absence of insulin, the body makes glucose from protein (gluconeogenesis). The excess glucose cannot be used by the cells and therefore accumulates in the blood. In essence, the diabetic body converts its protein to glucose that it cannot burn as fuel and then eliminates it in the urine. The body is "starving in the midst of plenty" (of glucose).
- *Glucosuria or glycosuria.* Glucose in the urine is called *glucosuria* or *glycosuria.* The hyperglycemia causes excess glucose to be eliminated in the urine.
- *Polyuria.* Excretion of a large volume of urine is called *polyuria.* Whenever the kidneys excrete a lot of glucose, they must also excrete a lot of water. Glucosuria therefore causes polyuria.
- *Polydipsia.* Excessive thirst is called *polydipsia.* Polyuria causes an excessive loss of body water, thereby stimulating the thirst mechanism in an attempt to replace the water lost in the urine.

- *Polyphagia.* Polyphagia refers to excessive eating. Despite plenty of glucose in the blood, the cells cannot use it; instead, the diabetic eats excessive amounts of food to fuel the cells. Despite the polyphagia, the diabetic person continues to lose weight.
- *Acidosis.* An excess of H^+ in the blood causes acidosis. Because the cells cannot burn glucose as fuel, they burn fatty acids instead. The rapid, incomplete breakdown of fatty acids produces strong acids (H^+) called *ketoacids*. This process causes a condition called *diabetic ketoacidosis*.

- *Fruity odor to the breath.* The rapid, incomplete breakdown of fatty acids causes the formation of acetone, a ketone body. Acetone smells fruity and makes the patient's breath smell like rotten apples. A fruity odor is a sign of ketoacidosis. Treatment of diabetic ketoacidosis requires the prompt administration of insulin and the correction of the fluid and electrolyte disturbances.

 Do You Know...

Why You Don't Die of Hypoglycemia between Meals?

After you eat a meal, the blood level of glucose rises as food is absorbed from the digestive tract into the blood. The increased blood glucose level signals the release of insulin; the insulin then causes the blood glucose level to decrease. As blood glucose levels decrease, however, insulin secretion decreases and other hormones such as growth hormone, epinephrine, and cortisol are secreted. These other hormones antagonize the effects of insulin by increasing the blood glucose level and preventing fatal hypoglycemia. Thus, you can fast for several weeks and not become hypoglycemic. Chances are that you will not die from fasting—it will only feel as if you are dying!

INSULIN RECEPTORS AND THE DIABETIC STATE

As indicated above, diabetes mellitus can be caused by a lack of insulin. However, some diabetics with adult-onset, or type 2, diabetes mellitus have excess insulin (hyperinsulinemia) and are still hyperglycemic. What's that about? Under normal conditions, insulin binds to the insulin receptors on the cell membrane. What if:

- The insulin receptors are damaged? The damaged receptors cannot respond to the insulin and the

person becomes hyperglycemic. The hyperglycemia then triggers the release of additional insulin and the person becomes hyperinsulinemic.

- There are a diminished number of receptors? The number of insulin receptors on the membrane can increase or decrease. Obesity and lack of exercise can cause the number of insulin receptors to decrease. This means that obese people can secrete plenty of insulin, but their cells cannot respond to that insulin. The good news is that weight loss and exercise increase the number of insulin receptors, thereby improving the insulin response and relieving the symptoms of diabetes.
- Excess fat (adipose) tissue secretes hormones that oppose the effects of insulin? Some cytokines antagonize insulin, causing a state of insulin resistance.

A strong link obviously exists among insulin resistance, obesity, and diabetes. A new term, *metabolic syndrome,* addresses this issue.

 Do You Know...

Who is Dawn and What Is Her Phenomenon?

Dawn refers to the early morning hours, as in sunrise. Diabetics are often hyperglycemic in the early morning hours (at dawn), despite insulin therapy and the lack of food intake during the night. Why? Throughout the night, the person secretes GH. GH stimulates gluconeogenesis and increases blood glucose; this accounts for the early morning hyperglycemia. An adjustment in the timing and type of insulin therapy generally corrects the dawn phenomenon.

GLUCAGON

Glucagon, a second pancreatic hormone, is secreted by the alpha cells of the islets of Langerhans. Its primary action is to increase blood glucose levels (see Figure 14-9). Glucagon raises the blood glucose level in two ways: by stimulating the conversion of glycogen to glucose in the liver and by stimulating the conversion of proteins into glucose (gluconeogenesis). Both these processes ensure a supply of glucose for the busy cells. Because of its effect on blood glucose levels, glucagon is used clinically to treat hypoglycemia. The stimulus for the release of glucagon is a decrease in blood levels of glucose.

GLUCAGON, INFECTION, AND DIABETES

A patient with diabetes is prone to infection. Infection increases glucagon secretion as well as the secretion of all stress hormones, including epinephrine, cortisol, and growth hormone. All these hormones elevate blood glucose levels, causing hyperglycemia. Thus, diabetic people with an infection always have difficulty in controlling their blood glucose levels; they require frequent blood glucose monitoring and additional insulin.

Do You Know...

When Diabetes Is Called "Insipidus"?

"Yuck! This urine is tasteless ... it's insipid!" growled the physician as he sipped his patient's urine. What is going on here? This patient has diabetes insipidus, a condition caused by a deficiency of ADH and characterized by the excretion of a large amount of pale dilute urine.

In the "good old days," physicians actually tasted the patient's urine as a way to diagnose disease. The pale, dilute urine of ADH deficiency is tasteless, in contrast to the sweet-tasting urine of a patient with insulin deficiency, or "sugar" diabetes. The word *diabetes* refers to diuresis (increased flow of urine), whereas the words *insipidus* and *mellitus* refer to the taste of the urine; *insipidus* refers to tasteless and *mellitus* refers to honey tasting. Fortunately, and none too soon, the "Taste Bud Assay" has given way to modern lab tests.

? **Re-Think**

1. Explain why an insulin deficiency causes hyperglycemia, glucosuria, and polyuria.
2. Compare the effects of insulin and glucagon on blood glucose.

2+2 **Sum It Up!**

A number of hormones, particularly those secreted by the pancreas, regulate blood glucose levels. Insulin works in two ways to decrease blood glucose levels: (1) it increases the transport of glucose from the blood into the cells, and (2) it stimulates the cells to burn glucose as fuel. Glucagon antagonizes the effects of insulin by increasing blood glucose levels. Insulin is the only hormone that decreases blood glucose levels.

GONADS

The gonads are the sex glands and refer to the ovaries in the female and to the testes in the male. The gonads not only produce ova (eggs) and sperm, but also secrete hormones. The gonads are therefore glands. The ovaries secrete two female sex hormones: estrogen and progesterone. A female appears female (i.e., size, hair, and fat distribution) primarily because of estrogen. The testes secrete testosterone; a male appears male primarily because of testosterone. (Reproductive anatomy and physiology are discussed in Chapters 26 and 27.)

THYMUS GLAND

The **thymus gland** lies in the thoracic cavity behind the sternum. The thymus gland is much larger in a child than in an adult. The gland involutes, or shrinks, as the child enters puberty. The thymus gland secretes hormones called *thymosins,* which play a role in the immune system (described in Chapter 21).

PINEAL GLAND

The **pineal** (PIN-ee-al) **gland** is a cone-shaped gland located close to the thalamus in the brain. It has been called the body's "biological clock," controlling many of its biorhythms. The pineal gland secretes a hormone called *melatonin,* which affects the reproductive cycle by influencing the secretion of hypothalamic-releasing hormones. In general, melatonin plays an important role in sexual maturation.

Melatonin is also thought to play a role in the sleep–wake cycle. The amount of melatonin secreted is related to the amount of daylight. Melatonin secretion is lowest during daylight hours and highest at night. As melatonin levels increase, the person becomes sleepy. Melatonin is therefore said to have a tranquilizing effect. Persons who work night shifts and sleep during the day have a reversed cycle of melatonin production. The reversal of the melatonin cycle is related to the fatigue experienced by night shift workers. Elevated melatonin levels have also been implicated in a type of depression called *seasonal affective disorder* (SAD). This condition occurs primarily in parts of the world where daylight hours are short in the winter, usually in areas far north and far south.

OTHER HORMONES

ORGAN-SPECIFIC HORMONES

The glands identified in Figure 14-1 make up the endocrine system, but numerous hormone-secreting cells are scattered throughout the body. These hormones usually control the activities of a particular organ. For example, hormone-secreting cells in the digestive tract secrete cholecystokinin and gastrin, which help regulate digestion. The kidneys secrete erythropoietin, which helps regulate red blood cell production. The liver secretes a number of hormones, including insulin-like growth factor (IGF-1). IGF-1 mediates the action of growth hormone. (Organ-specific hormones are described in later chapters.)

PROSTAGLANDINS

The prostaglandins (pross-tah-GLAN-dins) are hormones derived from a fatty acid called *arachidonic* (ah-RAK-i-don-ik) *acid*. The prostaglandins are produced by many tissues and generally act locally, near their site of secretion. The prostaglandins play an important role in the regulation of smooth muscle contraction and the inflammatory response. Prostaglandins are also thought to increase the sensitivity of nerve endings to pain. Drugs such as aspirin and ibuprofen block the synthesis of prostaglandins and are therefore useful in relieving pain and inflammation.

ADIPOSE TISSUE HORMONES

Excess adipose tissue acts as a gland—a very nasty gland—that secretes hormones called *cytokines*. First, a word about fat; there is bad fat and worse fat. How so? There's the bad fat that collects around the thighs, giving the person a pear-shaped appearance. There's also a worse fat that collects around the abdominal area ("ab flab"), creating an apple shape. The apple shape is also associated with excess visceral fat (surrounding the organs).

THE TAB OF AB FLAB

The cost is high with regard to heart disease, diabetes mellitus, cancer, and joint disease. Read on!

Heart and Blood Vessels

Most believe that obesity is a risk for heart disease merely because excess weight overburdens the heart. Although this is true, excess adipose tissue, through its cytokines, affects the heart and blood vessels in other ways. For example, adipose tissue contains many narrow blood vessels; in fact, miles of additional blood vessels may be required to carry blood throughout the excess fat. The additional narrowed blood vessels increase blood pressure and strain the heart. Adipose tissue secretes several cytokines that cause the blood vessels to become even narrower. The cytokines also stimulate the immune system, causing inflammation—an important risk factor for heart disease. In fact, inflammation plays a larger role in heart attacks than the narrowing of the coronary (heart) arteries by cholesterol. The cytokines also stimulate blood clotting. Blood clots, in turn, impair blood flow to the heart and brain, thereby predisposing the obese person to heart attack and stroke.

Diabetes Mellitus

Adipose tissue secretes several cytokines that adversely affect glucose metabolism and predispose the person to type 2 diabetes mellitus. First, the cytokines oppose the action of insulin, thereby decreasing the transport of glucose into the cells. Second, the cytokines stimulate the liver to make excess glucose. Both these actions increase blood glucose levels, causing hyperglycemia, a hallmark of diabetes mellitus. In short, cytokines make the obese person resistant to insulin.

Cancer

Fat cells secrete estrogen, a hormone that has been linked to several types of cancer, especially breast cancer.

Joint Disease

The added body weight puts additional stress on joints such as the knees. The joints simply cannot support the extra weight. (So lose the potato chips, get off the couch, and exercise!) An apology to cytokines is in order. Many cytokines cause undesirable effects, as noted previously, but most cytokines exert important and beneficial physiological effects (see Chapter 21).

 Re-Think

1. What is meant by organ-specific hormones?
2. Why is adipose tissue considered a "nasty gland"?

 Sum It Up!

The gonads are glands that include the ovaries in the female and the testes in the male. The ovaries secrete estrogens and progesterone; the testes secrete testosterone. Other endocrine glands include the thymus, liver, and pineal gland. The thymus gland plays an important role in the immune response. The pineal gland is thought to be the body's "biological clock," affecting reproduction and biorhythms. Other hormone-secreting cells are scattered throughout the body. Prostaglandins are chemical mediators of pain and inflammation and act locally. Excess adipose tissue functions as a nasty endocrine gland that contributes to the development of heart disease, diabetes, cancer, and joint disease.

As You Age

1. In general, age-related endocrine changes include an alteration in the secretion of hormones, circulating levels of hormones, metabolism of hormones, and biological activity of hormones.
2. Although most glands decrease their levels of secretion, normal aging does not lead to deficiency states. For example, although adrenal cortical secretion of cortisol decreases, negative feedback mechanisms maintain normal plasma levels of the hormones, thereby preserving water and electrolyte homeostasis.
3. Changes in the thyroid gland cause a decrease in the secretion of thyroid hormones, thereby decreasing the metabolic rate.
4. Decreased secretion of growth hormone causes a decrease in muscle mass and an increase in storage of fat.
5. A diminishment of circadian control of hormone secretion occurs.

MEDICAL TERMINOLOGY AND DISORDERS	Disorders of the Endocrine System

Medical Term	Word Parts	Word Part Meaning or Derivation	Description
Words			
adrenal	ad-	near	The **adrenal** glands sit atop the kidneys.
	-ren/o-	kidney	
	-al	pertaining to	
adenohypophyseal	aden/o-	gland	The **adenohypophysis** is *the anterior pituitary gland that is located under the hypothalamus.* The **neurohypophysis** (neur/o = nerve) is *the posterior pituitary gland; it is a downward extension of the hypothalamus.*
	-hypophysis-	From a Greek word meaning "to grow under"	
	-al	pertaining to	
adrenocorticotropic	adren/o-	adrenal gland	**Adrenocorticotropic hormone (ACTH)** stimulates the adrenal cortex to secrete steroids.
	-cortic/o-	cortex	
	-troph/o-	nourishment, development	
	-ic	pertaining to	
androgen	andr/o-	male	An **androgen,** such as testosterone, *stimulates the development of male or virilizing characteristics.*
	-gen	origin or production	
endocrine	endo-	within	**Endocrine** glands secrete hormones "within the body"; they are transported about the body by the blood.
	-crin/o-	to secrete	
gonadotropic	gonad/o-	gonad	**Gonadotropic** hormones (FSH and LH) target the gonads, the ovaries, and the testes.
	-troph/o-	nourishment or development	
	-ic	pertaining to	
hyperglycemia	hyper-	excessive	**Hyperglycemia** is *an increase in the amount of glucose in the blood.*
	-glyc/o-	glucose	
	-emia	condition of the blood	
Disorders			
Adrenal Gland Disorders			
adrenal cortical insufficiency and excess			Adrenal cortical deficiencies and excesses are described in the text.
pheochromocytoma	pheochromocyt/o-	catecholamine-secreting cell	**Pheochromocytoma** is *a benign tumor of the adrenal medulla that hypersecretes the catecholamines epinephrine and norepinephrine.*
	-oma	tumor	
Pituitary Gland Disorders			
somatotropic hormone imbalances	somat/o-	body	*Hypersecretion of somatotropic hormone (growth hormone [GH]).* The conditions are described in the text.
	-troph/o-	nourishment, development	
	-ic	condition of	

Continued

MEDICAL TERMINOLOGY AND DISORDERS   Disorders of the Endocrine System—cont'd

Medical Term	Word Parts	Word Part Meaning or Derivation	Description
diabetes insipidus	dia-	through	*A condition caused by a lack of ADH secretion (central diabetes insipidus) or by the lack of the response of the kidney to ADH (nephrogenic diabetes insipidus). Further described in the text.*
	-betes	From a Greek word *bainein,* meaning "to go or pass"	
	insipidus	Reference to the word *insipid,* meaning "tasteless"	
syndrome of inappropriate ADH (antidiuretic hormone) secretion	anti-	against	Abbreviated as **SIADH. SIADH** is caused by excess ADH secretion resulting in excess water reabsorption by the kidney, expansion of blood volume, and decreased plasma sodium.
	-diuretic	to increase the flow of urine	

Pancreatic Disorders

diabetes mellitus	dia-	through	*A deficiency or ineffectiveness of insulin.* There are several types of diabetes mellitus (DM), which is epidemic in the United States: **Type 1 DM,** also called **juvenile-onset diabetes,** usually develops in children and must be treated with insulin. **Type 2 DM** is called **adult-onset diabetes.** The typical adult-onset diabetic is older, obese, and sedentary. **Gestational diabetes mellitus** refers to the appearance of diabetic symptoms only during pregnancy. The symptoms usually subside when the baby is delivered. Unfortunately, in the United States, type 2 diabetes is appearing in children. The development of **MODY** (**m**aturity-**o**nset **d**iabetes in **y**outh) is related to lifestyle (diet, exercise, obesity). Further described in text.
	-betes	From the Latin word *bainein,* meaning "to go or pass"	
	mellitus	honey or sweet	

Parathyroid Gland Disorders

hyperparathyroidism	hyper-	above or excessive	*Refers to an excess secretion of parathyroid hormone (PTH) causing bone resorption and elevation of plasma calcium (hypercalcemia).* **Primary hyperparathyroidism** is caused by a hypersecretion of the parathyroid glands usually caused by a small tumor such as an adenoma. **Secondary hyperparathyroidism** occurs in response to low plasma calcium caused by vitamin D deficiency or chronic renal failure.
	-parathyroid/o-	parathyroid	
	-ism	condition of	
hypoparathyroidism	hypo-	below or deficient	*Refers to the diminished secretion of parathyroid hormone (PTH) causing low plasma levels of calcium (hypocalcemia). Further described in the text.*
	-parathyroid/o-	parathyroid	
	-ism	condition of	

Thyroid Gland Disorders

goiter	goiter	From a Latin word meaning "struma" (throat enlargement)	*An enlargement of the thyroid gland, which may or may not be functioning normally.* A **toxic nodular goiter** contains nodules that excrete excess T_3 and T_4, thereby causing a hyperthyroid state. A **nontoxic goiter,** such as a goiter induced by an iodine-deficient diet, does not secrete excess T_3 and T_4. The person is most often euthyroid or experiences mild hypothyroidism.

MEDICAL TERMINOLOGY AND DISORDERS   Disorders of the Endocrine System—cont'd

Medical Term	Word Parts	Word Part Meaning or Derivation	Description
hyperthyroidism	hyper-	above or excessive	Also called an "overactive thyroid"; **hyperthyroidism** is due to excess synthesis of thyroid hormones (T_3, T_4) by the thyroid gland. **Graves' disease** is the most common type and is described in the text. **Thyrotoxicosis,** which presents as severe hyperthyroidism, is due to an increase in the release of stored T_3 and T_4 from the thyroid gland. **Thyroid storm,** or **thyrotoxic crisis,** is an extreme and life-threatening manifestation of **thyrotoxicosis:** clinical presentation includes extreme elevation in body temperature and cardiac stimulation (tachycardia) progressing to heart failure.
	-thyroid/o-	thyroid	
	-ism	condition of	
hypothyroidism	hypo-	below or deficient	Also called a "sluggish thyroid" and **myxedema** in the adult (described in the text). **Myxedema coma** is *an extreme and life-threatening form of hypothyroidism.* **Cretinism** is *neonatal hypothyroidism;* insufficient treatment with thyroid hormones results in severe physical and mental developmental abnormalities.
	-thyroid/o-	thyroid	
	-ism	condition of	

Get Ready for Exams!

Summary Outline

The endocrine system and the nervous system are the two major communicating and coordinating systems in the body. The endocrine system communicates through chemical signals called *hormones.*

I. Hormones
  A. Classification of hormones
   1. Hormones are secreted by endocrine glands directly into the blood.
   2. Hormones are classified as proteins (protein-related substances) and steroids.
  B. Hormone receptors
   1. Hormones are aimed at receptors of target organs.
   2. Receptors are located on the outer surface of the membrane or inside the cell.
   3. Hormone secretion is controlled by three mechanisms: feedback control, biorhythms, and control by the central nervous system.

II. Pituitary Gland
  A. Hypothalamic-hypophyseal portal system
   1. The portal system is a system of capillaries that connects the hypothalamus and the anterior pituitary.
   2. The portal system transports releasing hormones from the hypothalamus to the anterior pituitary gland.
  B. Hormones of the anterior pituitary gland
   1. Growth hormone stimulates growth and maintains blood glucose levels during periods of fasting.
   2. Prolactin (lactogenic hormone) stimulates milk production by the breasts.
   3. Tropic hormones stimulate other glands to secrete hormones. These include thyroid stimulating hormone (TSH), adrenocorticotropic hormone (ACTH) and the gonadotropins (FSH, LH).
   4. Thyroid-stimulating hormone stimulates the thyroid gland.
   5. Adrenocorticotropic hormone (ACTH) stimulates the adrenal cortex.
   6. The gonadotropic hormones (FSH and LH) stimulate the gonads (ovaries and testes).
  C. Hormones of the posterior pituitary gland
   1. Antidiuretic hormone (ADH) stimulates the kidney to reabsorb water.
   2. Oxytocin stimulates the uterine muscle to contract for labor and stimulates the breast to release milk during suckling (milk let-down reflex).

III. Other Endocrine Glands
  A. Thyroid gland
   1. The follicular cells synthesize triiodothyronine (T_3) and tetraiodothyronine, or thyroxine (T_4). T_3 and T_4 regulate metabolic rate.
   2. The parafollicular cells secrete calcitonin. Calcitonin lowers blood calcium level.
  B. Parathyroid glands
   1. The parathyroid glands secrete parathyroid hormone (PTH).
   2. PTH stimulates the bones, kidneys, and intestines to increase blood calcium levels.
  C. Adrenal gland
   1. The adrenal medulla secretes the catecholamines epinephrine and norepinephrine and causes the "fight-or-flight" response.

2. The adrenal cortex secretes the steroids: glucocorticoids, mineralocorticoids, and sex hormones.

D. Pancreas
   1. The pancreas secretes insulin and glucagon.
   2. Insulin lowers blood glucose levels, whereas glucagon increases blood glucose levels.

E. Gonads
   1. The ovaries are stimulated by the gonadotropins and secrete estrogens and progesterone.
   2. The testes are stimulated by the gonadotropins and secrete testosterone.

F. The thymus gland plays an important role in the immune response.

G. The pineal gland houses the "biological clock" and secretes melatonin.

H. Other hormones include organ-specific hormones (cholecystokinin), prostaglandins, and hormones of adipose tissue.

Review Your Knowledge

Matching: Glands

Directions: Match the following words with their descriptions below. Some words may be used more than once.

a. pancreas
b. adrenal cortex
c. anterior pituitary gland
d. adrenal medulla
e. thyroid gland
f. parathyroid glands
g. posterior pituitary gland
h. hypothalamus

1. ___ Contains the beta cells of the islets of Langerhans
2. ___ Secrete glucocorticoids, mineralocorticoids, and androgens
3. ___ Its hormonal secretion is controlled by ACTH.
4. ___ Secretes iodine-containing hormones
5. ___ Secretes releasing hormones
6. ___ Secretes ACTH, TSH, prolactin, growth hormone, and the gonadotropins
7. ___ Its hormone moves calcium from the bone to the blood.
8. ___ Secretes both insulin and glucagon
9. ___ Part of the "fight-or-flight" system; secretes catecholamines
10. ___ The neurohypophysis; secretes ADH and oxytocin

Matching: Hormones

Directions: Match the following words with their descriptions in the right column. Some words may be used more than once.

a. aldosterone
b. insulin
c. prolactin
d. growth hormone
e. parathyroid hormone
f. epinephrine
g. T_3 and T_4
h. oxytocin
i. ACTH
j. ADH

1. ___ Stimulates osteoclastic activity to increase blood calcium
2. ___ Regulates metabolic rate
3. ___ Lowers blood glucose
4. ___ Cortisol is released in response to this hormone.
5. ___ Stimulates the breast to produce milk
6. ___ Catecholamine that participates in the "fight-or-flight" response
7. ___ The neurohypophyseal hormone that controls water balance
8. ___ Prednisone (cortisol) shuts down the secretion of this adenohypophyseal hormone.
9. ___ Also called *somatotropic hormone*
10. ___ The mineralocorticoid that is called the salt-retaining hormone

Multiple Choice

1. Which of the following is true about cortisol?
   a. It is a catecholamine.
   b. It is secreted by the adrenal cortex in response to ACTH.
   c. It stimulates the secretion of ACTH.
   d. It is released by the adrenal medulla in response to sympathetic nerve stimulation.

2. Aldosterone is
   a. a mineralocorticoid secreted by the adrenal cortex.
   b. the primary regulator of blood glucose.
   c. an adenohypophyseal hormone that stimulates the adrenal cortex to secrete cortisol.
   d. a neurohypophyseal hormone that causes the kidneys to reabsorb water.

3. The pancreas
   a. secretes steroids that are concerned with sugar, salt, and sex.
   b. is controlled by a hormone secreted by the anterior pituitary gland.
   c. secretes both insulin and glucagon.
   d. secretes hormones that only lower blood glucose levels.

4. Which of the following best describes the function of insulin?
   a. Regulates blood volume
   b. Stimulates cells to make glucose (gluconeogenesis)
   c. Causes ketone body formation and acidosis
   d. Lowers blood glucose

5. As plasma levels of calcium decrease,
   a. insulin is secreted.
   b. the parathyroid glands secrete calcitonin.
   c. the kidneys excrete calcium and phosphate.
   d. PTH is secreted, thereby stimulating osteoclastic activity.

6. Hypocalcemic tetany is
   a. a consequence of a deficiency of PTH.
   b. caused by calcitonin deficiency.
   c. a consequence of osteoclastic activity.
   d. of concern because it causes osteoporosis.

7. Which of the following is true of glucagon, epinephrine, growth hormone, and cortisol? All
   a. are secreted by the anterior pituitary gland.
   b. are secreted in response to hypocalcemia.
   c. raise blood glucose.
   d. are steroids.

8. Hyperglycemia, polyuria, polydipsia, polyphagia, and ketoacidosis are characteristic of a deficiency of
   a. cortisol.
   b. insulin.
   c. catecholamines.
   d. neurohypophyseal hormones.
9. Which of the following is not a steroid?
   a. Adrenal cortical hormones
   b. ACTH
   c. Estrogen
   d. Androgens
10. Which of the following is not true of antidiuretic hormone (ADH)?
   a. Secreted by the neurohypophysis
   b. Also called *vasopressin*
   c. Stimulates the kidney causing water reabsorption
   d. Is the salt-retaining hormone

Go Figure

1. **According to Figure 14-1**
   a. All endocrine glands are located in the abdominal cavity.
   b. No endocrine glands are located in the pelvic cavity.
   c. The pituitary gland is located within the thoracic cavity.
   d. The thyroid and parathyroid glands are located in the neck.

2. **According to Figure 14-4 which of the following is not true?**
   a. The adenohypophysis secretes TSH, growth hormone, prolactin, the gonadotropins, and ACTH.
   b. The posterior pituitary gland secretes ADH and oxytocin.
   c. The hypothalamic-hypophyseal portal system allows the anterior and posterior pituitary glands to "swap" hormones.
   d. Hypothalamic-releasing hormones control the secretion of the adenohypophysis.

3. **According to Figures 14-4 and 14-8**
   a. ACTH stimulates the secretion of catecholamines.
   b. Cortisol stimulates the adenohypophyseal secretion of ACTH.
   c. ACTH is a hypothalamic-releasing hormone.
   d. ACTH secretion decreases as plasma levels of cortisol increase.

4. **According to Figure 14-5**
   a. T_3 and T_4 are adenohypophyseal hormones.
   b. TSH stimulates the parathyroid glands.
   c. T_3 and T_4 stimulate the thyroid gland to secrete thyroxine.
   d. The secretion of TSH is inhibited by increased plasma levels of T_3 and T_4.

5. **According to Figures 14-6 and 14-7**
   a. PTH increases plasma calcium levels by its effects on bone, kidneys, and intestine.
   b. The stimulus for the release of PTH is hypercalcemia.
   c. Carpal spasm is a sign of hypercalcemia.
   d. As plasma levels of calcium increase, PTH levels increase.

6. **According to Figure 14-9**
   a. The pancreas secretes insulin and glucagon in response to hyperglycemia.
   b. Insulin is secreted in response to an increase in the blood glucose.
   c. Glucagon lowers the blood glucose level.
   d. Glucagon is secreted in response to hyperglycemia.

Key Terms

albumin (p. 285)
anemia (p. 286)
basophils (p. 294)
coagulation (p. 296)
eosinophil (p. 294)
erythrocytes (p. 285)
erythropoietin (p. 290)
fibrin (p. 296)

hematocrit (p. 285)
hemoglobin (p. 288)
hemolysis (p. 290)
hemopoiesis (p. 286)
hemostasis (p. 295)
leukocytes (p. 285)
lymphocytes (p. 286)
monocytes (p. 286)

neutrophil (p. 292)
plasma (p. 285)
platelets (p. 285)
red blood cells (p. 285)
reticulocyte (p. 287)
serum (p. 285)
thrombocytes (p. 285)
white blood cells (p. 285)

Objectives

1. Describe three functions of blood.
2. Describe the composition of blood, including:
   • Describe the three types of blood cells: erythrocytes, leukocytes, and thrombocytes.
   • Explain the formation of blood cells.
3. Explain the composition, characteristics, and functions of red and white blood cells and platelets, including

the breakdown of red blood cells and the formation of bilirubin.
4. Identify the steps of hemostasis.
5. Describe the four blood types.
6. Describe the Rh factor.

Long before modern medicine, blood was viewed as the part of the body that possessed the life force. This belief arose from the observation that severe bleeding episodes often ended in death, suggesting that the life force flowed out of the body with the blood. Blood was also credited with determining personality traits and emotions. For example, the wealthy were called *blue bloods*. Feuding groups often attributed the cause of the troubled relationship to bad blood. Anger was said to cause the blood to boil, whereas fear could generate blood-curdling screams. The qualities of blood seemed so magical that a sharing of a few drops of blood could make one's friend a blood brother. Although we no longer speak of blood in such terms, we do recognize that an adequate blood supply is essential for life. We are still fascinated by blood and have a fancy word for its study: hematology.

Blood flows through a closed system of blood vessels. The force that pushes the blood through the vessels is the pumping action of the heart (see Chapter 16).

WHAT BLOOD DOES

Blood performs three general functions: transport, regulation, and protection. First, the blood transports many substances around the body. For example, blood delivers oxygen from the lungs to every cell in the body. Blood picks up waste material from the cells and delivers the waste to organs that eliminate it from the body. Nutrients, ions, hormones, and many other substances use blood as the vehicle for movement throughout the body. Second, blood participates in the regulation of fluid and electrolyte balance, acid–base balance, and body temperature. Third, blood helps protect the body from infection. Blood also contains clotting factors, which help protect the body from excessive blood loss.

COMPOSITION OF BLOOD

CHARACTERISTICS

Blood is a type of connective tissue that has a liquid intercellular matrix. The color of blood varies from a bright red to a darker blue-red. The difference in color is caused by the amount of oxygen in the blood; well-oxygenated blood is bright red, whereas oxygen-poor blood is blue-red. The amount of blood varies, depending on body size, gender, and age. The average adult has 4 to 6 L of blood.

 Do You Know...

Why George Washington's 9 Pints of Blood Went Down the Drain?

You probably remember George Washington for chopping down the cherry tree, for his penchant for truth, and for being the first president—but here is something you probably didn't know about George's medical history. George had been quite ill with a long winter cold, pneumonia, and throat infection. Despite many home remedies and much attention, the infection lingered and worsened. Enter the "quacks"! Immediately before his death, George was bled of 9 pints of blood in an attempt to rid his body of disease. This commonly used procedure was called *bloodletting*.

The practice of bloodletting had been around since before the days of Hippocrates (a long, long time ago). Bloodletting grew out of the belief that health was the result of a balance of the four body humors (fluids): blood, phlegm, black bile, and yellow bile. Disease was therefore attributed to an imbalance of the humors. By draining George's blood, the bloodletter hoped to balance George's unbalanced humors. (Not funny!) The fact that George died immediately after being drained of 9 pints is not surprising. At a time when he needed all the help he could get from his blood, he was literally drained and probably plunged into a state of low-volume circulatory shock. Although the practice of bloodletting, as described in this case, has been discredited, the practice of bloodletting hasn't completely died out. It has, however, been cleaned up and refined. "Therapeutic phlebotomy," or the removal of blood for therapeutic purposes, is routinely performed in the treatment of polycythemia vera and hemochromatosis, conditions characterized by excess RBCs, iron, and blood volume. And our little leech on page 298 is a natural born phlebotomist when it comes to maintaining blood flow in edematous tissues.

We retain a friendly reminder of our former bloodletting ways in the barbershop pole. Barbers and surgeons were the early bloodletters, and the pole advertised their trade. The barbershop pole is striped red and white. Red represents blood, white represents the tourniquet, and the pole itself represents the stick that the patient squeezed to dilate the veins for easy puncturing. Fortunately, today's barbers go for your hair and not your jugular.

Other characteristics of blood include pH (normal, 7.35 to 7.45) and viscosity. Blood viscosity (vis-KOS-i-tee) refers to the thickness or stickiness of the blood and affects the ease with which blood flows through the blood vessels. Viscosity is best demonstrated by comparing the flow of water and molasses. If water and molasses are poured out of a bottle, the molasses flows more slowly. Molasses is said to be more viscous, or thicker, than water. Blood is normally three to five times more viscous than water. Although blood viscosity does not normally fluctuate widely, an increase in viscosity can thicken the blood so much that it puts an extra burden on the heart, thereby causing the pumping action of the heart to fail.

BLOOD HAS TWO PARTS

Blood is composed of two parts: the plasma and the formed elements (blood cells and cell fragments). The **plasma** is a pale yellow fluid composed mostly of water; it also contains proteins, ions, nutrients, gases, and waste. The plasma proteins consist of **albumin** (al-BYOO-min), various clotting factors, antibodies, and complement proteins. In general, the plasma proteins help regulate fluid volume, protect the body from pathogens, and prevent excessive blood loss in the event of injury. **Serum** is the plasma minus the clotting proteins.

The blood cells and cell fragments include the following:

- **Red blood cells** (RBCs) are also called **erythrocytes** (eh-RITH-roh-sytes) (from *erythro*, meaning "red"). RBCs are primarily involved in the transport of oxygen to all body tissues.
- **White blood cells** (WBCs) are also called **leukocytes** (LOO-koh-sytes) (from *leuko*, meaning "white"). WBCs protect the body from infection.
- **Platelets** (PLAYT-lets) are also called **thrombocytes** (THROM-boh-sytes). Platelets protect the body from bleeding.

The two parts of blood can be observed in a test tube. If a sample of blood is collected in a tube and spun in a centrifuge, two phases appear; the heavier blood cells appear at the bottom of the tube, whereas the lighter plasma accumulates at the top.

The separation of blood into two phases forms the basis of a blood test called the *hematocrit* (Hct) or *packed cell volume* (Figure 15-1). The **hematocrit** (hee-MAT-oh-krit) is the percentage of blood cells in a sample of blood. A sample of blood is normally composed of 45% blood cells and 55% plasma. The blood cells are

BLOOD SAMPLE

Plasma 55%

Buffy coat

Red blood cells (RBCs; erythrocytes)

Formed elements 45%

FIGURE 15-1 Hematocrit.

composed mainly of RBCs. A small layer of cells between the plasma and the RBCs is called the *buffy coat* and consists of WBCs and platelets. Because the buffy coat is so thin, any change in the Hct is generally interpreted as a change in the numbers of RBCs. For example, a person with a low Hct is considered to be anemic, with a lower than normal number of RBCs. A word of caution! Because the Hct is expressed as a percentage (%), any change in blood volume affects the Hct. For example, a dehydrated patient has a diminished blood volume. Thus, the ratio of RBCs to blood volume increases. The elevated Hct therefore represents not an increase in RBCs but a decrease in blood volume. Conversely, an expanded blood volume, as occurs in heart failure, decreases the Hct. The lowered Hct represents not a decrease in RBCs but an increase in blood volume. In essence, the RBCs have been diluted by the excess water in the blood. An expanded blood volume causes a "dilutional anemia."

> ### ? Re-Think
> 1. List the two parts of blood.
> 2. List the three types and functions of blood cells.
> 3. Describe the effect of dehydration on the hematocrit.

ORIGIN OF BLOOD CELLS

The process of blood cell formation is called **hemopoiesis** (hee-moh-POY-ess-iss). The three types of blood cells (RBCs, WBCs, and platelets) are made in hemopoietic tissue. The two types of hemopoietic tissue in the adult are the red bone marrow and the lymphatic tissue, which is found in the spleen, lymph nodes, and thymus gland.

Blood formation in the red bone marrow is called *myeloid hemopoiesis*. (Myeloid comes from the Greek word meaning "bone marrow.") Blood formation in the lymphatic organs (described in Chapter 21) is called *lymphoid hemopoiesis*. Red bone marrow is found primarily in the ends of long bones, such as the femur, and in flat and irregular bones, such as the sternum, cranial bones, vertebrae, and bones of the pelvis.

HEMOPOIESIS AND RED BONE MARROW

How does the red bone marrow produce three different types of blood cells? They are produced in the red bone marrow from the same cell, called a *stem cell*. Under the influence of specific growth factors, the stem cell differentiates into a RBC, a WBC, or a platelet. Note the stem cell in Figure 15-2. In line 1, the stem cell differentiates into the RBC (erythrocyte). In lines 2, 3, and 4, the stem cells form five different types of WBCs (leukocytes). The **lymphocytes** and **monocytes** originate in the bone marrow; some of the lymphocytes mature and reproduce in the lymphatic tissue. In line 5, the stem cell differentiates into a megakaryocyte (meg-ah-KAIR-ee-oh-syte), a large blood cell that breaks up into tiny cell fragments called *platelets* or *thrombocytes*.

BONE MARROW MISERY

BONE MARROW DEPRESSION

Cheer up! Even bone marrow gets depressed. Under certain conditions, the bone marrow cannot produce enough blood cells. Bone marrow depression is called *myelosuppression*. What happens if the bone marrow is depressed? Depressed bone marrow leads to a severe deficiency of RBCs, causing a serious form of anemia called *aplastic anemia*. Myelosuppression can also cause a deficiency of WBCs (leukocytes) called *leukopenia* (loo-koh-PEE-nee-ah). The leukopenic person is defenseless against infection and may die from a common cold. Depressed bone marrow may also produce inadequate numbers of platelets, or thrombocytes. This condition is called *thrombocytopenia* (throm-boh-sye-toh-PEE-nee-ah). The thrombocytopenic person is at high risk for hemorrhage. Why the concern for bone marrow depression? Because many drugs, especially cytotoxic cancer drugs, and certain procedures, such as radiation, depress the bone marrow, a person exposed to any of these therapies must be monitored for symptoms of myelosuppression. Clinically, this is a huge problem.

BONE MARROW OVERACTIVITY

Then, there is the hyperactive bone marrow known as *polycythemia vera*, or the overactivity and excess production of blood cells—bone marrow gone wild! The excess thickened blood (increased viscosity) burdens the heart, overwhelms the clotting system, and produces a beet-red, ruddy face (caused by the increase in RBC production). To help this condition, the patient may be given a drug that depresses the bone marrow or undergo therapeutic phlebotomy (fleh-BOHT-oh-mee) to remove excess blood. The myelosuppressed anemic patient appears pale and has a low RBC count, low hematocrit, and low hemoglobin. The patient with polycythemia vera has an elevated RBC count, elevated hematocrit, and an elevated hemoglobin, and has a ruddy or red face.

> ### ? Re-Think
> 1. Where does most hemopoiesis occur?
> 2. What are three consequences of myelosuppression?

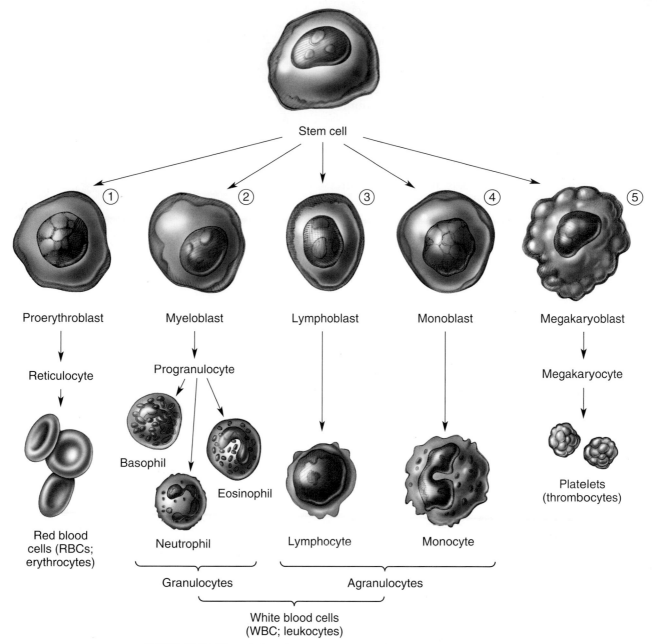

FIGURE 15-2 Differentiation of a stem cell into RBCs, WBCs, and platelets.

2+2 Sum It Up!

Blood is composed of plasma and blood cells. The RBCs (erythrocytes) carry oxygen; the WBCs (leukocytes) protect against infection and the platelets (thrombocytes) prevent bleeding. The hematocrit is a measure of the ratio of the blood cells to blood volume. Myelosuppression and polycythemia are two examples of altered bone marrow activity.

BLOOD CELLS

RED BLOOD CELLS

The RBCs are the most numerous of the blood cells. Between 4.5 and 6.0 million RBCs are in one microliter of blood. The rate of production by the red bone marrow is several million RBCs per second. The production of RBCs is called *erythropoiesis* (eh-rith-roh-poy-EE-sis). RBCs are primarily concerned with the transport of oxygen and carbon dioxide.

"RETICS"

The immature RBC is called a **reticulocyte** (reh-TIK-yoo-loh-syte) (clinical nickname, retics; see Figure 15-2). The number of reticulocytes in blood is normally very small (0.5% to 1.5%). Reticulocytes can develop into mature RBCs within 48 hours of release into the blood. Why measure the reticulocyte count? A high reticulocyte count may indicate blood loss or another iron-deficient state. Why? A loss of blood stimulates the bone marrow to make more RBCs. The greater the bone marrow activity, the higher the number of reticulocytes prematurely added to the circulation. The reticulocytes simply don't have time to mature in the bone marrow. Conversely, a low reticulocyte count might indicate that the patient's bone marrow is unable to make RBCs, as in myelosuppression or severe iron deficiency. Hence, changes in the reticulocyte count can provide valuable diagnostic clues.

SHAPE AND CONTENTS

What do RBCs look like? First, RBCs are large. The large RBCs stay in the blood vessels and do not roam around the tissue spaces, as do the WBCs. Second, RBCs are flexible disc-shaped cells that have a thick outer rim and a thin center (Figure 15-3). Because the RBC can bend, it can squeeze its way through tiny blood vessels. This flexibility allows the RBC to deliver oxygen to every cell in the body. The RBC's ability to bend is important. If the RBC were not able to bend, it would not fit through the tiny blood vessels, and tissue cells would be deprived of oxygen and die. Decreased oxygenation and cell death occur in a condition known as *sickle cell disease*. Instead of bending, the RBCs assume a sickle or C shape and block blood flow through the tiny blood vessels.

Red blood cell size and shape matter! While reading the results of a blood smear, you may come across the

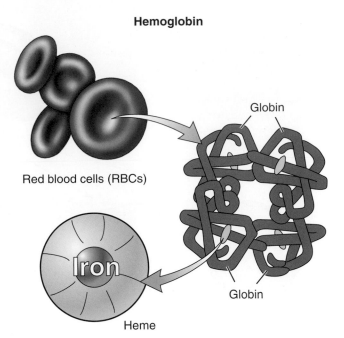

Hemoglobin

Red blood cells (RBCs)

Globin

Globin

Heme

Iron

FIGURE 15-4 Hemoglobin and iron.

Normal red
blood cells (RBCs)

B

RBCs in
sickle cell disease

C

FIGURE 15-3 **A,** The RBCs are large and doughnut shaped. **B,** The RBCs must bend to fit through the blood vessel. **C,** Sickled RBCs blocking the flow of blood through the blood vessel.

terms *anisocytosis* and *poikilocytosis*, which pertain to shape. Anisocytosis (ahn-ISS-oh-syte-OH-sis) refers to unequal-sized RBCs, whereas poikilocytosis (poy-KEE-loh-syte-OH-sis) refers to irregularly shaped RBCs. Both are found in anemia and other blood disorders (dyscrasias).

The content of the RBC is also unique. The RBC normally loses almost all its organelles as it develops. Having no mitochondria, the RBC is not powered aerobically; rather, it produces adenosine triphosphate (ATP) anaerobically. Think about it; the RBC does not metabolically use up the oxygen that it is transporting throughout the body. Also, the RBC, lacking a nucleus and DNA, cannot replicate; the "old" RBC is removed from the blood and replaced by a new RBC made in the bone marrow. We now know what the RBC does not contain, so what does it contain? It contains mostly hemoglobin. Read on.

HEMOGLOBIN

Red blood cells are filled with a large protein molecule called **hemoglobin** (Figure 15-4). Hemoglobin (hee-moh-GLOH-bin) consists of two parts: globin (protein) and heme, an iron-containing substance. Hemoglobin contains four globin chains, with each globin having a heme group. The hemoglobin molecule is responsible for RBC function.

What is so important about heme? As the RBCs circulate through the blood vessels in the lungs, oxygen (O_2) attaches loosely to the iron atom in the heme. The oxygenated hemoglobin is referred to as *oxyhemoglobin*. Then, as the blood flows to the various tissues in the body, the O_2 detaches from the hemoglobin. The unloaded oxygen diffuses from the blood to the cells, where it is used during cellular metabolism.

The globin portion of hemoglobin also plays a role in gas transport. Globin transports some of the carbon dioxide (CO_2) from its site of production in the metabolizing cells to the lungs, where it is excreted. The CO_2-hemoglobin complex is called *carbaminohemoglobin* (kahr-bam-ih-no-hee-moh-GLOH-bin). To repeat: Hemoglobin carries both O_2 and CO_2 but at different sites.

WHY BLOOD CHANGES ITS COLOR

The color of blood changes from bright red to blue-red. When hemoglobin is oxygenated, blood appears bright red. When hemoglobin is unoxygenated, blood assumes a darker blue-red color. Thus, blood coming from the lungs is well oxygenated and appears red. Blood leaving the tissues has given up its oxygen and appears blue-red. When a person is deprived of O_2, the blood is a blue-red color, causing the skin to look blue, or cyanotic. Cyanosis is a sign of hypoxemia, a deficiency of O_2 in the blood. Cyanosis is always cause for concern and should prompt a search for the underlying cause of the hypoxemia.

Oxygenated RBC   Unoxygenated RBC

Why can a person have cherry-red blood and be hypoxemic at the same time? It's a carbon monoxide (CO) thing. Blood is bright red when the hemoglobin is saturated with O_2. CO, like O_2, binds to the iron and also makes the blood appear bright cherry red. When CO occupies the iron site, however, no O_2 can be carried by the hemoglobin. Therefore, the person with CO poisoning can be both cherry red and hypoxemic. CO poisoning is deadly and very common. By the way, 20% of the hemoglobin of a cigarette smoker is unavailable for O_2 transport because of the presence of CO in the smoke.

SUBSTANCES ESSENTIAL FOR HEMOGLOBIN PRODUCTION

What does the body need to make adequate amounts of hemoglobin? In addition to healthy bone marrow, the body requires certain raw materials. Iron, vitamin B_{12}, folic acid, and protein are essential for hemoglobin synthesis. Recall that the heme, the O_2-carrying component of hemoglobin, contains iron. A diet deficient in iron can result in inadequate hemoglobin synthesis

and a condition called *iron deficiency anemia*. Young women are more prone to iron deficiency anemia than young men, as might be expected. Women not only are more apt to get caught up in rigorous and unhealthy dieting, but they also tend to lose more iron because of the blood loss associated with menstruation and fetal demands during pregnancy. Persons with a low income also have a higher incidence of iron deficiency anemia because iron-rich foods such as meat are expensive. The RBCs of a person with iron deficiency anemia are microcytic (small cell size) and hypochromic (pale).

Do You Know...

Why There Is a Needle in This Hip Bone?

Because the red bone marrow is the site of blood cell production, certain abnormalities of blood cells can be detected through a bone marrow biopsy. In this procedure, a needle is inserted into the red bone marrow, usually at the iliac crest (hip bone). A sample of bone marrow is withdrawn, or aspirated, and then studied microscopically. The analysis includes the numbers and types of blood cells and the specific developmental characteristics of each cell type.

A deficiency of other raw materials can cause other specific anemias. A deficiency of folic acid, for example, causes folic acid deficiency anemia. In addition to adequate dietary intake, raw materials must be absorbed from the digestive tract. Absorption of some of the raw materials requires special transport proteins. Adequate absorption of vitamin B_{12}, for example, requires a transport protein called *intrinsic factor*. Intrinsic factor is normally secreted by the lining of the stomach. The inability to secrete adequate intrinsic factor in some persons results in inadequate absorption of vitamin B_{12}. This condition results in a form of anemia called *pernicious anemia*. Why pernicious? Pernicious comes from the Latin word meaning "violent death," a reference to the painful neurological consequences of vitamin B_{12} deficiency. Today, pernicious anemia is easily treated with vitamin B_{12} and patients no longer die a violent death. Both folic acid deficiency and pernicious anemia are characterized by RBCs that are macrocytic (large RBCs) and normochromic (normal

RBC color). Note how the size and color of the RBCs can provide diagnostic clues about the different types of anemias.

REGULATION OF RBC PRODUCTION

New RBCs are constantly added to the circulation, and old, worn-out RBCs are constantly removed from the circulation. Figure 15-5 indicates that the RBC count is maintained through negative feedback control. When the O_2 in the body tissues decreases, the kidneys sense the need for additional O_2 and secrete a hormone called **erythropoietin** (eh-RITH-roh-POY-eh-tin). The erythropoietin (EPO) stimulates the bone marrow to produce additional RBCs. The increase in the number of RBCs causes an increase in the amount of oxygen transported to the tissues. As tissue O_2 increases, the stimulus for EPO release diminishes, and the bone marrow slows its rate of RBC production.

Three clinical thoughts about EPO follow:

- Note what happens in a person who is chronically hypoxemic, such as a person with emphysema (a chronic lung disorder). The low oxygen in the blood stimulates the secretion of excess EPO, causing additional RBC production. Thus, a person with emphysema often has polycythemia (excess RBCs) secondary to chronic lung disease. Similarly, a person who moves to a high-altitude location experiences a mild hypoxemia, which, in turn, stimulates EPO secretion and a rise in the RBC count. Both the emphysema-induced and altitude-induced polycythemias are called *secondary polycythemias*.
- Patients with bone marrow depression may be given EPO as a drug to increase RBC production. On a less upbeat note, athletes sometimes use EPO illegally. The drug increases RBC production, thereby increasing the amount of O_2 delivered to exercising muscle. The administration of EPO under this condition is a form of blood doping.
- Patients with declining kidney function do not produce enough EPO and therefore become anemic. This type of anemia is called the *anemia of chronic renal (kidney) failure*. It is treated with the administration of EPO.

REMOVAL AND BREAKDOWN OF RED BLOOD CELLS

How does the body know when an RBC needs to be removed from the circulation? The life span of a RBC is about 120 days. Because the mature RBC has no nucleus, it cannot reproduce and must be replaced as it wears out. The signal for RBC removal? With time, as it performs its job, the RBC eventually gets misshapen, ragged around the edges, and fragile; the poor thing looks worn out! The ragged RBC membrane is detected by the macrophages that line the spleen and liver. The macrophages, or big eaters, remove the RBCs from the circulation and phagocytose them. Sometimes, the RBCs are broken down very rapidly in a process called **hemolysis**, exceeding the rate of RBC replacement. This results in hemolytic anemia and jaundice. Why is the yellow hue called jaundice? Look in the "recycle bin" in Figure 15-6.

RECYCLE!

As the old, worn-out RBC is dismantled, its components are recycled. The hemoglobin is broken down into globin and heme (see Figure 15-6). The globin is broken down into various amino acids that are later used in the synthesis of other proteins.

The heme is further broken down into iron and bile pigments. The iron is stored in the liver until it is needed by the bone marrow for the synthesis of new hemoglobin. The liver removes bile pigments, especially bilirubin, from the blood and excretes them into the bile. Bile eventually flows into the intestines and is excreted from the body in the feces. What if RBC breakdown is excessive, as in hemolysis? The excess bilirubin in the blood, called *hyperbilirubinemia*, is deposited in the skin, causing it to appear yellow or jaundiced. Because the jaundice is caused by hemolysis, it is called *hemolytic jaundice*, as opposed to *obstructive jaundice* (described in Chapter 23).

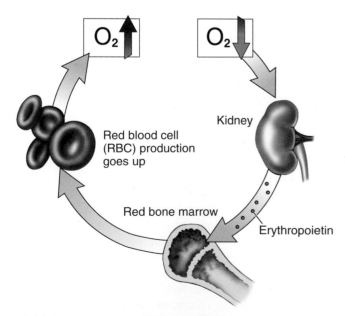

FIGURE 15-5 Regulation of RBC production by erythropoietin.

2+2 Sum It Up!

RBCs are filled with hemoglobin; the heme (iron) portion carries O_2 as oxyhemoglobin, while the globin portion carries CO_2 as carbaminohemoglobin. Normal RBCs are formed only in the presence of adequate raw materials, normal genetic information that directs hemoglobin synthesis, and healthy bone marrow. RBC production is regulated by erythropoietin, which in turn responds to tissue levels of oxygen. Hemoglobin is degraded into globin and bilirubin. The iron is recycled and the bilirubin is excreted in the bile.

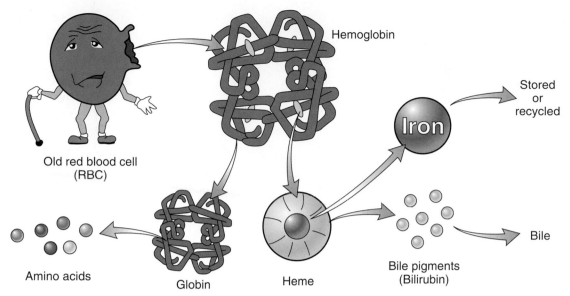

Hemoglobin

Iron

Stored or recycled

Old red blood cell (RBC)

Amino acids

Globin

Heme

Bile pigments (Bilirubin)

Bile

FIGURE 15-6 Breakdown of old RBCs. Note the recycling of amino acids and iron and the excretion of bilirubin.

 Do You Know...

Who This Little Yellow Bird Called *Icterus* Is?

The term *icterus* is a Greek word for "little yellow bird." Icterus is the same as jaundice. The ancient Greeks thought that a jaundiced person could be cured by gazing at the yellow bird. We now know that bird watching is not the cure. Jaundice is caused by an elevation of bilirubin in the blood (hyperbilirubinemia). The hyperbilirubinemia can be caused by excessive blood cell destruction (hemolysis) or the reduction in the elimination of bilirubin from the blood (via the liver and bile). When jaundice is present, it is essential to determine the cause of the hyperbilirubinemia. The cure? Treat the underlying cause of the jaundice.

THE ANEMIAS...AS A SUMMARY OF RED BLOOD CELL REQUIREMENTS AND CONDITIONS

Figure 15-7 is meant to draw attention to the various conditions and raw materials essential for RBC production. Failure to provide the necessary conditions and essential raw materials results in anemia, a deficiency of RBCs. For example, deficiencies of raw materials, such as iron, folic acid, and vitamin B_{12}, decrease the RBC count. Incorrect genetic information results in malformed and dysfunctional hemoglobin and

numerous types of anemia; the best known is sickle cell anemia. Impaired organ function, such as kidney disease and bone marrow depression, decreases the production of RBCs. Finally, anemias are caused by excess destruction (hemolytic anemia) or loss (bleeding) of RBCs (hemorrhagic anemia).

? Re-Think

1. Explain why excess hemolysis causes jaundice.
2. Why must you know the underlying cause of anemia before treating it? Provide three examples in your explanation.

WHITE BLOOD CELLS

White blood cells (WBCs), or leukocytes, are large round cells that contain nuclei. WBCs lack hemoglobin and are less numerous than RBCs. WBCs function primarily to protect the body by destroying disease-producing microorganisms (pathogens) and removing dead tissue and other cellular debris by phagocytosis. When an infection is present in the body, the numbers of WBCs generally increase. This increase in the number of WBCs is called *leukocytosis* (loo-koh-syte-OH-sis). A few infections cause leukopenia, a decrease in the numbers of WBCs. Leukocytes vary widely with respect to life span: granulocytes may live only a few hours, whereas some lymphocytes may live for years.

Normally, 1 µl (microliter) of blood contains 5000 to 10,000 WBCs (Table 15-1). This number is somewhat misleading because the WBCs spend less than 12 hours in the blood; they leave the blood vessels and migrate to connective tissue or to the site of an infection or inflammation, where they work and live out their lives (Figure 15-8). Thus, the number of WBCs distributed

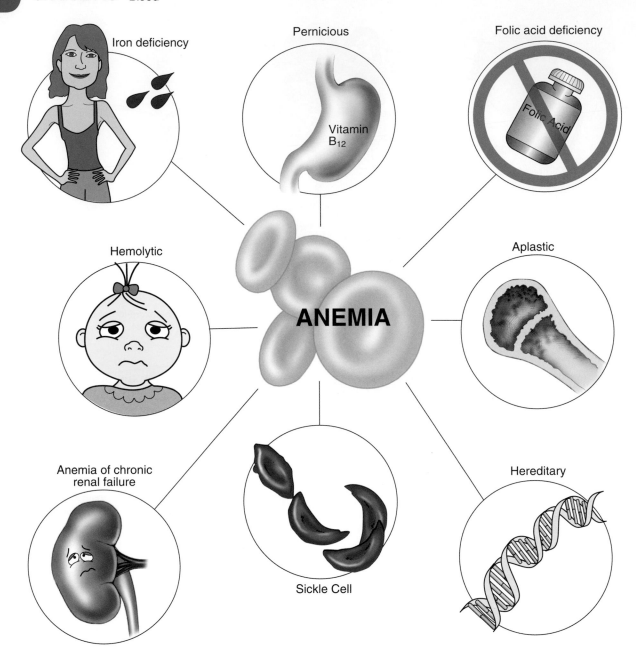

FIGURE 15-7 Summary of red blood cell formation and anemias.

throughout the body is much larger than what is suggested by the WBC count in the blood.

TYPES OF WHITE BLOOD CELLS

WBC production is called *leukopoiesis* (loo-koh-poy-EE-sis) (see Figure 15-2). Each of the five types of WBCs has a different name, appearance, and function (Table 15-2). How do we tell the difference? WBCs are classified according to granules in their cytoplasm. WBCs that contain granules are called *granulocytes*. Other WBCs do not have granules in their cytoplasm and are called *agranulocytes*. Granulocytes are produced in the red bone marrow and are classified according to their staining characteristics. The three types of granulocytes are neutrophils, basophils, and eosinophils.

NEUTROPHILS

The **neutrophil** (NOO-troh-fil) is the most common granulocyte. Neutrophils (which are pale or stain lavender) account for 55% to 70% of the total WBC population and usually remain in the blood for about 10 to 12 hours. The neutrophil's most important role is phagocytosis. These cells quickly move to the site of infection, where they phagocytose pathogens and remove tissue debris. The battle between the neutrophils and pathogens at the site of infection creates pus, a collection of dead neutrophils, parts of cells, and fluid.

Sometimes, the body can wall off the collection of pus from the surrounding tissue, forming an abscess. Abscess formation is one way that the body can prevent

Table 15-1 Types and Functions of Blood Cells

CELL TYPE	NORMAL RANGE	PRIMARY FUNCTION
Red blood cells (RBCs)	Men: 4.5–6.0 million/µL Women: 4.2–5.4 million/µL	Transport oxygen and carbon dioxide
Hemoglobin (Hgb)	Men: 13.5–17.5 g/100 mL Women: 12–16 g/100 mL	
Hematocrit (Hct)	Men: 40%–50% Women: 37%–47%	
Reticulocytes	0.5%–1.5%	
White blood cells (WBCs)*	5000–10,000/µL	Protect the body from infection
Platelets (thrombocytes)	150,000–450,000/µL	Help control blood loss from injured blood vessels

µL, Microliter.
*See Table 15-2 for the WBC differential count.

FIGURE 15-8 White blood cells are involved in phagocytosis.

the spread of infection. The neutrophil plays such an important role in the defense of the body that a deficiency of neutrophils (neutropenia or granulocytopenia) is considered life threatening. Unless resolved, the person may die from an overwhelming infection. Be sure that you understand these terms: *leukopenia, granulocytopenia,* and *neutropenia.* In what way are the terms similar and different?

Naming the Neutrophil
Because it plays such an important role in protecting the body from infection, the neutrophil is often the center of attention. Depending on its age, appearance, and its actions at the moment, the neutrophil has many nicknames.

Polys, Polymorphs, or Polymorphonuclear Leukocytes. The neutrophil is a round cell that contains a nucleus. The nucleus can have many shapes and different sizes. Because of the many-shaped (polymorphic) nucleus, neutrophils are called *polymorphs,* or *polymorphonuclear leukocytes* (PMNs). Sometimes, they are simply called *polys.*

Segs. The nucleus of the mature neutrophil appears segmented when viewed under a microscope. Mature neutrophils are therefore called *segs.*

Band Cells, Staff Cells, and Stab Cells. The nucleus of the immature neutrophil looks like a thick curved band—hence the name *band cells.* Because the band resembles the shape of a staff, the band cells are also called *staff cells.* Neutrophils are also called *stab cells.*

What Is a "Shift to the Left"?
This is a clinical phrase illustrating the response of the WBCs to a pathogen. As the body tries to mount an attack against a pathogen, it needs more neutrophils. The production of the neutrophils may be so rapid that the time for cells to mature is inadequate. A greater proportion of the neutrophils is therefore immature and appears banded. When immature neutrophils (bands) become prominent in the differential WBC count (lab test), the condition is termed a *shift to the left.* The term is derived from early studies that used tabular headings to report the numbers of each cell

Table 15-2 White Blood Cells (WBCs) (Differential Count)*

TYPE OF WBC	PERCENTAGE OF TOTAL WBC COUNT	FUNCTION OF CELL
Granulocytes		
Neutrophils	55–70	Phagocytosis
Eosinophils	1–3	Inflammatory responses, parasitic infection, allergies
Basophils	0–1	Inflammatory responses, release of heparin
Agranulocytes		
Lymphocytes	25–38	Immunity
Monocytes	3–8	Phagocytosis

*A differential WBC count indicates the percentage of each type of WBC.

type. The cell types were listed across the top of the printout, starting with bands on the left and the more mature neutrophils on the right. Thus, a shift to the left indicates an infection.

BASOPHILS

The second type of granulocytic WBCs, called baso-phils (BAY-so-fils), is normally present in small numbers. Basophils make up less than 1% of the WBCs and absorb a dark blue stain. The basophil plays a role in the inflammatory response, primarily through its release of histamine. The basophil also releases heparin, an anticoagulant. Because basophils are found in abundance in areas with large amounts of blood, such as the lungs and liver, the release of heparin is thought to reduce the formation of tiny blood clots.

EOSINOPHILS

The third type of granulocytic WBC is the eosinophil (ee-oh-SIN-oh-fil). The prefix eos- means rosy and refers to the staining characteristic of the eosinophil. Eosinophils are present in small numbers, constituting only 1% to 3% of the WBCs. They are involved in the inflammatory response, secreting chemicals that destroy certain parasites, engage in phagocytosis, and become elevated in persons with allergies.

AGRANULOCYTES

The two types of agranulocytes are lymphocytes and monocytes. The lymphocytes are produced in the red bone marrow; some migrate to, mature, and reproduce in the lymphoid tissue (lymph nodes, liver, spleen). Lymphocytes constitute 25% to 38% of the WBCs and perform an important role in the body's immune response. (Immunity will be discussed further in Chapter 21.) Monocytes are the second type of agranulocyte. Like the neutrophil, the monocyte is phagocytotic. Although the neutrophils are more abundant (55% to 70% of the WBCs), the monocytes (3% to 8% of the WBCs) are more efficient phagocytes.

Monocytes differentiate, or change, into macrophages. These macrophages become wandering or fixed. Wandering macrophages travel or wander about the body, patrolling for pathogens and cleaning up

debris. Wandering macrophages are particularly abundant under the mucous membranes and skin, where they destroy pathogens that gain entrance through cuts and abrasions. In contrast, fixed macrophages reside in a particular organ, such as the liver, spleen, lymph nodes, or red bone marrow. As blood or lymph flows through these organs, the fixed macrophages phagocytose pathogens. These same macrophages also phagocytose worn-out RBCs, thereby helping to remove them from circulation.

GOOD NEWS, BAD NEWS

The bad news is that clinically, you must know the names and classifications (granulocytes, agranulocytes) of the WBCs. The good news is that you can use the monkey business in Figure 15-9. "Naughty Little Monkeys Eat Bananas," says GRANpa BEN. "Naughty Little Monkeys Eat Bananas" identifies the type of WBCs—neutrophils, lymphocytes, monocytes, eosinophils, and basophils. GRANpa BEN indicates that the granulocytes are basophils, eosinophils, and neutrophils.

❓ Re-Think

1. Classify the neutrophil and identify its function.
2. Why can't you diagnose granulocytopenia or thrombocytopenia from a hematocrit reading?

PLATELETS

Platelets are tiny cell fragments of the larger mega-karyocytes. Normally, each microliter of blood contains between 150,000 and 450,000 platelets or thrombocytes. They are produced in the red bone marrow (see Figure 15-2) and have a life span of 5 to 9 days. The production of the platelet is called throm-bopoiesis (THROM-boh-poy-EE-sis).

Platelets prevent blood loss. (Platelet function is more fully described later in the "Hemostasis" section.) Failure of the bone marrow to replace platelets at an adequate rate results in a deficiency called thrombocy-topenia. This condition is characterized by petechiae—little pinpoint hemorrhages under the skin—and potentially lethal bleeding episodes.

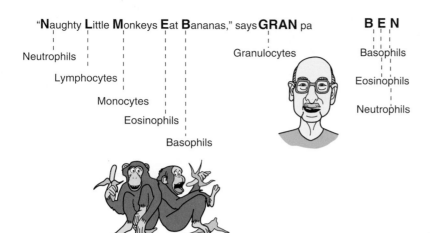

"**N**aughty **L**ittle **M**onkeys **E**at **B**ananas," says **GRAN** pa   **B E N**

Neutrophils

Lymphocytes

Monocytes

Eosinophils

Basophils

Granulocytes

Basophils

Eosinophils

Neutrophils

FIGURE 15-9 Naming white blood cells.

BLOOD COUNTS

A complete blood count (CBC) is a laboratory test that provides information about the composition of the blood. A CBC provides the normal range of the numbers of RBCs, WBCs, and platelets. In addition to the numbers of blood cells, the CBC provides information specific to each cell type. Relative to the RBC, the CBC indicates the normal hemoglobin content of the RBC, the normal Hct, and the percentage of the reticulocytes (the immature RBCs). With regard to information concerning the WBCs, a CBC indicates the percentage of each type of WBC (the differential WBC count).

DIFFERENTIAL COUNT

A differential WBC count indicates the percentage of each type of WBC (see Table 15-2). The differential count provides valuable diagnostic information because it indicates which specific WBC is involved. For example, one infection may cause an elevation primarily in the numbers of neutrophils, but a different infection may cause an elevation in the monocytes.

2+2 Sum It Up!

The WBCs (leukocytes) protect the body by destroying pathogens and removing dead tissue and other cellular debris by phagocytosis. The five types of WBCs are granulocytes (neutrophils, basophils, and eosinophils) and agranulocytes (lymphocytes and monocytes).

HEMOSTASIS: PREVENTION OF BLOOD LOSS

Injury to a blood vessel causes bleeding. Bleeding usually stops spontaneously when the injury is minor. What causes the bleeding to stop? The process that stops bleeding is called **hemostasis**, which literally means that the blood (hemo) stands still (stasis). Hemostasis involves three events: blood vessel spasm, the formation of a platelet plug, and blood clotting (Figure 15-10). (Do not confuse the words *hemostasis* and *homeostasis*.)

BLOOD VESSEL SPASM

When a blood vessel is injured, the smooth muscle in the blood vessel wall responds by contracting in a process called *vascular spasm*. (*Vascular* refers to blood vessels.) Vascular spasm causes the diameter of the blood vessel to decrease, thereby decreasing the amount of blood that flows through the vessel. In the smallest vessels, vascular spasm stops the bleeding completely. In the larger vessels, vascular spasm alone may slow bleeding but is generally insufficient to stop bleeding.

FORMATION OF A PLATELET PLUG

When a blood vessel is torn, the inner lining of the vessel activates the platelets. The platelets become sticky and adhere to the inner lining of the injured vessel and to each other. By sticking together, they form a platelet plug, which diminishes bleeding at the injured site. Over several minutes, the plug will be invaded by activated blood-clotting factors and will eventually evolve into a stable, strong blood clot. In addition to forming a plug, the platelets also release chemicals that further stimulate vascular spasm and help activate the blood-clotting factors. Thus, the platelets participate in all three phases of hemostasis. Good news! Exercise decreases platelet stickiness and the formation of deadly blood clots. Bad news? Stress increases platelet stickiness.

ANTIPLATELET DRUGS AND BLEEDING

Aspirin and other antiplatelet drugs such as clopidogrel (Plavix) slow vascular spasm and prevent platelet stickiness; they are commonly used to suppress

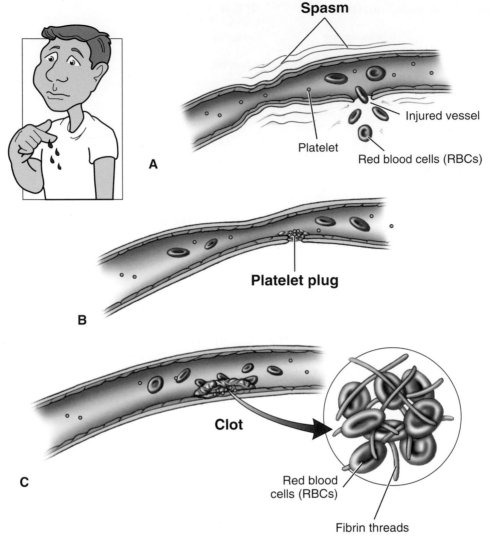

FIGURE 15-10 Steps in hemostasis. **A,** Blood vessel spasm. **B,** Formation of the platelet plug. **C,** Blood clotting (coagulation).

hemostasis. (A baby aspirin a day keeps the heart doctor away.) Excess antiplatelet therapy, however, can cause serious bleeding episodes, especially in a person who is thrombocytopenic or who is taking anticoagulant drugs.

BLOOD CLOTTING

Vascular spasm and a platelet plug alone are not sufficient to prevent the bleeding caused by a large tear in a blood vessel. With a more serious injury to the vessel wall, bleeding stops only if a blood clot forms. Blood clotting, or **coagulation**, is the third step in the process of hemostasis. A blood clot is formed by a series of chemical reactions that result in the formation of a netlike structure. The net, or framework, of the clot is composed of protein fibers called **fibrin**. As blood flows through the fibrin net, large particles in the blood, such as RBCs and platelets, become trapped within it. The fibrin net and the trapped

elements are called a *blood clot*. The blood clot seals off the opening in the injured blood vessel and stops the bleeding.

FORMATION OF THE BLOOD CLOT

How does the clot form? The clot is the result of a series of reactions in which a number of clotting factors are activated. The series of reactions in which one clotting factor activates another clotting factor is called the *clotting cascade*.

Follow the three stages of blood coagulation identified in Figure 15-11.

- *Stage I.* Injury to the blood vessel wall activates various clotting factors. These clotting factors normally circulate in the blood in their inactive form. When activated, the clotting factors produce prothrombin activator (PTA).
- *Stage II.* In the presence of calcium, platelet chemicals, and PTA, prothrombin is activated to form thrombin.

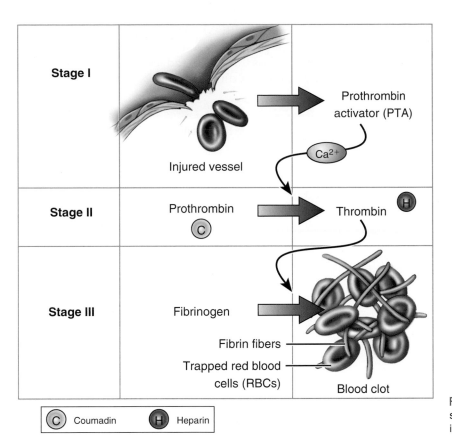

Stage I

Injured vessel

Prothrombin activator (PTA)

Ca²⁺

Stage II

Prothrombin Ⓒ → Thrombin Ⓗ

Stage III

Fibrinogen → Blood clot

Fibrin fibers

Trapped red blood cells (RBCs)

Ⓒ Coumadin Ⓗ Heparin

FIGURE 15-11 Three stages of blood clotting. The sites of Coumadin *(C)* and heparin *(H)* activity are indicated.

- *Stage III.* Thrombin activates fibrinogen. Activated fibrinogen forms the fibrin fibers, or fibrin net. The net traps other blood cells and particles to form the clot. Other factors then stabilize and strengthen the clot.

 Do You Know...

What Queen Victoria, the "Royal Disease," and Factor VIII Have in Common?

Hemophilia A is a bleeding disorder caused by the deficiency of a clotting factor called *factor VIII*, or the *hemophilic factor*. Hemophilia was common in the royal families of Europe; hence, it was called the "royal disease." Why was hemophilia so prevalent in the royal families? Hemophilia is genetically transmitted. Because of the tendency of the royals to intermarry (e.g., cousin marrying cousin), the gene carrying hemophilia was kept in the family and expressed frequently in the royal offspring. Queen Victoria of England carried the gene for hemophilia. Victoria, being both reproductively prolific and politically astute, placed a descendant on every throne in Europe. As each descendant married and intermarried, the incidence of hemophilia increased. (There are other forms of hemophilia, all caused by deficiencies of clotting factors and characterized by excessive bleeding. Hemophilia B is caused by a deficiency of factor IX, whereas hemophilia C is caused by a deficiency of factor XI.)

ANTICOAGULANTS

Although the body must be able to stop bleeding, it is equally essential for it to prevent excessive clot formation. Several natural mechanisms prevent clot formation. Two of the most important mechanisms are a smooth inner lining (endothelium) of the blood vessels and the secretion of heparin, an anticoagulant.

Endothelium

The inner lining (endothelium) of the blood vessels is smooth and shiny and allows blood to flow easily along its surface. If the surface of the endothelium becomes roughened or lined with cholesterol plaques, however, coagulation factors are activated and blood clots are apt to form.

Secretion of Heparin

Heparin is secreted by mast cells. Mast cells are basophils that are concentrated in and around the liver and lungs, sites where the blood is stagnant and therefore apt to clot easily. Heparin acts as an anticoagulant by removing thrombin from the clotting process. In other words, heparin is an antithrombin agent. Note in Figure 15-11 that the formation of thrombin in stage II is crucial for clot formation (the conversion of fibrinogen to fibrin).

This toe was accidentally severed from its owner. In reattaching the toe to the foot, the surgeon recognized that the toe graft would be successful only if the blood supply to the toe was good. Frequently, after surgery of this type, blood clots and edema (swelling) develop at the graft site, resulting in a decrease in blood flow. Leeches, or bloodsuckers, may be applied to the site of the graft. As the hungry leech attaches to the skin to feed, it injects a potent anticoagulant. The anticoagulant prevents blood clotting at the graft site, thereby maintaining a good blood flow and improving the chances for successful grafting. Enter the celebrities. The rich and famous have discovered that leeches "take away the years." Attach a hungry leech to some puffy *whatever* and presto, the swelling subsides. Leeches are making it big and bringing in big bucks!

Anticoagulant Medications

At times, the administration of anticoagulant drugs may be necessary. Anticoagulants are administered in an attempt to prevent the formation of a blood clot. The blood clot is called a *thrombus;* the process of blood clot formation is called *thrombosis*. The problem? A piece of the thrombus can break off, forming an embolus, a traveling blood clot. The embolus may lodge in the smaller blood vessels of other organs, blocking the flow of blood to the organ and resulting in organ damage, such as a pulmonary infarct (necrosis), heart attack, or brain attack (stroke). A common killer disorder, called *deep vein thrombosis* (DVT), is particularly lethal. A clot in the deep veins of the legs gives rise to an embolus. The embolus travels to the blood vessels of the lungs, where it blocks blood flow and often causes instant death.

Thrombosis may be prevented by the administration of two types of anticoagulants: heparin and warfarin (Coumadin). Heparin, designated "H" in Figure 15-11, acts as an antithrombin agent. Another anticoagulant, Coumadin (warfarin), also prevents clot formation. Like heparin, Coumadin interferes with the clotting scheme but does so at a different step. Coumadin, designated "C" in Figure 15-11, decreases the hepatic (liver) utilization of vitamin K in the synthesis of prothrombin, causing hypoprothrombinemia

(hye-poh-pro-THROM-ben-EE-mee-ah), a diminished amount of prothrombin in the blood. Less prothrombin means less thrombin, and less thrombin means that blood clotting is diminished.

Harry was diagnosed with DVT after a 15-hour nonstop flight on his broomstick. After a 3-day stay in the hospital with heparin therapy, he was discharged on Coumadin (warfarin) and directed not to eat spinach. Why no spinach? The drug Coumadin works by blocking the utilization of vitamin K in the hepatic synthesis of prothrombin. Because spinach contains a lot of vitamin K, it reduces the effectiveness of Coumadin, thereby reversing its anticoagulant effects. So leave the spinach to Popeye, Harry. Harry was also advised to lose the stick and walk.

Harry was also directed to have his prothrombin (PT) time measured regularly. The PT is a blood test that measures the time it takes for a sample of blood to clot. Coumadin blocks the synthesis of prothrombin, so it induces hypoprothrombinemia and prolongs the PT. Because Coumadin can prolong the PT, the person is at risk for bleeding. Conversely, too little Coumadin provides inadequate anticoagulation, predisposing the person to clot formation; hence, the need for regular monitoring. PT values are reported as international normalized ratio (INR) units in an attempt to standardize laboratory test results. Harry's physician would most likely aim for an INR between 2 and 3.

CLOT RETRACTION

What happens to the clot after it forms? It becomes smaller as water is squeezed out. This process is called *clot retraction*. As the clot retracts, the edges of the injured blood vessels are also pulled together. This pulling together slows bleeding and sets the stage for repair of the blood vessel.

CLOT BUSTING: FIBRINOLYSIS

Are you stuck with the clot forever? No! After the clot accomplishes its task, it is dissolved by a process called *fibrinolysis* (fye-brin-OL-is-sis) (Figure 15-12). A substance called *plasmin* dissolves the clot. Plasmin is formed from its inactive form, plasminogen (plaz-MIN-o-jen), which normally circulates within the blood. Tissue plasminogen activator (TPA), formed by injured tissue, activates plasminogen.

TPA can now be administered as a drug to persons with life-threatening conditions caused by clots. TPA is in a category of drugs called *clot busters* or *fibrinolytic agents*. These drugs have revolutionized the treatment of myocardial infarction (heart attacks caused by blood clots in the blood vessels of the heart) and brain attacks (blood clots in the blood vessels of the brain). Long before we started injecting clot-busting drugs, however, the vampire bat had figured out plasmin physiology and had perfected the technique. Vampire bat saliva contains a TPA-like substance that dissolves clots and facilitates its dining activities.

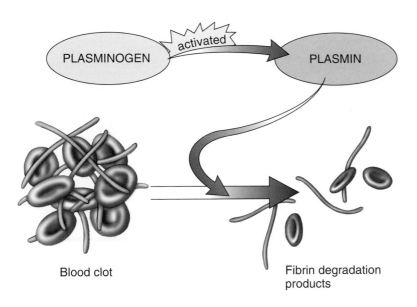

Blood clot

Fibrin degradation products

FIGURE 15-12 Fibrinolysis, also called "clot busting."

? Re-Think

1. Use the following words to explain the steps in coagulation: fibrinogen, thrombin, fibrin, PTA, and prothrombin.
2. Why might excessive doses of aspirin, heparin, Coumadin, and TPA cause bleeding?

2+2 Sum It Up!

The process that stops bleeding after injury is called *hemostasis*. Hemostasis involves three events: blood vessel spasm, the formation of a platelet plug, and blood clotting (coagulation). Clotting occurs when thrombin causes the conversion of fibrinogen into a fibrin clot. Blood clots are eventually dissolved by plasmin. Three major groups of drugs affect hemostasis: antiplatelet drugs, anticoagulants, and fibrinolytic or clot-busting drugs.

Do You Know...

About Miss Muffet, Her Curds, Whey, and Blood Clot?

As you know, little Miss Muffet sat on her tuffet eating her curds and whey—that is, her soured milk. (The lumps in soured milk are called *curds*, and the watery part is called *whey*. So much for Muffet's diet.) What does this have to do with blood? Thrombosis (blood clotting) is from a Greek word meaning "to curdle," as in the curdling of milk. Serum is from a Latin word that refers to whey or the watery residue left after milk has curdled. Miss Muffet didn't really have a blood clot, but her diet inspired blood-clotting vocabulary. Her tuffet and arachnophobic personality are another story!

BLOOD TYPES

The history of medicine has recorded attempted blood transfusions since its earliest days. Although some were successful, others were medical disasters. The earliest physicians recognized that a severely wounded person was in need of blood. They did not realize, however, that blood from one person cannot always be mixed with blood from another. These physicians unknowingly demonstrated by disaster the presence of different blood types.

ANTIGENS AND BLOOD TYPES

Blood is classified according to specific antigens on the surface of the RBC. An antigen is a substance that the body recognizes as foreign; the encounter evokes an immune response, thereby producing antibodies. As a foreign substance, an antigen stimulates an antigen–antibody response. This response is designed to attack and destroy the antigen.

The ABO grouping contains four blood types: A, B, AB, and O. The letters A and B refer to the antigen on the RBC. Table 15-3 shows what it means to be type A, B, AB, or O.

- A person with type A blood has the A antigen on the RBC.
- A person with type B blood has a B antigen on the RBC.
- A person with type AB blood has both A and B antigens on the RBC.
- A person with type O blood has neither A nor B antigen on the RBC.

Remember that the antigen is located on the RBC membrane.

Table **15-3** | ABO Blood Groups

BLOOD TYPE*	ANTIGEN (RBC MEMBRANE)	ANTIBODY (PLASMA)	CAN RECEIVE BLOOD FROM	CAN DONATE BLOOD TO
A (40%)	A antigen	Anti-B antibodies	A, O	A, AB
B (10%)	B antigen	Anti-A antibodies	B, O	B, AB
AB† (4%)	A antigen, B antigen	No antibodies	A, B, AB, O	AB
O‡ (46%)	No antigen	Both anti-A and anti-B antibodies	O	O, A, B, AB

*Number in parentheses indicates the percentage of the population with this blood type.
†Type AB, universal recipient.
‡Type O, universal donor.

ANTIBODIES AND BLOOD TYPE

In addition to the antigens on the RBCs, specific antibodies are found in the plasma of each blood type (see Table 15-3).

- A person with type A blood has anti-B antibodies in the plasma.
- A person with type B blood has anti-A antibodies in the plasma.
- A person with type AB blood has neither anti-A nor anti-B antibodies in the plasma.
- The person with type O blood has both anti-A and anti-B antibodies in the plasma.

ANTIGEN–ANTIBODY INTERACTION

Table 15-3 indicates that type A blood contains the A antigen and anti-B antibodies. What would happen if a person had the A antigen on his or her RBCs and anti-A antibodies in his plasma? The A antigen and the anti-A antibody would cause a clumping reaction much like the curdling seen when milk and vinegar are mixed together.

This clumping of the antigen–antibody interaction is called *agglutination*. Agglutination reactions cause the RBCs to burst or lyse, a process called *hemolysis*. If rapid hemolysis were to occur in the circulation, hemoglobin would be liberated from the RBCs, causing kidney failure and death.

COMPATIBILITY AND INCOMPATIBILITY OF BLOOD TYPES

The curdling, or agglutination, reaction has important implications for blood transfusions. Some blood types mix without undergoing agglutination reactions; they are said to be *compatible blood groups*. Other blood groups agglutinate, causing severe hemolysis. These blood groups are incompatible. To avoid giving a person incompatible blood, donor blood is first typed and cross-matched.

What do blood typing and cross-matching mean? First, the blood type (A, B, AB, or O) is determined. Then, a sample of donor blood (blood from the person who is donating it) is mixed (cross-matched) with a sample of recipient blood (blood from the person who is to receive the donated blood). Any evidence of agglutination indicates that the donor blood is incompatible with the recipient's blood.

Suppose a recipient of a blood transfusion has type A blood. She or he then can be given type A blood and type O blood (see Table 15-3). No antigen–antibody reaction (agglutination) would occur because type A donor blood has the A antigen and the recipient has only anti-B antibodies (plasma). The type O donor blood does not cause agglutination because that person's RBC has neither the A nor the B antigen. Type A and type O blood are therefore compatible with type A blood.

Note what happens, however, if the type A recipient receives type B blood (see Table 15-3). Type B donor blood has the B antigen on each RBC surface. The plasma antibodies of the recipient are anti-B antibodies. The B antigen and the anti-B antibodies cause agglutination; thus, type B blood is incompatible with type A blood. What happens if the type A recipient is given type AB blood? In this case, the RBC contains both A and B antigens. The plasma of the recipient contains anti-B antibodies. When types A and AB are mixed, an agglutination reaction then occurs; these blood groups are incompatible. The administration of incompatible blood groups forms the basis of hemolytic blood transfusion reactions. The presence or absence of antibodies dictates the compatibility/incompatibility characteristics of the four blood groups (see Table 15-3).

Note in Table 15-3 that type O blood can be given to people in all four blood groups. Type O blood is therefore called the *universal donor*. For this reason, blood banks stock a large supply of type O blood. Note also that someone with type AB blood can receive all four types of blood; this person is called a *universal recipient*. Table 15-3 also indicates the prevalence of the four blood types. Type A blood occurs in 40% of the population, 10% of the population has type B, 4% has type AB, and 46% has type O. Thus, type O is the most common and type AB is the least common. (What blood type are you?)

Plasma does not naturally carry anti-Rh antibodies. In two conditions, however, the plasma of an Rh-negative (−) person can develop anti-Rh antibodies.

 Do You Know...

About Bilirubin, Kernicterus, and Sulfa Drugs?

Normally, bilirubin is transported by the plasma proteins, especially albumin, in the blood. In pharmacology terms, bilirubin is said to be tightly bound to albumin. As long as the bilirubin is bound to the albumin, it is not free to leave the blood and stain the tissues yellow. Enter the sulfa drugs. If an infant (younger than 2 months old) is given a sulfa drug to treat an infection, the drug binds to the albumin and displaces or frees the bilirubin. The free bilirubin enters the tissues, staining them yellow. Because the blood–brain barrier of the infant is not fully developed, the bilirubin can enter the central nervous system (CNS), causing brain damage (kernicterus). The same thing happens when a pregnant woman is given a sulfa drug. The drug crosses the placental barrier, enters the fetal blood, and causes an excess of free bilirubin. Thus, the administration of sulfa drugs to an infant or to a pregnant or nursing mother is contraindicated.

 Re-Think

1. Why can't a person with type O blood safely receive a transfusion of type AB blood?
2. Why can't you change a person's blood type from type A to type O by giving him or her several transfusions of type O blood?

Rh CLASSIFICATION SYSTEM

Blood is also classified according to the Rh factor. The Rh factor is an antigen located on the surface of the RBC. The Rh factor was named for the rhesus monkey, in which it was first detected. If an RBC contains the Rh factor, the blood is said to be Rh-positive (+). If the RBC lacks the Rh factor, it is said to be Rh-negative (−). Thus, A+ blood refers to type A (A antigen) blood that also has the Rh factor, whereas A− blood is type A blood that does not have the Rh factor. Approximately 85% of the population is Rh positive (+).

The first condition involves the accidental administration of Rh-positive (+) blood to an Rh-negative (−) person. If Rh-positive (+) blood from a donor is administered to an Rh-negative (−) person (the recipient), the Rh antigen of the donor stimulates the recipient to produce anti-Rh antibodies. The recipient is now said to be sensitized. If the Rh-negative (−) person is later given a second transfusion of Rh-positive (+) blood, the anti-Rh antibodies in the plasma of the recipient will attack the Rh antigen of the Rh-positive (+) donor blood, causing agglutination and hemolysis.

The Rh factor may cause a serious problem in a second condition, that of an Rh-negative (−) pregnant mother who is carrying an Rh-positive (+) fetus (Figure 15-13). During this first pregnancy, the baby grows to term and is delivered uneventfully. During childbirth, however, some of the baby's Rh-positive (+) blood crosses the placenta and enters the mother's blood.

Rh– Red blood cell (RBC) of mother

Rh+ RBC of fetus with Rh antigen on surface

Anti–Rh antibody made against Rh+ RBC

Hemolysis of Rh+ RBC

FIGURE 15-13 Rh-negative (–) mother, Rh-positive (+) fetus.

The Rh antigen stimulates the mother's immune system to produce anti-Rh antibodies. In other words, the mother has become sensitized by her first baby. If the mother becomes pregnant for a second time with an Rh-positive (+) baby, the anti-Rh antibodies move from the mother's circulation into the baby's circulation. These anti-Rh antibodies attack the baby's RBCs, causing agglutination and hemolysis. In response, the baby becomes jaundiced and anemic as the RBCs undergo hemolysis.

This hemolytic condition is called *erythroblastosis fetalis*. The hemolysis causes a rapid rise in plasma levels of bilirubin. The hyperbilirubinemia (increased bilirubin in the blood), in turn, causes severe jaundice and a condition called *kernicterus*. Kernicterus (kehr-NIK-tehr-ahs), caused by the staining of a part of the brain with bilirubin, is characterized by severe retardation in mental development. The great tragedy is that kernicterus is preventable. Every woman should know her blood type and recognize the need for early prenatal care!

Erythroblastosis fetalis can be prevented by the administration of the drug RhoGAM. RhoGAM is administered to the Rh-negative mother during pregnancy and within 72 hours after delivery. RhoGAM surrounds, or coats, the baby's Rh-positive (+) antigens, thereby preventing them from stimulating the development of anti-Rh antibodies by the mother.

Other antigens in the maternal and fetal blood are capable of inducing hemolysis, hyperbilirubinemia, and jaundice. Consequently, a newer and more inclusive term than *erythroblastosis fetalis* is *hemolytic disease of the newborn* (HDN). HDN includes all antigen–antibody reactions, including the Rh factor, that cause hemolysis and jaundice.

Visit any newborn nursery and you will see a little yellow baby "sunbathing" in an isolette. What's that about? It has been known for years that ultraviolet radiation (sunlight) hastens the disappearance of jaundice. Phototherapy provides ultraviolet radiation, which helps break down the bilirubin deposited in the skin so that it can be eliminated from the body.

2+2 Sum It Up!

Blood is classified according to the antigens on the surface of the RBC. The ABO grouping contains four blood types: A (A antigens), B (B antigens), AB (A and B antigens), and O (neither A nor B antigens). An antigen–antibody reaction, called *agglutination*, occurs when blood is mismatched. Type AB blood is the universal recipient blood. Type O blood is the universal donor blood. The Rh factor is another type of antigen on the RBC. Rh-positive blood has the Rh factor on the RBC, whereas Rh-negative blood does not contain the Rh factor.

As You Age

1. The volume and composition of blood remain constant with age, so most laboratory values remain normal. Alterations in laboratory values for blood usually indicate alterations in other organ systems. For example, the fasting blood glucose level increases with aging. This alteration is not the result of changes in the blood, however. Rather, it is the result of age-related changes associated with insulin. The same is true regarding serum lipid levels. Serum lipid levels increase 25% to 50% after the age of 55, but the increase is caused by an altered metabolism and not by changes of the blood and blood-forming organs.

2. The amount of red bone marrow decreases with age. The total number of blood cells remains normal, but older persons take longer to form new blood cells and hence recover more slowly from bleeding episodes.

3. An age-related decline occurs in white blood cell (WBC) activity. Although WBC activity still increases in response to infection, it does so more slowly.

MEDICAL TERMINOLOGY AND DISORDERS   Disorders of the Blood

Medical Term	Word Parts	Word Part Meaning or Derivation	Description
Words			
ecchymosis	ecchy-	From the Greek word *eccym*, meaning "to pour out"	An **ecchymosis** is *a formation of escaped blood in the tissues from a blood vessel that has ruptured* (commonly called a bruise).
	-osis	condition or increase	
hematocrit	hemat/o-	blood	The **hematocrit** is *the ratio of the blood cells to the volume of the blood sample.*
	-crit	to separate	
normochromic	norm/o-	normal	**Normochromic** RBCs contain a normal amount of hemoglobin; therefore the color is normal.
	-chrom/o-	color	
	-ic	pertaining to	
myelodysplasia	myel/o-	bone marrow	Refers to *a group of disorders in which the bone marrow fails to produce blood cells, causing a reduction in RBCs, WBCs, and platelets.*
	-dys-	faulty	
	-plasia	formation	
petechiae		From an Italian word meaning "flea-bite," a reference to the appearance of petechiae	**Petechiae** are *tiny purple or red spots resulting from bleeding under the skin's surface.*
purpura		From a Latin word meaning "purple garment"	**Purpura** are *red or purple splotches under the skin or mucous membrane and are due to bleeding.*
Disorders			
anemia	an-	without	**Anemia** is *a deficiency of red blood cells (RBCs) or hemoglobin, diagnostically indicated by a low hematocrit.* The reduction in RBCs leads to varying degrees of hypoxemia, the basis for most of the signs and symptoms. The etiological classification is based on the causes of anemia. The anemias are described in the text.
	-emia	condition of the blood	

Continued

MEDICAL TERMINOLOGY AND DISORDERS   Disorders of the Blood—cont'd

Medical Term	Word Parts	Word Part Meaning or Derivation	Description
hemolytic disorders	hem/o-	blood	**Hemolytic** refers to *the breakdown of RBCs, which leak their contents (hemoglobin, bilirubin, K+) into the plasma.* There are many causes of hemolysis: infections, especially streptococcus and staphylococcus; antibody-inducing drugs; diseases such as sickle cell anemia (hemolytic crisis); the administration of incompatible blood; and hemolytic disease of the newborn (HDN).
	-lysis-	breakdown	
	-ic	pertaining to	
hemostatic disorders	hem/o-	blood	**Hemostatic** refers *to disorders that impair the ability of the blood to clot.* Disorders can be inherited or acquired (which is more common). **Thrombocytopenia,** *a reduction in platelets,* presents as spontaneous bleeding, such as hematuria, and prolonged bleeding from minor injuries. **Heparin-induced thrombocytopenia and thrombosis syndrome (HITTS),** also known as **white clot syndrome,** is of particular concern because of the frequent use of heparin as an anticoagulant. Heparin induces an immune response that causes platelet aggregation. **Hemophilia** refers to a group of bleeding disorders characterized by delayed coagulation and caused by a deficiency of a coagulation factor. **Hemophilia A,** the most common type, is due to a Factor VIII deficiency. Factor IX deficiency is called **hemophilia B** or **Christmas disease,** named for Stephan Christmas, the first patient diagnosed with factor IX deficiency. The chief symptom is bleeding, often into joints **(hemarthrosis).** Hemophilia (phil/o- = love) literally means "love of bleeding"; in this instance, love should be understood as a tendency to bleed. **Von Willebrand's disease** is the most common hereditary coagulation defect. It is a deficiency of von Willebrand factor, a protein that is necessary for platelet stickiness. **Disseminated intravascular coagulation (DIC),** despite its reference to coagulation, is characterized by excessive bleeding. An underlying condition stimulates accelerated clotting, depleting blood clotting factors and platelets and causing profuse hemorrhage.
	-stasis	stop or stand	
	-ic	pertaining to	
leukemias	leuk/o-	white	Also called *cancer of the blood,* **leukemia** is a hematological malignant condition in which there are excessive, immature ("blasts"), and abnormally functioning leukocytes. There are several classification systems. There are acute and chronic leukemias. There are also lymphocytic and myelocytic leukemias. The **lymphoblastic** or **lymphocytic leukemias** are caused by abnormal changes in bone marrow cells that give rise to B lymphocytes. The **myeloid** or **myelocytic leukemias** are caused by abnormal changes in bone marrow cells that give rise to RBCs, platelets, and some WBCs. Because the bone marrow becomes infiltrated with immature and abnormal leukocytes, hemopoiesis (blood formation) is severely impaired. The patient becomes anemic, thrombocytopenic, and neutropenic.
	-emia	blood condition	

| **MEDICAL TERMINOLOGY AND DISORDERS** | Disorders of the Blood—cont'd | | |

Medical Term	Word Parts	Word Part Meaning or Derivation	Description
hemorrhage	hem/o-	blood	**Hemorrhage** refers to *active bleeding*. The patient becomes symptomatic with a loss of 15% to 30% of the total blood volume. **Hemorrhage** is classified in stages depending on the amount of blood loss. Hemorrhage may be internal, as in the loss of blood from a ruptured aneurysm, or external as in bleeding from a laceration on the arm. With severe hemorrhage the patient can "bleed out" or "bleed to death." This is known in medical terminology as **exsanguinations** (*ex* = out of) and (*sanguis* = blood).
	-rrhage	to burst forth	
septicemia	sept-	rotten	Also called *blood poisoning* and refers to *the presence of harmful substances in the blood, such as pathogens and toxins.* Septicemia can cause a life-threatening septic shock.
	-emia	blood condition	

Get Ready for Exams!

Summary Outline

Blood has three main functions: it delivers oxygen to all cells; it helps regulate body functions, such as body temperature; and it protects the body from infection and bleeding.

 I. **Blood Functions**
   A. Transport (O_2, CO_2, nutrients)
   B. Regulation (fluid/electrolyte, acid–base, temperature)
   C. Protection (infection, blood loss)
 II. **Composition and Characteristics of Blood**
   A. Blood is composed of plasma and blood cells.
   B. The blood cells originate in the bone marrow and lymphoid tissue.
   C. Hemopoiesis: erythropoiesis, leukopoiesis, and thrombopoiesis
 III. **Blood Cells**
   A. Red blood cells (RBCs) or erythrocytes
     1. RBCs are filled with hemoglobin.
     2. Oxyhemoglobin transports oxygen and carbaminohemoglobin transports carbon dioxide.
     3. RBC production is regulated by erythropoietin (senses oxygen).
   B. White blood cells (WBCs)
     1. WBCs are classified as granulocytes and agranulocytes.
     2. The granulocytes are neutrophils, basophils, and eosinophils.
     3. The nongranulocytes are the lymphocytes and monocytes.
   C. Platelets
     1. Platelets are thrombocytes.
     2. Platelets are involved in hemostasis.

 IV. **Hemostasis**
   A. Stages of hemostasis
     1. The three stages of hemostasis are blood vessel spasm, formation of a platelet plug, and blood coagulation.
     2. The three stages of blood coagulation are summarized in Figure 15-11.
   B. Dissolving clots and preventing clot formation
     1. Eventually, the clot dissolves by a process called *fibrinolysis;* clot dissolution is achieved primarily by plasmin.
     2. Natural anticoagulant mechanisms include a smooth endothelial lining and heparin.
 V. **Blood Types**
   A. ABO blood types
     1. There are four types of blood: A, B, AB, and O.
     2. The A and B antigens are on the membrane of the RBC.
     3. Blood plasma contains anti-A and anti-B antibodies.
     4. Blood antigen and antibodies are summarized in Table 15-3.
   B. Rh factor
     1. An Rh-positive person has the Rh antigen on the RBC membrane; an Rh-positive person does not have anti-Rh antibodies in the plasma.
     2. The Rh factor must be considered when blood is transfused; an Rh-negative person cannot receive Rh-positive blood.
     3. An Rh-negative mother carrying an Rh-positive baby may give birth to a baby with hemolytic disease of the newborn (HDN).

Review Your Knowledge

Matching: Blood Cells

Directions: Match the following words with their descriptions below. Some words may be used more than once.

a. platelets
b. white blood cells
c. red blood cells

1. ___ Contains the antigens A and B
2. ___ Requires erythropoietin for production
3. ___ The reticulocyte is an immature cell of this type.
4. ___ Includes the neutrophil, eosinophil, and basophil
5. ___ A deficiency causes petechiae and bleeding
6. ___ Stickiness and plug both describe the functional role of this cell type.
7. ___ Primarily concerned with infection
8. ___ Measured as the hematocrit
9. ___ Classified as granulocytes and agranulocytes
10. ___ Primarily concerned with the delivery of oxygen

Matching: Blood Clots

Directions: Match the following words with their descriptions below. Some words may be used more than once.

a. embolus
b. plasmin
c. heparin
d. warfarin (Coumadin)
e. thrombus

1. ___ A blood clot in the leg
2. ___ Drug that interferes with the hepatic utilization of vitamin K in the synthesis of prothrombin
3. ___ A traveling or moving blood clot
4. ___ Enzyme that dissolves clots
5. ___ An anticoagulant that works by removing thrombin (antithrombin activity)

Matching: Blood Types

Directions: Match the following blood types with their descriptions below. Some may be used more than once.

a. A
b. B
c. AB
d. O

1. ___ The blood cells that contain neither the A antigen nor the B antigen
2. ___ The universal donor
3. ___ This blood type can receive type B and type A blood.
4. ___ This blood type contains only anti-B antibodies.
5. ___ This blood type contains both anti-A and anti-B antibodies.

Multiple Choice

1. The erythrocyte
   a. is phagocytic.
   b. contains hemoglobin and transports oxygen.
   c. initiates blood coagulation.
   d. produces antibodies that are involved in the immune response.

2. The neutrophil
   a. is a T lymphocyte.
   b. is a granulocytic phagocyte.
   c. secretes antibodies.
   d. activates plasmin.

3. Thrombin
   a. activates fibrinogen.
   b. is responsible for the formation of the platelet plug.
   c. is inactivated by vitamin K.
   d. is inactivated by prothrombin.

4. What statement is true regarding the administration of type A+ blood to a type O− recipient?
   a. The blood types are compatible; no hemolytic reaction is expected.
   b. Persons with O− blood are allergic to type A+ blood.
   c. The administration of type A+ blood to a type O− recipient causes hemolysis.
   d. Persons with type O− blood can safely receive type A+ blood.

5. Erythropoietin
   a. is synthesized by the kidneys.
   b. stimulates the bone marrow to make RBCs.
   c. is released by the kidney in response to hypoxemia.
   d. All of the above are true.

6. Which of the following is most likely to cause jaundice?
   a. Anemia
   b. A deficiency of erythropoietin
   c. A deficiency of intrinsic factor
   d. Hemolysis

7. Which of the following is a true statement?
   a. The reticulocyte is an immature thrombocyte.
   b. The neutrophil is a phagocytic granulocyte.
   c. The neutrophil, basophil, and eosinophil are fragments of the megakaryocyte.
   d. A deficiency of reticulocytes causes hypoprothrombinemia.

8. Hypoprothrombinemia and a prolonged prothrombin time is
   a. associated with bleeding.
   b. symptomatic of pernicious anemia.
   c. a consequence of heparin therapy.
   d. a consequence of thrombocytopenia.

9. Hyperbilirubinemia
   a. can be caused by hemolysis.
   b. causes jaundice.
   c. can cause kernicterus.
   d. All of the above are true.

10. Which of the following is least related to heme?
    a. Oxygen
    b. Phagocytosis
    c. RBC
    d. Iron

Go Figure

1. **According to Figure 15-2**
   a. The stem cell is also called the *reticulocyte*.
   b. Platelets give rise to megakaryocytes.
   c. Lymphocytes and monocytes are granulocytes.
   d. Stem cells can differentiate into RBCs, WBCs, and platelets.

2. **According to Figure 15-5**
   a. Erythropoiesis is stimulated by low levels of CO_2 in the blood.
   b. The secretion of erythropoietin increases as blood levels of O_2 decrease.
   c. Bilirubin stimulates the kidneys to secrete erythropoietin.
   d. Erythropoietin is secreted by the bone marrow in response to decreased blood levels of O_2.

3. **According to Figure 15-6, which of the following is not true?**
   a. Heme contains iron.
   b. Bilirubin is one of the degradation products of heme.
   c. Iron generated by the degradation of heme can be stored or recycled.
   d. Only the globin part of hemoglobin can produce bilirubin.

4. **According to Figures 15-11 and 15-12**
   a. PTA activates plasmin to plasminogen.
   b. Coumadin exerts an antithrombin effect.
   c. Both Coumadin and heparin exert an anticoagulant effect by decreasing the hepatic utilization of vitamin K in the synthesis of prothrombin.
   d. Heparin exerts an antithrombin effect, thereby delaying blood clotting.

5. **According to Figure 15-13**
   a. Anti-Rh antibodies are produced by the fetus.
   b. The mother is initially Rh+ and becomes Rh– as anti-Rh antibodies accumulate.
   c. The fetus is initially Rh+ and becomes Rh– as the disorder progresses.
   d. The mother is Rh– and the fetus is Rh+.

Anatomy of the Heart

Key Terms

aortic valve (p. 314)
atrioventricular valves (p. 313)
atrium (p. 311)
bicuspid valve (p. 314)
cardiology (p. 308)
chordae tendineae (p. 314)

coronary arteries (p. 316)
endocardium (p. 309)
epicardium (p. 308)
mitral valve (p. 314)
myocardium (p. 309)
pericardium (p. 310)

precordium (p. 308)
Purkinje fibers (p. 319)
semilunar valves (p. 313)
tricuspid valve (p. 314)
ventricles (p. 311)

Objectives

1. Describe the location of the heart.
2. Name the three layers and the covering of the heart.
3. Explain the function of the heart as two separate pumps.
4. Identify the four chambers and great vessels of the heart.
5. Explain the functions of the four heart valves.

6. Describe the physiological basis of the heart sounds.
7. Describe blood flow through the heart.
8. List the vessels that supply blood to the heart.
9. Identify the major components of the heart's conduction system.

Throughout history, many functions have been attributed to the heart. Some philosophers have called it "the seat of the soul." The ancient Egyptians, for example, weighed the heart after a person's death because they believed that the weight of the heart equaled the weight of the soul. The heart has also been described as the seat of wisdom and understanding; accordingly, it thinks and makes plans. More often than not, however, history has portrayed the heart as the seat of the emotions. An overly compassionate person is described as soft hearted, a generous person has a heart of gold, and a grief-stricken person is broken hearted. Every Valentine's Day card displays hearts, hearts, and more hearts to celebrate love. None focus on the heart as an efficient pump. Enter the modern-day heart specialist and the science of cardiology, the study of the heart.

FUNCTION, LOCATION, AND SIZE OF THE HEART

The heart is a hollow muscular organ. Its primary function is to pump and force blood through the blood vessels of the body, providing every cell in the body with vital nutrients and oxygen. The heart pumps an average of 72 times each minute for your entire lifetime. If you live until you are 75 years old, your heart

will beat in excess of 3 billion times. Puts the Energizer Bunny to shame!

The adult heart is about the size of a closed fist and weighs less than 1 pound. The heart sits in the chest within the mediastinum, between the two lungs (Figure 16-1). Two thirds of the heart is located to the left of the midline of the sternum, and one third is located to the right. The upper flat portion of the heart, called the *base,* is located at the level of the second rib. The lower, more pointed end of the heart is the apex; it is located at the level of the fifth intercostal space. The precordium refers to the area of the anterior chest wall overlying the heart and great vessels. You need to know the precise location of the heart because you will be asked to evaluate different heart sounds, accurately position electrodes for an electrocardiogram, and provide life-saving cardiopulmonary resuscitation (CPR).

LAYERS AND COVERING OF THE HEART

The heart is made up of three layers of tissue: endocardium, myocardium, and epicardium (Figure 16-2).

ENDOCARDIUM

The endocardium (en-doh-KAR-dee-um) is the heart's innermost layer. The endocardium also lines the valves

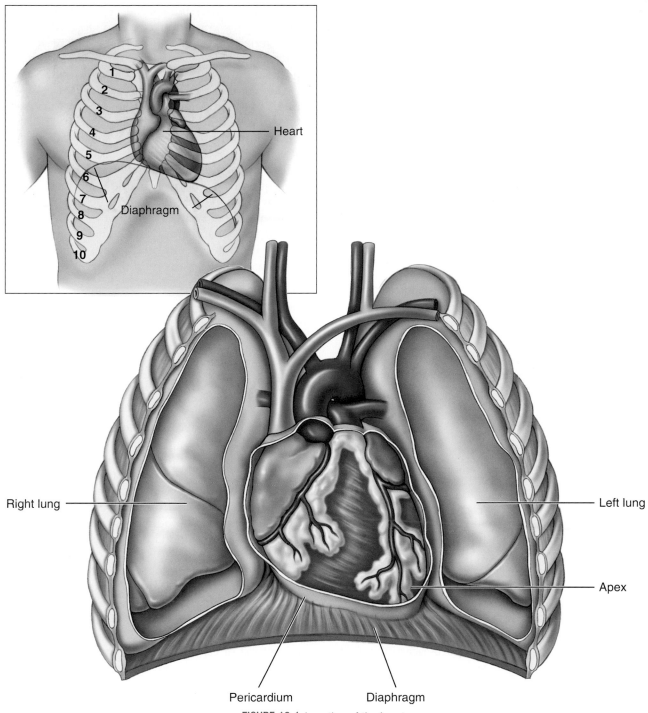

FIGURE 16-1 Location of the heart.

and is continuous with the blood vessels that enter and leave the heart. The smooth and shiny surface allows blood to flow over it easily.

MYOCARDIUM

The **myocardium** (my-oh-KAR-dee-um) is the middle layer of the heart. It is the thickest of the three layers. The myocardium is composed of cardiac muscle that contracts and pumps blood through the blood vessels. (Review muscle contraction in Chapter 9, especially the "sliding" of actin and myosin.)

Cardiac muscle

EPICARDIUM

The **epicardium** (ep-i-KAR-dee-um) is the thin outermost layer of the heart. The epicardium also helps form the pericardium.

FIGURE 16-2 Layers of the heart and pericardium.

PERICARDIUM

The heart is supported by a slinglike structure called the **pericardium**. The pericardium attaches the heart to surrounding structures, such as the diaphragm and the large blood vessels that attach to the heart. The pericardium has three layers. The innermost layer (closest to the heart) is the epicardium, also called the *visceral pericardium*. The visceral pericardium folds back and becomes the *parietal pericardium*. The parietal pericardium attaches to the outer fibrous pericardium that anchors the heart to its surrounding structures. Between the visceral pericardium and parietal pericardium is a space called the *pericardial space,* or *pericardial cavity*. The pericardial membranes are serous membranes that secrete a small amount of slippery serous fluid (10 to 30 mL) into the pericardial space. The pericardial fluid lubricates the surfaces of the membranes and allows them to slide past one another with little friction or rubbing.

At times, the pericardial membranes become inflamed; this condition is called *pericarditis* and is characterized by pain and a sound called a *friction rub*. The friction rub is similar to the sound of scratchy sandpaper and is best heard when the stethoscope is placed over the left sternal border, near the apex of the heart. The inflamed pericardial membranes also secrete excess serous fluid into the pericardial space. This collection of fluid in the pericardial space (called *pericardial effusion*) may compress the heart externally, making it difficult for the heart to relax and fill with blood. Consequently, the heart is unable to pump a sufficient amount of blood to the body. This life-threatening condition is called *cardiac tamponade* (TAM-pon-ade). Cardiac tamponade may be treated by inserting a long needle into the pericardial space and aspirating (sucking out) the serous fluid through the needle.

? Re-Think

1. Locate the heart with specific references to the sternum and ribs.
2. List the three layers of the heart. Identify the pumping layer.

A DOUBLE PUMP AND TWO CIRCULATIONS

The myocardium enables the heart to pump blood. The heart is a double pump that beats as one. The pumps are the right heart and the left heart (Figure 16-3). The right heart receives unoxygenated blood from the superior and inferior venae cavae, large veins that collect blood from all parts of the body. The right heart, which is colored blue because it contains unoxygenated blood, pumps blood to the lungs, where the blood is oxygenated.

The path that the blood follows from the right side of the heart to and through the lungs and back to the left side of the heart is called the *pulmonary circulation*. The function of the pulmonary circulation is to pump blood through the lungs in order to pick up oxygen and get rid of carbon dioxide. Oxygen diffuses from the lungs into the blood for delivery to the tissues, whereas carbon dioxide diffuses from the blood into the lungs for excretion.

The left heart receives the oxygenated blood from the lungs and pumps it to all the organs of the body. The left heart is colored red because it contains oxygenated blood. The path that the blood follows from the left heart to all the organs of the body and back to the right heart is called the *systemic circulation*. The systemic circulation is the larger of the two circulations.

? Re-Think

1. Why are the two circulations color-coded red and blue?
2. What is the difference between the pulmonary and systemic circulations?

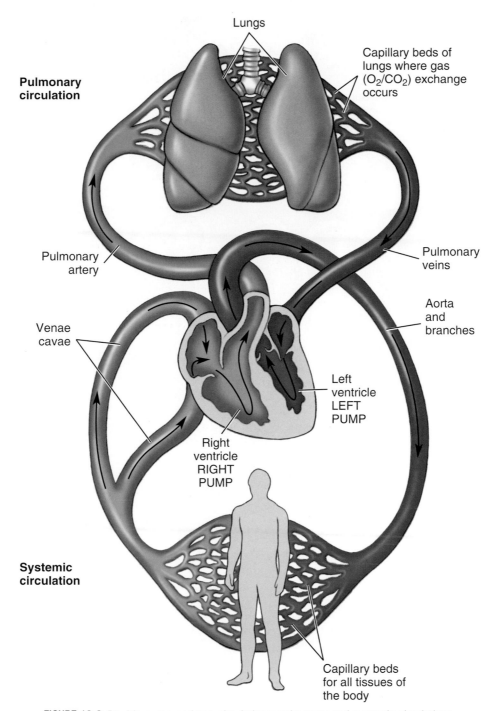

Pulmonary circulation

Lungs

Capillary beds of lungs where gas (O$_2$/CO$_2$) exchange occurs

Pulmonary artery

Pulmonary veins

Venae cavae

Aorta and branches

Left ventricle LEFT PUMP

Right ventricle RIGHT PUMP

Systemic circulation

Capillary beds for all tissues of the body

FIGURE 16-3 Double pump and two circulations: pulmonary and systemic circulations.

THE HEART'S CHAMBERS AND GREAT VESSELS

The heart has four chambers: two atria and two ventricles (Figure 16-4). The atria (sing., **atrium**) are the upper chambers and receive the blood into the heart; the **ventricles** (VEN-tri-kuls) are the lower chambers and pump blood out of the heart. The right and left hearts are separated from one another by two septa (sing., septum). The interatrial septum separates the two atria; the interventricular septum separates the two ventricles. Note the color coding. All structures that carry unoxygenated blood (right heart) are colored blue. All structures (left heart) that carry oxygenated blood are colored red.

RIGHT ATRIUM

The right atrium is a thin-walled cavity that receives unoxygenated blood from the superior and inferior venae cavae. The superior vena cava collects blood from the head and upper body region, whereas the inferior vena cava receives blood from the lower part of the body.

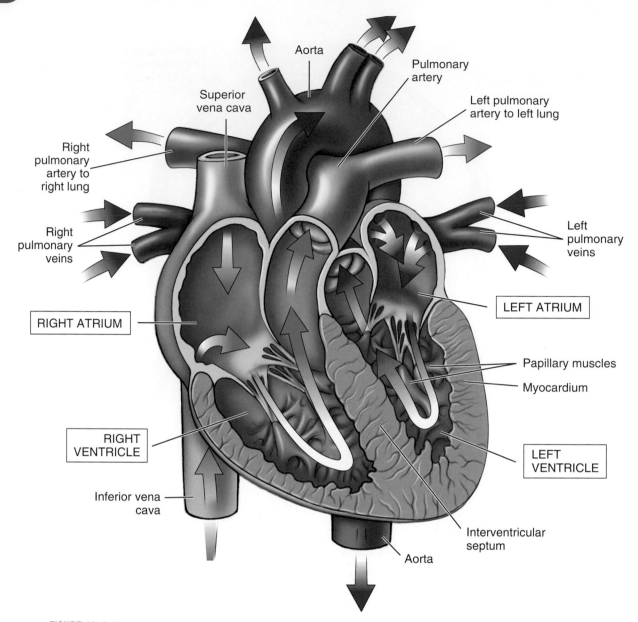

FIGURE 16-4 Chambers of the heart and the great vessels. The *arrows* indicate the blood flow through the heart.

RIGHT VENTRICLE

The right ventricle receives unoxygenated blood from the right atrium. The primary function of the right ventricle is to pump blood through the pulmonary arteries to the lungs.

LEFT ATRIUM

The left atrium is a thin-walled cavity that receives oxygenated blood from the lungs through four pulmonary veins.

LEFT VENTRICLE

The left ventricle receives oxygenated blood from the left atrium. The primary function of the left ventricle

is to pump blood into the systemic circulation. Blood leaves the left ventricle through the aorta, the largest artery of the body. Note the thickness of the myocardial layer of the ventricles as compared with the thinner atrial muscle. The thick muscle is needed to create enough force to pump blood out of the heart. Note also that the left ventricular myocardium is thicker than the right ventricular myocardium. This difference is the result of the greater amount of force required to pump blood into the systemic circulation (aorta).

As noted, the thickness of the myocardium reflects the amount of work performed by the myocardium. If a ventricle is forced to overwork, it will eventually enlarge—a condition called *ventricular hypertrophy*. For example, a chronically hypertensive (high blood pressure) person generally develops left ventricular

Bishop's mitre

Semilunar valves

Pulmonic valve

Aortic valve

Atrioventricular valves

Tricuspid valve

Chordae tendineae

Bicuspid (mitral valve)

FIGURE 16-5 Valves of the heart: semilunar valves and atrioventricular valves.

hypertrophy. Why? The high blood pressure in the aorta makes it more difficult for the left ventricle to pump blood into the aorta. The left ventricle works harder and therefore enlarges, or hypertrophies. If the blood pressure is not lowered, the left ventricle will eventually weaken and fail as a pump. For the same reason, a person with pulmonary artery hypertension develops right ventricular hypertrophy and right heart failure.

GREAT VESSELS OF THE HEART

The large blood vessels attached to the heart are called the *great vessels*. They include the superior and inferior venae cavae, pulmonary artery, four pulmonary veins, and the aorta.

2+2 Sum It Up!

The heart, a hollow muscular organ that pumps blood, is located within the mediastinum of the thoracic cavity. The heart has three layers: endocardium, myocardium, and epicardium. It is supported and anchored by a slinglike pericardium. The heart is a double pump; the right heart pumps blood to the pulmonary circulation, and the left heart pumps blood to the systemic circulation. The heart has four chambers: two atria and two ventricles. The upper atria are receiving chambers, and the lower ventricles are pumping chambers. The great blood vessels carry blood to and from the heart.

HEART VALVES

The heart has four valves (Figure 16-5). The purpose of the heart valves is to keep the blood flowing in a forward direction. The valves lie at the entrance and exit of the ventricles. Two of the valves are called **atrioventricular valves** (AV valves), which are located between the atria and the ventricles. Blood flows from the atria through the AV valves into the ventricles. AV valves, which look like basketball nets, are entrance valves because they allow blood to enter the ventricles.

The other two valves are classified as **semilunar valves**, so-named because the cusps of the valves resemble a half-moon (*semi-* means "half," *lunar* means "moon"). The semilunar valves control the outflow of blood from the right and left ventricles and are therefore exit valves.

ATRIOVENTRICULAR VALVES

The AV valves are located between the atria and the ventricles on each side of the heart. The AV valves have cusps, or flaps (see Figure 16-5). When the ventricles are relaxed, the cusps hang loosely within the ventricles; in this position, the valves are open and permit the flow of blood from the atria into the ventricles.

What closes the AV valves? Pressure! When the ventricles contract, the heart muscle compresses or squeezes the blood in the ventricles. The blood then gets behind and pushes the cusps upward toward the atria, into a closed position. The closed AV valves prevent the backward flow of blood from the ventricles to the atria.

Why are the cusps not pushed completely through the openings, into the atria, as the pressures within the ventricles increase during muscle contraction? The cusps are attached to the ventricular wall by tough fibrous bands of tissue called **chordae tendineae** (KOR-day ten-din-EE-ay). The chordae tendineae, in turn, are attached to papillary muscles in the ventricular walls. As blood pushes the cusps into a closed position, the papillary muscles contract, pulling on the chordae tendineae. The stretched chordae tendineae hold on to the cusps and prevent them from "blowing" through into the atria, like an inside-out umbrella.

The right AV valve is located between the right atrium and the right ventricle. The right AV valve is called the **tricuspid valve** because it has three cusps. When the tricuspid valve is open, blood flows from the right atrium into the right ventricle. When the right ventricle contracts, however, the tricuspid valve closes and prevents blood from flowing back into the right atrium. The valve ensures a forward flow of blood.

The left AV valve is located between the left atrium and the left ventricle. The left AV valve is called the **bicuspid valve** because it has two cusps. It is also known as the **mitral valve** because it resembles a bishop's mitre—a hat with two flaps. When the mitral valve is open, blood flows from the left atrium into the left ventricle. When the left ventricle contracts, the mitral valve closes and prevents the flow of blood from the left ventricle back into the left atrium.

SEMILUNAR VALVES

The two semilunar valves (exit valves) are the pulmonic and aortic semilunar valves (see Figure 16-5).

PULMONIC VALVE

The pulmonic semilunar valve is also called the *right semilunar valve*. It is located between the right

ventricle and the pulmonary artery. When the right ventricle relaxes, the valve is in a closed position. When the right ventricle contracts, thus increasing intraventricular pressure, blood from the ventricle forces the pulmonic valve open. Blood then flows into the pulmonary artery, the large vessel that carries the blood from the right ventricle to the lungs. When the right ventricle relaxes, the pulmonic valve snaps closed and prevents any blood from returning to the right ventricle from the pulmonary artery.

AORTIC VALVE

The aortic semilunar valve or the left semilunar valve is located between the left ventricle and the aorta. When the left ventricle relaxes, the valve is in a closed position. When the left ventricle contracts, thus increasing intraventricular pressure, blood from the ventricles forces the **aortic valve** open and flows into the aorta. When the left ventricle relaxes, the aortic valve snaps closed and prevents any backflow of blood from the aorta into the ventricle.

How and why do the semilunar valves close? Pressure! The semilunar valves close when the pressure in the pulmonary artery and the aorta becomes greater than the pressure in the relaxed ventricles. The blood in these large blood vessels gets behind the cusps of the valves, snapping them closed. The closed semilunar valves prevent the backward flow of blood from the pulmonary artery and aorta into the ventricles. To repeat: Valves open and close in response to the changing pressures within the heart chambers.

Valves are sometimes defective; they can become narrow or incompetent. Narrowing of the valve is called *stenosis*. A stenotic valve makes it difficult for a heart chamber to force blood through the stenosed valve, thereby increasing the work of the pumping chamber. Thus, aortic valve stenosis increases the work of the left ventricle, causing left ventricular hypertrophy and failure. What happens when a heart valve becomes leaky? A leaky, or incompetent, valve allows blood to leak back into the chamber from which it has just been pumped. For example, an incompetent aortic valve allows blood that has been pumped into the aorta to leak back into the left ventricle. The left ventricle must then pump the same blood again. Over time, stenotic and leaky valves damage the heart.

? Re-Think

1. List and locate the atrioventricular valves.
2. List and locate the semilunar valves.
3. Explain the reason for the following: When the ventricles contract, the AV valves close and the semilunar valves open.

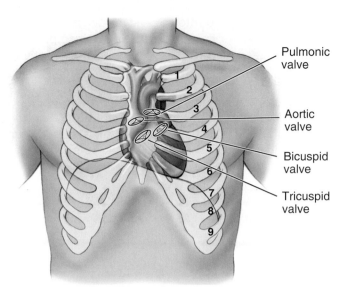

FIGURE 16-6 Areas on the precordium where valve sounds are best heard by stethoscope.

HEART SOUNDS

The heart sounds ("lubb-dupp, lubb-dupp") are made by the vibrations caused by the closure of the valves. When valves become faulty, the heart sounds change. Abnormal heart sounds are called *murmurs*.

The heart sounds can be heard through a stethoscope placed over the chest wall (Figure 16-6). The first heart sound (the "lubb") is called S_1. S_1 is caused by the closure of the AV valves at the beginning of ventricular contraction; it is best heard over the apex. The second heart sound (the "dupp") is called S_2. S_2 is caused by the closure of the semilunar valves at the beginning of ventricular relaxation. S_2 can be heard best at the base of the heart. Listening to S_1 and S_2 is like the sound made by drumming two fingers on a table. Sometimes extra sounds (called S_3 and S_4) can be heard; they are due to vibrations caused by the rapid flow of blood into the ventricles. When both S_3 and S_4 occur, a "gallop rhythm" is heard, which sounds like a galloping horse.

2+2 Sum It Up!

The purpose of the heart valves is to keep blood flowing forward. There are four heart valves. The two atrioventricular valves are the tricuspid (right heart) and the bicuspid or mitral valves (left heart). The two semilunar valves are the pulmonic (right heart) and aortic (left heart) semilunar valves. The heart sounds ("lubb dupp") are caused by the closure of the valves.

PATHWAY OF BLOOD FLOW THROUGH THE HEART

The arrows in Figure 16-4 indicate the pathway of blood as it flows through the heart. Unoxygenated blood enters the right atrium from the superior and inferior venae cavae. The blood flows through the tricuspid valve into the right ventricle. From the right ventricle, the blood flows through the pulmonic valve into the pulmonary artery. The pulmonary artery branches into the right and left pulmonary arteries. The right and left pulmonary arteries carry unoxygenated blood to the right and left lungs for gas exchange. The blood releases carbon dioxide as waste and picks up a fresh supply of oxygen. Note the blue color coding of the right heart structures.

The oxygenated blood flows through four pulmonary veins from the lungs into the left atrium. From the left atrium, the blood flows through the bicuspid, or mitral, valve into the left ventricle. Left ventricular contraction forces blood through the aortic valve into the aorta for distribution to the systemic circulation. The pathway of blood flow through the heart and pulmonary circulation is summarized in Figure 16-7.

BLOOD FLOW AND SHUNTS

Normally, blood flows through four separate chambers, from the right side of the heart to the lungs and back to the left side of the heart. Congenital heart defects often detour, or shunt, blood so that the normal pathway is disrupted. Let's see how this happens. Keep in mind the following points as we analyze the effects of shunts:

- The right and left hearts are separated by the interatrial and interventricular septa.
- Blood flows in response to a pressure gradient (from high pressure to low pressure).
- Pressure is higher in the left heart than in the right heart.
- Blood in the left heart is oxygenated and is bright red, whereas blood in the right heart is unoxygenated and is bluish-red.

SHUNTS

A shunt is a passageway that diverts blood from its normal pathway. There are two types of shunts: a left-to-right shunt and a right-to-left shunt.

Left-to-Right Shunt

A left-to-right shunt diverts blood from the left heart to the right heart; it can be illustrated by a child with a hole in the interventricular septum. The ventricular septal defect (VSD) causes the left ventricle to do two things. It pumps blood into the aorta; it also pumps blood into the right ventricle through the hole in the septum. Because blood is shunted from the left heart to the right heart, it is called a *left-to-right shunt*. The child is acyanotic (not cyanotic) because the left ventricle is pumping oxygenated blood to the systemic circulation. A VSD is thus described as a left-to-right shunt that is acyanotic.

Right-to-Left Shunt

A right-to-left shunt diverts blood from the right to the left heart; it is illustrated by a child who has a VSD and

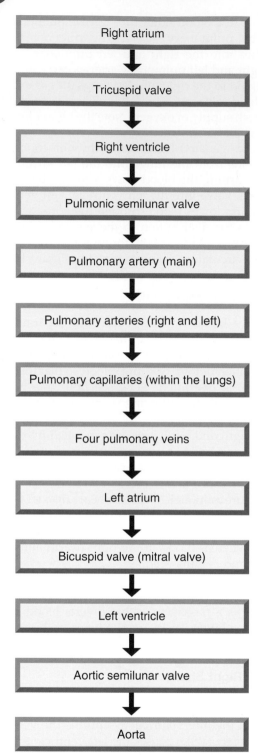

Right atrium

↓

Tricuspid valve

↓

Right ventricle

↓

Pulmonic semilunar valve

↓

Pulmonary artery (main)

↓

Pulmonary arteries (right and left)

↓

Pulmonary capillaries (within the lungs)

↓

Four pulmonary veins

↓

Left atrium

↓

Bicuspid valve (mitral valve)

↓

Left ventricle

↓

Aortic semilunar valve

↓

Aorta

FIGURE 16-7 Blood flow through the heart and pulmonary circulation.

a stenotic (narrowed) pulmonic semilunar valve. Pulmonary valve stenosis increases the pressure within the right ventricle. The elevated right ventricular pressure pumps blood into the left ventricle through the ventricular septal defect. Because blood is shunted from the right heart to the left heart, it is called a *right-to-left shunt*. Note that the left ventricle now contains unoxygenated blood. The left ventricle pumps

unoxygenated blood into the systemic circulation and the child appears cyanotic. This is an example of a cyanotic right-to-left shunt. A VSD can be acyanotic or cyanotic, depending on other complicating factors, such as pulmonic semilunar valve stenosis.

Numerous congenital heart defects result in shunting of blood. You must be able to analyze the defect(s) in terms of the direction (pressure gradients) of the shunt and its implication for blood oxygen content (oxygen saturation).

❓ Re-Think

1. Describe the path of the flow of blood through the right heart. Describe the path of the flow of blood through the left heart.
2. Describe the path of the flow of blood in a child with a ventricular septal defect (VSD).

BLOOD SUPPLY TO THE MYOCARDIUM

Although blood constantly flows through the chambers of the heart, this blood does not nourish the myocardium. The blood supply that nourishes and oxygenates the myocardium is provided by the coronary arteries (Figure 16-8). The arteries supplying the myocardium are called **coronary arteries** because they resemble a crown encircling the heart. The coronary arteries arise from the base of the aorta, just distal to the aortic semilunar valve.

The two main coronary arteries are the left and right coronary arteries. The right coronary artery nourishes the right side of the heart, especially the right ventricle. It also supplies blood to the parts of the electrical conduction system, including the sinoatrial (SA) node and the atrioventricular (AV) node. These nodes are important in establishing the normal heart rate and rhythm and will be described more fully later in the chapter. The left coronary artery branches into the left anterior descending (LAD) artery and the circumflex artery. These arteries carry blood to the left side of the heart, especially the left ventricular wall and interventricular septum. Small branches of the right and left coronary arteries fuse, forming interconnections that help maintain an adequate blood supply to the myocardium, despite pressure fluctuations within the heart. The coronary veins collect the blood that nourishes the myocardium. The coronary veins carry the blood to the coronary sinus, which empties the blood into the right atrium.

Coronary blood flow has three important characteristics:

- Coronary blood flow can increase. The heart must have a constant supply of oxygenated blood. Under resting conditions, the heart muscle removes almost all the oxygen from the blood flowing through the coronary arteries. Thus, if the heart needs more oxygen, coronary arteries dilate and blood flow increases. With exertion, coronary blood flow

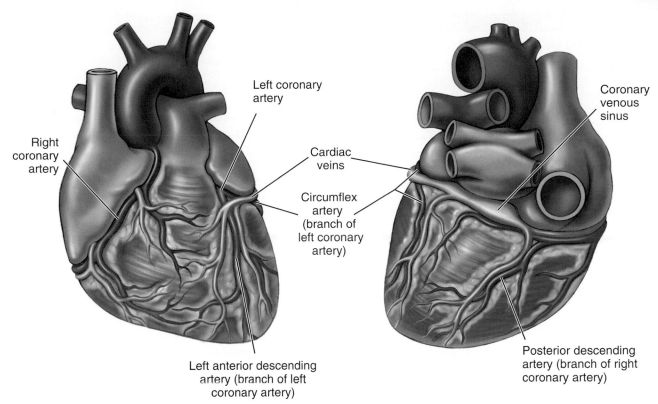

FIGURE 16-8 Blood supply to the myocardium: coronary blood vessels.

can increase up to nine times in the normal heart. However, coronary arteries that have severe fatty plaque buildup are usually maximally dilated at rest. With exertion, coronary blood flow cannot increase and the myocardium experiences oxygen deprivation. Thus, patients with coronary artery disease will often experience pain (angina) with exertion.

- Coronary blood flow is greatest during myocardial relaxation. Why? Because contraction of the myocardium externally compresses or squeezes the coronary arteries, thereby cutting off blood flow. When the heart muscle relaxes, the coronary arteries open, thereby restoring blood flow. When the relaxation phase is shortened, as in a "racing heart," coronary blood flow decreases and the myocardial cells may experience signs of oxygen deprivation, causing chest pain (angina).
- Coronary arteries can form anastomoses, or multiple connections between the arteries. An anastomosis allows blood to flow around an artery that is blocked. Additional collateral blood vessels develop in response to chronic diminished coronary blood flow, as often occurs with aging and chronic coronary artery disease. For this reason, older persons often experience less myocardial damage from a heart attack than younger persons.

> **? Re-Think**
>
> 1. Why is coronary blood flow highest when the myocardium is relaxed?
> 2. Explain why a rapid heart rate can cause chest pain.

ISCHEMIA AND INFARCTION

If coronary blood flow diminishes, the myocardium experiences oxygen deprivation (ischemia) and soon informs its owner of the situation. For example, a coronary artery may become partially occluded by fatty plaque or blood vessel spasm, thereby diminishing coronary blood flow. The person experiences chest pain that often radiates to the left shoulder and down the left arm into the fingers (referred pain). "Pain at the pump"? Think angina. Angina is often relieved by rest and the administration of drugs such as nitroglycerin and beta-adrenergic blockers that decrease the work of the heart.

Do You Know...

About Balloons and CABGs as Treatment for Coronary Artery Disease?

Angina is usually caused by the accumulation of fatty plaque within the coronary arteries. Coronary artery occlusion is often treated with balloon therapy. A deflated balloon is inserted into the coronary artery. It is then inflated against the fatty plaque, flattening the plaque against the arterial wall and restoring coronary blood flow. A stent is then inserted to maintain the opening of the coronary vessel. A stent is a hollow, wire mesh cylinder that looks like a tiny Slinky. Improved cardiac blood flow improves myocardial oxygenation, reduces chest pain, and prevents myocardial damage. A patient may not be a suitable candidate for balloon angioplasty and stent; instead, he or she may require a CABG (pronounced like the vegetable, cabbage). CABG refers to a *coronary artery bypass graft*, whereby the surgeon bypasses the obstructions in the coronary vessels with donor blood vessels.

Sometimes, the coronary artery occlusion worsens when a platelet-containing fatty plaque ruptures and completely blocks coronary blood flow. The oxygen-deprived myocardial cells die, causing a myocardial infarction (MI), or heart attack. A man having a heart attack often experiences nausea and vomiting, diaphoresis (profuse sweating), and severe crushing chest pain. With a fist clenched over his heart, he may complain that the pain feels as though an elephant is sitting on his chest. Occlusion of the left anterior descending artery (LAD) is particularly devastating because it oxygenates so much of left ventricle. For this reason occlusion of the LAD is called the "widow maker."

Older people and women who experience an MI may present a very different clinical picture. For example, many do not experience crushing chest pain and diaphoresis. They often complain of fatigue and digestive symptoms, such as heartburn and upset stomach. Depending on the severity and location of the infarction, the person may recover uneventfully or experience a lethal electrical disturbance (dysrhythmia), cardiogenic shock, or heart failure. Time to treatment is crucial! Cardiologists have a saying: "Time is muscle." The faster the intervention, the less myocardial damage is sustained.

CARDIAC ENZYMES AND LEAKY CELLS

The dead myocardial cells leak enzymes into the blood, causing plasma elevations of cardiac enzymes such as creatine phosphokinase (CPK), aspartate aminotransferase (AST), and lactic dehydrogenase (LDH). A regulator myocardial protein, called *troponin*, also leaks out of the necrotic myocardium into the blood. Thus, plasma elevations of CPK, AST, LDH, and troponin are indicative of MI. The leaked enzymes thus provide a valuable diagnostic tool for heart attacks.

2+2 Sum It Up!

Blood flows from the right atrium to the right ventricle, where it is pumped to the lungs for oxygenation (pulmonary circulation). Oxygenated blood returns to the left atrium and then to the left ventricle where it is pumped into the aorta and systemic circulation. Shunts, usually congenital, divert the path of blood flow through the heart. The myocardium (pump) is nourished by the left and right coronary arteries. Coronary blood flow must be maintained if the heart is to function normally. Coronary blood flow is greatest during ventricular relaxation. Occlusion of the coronary arteries is a major cause of disability and death.

CARDIAC CONDUCTION SYSTEM

How does the heart know when to contract (pump) and when to relax? The heart's conduction system initiates an electrical signal and then moves that signal along a special pathway through the heart. The cardiac conduction system not only provides the stimulus (cardiac impulse) for muscle contraction, but also coordinates the pumping activity of the atria and ventricles. First, both atria must contract, forcing blood into the relaxed ventricles. Then, the ventricles contract, forcing blood out of the heart. The cardiac conduction system gets it going and keeps it organized!

PARTS OF THE CARDIAC CONDUCTION SYSTEM

The conduction system is located within the walls and septum of the heart. The conduction system consists of the following structures: the sinoatrial node, the atrial conducting fibers, the atrioventricular node, and the His-Purkinje system (Figure 16-9).

SINOATRIAL NODE

The sinoatrial (SA) node is located in the upper posterior wall of the right atrium. An electrical signal originates within the SA node. The electrical signal is called the *action potential* or the *cardiac impulse*. In this chapter, we use the term *cardiac impulse*.

The SA node fires a cardiac impulse 60 to 100 times per minute (average, 72 times/min). Because the firing of the SA node sets the rate at which the heart beats, or contracts and relaxes, the SA node is called the *pacemaker* of the heart. The heart rate is set by this pacemaker, just as the speed of a race is set by the pace car.

Pace car

FIGURE 16-9 Conduction system of the heart.

ATRIAL CONDUCTING FIBERS

The cardiac impulse spreads from the SA node through both atria along the atrial conducting fibers. The signal also spreads to the AV node.

ATRIOVENTRICULAR NODE

The atrioventricular (AV) node is located in the floor of the right atrium, near the interatrial septum. The purpose of the AV node is twofold: (1) it acts as a path for the cardiac impulse to travel from the atrial conducting fibers into the ventricular bundle of His, and (2) the AV node slows the cardiac impulse as it moves through the AV node into the bundle of His.

The slowing of the cardiac impulse by the AV node is important because it delays ventricular activation and allows the relaxed ventricle time to fill with blood during atrial contraction.

NOTE: Do not confuse the AV node with the AV valve.

HIS-PURKINJE SYSTEM

The cardiac impulse next enters the bundle of His, specialized conduction tissue located in the interventricular septum. The bundle of His divides into two branches: the right and left bundle branches. These branches send out numerous long fibers called **Purkinje fibers**. Purkinje (pur-KIN-jee) fibers are distributed throughout the ventricular myocardium. Purkinje fibers conduct the cardiac impulse very rapidly throughout the ventricles, thereby ensuring a coordinated contraction of both ventricles. The pathway followed by the cardiac impulse is summarized in Figure 16-10. Be sure you can trace the path of the cardiac impulse from its origin, the SA node, to its destination, the Purkinje fibers.

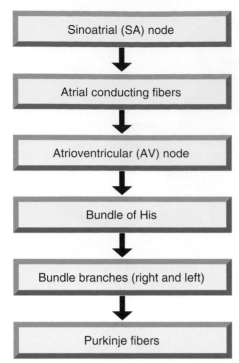

FIGURE 16-10 Pathway followed by a cardiac impulse.

AUTOMATICITY AND RHYTHMICITY

Your heart has automaticity and rhythmicity. Automaticity refers to the ability of cardiac pacemaker cells to generate their own electrical signal with no help from extrinsic nerves coming from the central nervous system. The signal arises automatically (see the "Ramp It Up!" box on Pacemaker Cells). Because cardiac tissue fires a cardiac impulse regularly, the heart is said to have rhythmicity. Feel the rhythmicity of your heart rate at the radial (wrist) pulse.

NORMAL, SLOW, AND SLOWER

Not all pacemaker cells fire at the same rate. The SA node is *the* pacemaker of the heart; it sets the heart rate between 60 and 100 beats/min. There are many other pacemaker cells within the heart, but they fire at a slower rate. For example, when the SA node fails to function as a pacemaker, the AV takes over and fires at a slower rate of 40 to 60 beats/min. Sometimes the ventricles assume the pacemaker role and fire at a much slower rate of 30 to 40 beats/min. Impaired pacemaker activity often requires the insertion of an artificial pacemaker.

At times, the rhythm of the heart is disturbed; the heart is then said to be dysrhythmic (difficulty with rhythm). Some dysrhythmias are relatively harmless; others are life threatening and demand immediate attention. For example, ventricular fibrillation is a life-threatening dysrhythmia because it causes the ventricular myocardium to fibrillate. A fibrillating muscle merely quivers and is unable to contract and pump

blood. Dysrhythmias that are caused by excess electrical activity are called *tachydysrhythmias*, whereas dysrhythmias characterized by diminished electrical activity are called *bradydysrhythmias*.

? Re-Think

1. Trace the electrical signal (cardiac impulse) from its origin to the ventricles.
2. Why is it important that the AV node slows the conduction of the cardiac impulse from the atria to the ventricles?
3. What happens if the AV nodal rate exceeds the rate of the SA node?

ELECTROCARDIOGRAM

The cardiac impulse that stimulates muscle contraction is an electrical signal. The entire electrical activity of the heart is measured by placing electrodes on the surface of the chest and attaching the electrodes to a recording device. The record of these electrical signals is called an *electrocardiogram* (ECG) (Figure 16-11).

The components of the ECG include a P wave, a QRS complex, and a T wave. The P wave reflects the electrical activity associated with atrial depolarization.

FIGURE 16-11 Electrocardiogram (ECG).

Depolarization precedes and triggers contraction of the heart muscle. (See Chapter 10 for a review of polarization, depolarization, and repolarization.) The QRS complex reflects the electrical activity associated with ventricular depolarization. The T wave reflects the electrical activity associated with ventricular repolarization.

In addition to identifying areas of depolarization and repolarization, the P, QRS, and T deflections (waves) of the ECG provide other useful information. For example, the P-R interval represents the time it takes for the cardiac impulse to travel from the atria (P wave) to the ventricles (QRS complex). Other measurements include the width of the QRS complex and the length of the S-T interval. Normal sinus rhythm (NSR) means that the ECG appears normal and that the impulse originates in the SA node. If the electrical signal originates outside of the SA node, it is referred to as *ectopic*.

Note that the ECG is recorded on special graph paper that allows electrical events to be timed. The clinician can determine whether the electrical signals are moving too fast, too slow, or generating an irregular pattern.

Ramp It Up!

Panel A: Nerve action potential

Panel B: SA node action potential

Pacemaker Cells

What is a pacemaker cell? This is best understood by first comparing pacemaker cells with the nerve action potential illustrated in Panel A.

Panel A shows a nerve action potential. The nerve action has a resting membrane potential of −90 mV, reflecting the internal negativity of the cell. When the nerve cell is stimulated, the cell membrane depolarizes to a point called the *threshold potential* (−65 mV). When the threshold potential is reached, the cell fires an action potential; it depolarizes to +20 mV and then very quickly returns to its resting state (repolarization). The cell does not fire another action potential until stimulated again.

Panel B shows the action potential of the SA node (pacemaker) cell. The SA node does not have a stable resting membrane potential (RMP); the cell momentarily rests at −60 mV. The membrane immediately and spontaneously depolarizes to its threshold potential (−40 mV) and fires an action potential. The important term is *spontaneous depolarization*. The slope of the spontaneous depolarization is called the *pacemaker potential*. Repolarization resets the action potential to −60 mV. The spontaneous depolarization immediately begins again, thereby firing a second action potential. Note that a pacemaker cell is not stimulated to fire an action potential (like the nerve cell)—it fires "on its own."

Can the rate of spontaneous depolarization change?

Yes. The faster the rate of spontaneous depolarization, the faster the heart rate. The slower the rate of spontaneous depolarization, the slower the heart rate. Several factors affect the rate of spontaneous depolarization. First, autonomic nerve stimulation affects the rate of spontaneous depolarization. Sympathetic nerve stimulation increases the rate of spontaneous depolarization, thereby increasing heart rate. Excessive sympathetic stimulation can cause tachycardia and tachydysrhythmias. Parasympathetic or vagal simulation slows the rate of spontaneous depolarization, thereby slowing heart rate. Intense vagal discharge, in fact, can cause bradycardia and heart block, and even cardiac standstill. Hormones and drugs also affect the rates of depolarization.

Continued

Ramp It Up!—cont'd

Panel C: SA and AV node action potentials

SA node

AV node

Membrane potential (mV)

0

Threshold potential

Pacemaker potential

Pacemaker potential

−50

−100

0   0.15   0.30   0.45

Time (sec)

Panel C shows a comparison of the action potential of the SA and AV nodes. Note that both the SA and AV nodes can both spontaneously depolarize to threshold potential. Thus, both cells have pacemaker capabilities. The SA node, however, is *the* pacemaker. Why? The SA node spontaneously depolarizes at a faster rate than the AV node. Once the SA node depolarizes, it sends an electrical signal throughout the conduction system of the heart, including the AV node. Consequently, all cells, including the AV node, must repolarize and thus reset to the RMP. Why isn't the AV node the pacemaker? The SA depolarizes at a faster rate.

Can the AV node ever become the pacemaker?

Yes. If the rate of SA node activity slows too much or if the rate of the AV node increases too much, the AV node can assume the role of pacemaker activity. This is called *nodal rhythm*. For example, a diseased SA node, such as in sick sinus syndrome or scarring of the conduction pathway, can seriously depress SA node activity, thereby allowing the AV to take over as pacemaker. Typically, the slower nodal rhythm generates a heart rate of 40 to 50 beats/min.

There are even pacemaker cells in the conduction tissue of the ventricles. These ventricular pacemaker cells spontaneously depolarize very slowly and therefore rarely function as the pacemaker. However, in complete heart block, a condition in which no electrical signal crosses the AV node into the His-Purkinje system, the ventricular pacemaker cells take over as the pacemaker, typically generating a heart rate of 30 to 40 beats/min. This excessively slow heart rate decreases cardiac output and requires the implantation of an artificial pacemaker. An artificial pacemaker "drives" the ventricles at a higher rate, thereby increasing cardiac output.

 Sum It Up!

Heart muscle contracts in response to an electrical signal called the *cardiac impulse,* which spreads throughout the heart, coordinating cardiac muscle contraction. The cardiac impulse normally arises within the SA node and spreads throughout both atria over specialized conduction tissue. The cardiac impulse then enters the AV node, where it is momentarily delayed before entering the His-Purkinje system in the ventricles. Cardiac conduction tissue displays automaticity and rhythmicity. The electrical events are recorded as the electrocardiogram (ECG).

Note: The As You Age box and the Medical Terminology and Disorders table appear in Chapter 17.

Get Ready for Exams!

Summary Outline

The heart is a four-chambered pump that delivers blood to the pulmonic and systemic circulations.

I. Function, Location, and Size of the Heart
   A. The heart (size of a fist) is located in the mediastinum, toward the left side of the sternum.
   B. Located between the second rib and fifth intercostal space

   C. The heart pumps blood throughout the body, delivering oxygen and nutrients and picking up waste.

II. The Heart's Layers and Covering
   A. The heart has three layers: endocardium, myocardium, and epicardium.
   B. The heart is supported by a slinglike pericardium.
   C. Two layers of the pericardium form the pericardial space (contains serous fluid).

III. **A Double Pump and Two Circulations**
   A. The right heart pumps blood to the lungs for oxygenation (called the *pulmonary circulation*).
   B. The left heart pumps blood throughout the rest of the body (called the *systemic circulation*).

IV. **The Heart's Chambers and Great Vessels**
   A. The heart has four chambers: two atria and two ventricles.
   B. The atria receive the blood and the ventricles pump the blood to the pulmonary and systemic circulations.

V. **Heart Valves**
   A. The purpose of heart valves is to keep blood flowing in a forward direction.
   B. Two atrioventricular (AV) valves are the tricuspid valve (right heart) and the bicuspid (mitral) valve (left heart).
   C. The two semilunar valves are the pulmonic valve (right heart) and the aortic valve (left heart).

VI. **Heart Sounds**
   A. The heart sounds ("lubb-dupp") are made by the vibrations caused by closure of the valves.
   B. The "lubb" (S$_1$) is caused by the closure of the AV valves at the beginning of ventricular contraction. The "dupp" (S$_2$) is caused by the closure of the semilunar valves at the beginning of ventricular relaxation.

VII. **Pathway: Blood Flow through the Heart**
   A. The right heart receives blood from the venae cavae and pumps it to the lungs for oxygenation. The left heart receives oxygenated blood from the lungs and pumps it to the systemic circulation.
   B. Blood flow through the heart is summarized in the flow chart (see Figure 16-7).
   C. Shunts alter the path of blood flow through the heart.

VIII. **Blood Supply to the Myocardium**
   A. The left and right coronary arteries supply the myocardium with oxygen and nutrients.
   B. The coronary veins drain the unoxygenated blood and empty it into the coronary sinus, which empties into the right atrium.

IX. **Cardiac Conduction System**
   A. The SA node generates an electrical signal (cardiac impulse) that moves throughout the heart in a coordinated way. The electrical signal causes the myocardium to contract.
   B. The pathway followed by the cardiac impulse is summarized in Figure 16-10.
   C. Cardiac muscle displays automaticity and rhythmicity.
   D. The SA node is the pacemaker of the heart. Pacemaker cells throughout the heart fire at different rates: normal, slow, and slower.
   E. The electrical activity of cardiac muscle is recorded as an electrocardiogram.

Review Your Knowledge

Matching: Structures of the Heart
Directions: Match the following words with their descriptions below. Some words may be used more than once.
a. left ventricle
b. coronary arteries
c. right atrium
d. left atrium
e. right ventricle
f. myocardium
g. pericardium
h. precordium

1. ___ Slinglike structure that supports the heart
2. ___ Delivers oxygenated blood to the myocardium
3. ___ Layer of the heart that contains actin and myosin; arranged in sarcomeres
4. ___ Chamber that receives unoxygenated blood from the venae cavae
5. ___ Chamber that receives oxygenated blood from the four pulmonary veins
6. ___ Chamber that pumps blood into the aorta
7. ___ Chamber that has the thickest myocardium
8. ___ Chamber that pumps blood into the pulmonary artery
9. ___ The left ventricle receives oxygenated blood from this chamber.
10. ___ Refers to the area of the chest that overlies the heart

Matching: Valves
Directions: Match the following words with their descriptions below. Some words may be used more than once.
a. aortic
b. tricuspid
c. bicuspid
d. pulmonic

1. ___ The semilunar valve through which blood exits the right ventricle
2. ___ The exit valve for the right ventricle
3. ___ The atrioventricular valve that "sees" unoxygenated blood
4. ___ The valve that is also called the mitral valve
5. ___ The semilunar valve through which blood exits the left ventricle
6. ___ The AV valve that "sees" oxygenated blood
7. ___ The AV valve located between the left atrium and left ventricle
8. ___ If "leaky," this valve allows blood to flow backward from the pulmonary artery.
9. ___ This valve is located in the right heart and does not have chordae tendineae.
10. ___ This valve is located in the left heart and has chordae tendineae.

Multiple Choice
1. Which of the following is not true of the heart?
   a. The heart is located within the mediastinum.
   b. The apex is located to the left of the sternal midline at the level of the fifth intercostal space.
   c. The base of the heart is located at the level of the second rib.
   d. The precordium is composed of cardiac muscle.

2. Which of the following is descriptive of the myocardium?
   a. Composed of contractile proteins (actin and myosin)
   b. Thicker in the ventricles than the atria
   c. Thicker in the left ventricle than the right ventricle
   d. All of the above.
3. Which of the following is the function of a valve?
   a. Regulates the direction of the flow of blood through the heart
   b. Regulates the amount of oxygen bound to hemoglobin
   c. Regulates heart rate
   d. Directs the progression of the cardiac impulse
4. Which of the following is true regarding the structures of the electrical conduction system?
   a. The AV node is the pacemaker.
   b. In normal sinus rhythm, the electrical signal arises within the SA node.
   c. The His-Purkinje system spreads the electrical signal from the right atrium to the left atrium.
   d. The purpose of the AV node is to increase the speed at which the cardiac impulse moves from the atria to the ventricles.
5. Which of the following is least true of the aortic valve?
   a. "Sees" oxygenated blood
   b. Causes left ventricular hypertrophy if the valve is stenotic
   c. Allows blood to flow from the ventricle into the pulmonary artery
   d. Classified as a semilunar valve
6. Pacemaker cells fire at a faster rate in the
   a. left coronary artery.
   b. SA node.
   c. ventricular myocardium.
   d. AV node.
7. The coronary arteries
   a. exit the aorta at a point immediately distal to the aortic semilunar valve.
   b. fill the right atrium with blood with each myocardial contraction.
   c. are color-coded blue.
   d. deliver most O_2 and nutrients while the myocardium is contracted.
8. Which of the following blood flow statements is true?
   a. Blood is pumped by the right atrium through the mitral valve.
   b. Blood is pumped by the right ventricle into the pulmonary artery.
   c. Blood is pumped by the left ventricle through the mitral valve.
   d. An incompetent or leaky tricuspid valve allows blood to flow from the pulmonary artery to the right ventricle.
9. The structure(s) that is/are color-coded red:
   a. Right ventricle
   b. Both AV valves
   c. Both semilunar valves
   d. Pulmonary veins
10. The chordae tendineae are necessary for the proper functioning of the
    a. SA node.
    b. pericardium.
    c. pulmonic semilunar valve.
    d. mitral valve.

Go Figure

1. **According to Figure 16-1**
   a. The apex (tip) of the heart is at the level of the 10th intercostal space.
   b. The apex of the heart is located left of the midsternal line.
   c. The ascending aorta is located to the right of the midsternal line.
   d. The base of the heart is located at the level of the fifth intercostal space.

2. **According to Figure 16-3**
   a. The left heart pumps blood to the lungs for oxygenation.
   b. The right heart pumps blood into the systemic circulation.
   c. The systemic circulation delivers blood to the brain, liver, feet, and digestive tract.
   d. The right heart is color-coded blue because it carries oxygenated blood.

3. **According to Figure 16-4**
   a. Pulmonary veins are color-coded red, meaning that they carry oxygenated blood.
   b. All arteries carry oxygenated blood.
   c. The venae cavae carry blood to the left side of the heart.
   d. The left side of the heart carries unoxygenated blood.

4. **According to Figures 16-5 and 16-6**
   a. All AV valves are located in the right heart.
   b. All semilunar valves are located in the left heart.
   c. Both AV valves contain cusps and are attached to papillary muscles of the ventricular wall by chordae tendineae.
   d. All valvular sounds are best heard at the second intercostal space.

5. **According to Figure 16-9**
   a. The sinoatrial node is located within the interatrial septum and is the pacemaker of the heart.
   b. The AV node is located on the cusps of the AV valves.
   c. Fast-conducting Purkinje fibers are located within the ventricular myocardium.
   d. NSR (normal sinus rhythm) implies that the electrical signal arises within the AV node and acts as pacemaker.

Function of the Heart

Key Terms

afterload (p. 331)
cardiac cycle (p. 325)
cardiac reserve (p. 329)
chronotropic effect (p. 331)
diastole (p. 325)

dromotropic effect (p. 331)
ejection fraction (p. 330)
heart failure (p. 327)
inotropic effect (p. 329)
preload (p. 330)

pulmonary edema (PE) (p. 332)
Starling's law of the heart (p. 329)
stroke volume (p. 329)
systole (p. 325)

Objective

1. Define *cardiac cycle* with respect to systole and diastole.
2. Describe the autonomic innervation of the heart, including:
   • Define *cardiac output.*
   • Describe the effect of Starling's law of the heart on myocardial contraction.
   • Describe the inotropic effect on myocardial contraction.
   • Explain how changes in heart rate and/or stroke volume change cardiac output.

3. Define specific clinical vocabulary used to describe cardiac function, including:
   • Define *preload* (end diastolic volume) and explain how it affects cardiac output.
   • Define *afterload* and identify the major factor that determines afterload.
4. Define *heart failure* and differentiate between right-sided and left-sided heart failure.

The heart functions as a pump that supplies blood to every cell in the body. Moreover, the heart is an adaptable pump. For example, the heart alters its pumping activity to meet the demands of day-to-day physiological functions such as eating, exercise, and responding to changes in environmental temperature; it also adapts to disease. How does the heart know when to beat faster or slower, or weaker or stronger? The coordinated and adaptable heart is the focus of the first part of this chapter, "The Coordinated and Adaptable Pump." The second part of this chapter, "Heart Talk," defines terminology that is commonly used in clinical situations. The third part, "The Failing Heart: When the Heart Can't Pump," describes the failing heart.

THE COORDINATED AND ADAPTABLE PUMP

CARDIAC CYCLE

The cardiac cycle is the sequence of events that occurs during one heartbeat. A cardiac cycle is a coordinated contraction and relaxation of the chambers of the heart. Contraction of the heart muscle (myocardium) is called systole (SIS-toh-lee). Contraction of the heart muscle during systole pumps blood out of a chamber. Relaxation of the myocardium is called diastole (dye-ASS-toh-lee). Blood fills a chamber during diastole.

Atrial and ventricular muscle activity is closely coordinated. For example, during atrial systole, the ventricles are in diastole. In this way, when the atria contract, they pump blood into the relaxed ventricles.

The cardiac cycle has three stages (Figure 17-1):
• *Atrial systole.* The atria contract (systole) and pump blood into the ventricles. During atrial systole, the atrioventricular (AV) valves are open and the ventricles are relaxed.
• *Ventricular systole.* At the end of atrial systole, the ventricles contract; this is called *ventricular systole.* As ventricular contractions begin, blood is forced against the AV valves, causing them to snap shut. The blood pushes the semilunar valves open, allowing blood to flow into the pulmonary artery and aorta.
• *Diastole.* For a brief period during the cardiac cycle, both the atria and the ventricles are in diastole. As the chambers relax, blood flows into the atria. Because the AV valves are open at this time, much of this blood also flows passively into the ventricles. The period of diastole therefore is a period of filling (of blood); atrial systole follows. The cycle then repeats itself.

How long does the cardiac cycle last? With a heart rate of 70 beats/min, the duration of the cardiac cycle is 0.8 second. All chambers rest for 0.4 second. As heart rate increases, the duration of the cardiac cycle

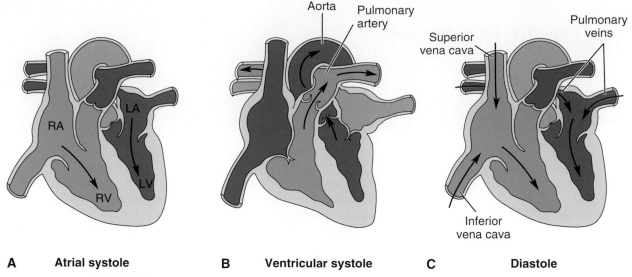

FIGURE 17-1 Stages of the cardiac cycle. **A,** Atrial systole. **B,** Ventricular systole. **C,** Diastole.

shortens. With a dramatic increase in heart rate, the period of rest (diastole) may shorten so much that cardiac function is compromised. Why? First, because of a decreased filling time, the amount of blood that enters the ventricles decreases so that less blood is pumped. Second, because coronary blood flow to the myocardium occurs during diastole, the diminished period of diastole decreases coronary blood flow.

NOTE: The valves of the heart open and close in response to pressure changes. Think of the valves during the three stages of the cardiac cycle. Are they open or closed?

? Re-Think

1. Define systole and diastole.
2. Why is it important that the atria and ventricles do not contract and relax at the same time?

2+2 Sum It Up!

The cardiac cycle is the sequence of events that occurs during one heartbeat. The cardiac cycle has three stages: atrial systole, ventricular systole, and diastole. Cardiac muscle contraction is called *systole;* cardiac muscle relaxation is called *diastole.* The duration of the cardiac cycle (resting heart) is 0.8 second; duration changes with a change in heart rate.

AUTONOMIC CONTROL OF THE HEART

The autonomic nervous system (ANS) plays an important role in coordinating and adapting cardiac function.

WHY THE AUTONOMIC NERVOUS SYSTEM?

In the previous chapter, we learned that specialized cardiac tissue displays automaticity and rhythmicity. The electrical signal, the cardiac impulse, arises within the sinoatrial (SA) node and then spreads throughout the heart, causing the heart muscle to contract. If the heart is capable of initiating its own cardiac impulse, why are the autonomic nerves needed? Although the ANS does not cause the cardiac impulse, it can affect the rate at which the cardiac impulse is fired and the speed at which it travels throughout the heart. The ANS can also make the heart muscle contract more forcefully; thus, the ANS can change the pumping activity of the heart. For example, if a person suddenly sprints down the street, his or her heart autonomically or automatically responds to the increased need for more oxygenated blood; it beats faster and stronger.

AUTONOMIC WIRING

As described in Chapter 12 the ANS has two branches: the sympathetic and parasympathetic branches. Refer to Figure 17-2 and note the autonomic wiring of the heart. Sympathetic nerves supply the SA node, AV node, and ventricular myocardium (the sarcomere represents heart muscle). Parasympathetic nerves, also called the *vagus nerve,* innervate the SA node and the AV node; there is no parasympathetic innervation of the ventricular myocardium.

AUTONOMIC FIRING

What happens when the ANS fires?

Sympathetic Stimulation

- Increases SA node activity, thus increasing heart rate
- Increases the speed at which the cardiac impulse travels from the SA node throughout the His-Purkinje system
- Increases the force of myocardial contraction

There are four clinically important points regarding excess sympathetic activity on the heart and blood vessels:

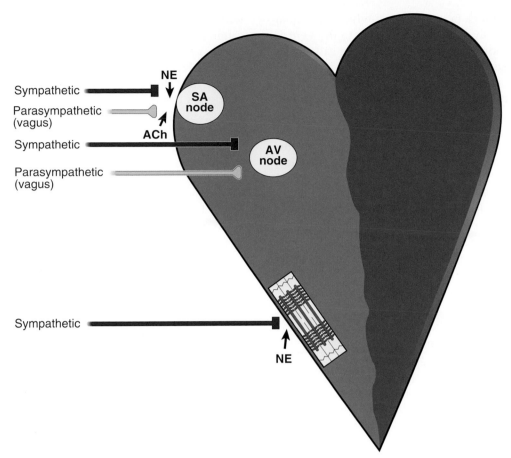

FIGURE 17-2 Autonomic innervation of the heart.

- Excess sympathetic activity produces the "fight-or-flight" response. You will often observe these symptoms (racing and pounding heart) in people who are very anxious, such as during panic attacks. The symptoms are frightening, and the person is convinced of an impending heart attack. Many trips to the emergency room (ER) are panic related.
- Excess sympathetic activity plays a key role in some disease states. For example, most of the signs and symptoms of circulatory shock are caused by excess sympathetic firing. Similarly, the progressive deterioration of patients with **heart failure** is in large measure caused by persistent sympathetic nerve stimulation. Some of the drugs used to treat heart failure are aimed at minimizing the sympathetic effects.
- Excess sympathetic activity often causes tachydysrhythmias ("fast" rhythm disorders).
- You will be giving drugs that resemble or block the effects of sympathetic activity. For example, epinephrine (Adrenalin) and dopamine increase heart rate and myocardial contractile force. Because the effects mimic stimulation of the sympathetic nervous system (SNS), these drugs are called *sympathomimetic drugs*. You will also be giving drugs that block the sympathetic effects, including beta- and alpha-adrenergic blockers.

Parasympathetic (Vagus Nerve) Stimulation
- Decreases SA node activity, thereby decreasing heart rate
- Decreases the speed at which the cardiac impulse travels from the SA node to and through the AV node
- Exerts no effect on the strength of myocardial contraction because there are no parasympathetic (vagal) fibers innervating the ventricular myocardium

There are three clinically important points about parasympathetic (vagal) nervous system activity:
- In the resting heart, vagal tone is more intense than sympathetic activity. For example, the SA node would like to fire at a rate of 90 beats/min. However, the "braking" or inhibiting effect of the vagus nerve slows SA node firing to a rate of 72 beats/min, the normal resting heart rate. If the vagus nerve were interrupted, the heart rate would increase to 90 beats/min.
- Certain conditions (heart attack) and drugs (digoxin) can cause excess vagal discharge. Excess vagal discharge causes *bradycardia* (bray-dee-KAR-dee-ah) (<60 beats/min) and increases the tendency of the heart to develop life-threatening electrical rhythm disturbances. Excess vagal discharge also slows the conduction of the cardiac impulse through the heart,

causing heart block (a condition in which the signal has difficulty traveling from the atria to the ventricles). The abnormally slow rhythms are called *bradydysrhythmias* (bray-dee-diss-RITH-mee-ahs).

- You will be giving drugs that alter the effects of vagal activity. For example, digoxin decreases the heart rate and slows the speed at which the cardiac impulse travels from the atria to the ventricle. Because the effects of digoxin "mimic" vagal stimulation, it is called a *vagomimetic* (vag-oh-mihm-EHT-ik) *drug*. Vagomimetic drugs are also called *parasympathomimetic drugs*. A drug may also produce effects that are similar to an inhibition of vagal discharge. For example, atropine is used to relieve bradycardia (following a heart attack) because it blocks the effects of vagal stimulation and increases heart rate. Because of its effects on the vagus nerve, atropine is called a *vagolytic* (vag-oh-LIT-ik) *drug*.

 Do You Know...

Why a Patient May "Brady-Down"?

Sometimes a patient may respond to fear or anxiety by an intense discharge of the parasympathetic (vagus) nerves. Vagal discharge to the heart causes a dangerous bradycardia and decline in cardiac output and blood pressure. The administration of a vagolytic drug, such as atropine, relieves the vagal effects and restores the heart rate to normal.

 Re-Think

1. If the electrical signal (cardiac impulse) arises within the SA node spontaneously, why is the heart innervated by the ANS?
2. Describe a sympathomimetic effect on heart rate and force of myocardial contraction.
3. Describe a vagomimetic effect on heart rate.

CARDIAC OUTPUT

To understand how the heart alters its pumping activity, you must understand cardiac output. Cardiac output is the amount of blood pumped by each ventricle in 1 minute. The normal cardiac output is about 5 L/min. Because the total blood volume is about 5 L (5000 mL), the entire blood volume is pumped through the heart every minute.

Two factors determine cardiac output: heart rate and stroke volume.

Cardiac Output = Heart Rate × Stroke Volume

Heart Rate

The heart rate (HR) is the number of times the heart beats each minute. The heart rate is caused by the rhythmic firing of the SA node. The normal adult resting heart rate is between 60 and 100 beats/min, with an average of 72 beats/min. Resting heart rates differ for many reasons, including size, gender, and age.

- *Size.* Size affects heart rate; generally, the larger the size, the slower the rate. Our feathered and furry friends dramatically illustrate this point. The heart rate of a hummingbird, for example, is more than 200 beats/min, whereas that of a grizzly bear is only about 30 beats/min. Why do heart rates differ? The small hummingbird has a very high metabolism and therefore requires a large amount of oxygen. The metabolism of a grizzly is much slower, requiring less oxygen. Similarly, a tiny baby has a faster heart rate than a larger adult.
- *Gender.* Women have slightly faster heart rates than men.
- *Age.* Generally, the younger the person, the faster the rate. The normal adult heart rate, for example, is 70 to 80 beats/min, whereas a normal child's heart rate is around 100 beats/min. An infant's heart rate is about 120 beats/min, and fetal heart rates are about 140 beats/min.

In addition to the variation in heart rate according to size, age, and gender, a person's heart rate can change for a variety of other reasons, such as exercise, stimulation of the autonomic nerves, hormonal influence, pathology, and various medications.

- *Exercise.* Exercise increases heart rate. Check your pulse as you exercise and note the increase; also note the decrease in pulse when you rest. At rest, the heart rate may be 65 beats/min but may increase to well over 100 beats/min with exercise.
- *Stimulation of the autonomic nerves.* Firing of the sympathetic nerve stimulates the SA node, causing an increase in heart rate. Stimulation of the parasympathetic (vagus) nerve slows the rate.
- *Hormonal influence.* Several hormones affect heart rate. Epinephrine and norepinephrine (adrenal gland hormones) and thyroid hormone increase heart rate.
- *Pathology.* Certain disease states can affect heart rate. For example, a sick SA node may fire too slowly, thereby slowing the heart too much. Vagal discharge following a heart attack (myocardial infarction) slows the rate, predisposing the heart to lethal rhythm disorders. A high fever and persistent sympathetic activity can increase heart rate, overworking the heart and causing it to fail.
- *Medications.* Certain drugs can affect heart rate. Digoxin slows heart rate, whereas epinephrine and dopamine increase heart rate. Heavy coffee drinkers often experience palpitations (the heart feels "jumpy," as if it has extra beats) because of the stimulatory effect of caffeine on the heart. Because some drugs can profoundly alter heart rate, heart rate must be monitored when these drugs are used. For example, digoxin should not be administered if the heart rate is less than 60 beats/min.

Stroke Volume

Stroke volume is the second factor affecting cardiac output. **Stroke volume** is the amount of blood pumped by the ventricle per beat. An average resting stroke volume is 60 to 80 mL/beat (about 2 ounces). At rest, the ventricles pump out only about 67% of the blood in the ventricles. Therefore, if the ventricles can be made to contract more forcefully, a greater percentage of the blood can be pumped per beat. In other words, a greater force of contraction can increase stroke volume.

Re-Think

1. What two factors determine cardiac output?
2. Explain why cardiac output can remain unchanged if heart rate changes.

How to Change Stroke Volume

The stroke volume can be altered in two ways: through Starling's law of the heart and through an inotropic effect.

Starling's Law of the Heart. **Starling's law of the heart** depends on the degree of stretch of the myocardial fibers. The greater the stretch, the stronger the force of contraction. For example, an increase in the amount of blood entering the ventricle, the venous return, causes the ventricle to stretch (Figure 17-3). Stretch increases the force of contraction, which in turn increases stroke volume. Conversely, a decrease in the amount of blood entering the ventricles causes less stretch. As a result, the force of contraction decreases, thereby decreasing stroke volume.

What is the purpose of Starling's law of the heart? It allows the heart to pump out the same amount of blood it receives. In other words, Starling's law allows the heart to match cardiac output with venous return (of blood).

Do You Know...

About Atrial Kick?

About 70% of blood flows passively from the atria into the ventricles. Atrial contraction (systole) accounts for the remaining 30%; it is called the *atrial kick*. With atrial fibrillation the contribution from atrial kick is missing and cardiac output declines. Atrial kick—it's a good thing!

Inotropic Effect. A second way to increase stroke volume is by strengthening the force of myocardial contraction without stretching the myocardial fibers. This is called a positive **inotropic** (in-o-TROH-pik) **effect.** Stimulation of the heart muscle by sympathetic nerves causes a positive inotropic effect. Certain hormones and drugs, such as epinephrine, also cause this effect. Digoxin is the most famous of the positive inotropic drugs. Some medications cause a negative inotropic effect. A negative inotropic effect is a decrease in the force of contraction, resulting in a weaker myocardial contraction. Excessive dosing with a negative inotropic agent can depress the myocardium to the point of failure.

CHANGING CARDIAC OUTPUT

Because cardiac output is determined by heart rate and stroke volume, cardiac output can be altered by changing either or both. The healthy heart can increase cardiac output four to five times the resting cardiac output; an Olympic athlete can do even better! The capacity to increase cardiac output above the resting cardiac output is called the **cardiac reserve.** A person with a diseased heart may have little cardiac reserve and therefore becomes easily fatigued with mild exercise.

FIGURE 17-3 Starling's law of the heart, matching venous return with cardiac output. **A,** A large venous return. **B,** A smaller venous return.

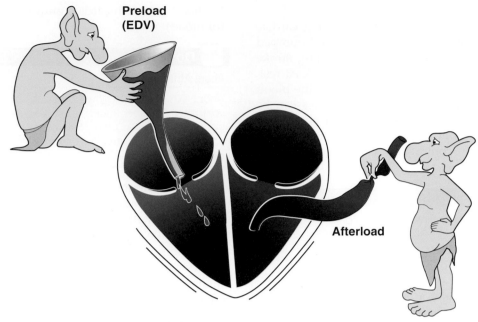

FIGURE 17-4 Preload and afterload.

? Re-Think

1. Explain how a Starling effect changes force of myocardial contraction.
2. Explain how an inotropic effect changes force of myocardial contraction.

2+2 Sum It Up!

Cardiac output is determined by multiplying heart rate by stroke volume. The heart rate is the number of times the heart beats each minute. The normal adult resting heart rate is between 60 and 100 beats/min (average, 72 beats/min). Heart rates differ for three main reasons: size, gender, and age. A person's heart rate may also change in response to exercise, stimulation of the ANS, hormonal influence, pathology, and various medications. Stroke volume is the amount of blood ejected by the ventricle in one beat. Stroke volume can be altered through Starling's law of the heart or an inotropic effect.

The following major sections, "Heart Talk" and "The Failing Heart: When the Heart Can't Pump," are clinically focused and may be omitted in nonmedical courses.

HEART TALK

HEART TALK: CLINICAL TERMS

Clinically, cardiac function is described using special vocabulary.

END-DIASTOLIC VOLUME

The end-diastolic volume (EDV) refers to the amount of blood in the ventricle at the end of its resting phase (diastole). Remember that the ventricle fills with blood during diastole. The EDV determines how much the ventricle is stretched and is the basis of Starling's law of the heart.

PRELOAD

The **preload** is the amount of blood in the ventricles at the end of diastole; this is the same as the EDV. Note in Figure 17-4 that the filling of the right heart by the funnel illustrates preload. An increased preload stretches the ventricles, causing a stronger force of contraction. The stronger contraction increases stroke volume and cardiac output. Drugs can also affect preload. For example, a drug may dilate the veins, causing blood to pool in the veins and decreasing the amount of blood returned to the heart, thus decreasing preload, stroke volume, and cardiac output. Another drug may constrict the veins; this increases blood flow to the ventricles, thereby increasing preload, stroke volume, and cardiac output.

? Re-Think

Explain why EDV, preload, and the Starling effect "make" the same point?

EJECTION FRACTION

When the ventricle contracts, it pumps about 67% of its volume (EDV); therefore, some blood remains in the ventricle. The percentage of the EDV that is pumped is called the **ejection fraction**. The ejection fraction is an indication of cardiac health. For example, a healthy heart can increase its ejection fraction to 90% with exercise. A weakened failing heart is characterized by a decrease in ejection fraction, perhaps as low as 30%.

AFTERLOAD

Afterload refers to resistance or opposition to the flow of blood. For example, for the left ventricle to pump blood into the aorta, it must push against blood that is already in the aorta. The aortic blood pressure is the resistance or the afterload. Note in Figure 17-4 that the pinched aorta represents an increased afterload, demanding that the left ventricle work harder to overcome the resistance. The pinched aorta can represent a number of clinical conditions such as aortic valve stenosis and systemic hypertension. If the person develops high blood pressure, afterload increases and the ventricle must work harder to pump blood into the aorta. Like any other muscle that overworks, the left ventricular myocardium enlarges or hypertrophies. The enlarged left ventricle will eventually fail as a pump.

What about afterload and the right ventricle? Its afterload is determined by the pressure within the pulmonary artery. If pulmonary artery pressure rises (increased afterload), the right ventricle must work harder to pump blood and therefore hypertrophies. Right ventricular hypertrophy frequently occurs in response to chronic lung diseases such as emphysema and asthma. The elevation in pulmonary artery pressure and right ventricular hypertrophy is called *cor pulmonale* (kohr pul-mah-NAL-ee). Cor pulmonale often causes the right ventricle to fail as a pump.

Afterload can be altered by drugs. For example, a drug that relaxes and dilates the blood vessels in the peripheral circulation can lower blood pressure and therefore decrease the afterload. The reduction in afterload reduces the work of the heart. Conversely, a drug that constricts blood vessels in the periphery increases afterload, thereby increasing the workload of the heart.

INOTROPIC EFFECT

An inotropic effect is a change in myocardial contraction that is not caused by stretch. A positive inotropic effect is an increase in contractile force, whereas a negative inotropic effect is a decrease in contractile force. Sympathetic nerve stimulation and hormones such as epinephrine and norepinephrine cause a positive inotropic effect.

CHRONOTROPIC EFFECT

A chronotropic (KRON-oh-TROH-pik) effect is a change in heart rate. Anything that increases heart rate exerts a positive chronotropic effect, whereas anything that decreases heart rate exerts a negative chronotropic effect. Sympathetic nerve stimulation causes a positive chronotropic effect, whereas vagal (parasympathetic) stimulation causes a negative chronotropic effect.

DROMOTROPIC EFFECT

A dromotropic (DROM-oh-TROH-pik) effect is a change in the speed at which the cardiac impulse travels from the SA node through the AV node and the His-Purkinje system. If the speed of the cardiac impulse increases, it is called a positive dromotropic effect; a decrease in the speed causes a negative dromotropic effect. Sympathetic nerve stimulation causes a positive dromotropic effect, whereas vagal (parasympathetic) stimulation causes a negative dromotropic effect. The negative dromotropic effect may be so pronounced that the person develops a heart block.

HEART TALK: RECEPTOR LANGUAGE

Heart talk often involves the autonomic receptors of the heart and their responses to autonomic stimulation and to drugs. (Review Chapter 12.)

BETA$_1$-ADRENERGIC RECEPTOR ACTIVATION

The sympathetic nerves innervate the SA node, AV node, His-Purkinje system, and ventricular myocardium. The neurotransmitter for the adrenergic neuron is norepinephrine. The cardiac adrenergic receptors for norepinephrine are called *beta$_1$-adrenergic receptors*. Activation of the beta$_1$ receptors causes a positive chronotropic effect, a positive dromotropic effect, and a positive inotropic effect. The increase in heart rate and stroke volume increases cardiac output. A drug that activates beta$_1$-adrenergic receptors is called a *beta$_1$-adrenergic agonist*. Examples include dopamine and epinephrine. Note that beta$_1$-adrenergic receptor activation is the same as a sympathomimetic effect.

BETA$_1$-ADRENERGIC RECEPTOR BLOCKADE

Blockade of the beta$_1$-adrenergic receptors prevents cardiac beta$_1$-adrenergic receptor activation. People taking beta$_1$-adrenergic blockers, such as propranolol, will not increase their heart rate when their sympathetic nerves fire as in exercise or stress. If a person is tachycardic (heart rate >100 beats/min) from excessive sympathetic nervous stimulation, a beta$_1$-adrenergic blocker can decrease the heart rate and the force of myocardial contraction; this results in a decrease in cardiac output and blood pressure.

? Re-Think

1. Why is a beta$_1$-adrenergic agonist called a *sympathomimetic drug*?
2. What is the name of the neurotransmitter that activates a beta$_1$-adrenergic receptor?

MUSCARINIC (CHOLINERGIC) RECEPTOR ACTIVATION

The parasympathetic (vagus) nerves supply the SA and the AV nodes. The neurotransmitter for the cholinergic neuron is acetylcholine (ACh). The cardiac cholinergic receptors for ACh are called *muscarinic receptors*. Activation of the muscarinic receptors causes a negative chronotropic effect and a negative dromotropic effect. There is no effect on myocardial contractile force because there is no parasympathetic innervation to the ventricular myocardium. The administration of a cholinergic (muscarinic) agonist drug causes a negative chronotropic effect and a negative dromotropic effect. Note that muscarinic receptor activation is the same as a parasympathomimetic or vagomimetic effect.

MUSCARINIC (CHOLINERGIC) RECEPTOR BLOCKADE

The muscarinic receptors can also be blocked. Muscarinic-blocking drugs act by blocking the effects of ACh at the muscarinic receptors. Muscarinic blockade relieves the inhibiting effects of ACh at the receptors, thereby increasing heart rate and increasing the speed of the cardiac impulse from the atria to the ventricles. Atropine is an example of a muscarinic blocker that is often used to relieve bradycardia and heart block.

Note the duplication in terminology (your worst terminology nightmare!). The muscarinic receptors are activated by ACh. Because ACh is secreted by a cholinergic fiber, a muscarinic agonist is also called a *cholinergic agonist*. A muscarinic blocker is also called an *antimuscarinic agent,* a *cholinergic blocker,* or an *anticholinergic agent.* Unfortunately this terminology is used frequently in pharmacology, so you need to start building your vocabulary now.

? | **Re-Think**

1. Why is a muscarinic agonist called a *vagomimetic drug?*
2. What is the name of the neurotransmitter that activates the muscarinic receptors?

2+2 | **Sum It Up!**

Cardiac function is often described using special vocabulary, such as EDV, preload, ejection fraction, and afterload. Inotropic, chronotropic, and dromotropic effects describe changes in cardiac contractile force, heart rate, and conduction velocity through the heart. Cardiac function is also described in receptor terminology, specifically the beta$_1$-adrenergic and muscarinic receptors.

THE FAILING HEART: WHEN THE HEART CAN'T PUMP

The heart functions as a double pump. The right ventricle pumps blood to the lungs for oxygenation and the left ventricle pumps blood into the aorta for distribution to the systemic circulation. What happens when either or both pumps fail?

 Do You Know...

Why BNP Is Used in the Assessment of Heart Failure?

Brain natriuretic peptide (BNP) is secreted by the walls of the ventricles in response to stretch. The failing heart is characterized by pooling of blood in the cardiac chambers (cardiac dilation), thereby increasing the secretion of BNP.

A new class of drugs that mimic BNP is also used to treat heart failure. The BNP-like drug increases the excretion of sodium in the urine, suppresses the renin-angiotensin system, and decreases sympathetic activity.

LEFT HEART FAILURE

When the left ventricle fails to pump blood into the aorta, two things happen: blood backs up in the lungs, and the heart is unable to pump a sufficient amount of blood to the systemic circulation.

BACKWARD FAILURE

What happens when the blood backs up (Figure 17-5)? The blood backs up into the structures "behind" the left ventricle—namely, the left atrium, pulmonary veins, and, most importantly, the pulmonary capillaries. The pooled blood increases the pressure within the pulmonary capillaries and forces fluid into the lungs. The presence of fluid in the lungs impairs oxygenation of blood. The accumulation of fluid within the lungs is called **pulmonary edema (PE)**. The signs and symptoms of PE are exertional dyspnea (difficulty breathing upon exertion), cyanosis (bluish appearance), blood-tinged sputum and cough, orthopnea (or-THOP-nee-ah) (inability to breathe while lying down), tachycardia, and restlessness. Because these symptoms are largely caused by the backup of blood behind the failed ventricle, the condition is called *backward failure.* Note that the signs and symptoms of left-sided heart failure are predominantly respiratory!

 Do You Know...

About Two- and Three-Pillow Dyspnea?

A patient with heart failure may develop pulmonary edema and dyspnea. There is a simple way to determine the severity of the dyspnea: ask the patient how many pillows he uses at night. A patient with no pulmonary edema can lie flat and use a single pillow. As fluid collects in the alveoli (lungs), a patient must sit up to breathe (orthopnea). Thus, he tends to use two or three pillows, depending on the severity of the edema and dyspnea—hence the name *two-* or *three-pillow dyspnea.*

FORWARD FAILURE

There is also a "forward" component to left heart failure. For example, if the damaged left ventricle cannot pump enough blood to the systemic circulation, all the organs of the body receive inadequate oxygen. The decreased cardiac output causes additional signs and symptoms to develop. For example, the kidneys

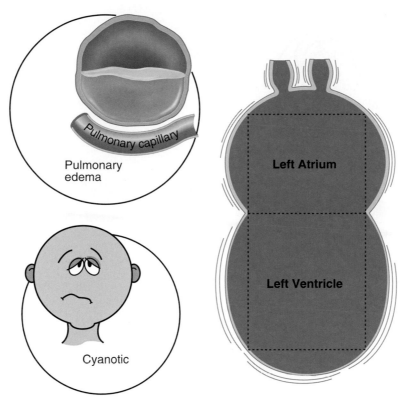

FIGURE 17-5 Left-sided heart failure.

filter less water for excretion as urine. The kidneys also reabsorb excess salt and water, causing an increase in blood volume and edema formation. The decrease in cardiac output also stimulates the sympathetic nervous system. Sympathetic activity stimulates the heart and blood vessels in a way that temporarily improves cardiac output. Over time, however, the improvement diminishes and additional signs of heart failure develop. The heart begins to show the wear and tear of continuous and excessive sympathetic activity.

What usually causes the left heart to fail? Two common causes are myocardial infarction (MI) and chronic hypertension (increased blood pressure). If a person suffers an acute MI, a part of the left ventricular myocardium may be destroyed. The damaged myocardium is unable to contract and fails as a pump. More commonly, the left heart fails in response to chronic hypertension. Increased blood pressure overworks the heart, eventually causing the left ventricle to enlarge (left ventricular hypertrophy) and then fail.

? Re-Think

1. Why does left-sided heart failure cause pulmonary edema?
2. Differentiate between forward and backward heart failure.
3. Explain why a positive inotropic drug, such as digoxin, relieves backward and forward heart failure.

RIGHT HEART FAILURE

When the right ventricle fails (Figure 17-6), blood backs up into the veins that return blood to the right heart. Blood backs up into the superior vena cava, thereby slowing venous drainage from the head via the jugular veins. The congestion of the jugular veins causes jugular vein distention (JVD), which is visible as the veins in the neck pulsate. Blood also backs up into the veins that drain the liver, spleen, and digestive organs, causing hepatomegaly (enlarged liver), splenomegaly (enlarged spleen), and digestive symptoms. Right-sided failure is also characterized by ankle, or pedal, edema; ankle edema can be so severe that the skin remains indented when you depress an area of skin with your thumb. This "indentation" response is called *pitting edema*.

The right heart most often fails as a consequence of left-sided failure; when one side of the heart fails, the other side will eventually fail. Another common cause is chronic lung disease, such as emphysema. The diseased lungs make it difficult for the right ventricle to pump blood into the pulmonary circulation. The overworked right ventricle becomes enlarged (right ventricular hypertrophy) and eventually fails.

? Re-Think

1. Why does right-sided heart failure cause JVD, hepatomegaly, and pedal edema rather than pulmonary edema?
2. Translate this into lay terminology. A patient with an ejection fraction of 35% was given a drug (digoxin) that exerted positive inotropic, negative dromotropic, and negative chronotropic effects.

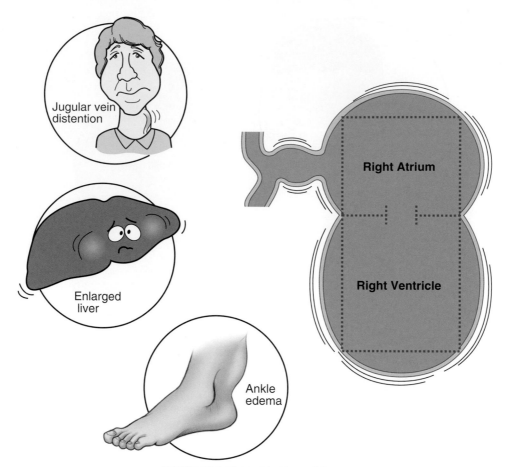

FIGURE 17-6 Right-sided heart failure.

 Do You Know...

Why CVP Is Elevated in Heart Failure?

Central venous pressure (CVP) is considered a direct measurement of the pressure in the right atrium and superior vena cava (the large vein that empties blood into the right atrium). The CVP reading is obtained by threading a catheter through the subclavian vein into the superior vena cava. When the heart fails, blood backs up in the vena cava, thereby elevating venous pressure. Thus, an elevated CVP is indicative of a failing heart.

Let's see if you can follow the rationale for the treatment in the following case studies.

- *Case 1.* A patient in left-sided heart failure and pulmonary edema is given a positive inotropic drug, a potent diuretic, oxygen, and morphine. The rationale for this is that the failing heart muscle contracts weakly. A positive inotropic drug such as digoxin or dopamine strengthens myocardial contraction. The increased force of contraction results in an increased cardiac output, decreased pooling of blood in the pulmonary capillaries (decreases pulmonary edema), and increased blood flow to the kidney, which results in greater excretion of urine. A potent diuretic, such as furosemide (Lasix), blocks the absorption of sodium and water by the kidney,

thereby ridding the body of excess water and decreasing the edema. The oxygen and morphine improve oxygenation and relieve the anxiety caused by poor oxygenation.

- *Case 2.* An older patient with symptoms of right-sided failure and a fast heart rate is given a beta$_1$-adrenergic blocker. The rationale for this is that heart failure is characterized by excess sympathetic nerve stimulation. Long-term sympathetic stimulation damages the heart, causing the heart to fail eventually. The administration of a beta$_1$-adrenergic receptor blocker diminishes the response to sympathetic activity and protects the heart from further damage.

- *Case 3.* An older patient has mild right-sided failure and is given an angiotensin-converting enzyme (ACE) inhibitor. An ACE inhibitor decreases afterload, acts like a diuretic, and decreases the secretion of aldosterone from the adrenal cortex. The decreased afterload decreases the workload of the heart. The diuretic effect excretes water and relieves the edema. The decrease in the secretion of aldosterone has two effects: it causes diuresis, and it prevents myocardial damage. (Chronic secretion of aldosterone causes structural damage, called *remodeling,* to the heart muscle.)

Clearly, the healthy heart is a magnificent, adaptable pump. Pump failure adversely affects the functioning of every organ system and is a common cause of disability and death.

2+2 Sum It Up!

The heart functions as a double pump. Either or both pumps can fail. When the left heart fails, fluid backs up into the lungs, causing pulmonary edema. The failing left heart is also unable to pump sufficient blood to the organs of the body; the result is poor tissue oxygenation. Right-sided failure causes JVD, ankle edema, and congestion of the abdominal organs. The treatment of heart failure is aimed at strengthening of myocardial contractile force, removing excess water, decreasing the work of the heart, and protecting the heart from excess sympathetic nerve activity.

As You Age

1. Contrary to popular opinion, no significant age-related decline occurs in resting cardiac output. When cardiac output declines, it is a result of age-related disease processes such as arteriosclerosis.
2. An age-related decline occurs in exercise cardiac output. The heart cannot respond as quickly or as forcefully to the increased workload of the exercised heart. Exertion, sudden movements, and changes in position may cause a decrease in cardiac output, resulting in dizziness, loss of balance, and falls.
3. Several structural changes in the heart contribute to the impaired response to exercise: heart muscle loses elasticity and becomes more rigid; heart valves become thicker and more rigid; the number of pacemaker cells decreases; and the aging heart cells have a decreased ability to use oxygen.
4. An age-related increase occurs in blood pressure, which increases the work the heart must do to pump blood into the systemic circulation.

MEDICAL TERMINOLOGY AND DISORDERS   Disorders of the Heart

Medical Term	Word Parts	Word Part Meaning or Derivation	Description
Words			
bradycardia	brady-	abnormally slow	**Bradycardia** is *an abnormally slow heart rate (<60 beats/min).*
	-cardi/o-	heart	
	-ia	condition of	
cardiogram	cardi/o-	heart	A **cardiogram** is *a recording of the electrical events of the heart.*
	-gram	record	
ectopic	ec-	out of	An ectopic beat is one that originates outside the SA node. Examples include premature atrial and ventricular beats.
	-top/o-	place	
	-ic	condition of	
pericardium	peri-	around	The **pericardium** is *a slinglike membrane that surrounds the heart.*
	-cardi/o-	heart	
	-ium	tissue or structure	
tachycardia	tachy-	fast	**Tachycardia** is *an abnormally fast heart rate (>120 beats/min).*
	-cardi/o-	heart	
	-ia	condition of	
Disorders			
angina pectoris	angina	From the Greek word *ankhone,* meaning "to strangle"	**Angina pectoris,** also called *chest pain,* signals a diminished coronary blood flow to the heart. There are three forms of angina pectoris: 1. **Chronic stable angina (or exertional angina)** is triggered by physical activity and/or emotional excitement. The decreased coronary flow is due to changes associated with fatty plaque buildup (atherosclerosis).
	pectoris	From the Latin word *pectus,* meaning "chest"	2. **Variant angina (Prinzmetal's angina, vasospastic angina)** is caused by diminished blood flow resulting from spasm of the coronary arteries. 3. **Unstable angina** is a medical emergency; the diminished blood flow is due to severe coronary artery disease and complicated by vasospasm, rupture of the plaques, and formation of thrombi.

Continued

MEDICAL TERMINOLOGY AND DISORDERS	Disorders of the Heart—cont'd

Medical Term	Word Parts	Word Part Meaning or Derivation	Description
coronary artery disease and atherosclerosis	coronary	Related to the veins and arteries	Also referred to as **CAD**, or **coronary heart disease (CHD)**. Coronary blood flow is reduced because of a progressive narrowing of the coronary blood vessels that deprives the myocardium of O_2 and nutrients. Diminished coronary blood flow is most often caused by **atherosclerosis**, an inflammation-induced accumulation of fatty plaques on the inner lining of the coronary blood vessels. With time the fatty plaques reduce the elasticity of the arteries, causing them to thicken and harden *(sclerosis)*; the plaque reduces coronary blood flow and can eventually rupture, causing thrombotic occlusion of the coronary artery. Untreated, atherosclerosis commonly progresses to myocardial infarction. A **myocardial infarction (MI)**, or **"heart attack,"** refers to *the death or necrosis **(infarction)** of the heart muscle* **(myocardium)** *caused by insufficient oxygenated blood.*
	athero/o-	From the Greek word *ather/o,* meaning "oatmeal" or "gruel"	
	-scler/o-	harden	
	-osis	condition of	
carditis	cardi/o-	heart	**Carditis** is *inflammation of the heart;* this includes the following conditions: endocarditis, myocarditis, and pericarditis. **Endocarditis** is *an inflammation of the endocardium, the inner lining of the heart and valves.* It is most often caused by bacterial infection; bacteria enter the blood from any infected part of the body, particularly infected gums and dental procedures. **Myocarditis** is *an inflammation of the heart muscle and is most often associated with viral infection.* **Pericarditis** is *an inflammation of the outer lining of the heart (pericardium).* Pericarditis may be accompanied by the accumulation of serous or purulent exudates in the pericardial space, which, in turn, may cause **cardiac tamponade** *(external compression of the heart)* and heart failure.
	-itis	inflammation	
cardiomegaly	cardi/o-	heart	**Cardiomegaly,** *an enlarged heart,* is not a disease, but a consequence of an underlying disorder. There are two types of cardiomegaly: 1. **Dilative cardiomegaly** develops when the heart weakens and becomes dilated by the increased blood volume, as in heart failure. 2. **Hypertrophic cardiomegaly** refers to the hypertrophy (growth in size) of the myocardium in response to an increased workload.
	-megal/o-	large	
	-y	condition of	
cardiomyopathy	cardi/o-	heart	**Cardiomyopathy** is *a disease of the heart muscle that results in weak and insufficient pumping activity.* In its earliest stage, cardiomyopathy is often asymptomatic, but it gradually progresses to cardiomegaly and heart failure. There are four types: 1. In **dilated cardiomyopathy,** the cardiac chambers dilate. 2. In **hypertrophic cardiomyopathy,** the myocardium thickens or hypertrophies. 3. In **ischemic cardiomyopathy,** the myocardium thins and weakens because of a poor blood supply. 4. In **restrictive cardiomyopathy,** the thickened myocardium prevents ventricular filling.
	-my/o-	muscle	
	-path	disease of	
	-y	condition of	
congenital heart defects	con-	together or with	*Heart and defects of the great vessels that are present from birth are called* **congenital heart defects.** The term includes structural defects, such as septal defects, valvular disorders, absence or incomplete development of cardiac structures, and disturbances in cardiac rhythm. Congenital heart defects are also classified as **cyanotic** or **acyanotic,** depending upon the degree of O_2 saturation. Examples of congenital heart defects are septal defects, patent ductus arteriosus, tetralogy of Fallot, transposition of the great vessels, tricuspid atresia, and coarctation of the aorta. Septal defects create **shunts** (left-to-right, right-to-left) because of the pressure differences within the chambers. A **ventriculoseptal defect (VSD)** is the most common congenital heart defect.
	-gen/o-	origin	
	-al	pertaining to	

MEDICAL TERMINOLOGY AND DISORDERS Disorders of the Heart—cont'd

Medical Term	Word Parts	Word Part Meaning or Derivation	Description
dysrhythmia	dys-	faulty	*Any disturbance in normal cardiac rhythm* is referred to a **dysrhythmia.** Dysrhythmias are classified in several ways. According to rate: normal sinus rhythm, bradycardia, and tachycardia. According to mechanism: automaticity, reentry, junctional, and fibrillation. According to origin: atrial, junctional, ventricular, heart blocks, and arrhythmias that cause sudden death. **Bradydysrhythmias** (*brady-* = slow) are *rhythm disturbances that are characterized by excessively slow activity.* Slow electrical conduction through the heart causes varying degrees of heart block (first, second, complete). **Tachydysrhythmias** (*tachy-* = fast) are *rhythm disturbances that are characterized by excessive electrical activity.* Fast rhythm disorders include tachycardia, flutter, and fibrillation. These dysrhythmias may be atrial, ventricular, or both. Generally the ventricular rhythm disorders are more acute, demanding prompt attention.
	-rhythm/o-	rhythm	
	-ia	condition of	
heart failure			**Described in the text.**
valvular disorders	valvul/o-	valve	Some examples of **valvular disorders** include semilunar and AV valves, which are incompletely formed, too narrow, or incompetent. Tricuspid atresia is an example of an incompletely formed valve. **Valvular stenosis** (i.e., mitral valve stenosis) is a narrowing of a valve restricting the flow of blood. An **incompetent valve** is a leaky valve; it does not do its job, which is to prevent backflow of blood.
	-ar	pertaining to	

Get Ready for Exams!

Summary Outline

The heart pumps blood through the blood vessels, supplying the cells of the body with oxygen and nutrients, and carrying away the waste products of metabolism. The heart functions in a coordinated and adaptable manner to perform its tasks.

I. **The Coordinated and Adaptable Pump**
   A. Cardiac Cycle
      1. The cardiac cycle is a sequence of events that occurs during one heartbeat.
      2. The events of the cardiac cycle include atrial and ventricular systole (contraction) and diastole (relaxation).
   B. Heart: Autonomic Control
      1. The autonomic nervous system (ANS) allows the heart to respond to changing body needs.
      2. Stimulation of the sympathetic nerves increases heart rate (SA node), conduction velocity (AV node), and contractile force (myocardium).
      3. Stimulation of the parasympathetic nerves (vagus) decreases heart rate and conduction velocity.
   C. Cardiac Output (CO)
      1. CO is the amount of blood pumped by the ventricle in 1 minute.
      2. CO is determined by heart rate (HR) and stroke volume (SV).
      3. Many factors can change HR and/or SV.
   D. How Stroke Volume Can Be Changed
      1. SV can be changed by Starling's law of the heart (stretch).

      2. SV can be changed by an inotropic effect (nonstretch).

II. **Heart Talk**
   A. Heart Talk: Clinical Terms
      1. Includes the definition and description of commonly used clinical terms such as *preload, afterload, ejection fraction, inotropic effect, chronotropic effect,* and *dromotropic effect*
   B. Heart Talk: Receptor Terminology
      1. Includes the definitions of *beta$_1$-adrenergic receptor activation, beta$_1$-adrenergic receptor blockade, muscarinic receptor activation,* and *muscarinic receptor blockade*

III. **The Failing Heart: When the Heart Can't Pump**
   A. Left Heart Failure
      1. The left heart can fail, producing symptoms caused by a backup of blood into the pulmonic circulation (pulmonary edema); referred to as *backward failure.*
      2. The failing left heart is unable to pump enough blood to the systemic circulation, producing symptoms related to poor tissue oxygenation; referred to as *forward failure.*
   B. Right Heart Failure
   C. Blood backs up behind the failed right ventricle, causing jugular vein distention, hepatomegaly, splenomegaly, digestive problems, and ankle edema.

Review Your Knowledge

Matching: Cardiac Function Terms

Directions: Match the following words with their descriptions below. Some words may be used more than once.

a. inotropic effect
b. cardiac output
c. stroke volume
d. diastole
e. systole
f. Starling's law of the heart

1. ___ 5000 mL/min
2. ___ 70 mL/beat
3. ___ Stroke volume times heart rate
4. ___ Phase of the cardiac cycle that refers to myocardial contraction
5. ___ Phase of the cardiac cycle during which the ventricles fill with blood
6. ___ Phase of the cardiac cycle that refers to myocardial relaxation
7. ___ Change in myocardial contraction that is caused by stretching of the heart muscle
8. ___ Change in myocardial contraction that is not caused by stretching of the heart muscle
9. ___ Amount of blood pumped by the ventricle in one beat
10. ___ Amount of blood pumped by the ventricle in 1 minute

Matching: Loads and Effects

Directions: Match the following words with their descriptions below. Some words may be used more than once.

a. afterload
b. preload
c. ejection fraction
d. dromotropic effect
e. chronotropic effect

1. ___ Amount of blood in the ventricle at the end of its resting phase
2. ___ Percentage of the end-diastolic volume (EDV) pumped by the ventricle
3. ___ Arteriolar constriction and hypertension cause this to increase.
4. ___ Forms the basis of Starling's law of the heart
5. ___ The effect of a drug that changes heart rate
6. ___ Digoxin slows the speed of the cardiac impulse through the conduction system, thereby causing a heart block.
7. ___ Same as end-diastolic volume (EDV)
8. ___ May decline from 67% to 30% in the failing heart

Multiple Choice

1. Which of the following statements is correct about cardiac output?
   a. Cardiac output is determined by the heart rate and pulse.
   b. Stimulation of the sympathetic nerves decreases cardiac output.
   c. Vagal discharge increases cardiac output.
   d. Cardiac output is determined by heart rate and stroke volume.

2. Which statement is true of ventricular diastole?
   a. Blood is ejected from the ventricles.
   b. The semilunar valves are open.
   c. The atrioventricular valves are closed.
   d. Blood fills the ventricles.

3. Increased return of blood to the heart stretches the heart muscle, thereby
   a. stimulating the vagus nerve.
   b. increasing stroke volume.
   c. closing the atrioventricular valves.
   d. increasing coronary blood flow.

4. Ventricular systole refers to
   a. ventricular depolarization.
   b. the opening of the valves of the ventricles.
   c. ventricular filling.
   d. contraction of the ventricular myocardium.

5. Which of the following is least related to the vagus nerve?
   a. Parasympathetic
   b. Slows heart rate
   c. Positive inotropic effect
   d. Autonomic nerve

6. Which of the following is least characteristic of sympathetic nerve stimulation?
   a. Negative inotropic effect
   b. Increased heart rate
   c. Increased stroke volume
   d. Increased cardiac output

7. Which of the following is least related to bradycardia?
   a. <60 beats/min
   b. Vagal discharge
   c. Negative chronotropic effect
   d. $Beta_1$-adrenergic receptor activation

8. Which of the following is least apt to increase cardiac output?
   a. Increased heart rate
   b. Increased stroke volume
   c. Increased venous return (Starling's law of the heart)
   d. Vagal discharge

Go Figure

1. According to Figure 17-1
   a. The semilunar valves are open during atrial systole.
   b. The AV valves are closed during ventricular systole.
   c. Blood is pumped out of the atria during ventricular systole.
   d. The AV valves remain closed during atrial systole.

2. According to Figure 17-2
   a. The neurotransmitter for the vagus nerve is norepinephrine.
   b. The vagus nerve is a sympathetic nerve.
   c. The ventricular myocardium is innervated only by a sympathetic nerve.
   d. The SA node is subject only to vagal effects.

3. **According to Figure 17-2, the postganglionic parasympathetic fiber**
   a. secretes NE.
   b. secretes a transmitter that binds to a beta$_1$-adrenergic receptor.
   c. is cholinergic.
   d. is adrenergic.

4. **According to Figure 17-2**
   a. Sympathetic firing affects force of myocardial contraction.
   b. The AV node can be stimulated only by ACh.
   c. The SA node contains receptors that respond only to ACh.
   d. The fibers that are color-coded red are cholinergic.

5. **According to Figures 17-3 and 17-4**
   a. An increase in venous return stretches the ventricular myocardium.
   b. A decrease in venous return increases preload.
   c. Chronic hypertension is expressed as a decrease in afterload.
   d. All of the above are true.

6. **According to Figure 17-4**
   a. Increased venous return increases preload.
   b. Increased venous return decreases EDV.
   c. Increased EDV increases afterload.
   d. Dilation of the aorta and peripheral blood vessels increases afterload.

7. **According to Figures 17-5 and 17-6**
   a. Right ventricular failure causes orthopnea.
   b. Left ventricular failure causes jugular vein distention and ankle edema.
   c. Left-sided heart failure causes pulmonary edema.
   d. Jugular vein distention, liver congestion, and ankle edema cause right-sided failure.

Anatomy of the Blood Vessels

Key Terms

aorta (p. 343)
arteries (p. 341)
arterioles (p. 341)
capacitance vessels (p. 343)
capillaries (p. 341)

conductance vessels (p. 342)
exchange vessels (p. 343)
pulmonary circulation (p. 340)
resistance vessels (p. 342)
splanchnic circulation (p. 350)

systemic circulation (p. 340)
veins (p. 341)
venae cavae (p. 346)
venules (p. 341)

Objective

1. Describe the pulmonary and systemic circulations.
2. Describe the structure and function of arteries, capillaries, and veins, including:
   - List the three layers of tissue found in arteries and veins.
   - Explain the functions of conductance, resistance, exchange, and capacitance vessels.

3. List the major arteries of the systemic circulation that are branches of the ascending aorta, aortic arch, and descending aorta.
4. List the major veins of the systemic circulation.
5. Describe the following special circulations: blood supply to the head and brain, hepatic circulation, and fetal circulation.
6. Explain pulse and its use as an assessment tool.

The circulatory system consists of the heart and blood vessels. The historical description of the heart and blood vessels is intriguing. The ancients knew that the heart played an important role in pumping blood through the body, but no one described the intricate role of the blood vessels. The ancient Greeks thought that blood moved throughout the body like an ocean tide. Blood was seen as washing out from the heart through a series of blood vessels and then ebbing back to it through those same blood vessels, with impurities removed from the blood as it washed through the lungs. Not until the seventeenth century did the English physician William Harvey, described as a crackpot by his fellow scientists, identify the system of blood vessels and thus provide the first accurate description of the circulation.

CIRCLES, CIRCUITS, AND CIRCULATIONS

The blood vessels are a series of connected hollow tubes that begin and end in the heart. The blood vessels form a path through the body, much like the system of highways and roads that enables us to travel from place to place. Note the path of the delivery truck in Figure 18-1. Leaving the bakery, the truck travels on a major highway and exits onto a smaller road. The truck then arrives at a grocery store, where it makes a delivery. The empty truck returns to the bakery through a number of connecting roads. Note the circle, or circuit, from bakery to grocery store to bakery.

The heart and blood vessels also form a circuit. The heart pumps blood into the large artery. The blood flows through a series of blood vessels back to the heart. Moving from heart to blood vessels to heart, the blood forms a circuit, or circulation. This arrangement ensures a continuous one-way movement of blood. As Chapter 16 explained, the two main circulations are the pulmonary circulation and the systemic circulation.

The **pulmonary circulation** carries blood from the right ventricle of the heart to the lungs and back to the left atrium of the heart (see Figure 16-3). The pulmonary circulation transports unoxygenated blood to the lungs, where oxygen is loaded and carbon dioxide is unloaded. Oxygenated blood then returns to the left side of the heart to be pumped into the systemic circulation.

The **systemic circulation** is the larger circulation; it provides the blood supply to the rest of the body. The systemic circulation carries oxygen and other nutrients to the cells and picks up carbon dioxide and other waste.

FIGURE 18-1 A circuit or route: the circulatory system.

BLOOD VESSELS

NAMING THE BLOOD VESSELS

Note the different types of blood vessels (Figure 18-2), their relationship to the heart, and the color coding. The blood vessels are the body's highways and byways; they are anatomically classified as arteries, capillaries, and veins (Table 18-1).

ARTERIES

Arteries are blood vessels that carry blood away from the heart. The large arteries repeatedly branch into smaller and smaller arteries as they are distributed throughout the entire body. As they branch, the arteries become much more numerous but smaller in diameter. The smallest arteries are called arterioles (ar-TEER-ee-ohls). The arteries are red in Figure 18-2 because they carry oxygenated blood.

CAPILLARIES

Blood flows from the arterioles into the capillaries. The capillaries (KAP-i-lair-ees) are the smallest and most numerous of all the blood vessels. They connect the arterioles with the venules. Because the body has so many of them, a capillary is close to every cell in the body. This arrangement provides every cell with a continuous supply of oxygen and other nutrients. The capillaries are colored from red to purple to blue. Why? At the capillary level, the blood gives up its oxygen to the tissues; the unoxygenated blood leaving the tissues is therefore bluish.

VEINS

Blood flows from the capillaries into the veins. Veins are blood vessels that carry blood back to the heart. The smallest veins are called venules (VEN-yools). The small venules converge to form fewer but larger veins. The largest veins empty the blood into the right atrium of the heart. The veins are colored blue because they transport unoxygenated blood.

BLOOD VESSEL WALLS: THE LAYERED LOOK

With the exception of the capillaries, the blood vessels are composed of three layers (or tunics) of tissue (see Figure 18-2): tunica intima, tunica media, and tunica adventitia.

1. *Tunica intima.* The tunica (TOO-nik-kah) intima is the innermost layer, an endothelium. The endothelial lining forms a slick shiny surface continuous with the endocardium, the inner lining of the heart. Blood flows easily and smoothly along this surface.
2. *Tunica media.* The tunica media is the middle layer. It is the thickest layer and is composed primarily of elastic tissue and smooth muscle; the thickness and composition vary according to the function of the blood vessel. The large arteries, for example, contain considerable elastic tissue so that they can stretch in response to the pumping of blood by the heart. The smallest of the arteries, the arterioles, are composed primarily of smooth muscle. The muscle allows the arterioles to contract and relax, thereby changing the diameter of the arteriole.

FIGURE 18-2 Blood vessel wall layers: the tunica intima, tunica media, and tunica adventitia.

3. *Tunica adventitia.* The outer layer is called the tunica adventitia (ad-ven-TEESH-ah). Composed of tough connective tissue, its main function is to support and protect blood vessels.

BLOOD VESSELS: WHAT THEY DO

Note how the structure of the blood vessels changes from artery to capillary to vein (see Figure 18-2 and Table 18-1). As always, the structure is related to its function. The following is a functional classification of blood vessels.

ARTERIES

The walls of the large arteries are thick, tough, and elastic because they must withstand the high pressure of the blood pumped from the ventricles. Because the primary function of the large arteries is to conduct blood from the heart to the arterioles, the large arteries are called **conductance vessels**.

ARTERIOLES

The arterioles are the smallest of the arteries. They are composed primarily of smooth muscle and spend most of their time contracting and relaxing. By changing their diameter, the arterioles affect resistance to the flow of blood. A narrow (constricted) vessel offers an increased resistance to blood flow; a wider (dilated) vessel offers less resistance. Because of their effect on resistance, the arterioles are called **resistance vessels**.

CAPILLARIES

The capillaries have the thinnest walls of any of the blood vessels. The capillary wall is made up of a single layer of endothelium lying on a delicate basement membrane. The thin capillary wall enables water and dissolved substances, including oxygen, to diffuse from the blood into the tissue spaces, where they become available for use by the cells. The capillary also allows waste from the metabolizing cell to diffuse from the tissue spaces into the capillaries for transport by

Table 18-1	Structure and Function of Blood Vessels	
VESSEL	**STRUCTURE**	**FUNCTION**
Artery	Thick wall with three layers: tunica intima (endothelial lining), tunica media (elastic tissue and smooth muscle), and tunica adventitia (connective tissue)	Called *conductance vessels* because they carry blood from the heart to the arterioles
Arteriole	Small artery but with three layers, mostly smooth muscle	Called *resistance vessels* because the contraction and relaxation of the muscle changes vessel diameter, which alters resistance to blood flow
Capillary	Layer of endothelium on a basement membrane	Called *exchange vessels* because nutrients, gases, and wastes exchange between the blood and interstitial fluid
Venule	Thin wall with less smooth muscle and elastic tissue than an artery or arteriole	Venules and veins collect and return blood from the tissues to the heart. They are called *capacitance vessels* because they hold or store blood.
Vein	Three layers (intima, media, and adventitia), but thinner and less elastic than an artery; contain valves	

the blood to the organs of excretion. The capillaries are called **exchange vessels** because they allow for an exchange of nutrients and waste.

? Re-Think

1. Why are the layers of the arteries thicker than those of the capillaries?
2. Explain the color coding of arteries, capillaries, and veins.

VEINS AND VENULES

As the capillaries begin to converge to form venules, the structure of the wall changes again. The venule wall is slightly thicker than the capillary wall. As the venules converge to form larger veins, the walls become even thicker. The tunica media of the vein, however, is much thinner than the tunica media of the artery. This difference is appropriate, because pressure in the veins is much less than the pressure in the arterial blood vessels.

In addition to thinner walls, the veins differ in another way; most veins contain one-way valves. These valves direct the flow of blood toward the heart. The valves are most numerous in the veins of the lower extremities, where they prevent backflow, helping move blood up and away from the ankles.

In addition to carrying blood back to the heart, the veins play another role. The veins store blood. In fact, about 70% of the total blood volume is found on the venous side of the circulation. Because the veins store blood, they are called **capacitance vessels**. (*Capacitance* refers to storage.) When this stored blood is needed, the veins constrict (venoconstriction) and move blood to the heart for circulation.

? Re-Think

1. Why are the arterioles called *resistance vessels*?
2. Why are the capillaries called *exchange vessels*?
3. Why are the large arteries and veins not suitable for exchange?
4. Why do the veins, but not the arteries, contain valves?

2+2 Sum It Up!

The blood vessels are a series of connected hollow tubes that form a circuit. There are two circulations: the pulmonary circulation and the systemic circulation. The three types of blood vessels are arteries (conductance), capillaries (exchange), and veins (capacitance). The arterioles are tiny arteries called *resistance vessels*.

MAJOR ARTERIES OF THE SYSTEMIC CIRCULATION

The major arteries of the systemic circulation include the aorta and the arteries arising from the aorta.

AORTA

The **aorta** (ay-OR-tah) is the mother of all arteries; its average diameter is that of a garden hose. The aorta originates in the heart's left ventricle (Figure 18-3), extends upward from the left ventricle, curves in an archlike fashion, and then descends through the thorax (chest) and abdomen. The aorta ends in the pelvic cavity, where it splits into two common iliac arteries.

The aorta is divided into segments, each named according to two systems. One system is the path that the aorta follows as it courses through the body. In this

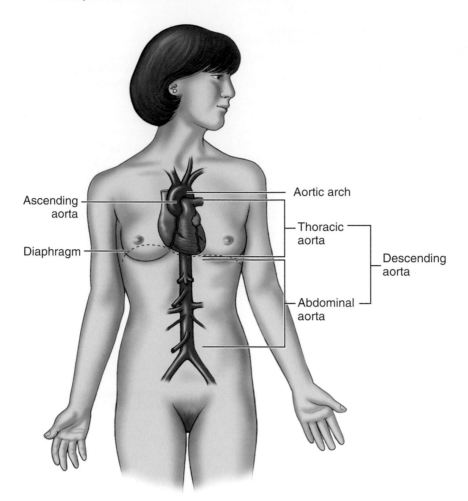

FIGURE 18-3 Naming the parts of the aorta.

system, the aorta is divided into the ascending aorta, the arch of the aorta, and the descending aorta. In the second naming system, the aorta is named according to its location within the body cavities. Thus, we have the thoracic aorta and the abdominal aorta. This text, like most texts, uses both naming systems.

 Re-Think

List five words that describe parts of the aorta.

BRANCHES OF THE AORTA

All systemic arteries are direct or indirect branches of the aorta. In other words, the arteries arise directly from the aorta or they arise from vessels that are themselves branches of the aorta. For example, the coronary arteries arise directly from the ascending aorta. The brachial artery in the right arm, however, arises from the axillary artery. The axillary artery has its origin in the subclavian artery, an extension of the brachiocephalic artery, which arises from the arch of the aorta. The brachial artery therefore arises indirectly from the aorta.

The systemic arteries are described in the order in which they arise from the aorta. Refer to Figure 18-4 as you read the text to identify the arteries and the structures that they supply.

BRANCHES OF THE ASCENDING AORTA

The ascending aorta arises from the left ventricle of the heart. It begins at the aortic semilunar valve and extends to the aortic arch. The right and left coronary arteries branch from the ascending aorta. The coronary arteries are distributed throughout the heart and supply oxygenated blood to the myocardium.

BRANCHES OF THE AORTIC ARCH

The aortic arch extends from the ascending aorta to the beginning of the descending aorta. The following three large arteries arise from the aortic arch:

• The brachiocephalic artery is a large artery on the right side of the body. It supplies blood to the right side of the head and neck, right shoulder, and right upper extremity. Refer to Figure 18-4 for the names of the arteries that extend from, or branch off, the brachiocephalic artery. These arteries supply the right side of the head and neck and the arm and

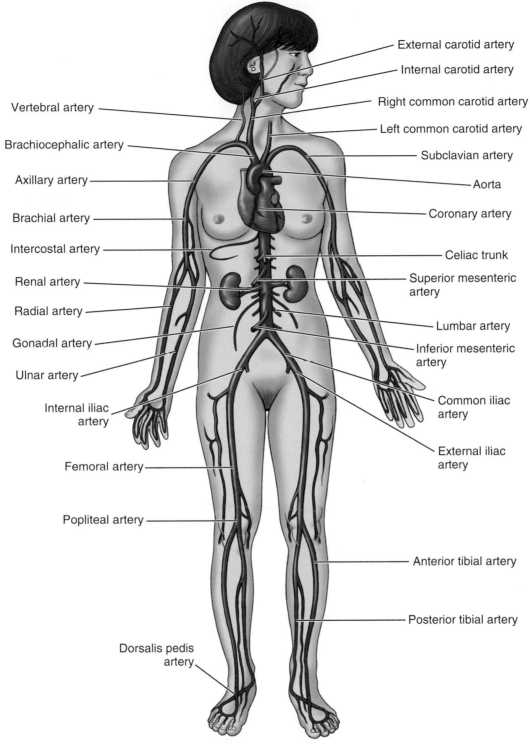

External carotid artery

Internal carotid artery

Right common carotid artery

Left common carotid artery

Subclavian artery

Aorta

Coronary artery

Celiac trunk

Superior mesenteric artery

Lumbar artery

Inferior mesenteric artery

Common iliac artery

External iliac artery

Anterior tibial artery

Posterior tibial artery

Vertebral artery

Brachiocephalic artery

Axillary artery

Brachial artery

Intercostal artery

Renal artery

Radial artery

Gonadal artery

Ulnar artery

Internal iliac artery

Femoral artery

Popliteal artery

Dorsalis pedis artery

FIGURE 18-4 Major arteries.

hand regions. (There is no left brachiocephalic artery.)

- The left common carotid artery extends upward from the highest part of the aortic arch and supplies the left side of the head and neck. Note that the left common carotid artery arises directly from the aorta, whereas the right common carotid arises from the brachiocephalic artery.

- The left and right subclavian arteries supply blood to the shoulders and upper arms.

BRANCHES OF THE DESCENDING AORTA (THORACIC AORTA)

The thoracic aorta is the upper portion of the descending aorta. It extends from the aortic arch to the diaphragm. Intercostal arteries arise from the aorta and supply the intercostal muscles between the ribs. Other small arteries supply the organs in the thorax.

BRANCHES OF THE DESCENDING AORTA (ABDOMINAL AORTA)

The abdominal aorta extends from the thoracic aorta to the lower abdomen. Branches of the abdominal aorta include the following:

- The celiac trunk is a short artery that further divides into three smaller arteries: the gastric artery supplies the stomach, the splenic artery supplies the spleen, and the hepatic artery supplies the liver.
- Two mesenteric (MEZ-en-tair-ik) arteries are the superior and inferior segments. The superior mesenteric artery supplies blood to most of the small intestine and part of the large intestine. The other part of the large intestine receives its blood supply from the inferior mesenteric artery.
- Two renal arteries supply blood to the right and left kidneys. Other branches of the abdominal aorta include the gonadal arteries and the lumbar arteries.

The distal abdominal aorta splits into the right and left common iliac arteries that supply the pelvic organs, thigh, and lower extremities. Refer to Figure 18-4 and identify the major arteries of the thigh and leg: external iliac arteries and the femoral, popliteal, anterior, and posterior tibial arteries. The anterior and posterior tibial arteries give rise to arteries that supply the foot. The anterior tibial artery becomes the dorsalis pedis artery in the foot.

? Re-Think

1. Identify the origin of the right and left common carotid arteries.
2. List five arteries that emerge *directly* from the aorta.
3. Trace a drop of blood from the left ventricle to the left foot.

MAJOR VEINS OF THE SYSTEMIC CIRCULATION

If you look at the back of your hand, you can see several veins but no arteries. Why? The arteries are usually located in deep and well-protected areas. Many of the veins, however, are located more superficially and can be seen. These are called *superficial veins.* Deep veins are located more deeply and usually run parallel to the arteries. With few exceptions, the names of the deep veins are the same as the names of the companion arteries. For example, the femoral artery is accompanied by the femoral vein. In Figures 18-4 and 18-5, note the similarity in the names of many of the arteries and veins. Good news! If you learn the names of the arteries, you'll also know most of the names of the veins.

VENAE CAVAE

The veins carry blood from all parts of the body to the venae cavae for delivery to the heart. The venae cavae are the main veins. They are divided into the superior vena cava (SVC) and the inferior vena cava (IVC). Veins draining blood from the head, shoulders, and upper extremities empty into the SVC. Veins draining the lower part of the body empty into the IVC. The SVC and IVC empty into the right atrium.

 Do You Know...

Why Your Veins May Hum?

About 20% of the cardiac output flows to the brain and must therefore be returned to the right side of the heart. The large flow of blood through the jugular veins causes the walls of the veins to vibrate; the vibration can be heard as a venous hum in the upper chest near the clavicle (collarbone). The condition is benign but may be confused with a heart murmur. How do we differentiate between a heart murmur and venous hum? The venous hum disappears when the patient is placed in a supine position or if the clinician presses on the jugular vein. A true heart murmur is not affected by a change of position or compression of the jugular vein.

VEINS THAT EMPTY INTO THE SUPERIOR VENA CAVA

The SVC receives blood from the head, shoulder, and upper extremities. Veins may drain directly or indirectly into the SVC. For example, the brachiocephalic veins empty directly into the SVC. The axillary vein, however, drains into the subclavian vein, which drains into the brachiocephalic vein, which in turn drains into the SVC. Refer to Figure 18-5 to help trace the flow of venous blood from a distal site to the vena cava, as follows:

- The cephalic vein is a superficial vein that drains the lateral arm region and carries blood to the axillary vein toward the SVC.
- The basilic vein is a superficial vein that drains the medial arm region. The cephalic and basilic veins are joined by the median cubital vein (anterior aspect of the elbow). Blood samples are often drawn from the median cubital vein.
- The subclavian veins receive blood from the axillary veins and from the jugular veins. Blood is carried by these veins to the brachiocephalic veins, which empty into the superior vena cava.
- The jugular veins drain blood from the head and drain into the subclavian veins. The external jugular veins drain blood from the face, scalp, and neck. The internal jugular veins drain blood from the brain. The internal jugular vein, in fact, is the main vein that drains the brain. Because the jugular veins are so close to the heart (right atrium), the pressure in the jugular veins reflects the pressure of blood in the

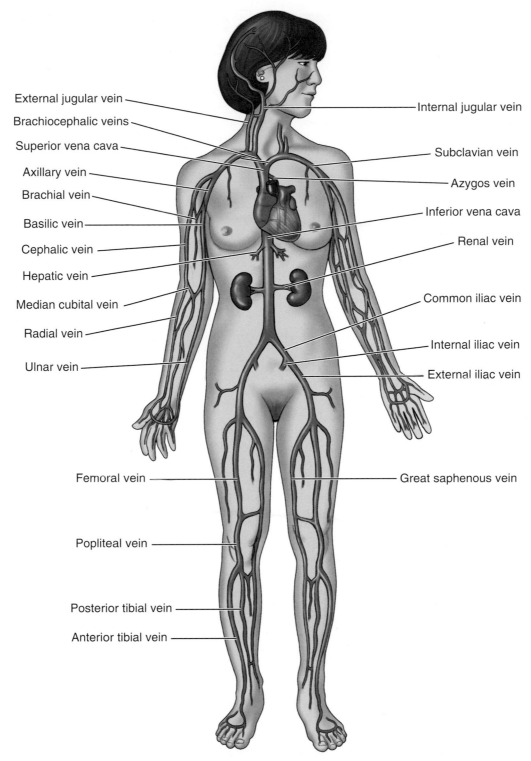

External jugular vein

Brachiocephalic veins

Superior vena cava

Axillary vein

Brachial vein

Basilic vein

Cephalic vein

Hepatic vein

Median cubital vein

Radial vein

Ulnar vein

Internal jugular vein

Subclavian vein

Azygos vein

Inferior vena cava

Renal vein

Common iliac vein

Internal iliac vein

External iliac vein

Femoral vein

Popliteal vein

Posterior tibial vein

Anterior tibial vein

Great saphenous vein

FIGURE 18-5 Major veins.

right side of the heart. A person in right-sided heart failure has a higher-than-normal pressure in the right heart. This is observed clinically as pulsating jugular veins and is referred to as *jugular vein distention* (JVD). As a clinician, you will be observing, measuring, and recording JVD.

- The brachiocephalic veins are large veins formed by the union of the subclavian and internal jugular veins. The right and left brachiocephalic veins drain into the SVC.
- The azygos vein is a single vein that drains the thorax and empties directly into the SVC.

Do You Know...

What the Subclavian Stole?

"Thou shalt not steal." Good advice! It even applies to blood, with a condition called *subclavian steal syndrome*. This is how the heist goes down. A person develops an occlusion in the subclavian artery proximal to the origin of the vertebral artery. (Remember, the vertebral artery supplies blood to the posterior brain and the subclavian artery supplies blood to the shoulder and arm.) When the affected arm is exercised, the subclavian artery is unable to supply enough blood. Blood pressure in the exercising shoulder and arm decreases, causing a retrograde (backward) flow of blood from the vertebral artery to the subclavian artery. The subclavian artery robs the posterior brain of blood, causing neurological symptoms such as impaired vision, dizziness, and syncope (fainting).

VEINS THAT EMPTY INTO THE INFERIOR VENA CAVA

The IVC returns blood to the heart from all regions of the body below the diaphragm. Follow the venous drainage from the leg to the right atrium in Figure 18-5.

- The tibial veins drain the calf and foot regions. The posterior tibial vein drains into the popliteal vein (behind the knee) and then the femoral vein (in the thigh). The femoral vein enters the pelvis as the external iliac vein; it joins with the internal iliac vein and continues as the common iliac vein. The common iliac vein continues as the IVC.
- The great saphenous (SAF-en-us) veins are the longest veins in the body. They begin in the foot, ascend along the medial side, and merge with the femoral vein to become the external iliac vein. These veins receive drainage from the superficial veins of the leg and thigh region. The great saphenous veins also connect with the deep veins of the leg and thigh. Thus, blood can return from the lower extremities to the heart by several routes. The great saphenous veins are sometimes "borrowed" by cardiac surgeons. Portions of a vein are surgically removed and transplanted into the heart to bypass clogged coronary arteries.
- The renal veins drain the right and left kidneys, emptying blood directly into the IVC.
- The hepatic veins drain the liver, emptying blood directly into the upper IVC. Because the hepatic veins are so close to the heart, congestion of the right heart often causes congestion in the hepatic veins and liver.

? **Re-Think**

1. Why aren't all veins colored blue?
2. List five veins that empty directly into the venae cavae.
3. Trace a drop of blood from the left hand to the right atrium.

 Do You Know...

What Varicose Veins Look Like?

Varicose veins are distended and twisted veins, usually involving the superficial veins in the legs. Varicosities can develop in other veins. Hemorrhoids, for example, are varicose veins that affect the veins in the anal region. Persons who are alcoholic often develop varicose veins at the base of the esophagus—esophageal varices. These varices are apt to rupture, causing a massive life-threatening hemorrhage.

Varicose veins

2+2 **Sum It Up!**

The arrangement and names of the major arteries and veins are summarized in Figures 18-4 and 18-5. All systemic arteries are direct or indirect branches of the aorta, the main artery that arises from the left ventricle. Most veins drain directly or indirectly into the superior and inferior venae cavae and then into the right atrium of the heart.

SPECIAL CIRCULATIONS

Most organs receive oxygen-rich blood from a single large artery, whereas oxygen-poor blood is drained by large veins. Several organs have circulations that are arranged differently. They include the blood supply to the head and brain, the blood supply to the liver, and the arrangement of the blood vessels in the unborn child (fetal circulation).

BLOOD SUPPLY TO THE HEAD AND BRAIN

The brain requires a continuous supply of blood; even a few minutes without oxygen causes brain damage. To ensure a rich supply of blood, the head is supplied by two pairs of arteries: carotid arteries and vertebral arteries (Figure 18-6, *A*).

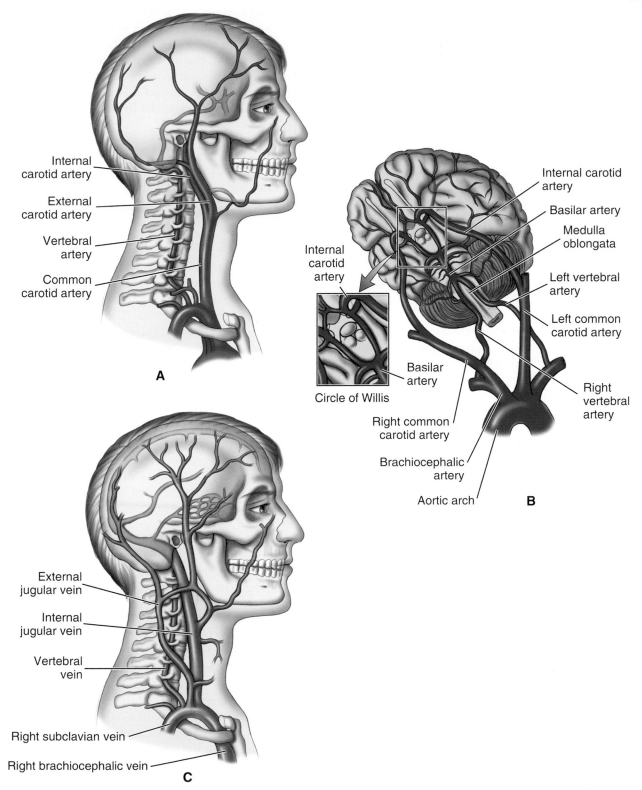

FIGURE 18-6 Blood supply to the head and the brain. **A,** The head is supplied by the common carotid and the vertebral arteries. **B,** The circle of Willis. **C,** Venous drainage of the brain and head.

ARTERIES OF THE HEAD AND NECK

The right common carotid artery arises from the brachiocephalic artery and the left common carotid artery arises directly from the aortic arch (see Figure 18-6, *B*) and ascends in the anterolateral neck. At about the level of the mandible, the common carotid arteries split to form the external and internal carotid arteries. The external carotid arteries supply the superficial areas of the neck, face, and scalp. The internal carotid arteries extend to the front part of the brain. Once inside the cranium, the internal carotid artery divides, sending numerous branches to various parts of the brain and to the basilar artery at the base of the brain. The internal carotid arteries supply most of the blood to the brain.

Vertebral arteries pass upward in the posterolateral neck from the subclavian arteries toward the brain. As the vertebral arteries extend up into the cranium, they join to form a single basilar artery (see Figure 18-6, *B*). Numerous branches from the basilar artery supply areas of the brain around the brain stem and cerebellum. Other branches of the basilar artery connect with branches of the internal carotid arteries.

The branches from the internal carotid arteries and basilar artery form a circle of arteries at the base of the brain. This circular arrangement of arteries is an anastomosis, or connection, called the *circle of Willis* (see Figure 18-6, *B*). Arising from the circle of Willis are many arteries that penetrate the brain and maintain its rich supply of blood.

Most of the blood supply to the brain runs through the internal carotid arteries. What about knotted or clotted carotids? If the carotid arteries become blocked, the vertebral arteries cannot supply sufficient blood to the brain, which results in impaired brain function. Impaired brain function is most often observed as a cognitive (thinking) impairment and dizziness.

VENOUS DRAINAGE OF THE HEAD AND BRAIN

The external and internal jugular veins are the two major veins that drain blood from the head and neck (see Figure 18-6, *C*). The external jugular veins are more superficial and drain blood from the posterior head and neck region. They empty into the subclavian veins. The internal jugular veins drain the anterior head, face, and neck. The deep internal jugular veins drain most of the blood from the venous sinuses of the brain. The internal jugular veins on each side of the neck join with the subclavian veins to form the brachiocephalic veins. The brachiocephalic veins empty blood into the SVC.

> **? Re-Think**
>
> 1. Explain the formation of the circle of Willis by the carotid and vertebral arteries.
> 2. What is the role of the jugular and subclavian veins?

BLOOD SUPPLY TO THE LIVER AND THE HEPATIC PORTAL CIRCULATION

The purpose of the hepatic portal circulation is to carry blood rich in digestive end products from the organs of digestion to the liver. Because it plays such a critical role in metabolism, the liver needs easy access to the digestive end products. As the blood flows through the liver, many of the nutrients are extracted from the

blood and modified in some way. For example, the liver prevents nitrogen from entering the general circulation as ammonia. Instead, the nitrogen is excreted by the liver into the blood in the form of urea. Urea is less toxic than ammonia and is easily eliminated by the kidneys. Thus, it is crucial that blood from the digestive organs first goes to the liver!

HEPATIC BLOOD VESSELS

The blood vessels of the liver have a unique arrangement. Three groups of blood vessels are associated with hepatic circulation: the portal vein, the hepatic veins, and the hepatic artery.

The portal vein is a large vein that carries blood from the organs of digestion to the liver (Figure 18-7). It is formed by the union of two large veins: the superior mesenteric vein and the splenic vein. The superior mesenteric vein receives blood from the small intestine (where most digestion and absorption occur) and the first part of the large intestine. The splenic vein receives blood from the stomach, spleen, and pancreas. In addition, the splenic vein receives blood from the inferior mesenteric vein, which drains the last part of the large intestine.

In addition to the portal vein, the liver has two other blood vessels: the hepatic artery and the hepatic veins. The hepatic artery is a branch of the celiac trunk, a large artery that branches off the abdominal aorta. The hepatic artery carries oxygen-rich blood to the liver. The hepatic veins drain blood from the liver and deliver it to the inferior vena cava.

Note that both the hepatic artery and portal vein carry blood toward the liver. The hepatic artery carries oxygen-rich blood, and the portal vein carries blood rich in the products of digestion to the liver but poor in oxygen content. Two thirds of the hepatic blood flow is unoxygenated blood and is delivered by the portal vein.

HEPATIC PORTAL CIRCULATION: A PART OF THE SPLANCHNIC CIRCULATION

The blood flow to the stomach, spleen, pancreas, intestines, and liver is referred to as the splanchnic circulation. The splanchnic circulation is very adjustable. Blood flow may increase up to eight times following a meal. When digestion is complete, the blood can then be diverted from the splanchnic blood vessels to other organs such as exercising skeletal muscles. Your mother was right: Do not go for a vigorous swim immediately after eating! Your splanchnic blood vessels are using the blood that your swimming skeletal muscles need. Cramping and drowning are possible. The splanchnic circulation also responds vigorously to a severe hemorrhage; the vessels constrict so intensely that they cause an ischemic or blood-deprived gut (intestines). The damaged gut is characterized by bloody diarrhea and absorption of toxins from the intestine into the blood, which is potentially lethal.

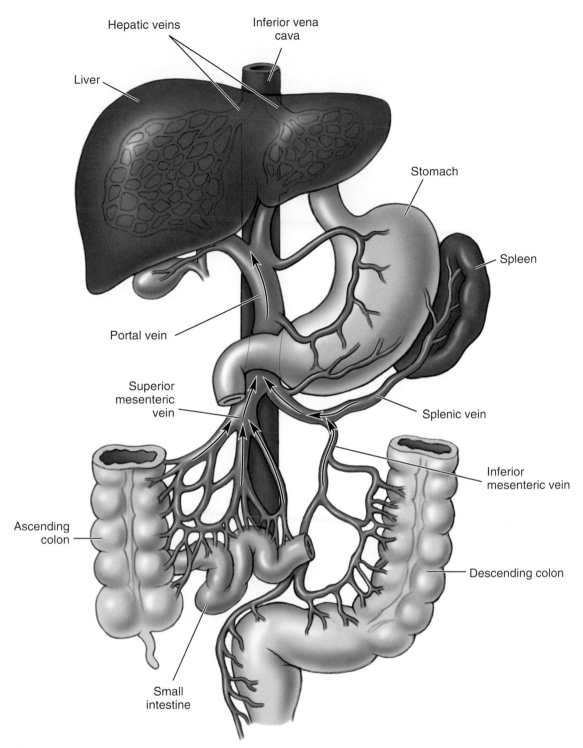

FIGURE 18-7 Hepatic portal circulation.

FETAL CIRCULATION

Look at your "belly button," or umbilicus. At one time, you had a long umbilical cord, a lifeline that attached

you to a structure called the *placenta* embedded in the wall of your mother's uterus. Why was this attachment necessary? As a fetus, you were submerged in amniotic fluid and were unable to eat or breathe. All your nutrients and oxygen had to be supplied by your mother. Your mother also absorbed much of the waste produced by your tiny body and eliminated it through her excretory organs. The exchange of your nutrients, gases, and waste occurred at the placenta.

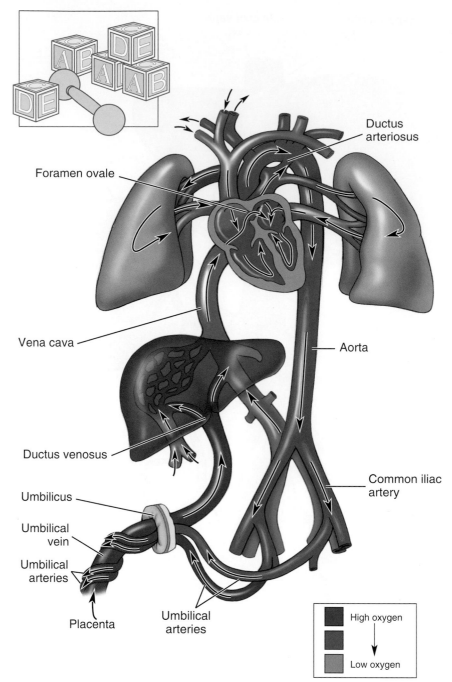

Ductus arteriosus

Foramen ovale

Vena cava

Aorta

Ductus venosus

Common iliac artery

Umbilicus

Umbilical vein

Umbilical arteries

Placenta

Umbilical arteries

High oxygen

Low oxygen

FIGURE 18-8 Fetal circulation.

Because of these special needs, the fetal heart and circulation have several modifications that make them different from "life on the outside" (Figure 18-8). The following modifications are described and summarized in Table 18-2:

- *Umbilical blood vessels.* The umbilical cord contains three blood vessels: one large umbilical vein and two smaller umbilical arteries. The umbilical vein carries blood rich in oxygen and nutrients from the placenta to the fetus. The two umbilical arteries carry carbon dioxide and other waste from the fetus to the placenta. NOTE: In the fetal circulation, the umbilical vein carries oxygen-rich blood, whereas it

is the umbilical arteries that carry oxygen-poor blood.

- *Ductus venosus.* Blood flows through the umbilical vein into the fetus. Within the body of the fetus, the umbilical vein branches. Some blood flows through one branch to the fetal liver. Most of the blood, however, bypasses the liver and flows through the ductus venosus into the IVC. After birth, the ductus venosus closes and serves no further purpose.

Because the deflated fetal lungs are not used for gas exchange, they have no need for blood to be pumped through the pulmonary circulation. Two modifications in the fetal heart and large vessels reroute most of the

Table 18-2	Special Features in the Fetal Circulation	
STRUCTURE	**LOCATION**	**FUNCTION**
Umbilical arteries (two)	Umbilical cord	Transport unoxygenated blood from fetus to the placenta
Umbilical vein (one)	Umbilical cord	Transports oxygenated blood from the placenta to the fetus
Ductus venosus	Between the umbilical vein and inferior vena cava	Carries blood from the umbilical vein to the inferior vena cava; allows some of the blood to bypass the liver
Foramen ovale	Septum between the right and left atria	Allows blood to flow directly from the right atrium into the left atrium to bypass the pulmonary circulation
Ductus arteriosus	Between the pulmonary artery and aorta	Allows blood in the pulmonary artery to flow directly into the descending aorta to bypass the pulmonary circulation

blood past the lungs. These are the foramen ovale and the ductus arteriosus:

- *Foramen ovale.* The foramen ovale (foh-RAY-men oh-VAL-ee) is an opening in the interatrial septum of the heart. This opening allows most of the blood to flow from the right atrium directly into the left atrium.
- *Ductus arteriosus.* Although most blood flows through the foramen ovale into the left atrium, some blood enters the right ventricle and is pumped into the pulmonary artery. How does this blood bypass the lungs? The fetal heart has a short tube called the *ductus arteriosus* (DUK-tus ar-teer-ee-OH-sus) that connects the pulmonary artery with the aorta. Blood pumped into the pulmonary artery bypasses the lungs by flowing through the ductus arteriosus directly into the aorta. After birth, these fetal structures close.

Why is it not a good idea for a pregnant woman to take aspirin or a similar drug, such as indomethacin? Naturally secreted prostaglandins help keep the ductus arteriosus open. Drugs such as aspirin and indomethacin block prostaglandin synthesis, thereby causing a premature closure of the ductus arteriosus. This can be lethal for the baby!

Occasionally, the fetal structures do not close after birth and appear as congenital heart defects. For example, the ductus arteriosus may fail to close, thereby allowing blood to shunt continuously from the aorta to the pulmonary artery. A patent ductus arteriosus (PDA) creates a left-to-right shunt. Fortunately, a PDA is easily corrected.

See Figure 18-8 for color coding of the fetal veins and arteries. Blood vessels carrying oxygenated blood are in red; these are usually the arteries. Vessels carrying unoxygenated blood are in blue; these are usually veins. Note, however, that the umbilical vein is red, indicating oxygenated blood. The umbilical arteries are blue, indicating unoxygenated blood.

Note the color of the upper portion of the vena cava. The adult venae cavae are colored blue because they contain unoxygenated blood. The fetal venae cavae,

however, are violet, indicating that the blood is a mixture of unoxygenated blood (coming from the metabolizing fetal tissue) and oxygenated blood (coming from the umbilical vein). Note also the color of the blood in the fetal aorta; it is not the bright red that is characteristic of the adult aorta. The adult aorta carries only oxygenated blood, but the fetal aorta mixes oxygenated and unoxygenated blood.

? Re-Think

1. List three structural modifications of the fetal circulation.
2. To what maternal structure do the umbilical blood vessels attach?

PULSE

WHAT IS A PULSE?

The ventricles pump blood into the arteries about 72 times/min. The blood causes an alternating expansion and recoil of the arteries with each beat of the heart. This alternating expansion and recoil creates a pressure wave (similar to vibration), which travels through all the arteries. This wave is called the *pulse.*

Because it is caused by the rhythmic contraction of the ventricles of the heart, the pulse is often described as a "heartbeat that can be felt at the wrist." Although a pulse can be felt in any artery lying close to the surface of the body, the site most often used to feel the pulse is the radial artery in the wrist area. Determine your own radial pulse and then try feeling a pulse at any of the nine "pulse points" identified in Figure 18-9.

WHAT CAN YOU LEARN ABOUT A PATIENT BY FEELING THE PULSE?

By feeling a person's pulse, you can determine the heart rate. A normal heart rate is about 72 beats/min. You can also determine if the heart is beating regularly (rhythmically) or irregularly.

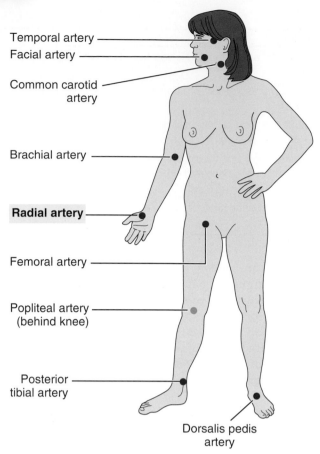

Temporal artery

Facial artery

Common carotid
artery

Brachial artery

Radial artery

Femoral artery

Popliteal artery
(behind knee)

Posterior
tibial artery

Dorsalis pedis
artery

FIGURE 18-9 Pulse points.

You can also assess the pulse for its strength. Does the pulse feel strong or weak? At times, the heart contracts so weakly that the heartbeat cannot be felt over the radial artery; this happens in a person who has lost a lot of blood and is in shock. A pulse may also be described as full or bounding as happens in a person with excess blood volume. It is also possible that you may not be able to detect a pulse in a particular artery. The pulse may be absent if the artery is blocked or occluded. For example, if a person has poor arterial circulation to the feet, as occurs with many diabetic persons, the dorsalis pedis pulse may be undetectable. Thus, a correct assessment of the pulse can provide much useful information about the patient's condition.

2+2 Sum It Up!

There are three special circulations: circulation to the head and brain, the hepatic portal circulation, and the fetal circulation. The brain receives oxygen-rich blood from the circle of Willis, formed by branches of the internal carotid and basilar artery (merger of the vertebral arteries). The purpose of the hepatic portal circulation is to deliver blood rich in digestive end products to the liver for metabolic processing. The fetal circulation has three modifications that allow the fetus to "live under water": the ductus venosus, foramen ovale, and ductus arteriosus. The fetus "breathes and feeds" at the placenta. The pulse is described as a "heartbeat that can be felt at the wrist." Numerous pulse points can be used to assess the pulse.

Note: The As You Age box and the Medical Terminology and Disorders table appear in Chapter 19.

Get Ready for Exams!

Summary Outline

The circulatory system is a series of blood vessels that begin and end in the heart. The circulatory system delivers blood to all the body's cells and then returns the blood to the heart.

I. Circles, Circuits, and Circulations
  A. The heart and blood vessels form a circle.
  B. There are two circulations: pulmonic and systemic.

II. Blood Vessels
  A. Naming the blood vessels
    1. Arteries carry blood away from the heart; the smallest arteries are the arterioles.
    2. Capillaries connect arteries and veins; a capillary is close to every cell in the body.
    3. Veins carry blood back to the heart; small veins are called *venules*.
  B. Layers of blood vessels
    1. The tunica intima is the smooth, innermost layer.
    2. The tunica media is the middle layer, which contains elastic tissue and smooth muscle.

  3. The tunica adventitia is the outermost layer of connective tissue.
  C. Blood vessels: what they do
    1. Arteries conduct blood from the heart to the organs and are called *conductance vessels*.
    2. The arterioles constrict and dilate, thereby determining resistance to the flow of blood. The arterioles are called *resistance vessels*.
    3. Capillaries are concerned with the exchange of water and dissolved substances between the blood and tissue fluid. Capillaries are called *exchange vessels*.
    4. Veins and venules return blood to the heart from the body. The veins also store blood and are therefore called *capacitance vessels*. Veins also contain valves.

III. Major Arteries of the Systemic Circulation
  A. The major arteries include the aorta and the arteries arising directly and indirectly from the aorta.
  B. See Figure 18-4 for the names and locations of the major arteries.

IV. Major Veins of the Systemic Circulation
   A. The major veins include the venae cavae and the veins that directly and indirectly empty into the superior and inferior venae cavae.
   B. See Figure 18-5 for the names and locations of the major veins.

V. Special Circulations
   A. The head and brain are supplied by two sets of arteries: the carotid arteries and the vertebral arteries. The internal carotid arteries and the basilar artery (merger of the vertebral arteries) form the circle of Willis. Blood from the head and brain drains into the jugular veins.
   B. The blood supply of the liver is composed of the portal vein, hepatic artery, and hepatic veins. The hepatic artery brings oxygen-rich blood to the liver. The portal vein carries blood from the digestive tract to the liver. The hepatic veins carry blood from the liver to the inferior vena cava.
   C. The fetal circulation has several unique features. The fetus uses the placenta as lungs. The umbilical blood vessels carry blood between the placenta and the fetus. Three special structures (modifications) are the ductus venosus, foramen ovale, and ductus arteriosus.

VI. The Pulse
   A. The pulse is caused by the alternating expansion and recoil of the artery creating a pressure wave.
   B. The pulse is often described as a "heartbeat that can be felt at the wrist."
   C. Figure 18-9 identifies the pulse points.

Review Your Knowledge

Matching: Blood Vessels: Structure and Function
Directions: Match the following words with their descriptions below. Some words may be used more than once.
a. large arteries
b. arterioles
c. capillaries
d. veins

1. ___ Exchange vessels
2. ___ Resistance vessels
3. ___ Composed of a single layer of epithelium sitting on a basement membrane
4. ___ The most numerous of the blood vessels
5. ___ Capacitance vessels
6. ___ Blood pressure is lowest in these blood vessels.
7. ___ Generally colored blue and contain valves
8. ___ These are the strongest of the blood vessels.
9. ___ Blood pressure is highest in these blood vessels.
10. ___ Connect the arteries and veins

Matching: Names of Blood Vessels
Directions: Match the following words with their descriptions below. Some words may be used more than once.
a. aorta
b. inferior vena cava
c. carotids
d. circle of Willis
e. portal vein
f. hepatic artery
g. jugular
h. brachial artery
i. renal artery
j. median cubital vein
k. saphenous
l. radial artery
m. coronaries

1. ___ Carries oxygen-rich blood to the liver
2. ___ Carries oxygen-rich blood to the kidneys
3. ___ Carries blood that is rich in digestive end products to the liver
4. ___ Classified as ascending, arch, and descending
5. ___ The superior mesenteric and splenic veins merge to form this vein.
6. ___ Classified as thoracic and abdominal
7. ___ Vein in the arm that is used to "draw" a sample of blood
8. ___ Main vein that drains the brain
9. ___ Arterial blood supply at the base of the brain
10. ___ Arteries that ascend along the anterolateral neck to the brain
11. ___ Longest superficial vein in the thigh and leg
12. ___ The common iliac veins drain into this blood vessel.
13. ___ Blood pressure is usually taken over this artery.
14. ___ This artery is usually used in "taking a pulse."
15. ___ These arteries supply the myocardium.

Matching: Fetal Circulation
Directions: Match the following words with their descriptions below.
a. umbilical arteries
b. umbilical vein
c. ductus arteriosus
d. ductus venosus
e. foramen ovale

1. ___ Carry blood from the fetus to the placenta
2. ___ Opening that connects the right and left atria in the fetal circulation
3. ___ Structure that connects the pulmonary artery and the aorta in the fetal circulation
4. ___ Structure that partially bypasses the fetal liver
5. ___ Carries oxygen-rich blood from the placenta to the fetus

Multiple Choice
1. Which of the following is not true about the capillaries?
   a. They are called the *exchange vessels*.
   b. Capillary membranes have holes or pores.
   c. They connect the arteries and the veins.
   d. They have valves.

2. The common carotid
   a. supplies oxygenated blood to the brain.
   b. is the main vein that drains the brain.
   c. is part of the hepatic portal system.
   d. ascends along the posterolateral neck to the brain to form the basilar artery.
3. The purpose of the hepatic portal system is to
   a. provide the fetus with oxygenated blood.
   b. deliver blood that is rich in digestive end products to the liver.
   c. drain unoxygenated blood from the brain.
   d. deliver oxygenated blood to the liver.
4. Which statement is true about the fetal circulation?
   a. The umbilical arteries deliver oxygenated blood to the fetus.
   b. The umbilical vein delivers oxygenated blood to the fetus.
   c. The ductus venosus connects the right and left fetal atria.
   d. The ductus arteriosus bypasses the fetal liver.
5. Which of the following is descriptive of the aorta?
   a. It is the largest and strongest of the arteries.
   b. It carries unoxygenated blood and is therefore colored blue.
   c. It is lined with large valves.
   d. Blood pressure in the aorta is lower than blood pressure in the veins.
6. The portal vein, hepatic vein, and celiac trunk are most associated with the
   a. stomach.
   b. pancreas.
   c. small intestine.
   d. liver.
7. The superior mesenteric vein and the splenic vein
   a. drain directly into the superior vena cava.
   b. drain the brain.
   c. merge to form the portal vein.
   d. carry venous blood from the liver to the inferior vena cava.
8. The common iliac arteries, renal arteries, and celiac trunk
   a. are branches of the descending aorta.
   b. are branches of the abdominal aorta.
   c. carry oxygenated blood.
   d. All of the above are true.
9. The median cubital vein, brachial vein, and radial vein
   a. carry oxygenated blood.
   b. are color-coded red.
   c. are located in the upper extremities.
   d. are prone to varicosities.
10. Both the brachiocephalic artery and the left common carotid artery
    a. arise from the arch of the aorta.
    b. arise from the abdominal aorta.
    c. drain into the superior vena cava.
    d. receive blood from the jugulars.

Go Figure

1. **According to Figures 18-1 and 18-2**
   a. Blood is pumped by the heart to arteries → veins → capillaries → back to the right side of the heart.
   b. The capillaries are closer to the individual cells than is the aorta.
   c. Capillaries have a more elastic wall than the aorta.
   d. The venae cavae deliver blood to the capillaries.

2. **According to Figures 18-3 and 18-4**
   a. The ascending aorta gives rise to the common iliac arteries.
   b. Both common carotid arteries arise directly from the arch of the aorta.
   c. The abdominal aorta is part of the descending aorta.
   d. The thoracic aorta gives rise to the renal arteries.

3. **According to Figures 18-5 and 18-7**
   a. The portal vein bypasses the liver and drains directly into the inferior vena cava.
   b. The superior mesenteric vein and splenic vein merge to form the portal vein.
   c. The hepatic vein drains into the portal vein.
   d. The inferior vena cava delivers blood to the saphenous veins.

4. **According to Figure 18-6**
   a. The jugulars are part of the circle of Willis.
   b. The vertebral arteries carry blood to the facial structures.
   c. The internal carotids deliver oxygenated blood to the circle of Willis.
   d. All blood delivered to the circle of Willis comes from the internal carotid arteries.

5. **According to Figure 18-8**
   a. The ductus venosus is the hole in the fetal interatrial septum.
   b. The umbilical vein carries oxygenated from the placenta to the fetus.
   c. The foramen ovale is the fetal structure that connects the pulmonary artery with the aorta.
   d. The fetal heart is color-coded blue and red as in the adult heart.

Functions of the Blood Vessels

Key Terms

baroreceptor reflex (p. 362)
blood pressure (p. 357)
capillary exchange (p. 364)
diastolic pressure (p. 358)
hypertension (p. 358)
hypotension (p. 358)

ischemia (p. 357)
Korotkoff sounds (p. 358)
oncotic pressure (p. 365)
pulse pressure (p. 358)
systemic vascular resistance
    (p. 360)

systolic pressure (p. 358)
vasoconstriction (p. 361)
vasodilation (p. 361)
vasopressor (p. 364)

Objective

1. List the five functions of the blood vessels.
2. Discuss blood pressure, including:
   - Describe the measurement of blood pressure.
   - Explain the variance of blood pressure in different blood vessels.
   - Describe the factors that determine blood pressure.
   - Explain the mechanisms involved in regulation of blood pressure, including the baroreceptor reflex.

3. Explain how blood vessels act as exchange vessels, including:
   - Describe the factors that determine capillary exchange.
   - Describe the mechanisms of edema formation.
4. Explain how the blood vessels respond to changing body needs.
5. Describe the role of the blood vessels in the regulation of body temperature.

As mentioned earlier in this text, it took seemingly forever for the ancients to "connect" the heart and the peripheral blood vessels. After that connection was made, scientists realized that blood was pumped out of the left heart, circulated around the body, and returned to the right side of the heart. However, we still had no real understanding of the functions (physiology) of the peripheral blood vessels.

Today, we know that the blood vessels do more than allow blood to run around in circles. The blood vessels perform five important functions:
1. Act as a delivery system
2. Regulate blood pressure
3. Engage in the exchange of nutrients and waste between the capillaries and cells
4. Redistribute blood in response to changing body needs
5. Help regulate body temperature

BLOOD VESSELS DELIVER

The primary purpose of the cardiovascular system is to deliver blood that is rich in oxygen, hormones, nutrients, and water to the cells; the blood also collects cellular waste and delivers it to organs of excretion, such as the kidneys. The delivery of oxygen is especially critical. All cells need oxygen; without oxygen,

they die. Impaired blood flow and oxygen deprivation is called ischemia; the consequences of ischemia are tissue damage, pain, and gangrene.

BLOOD VESSELS REGULATE BLOOD PRESSURE

Why do you need a blood pressure? Blood pressure is needed to push blood through the blood vessels to an organ. No blood pressure means no organ perfusion! Blood pressure is the force that blood exerts against the walls of the blood vessels. Blood pressure is determined by the pumping action of the heart and the diameter of the blood vessels.

MEASUREMENT OF BLOOD PRESSURE

116/72 mm Hg: WHAT IT MEANS

You just had a physical examination. The physician nodded approvingly that your blood pressure is normal at 116/72 mm Hg. Although you are thrilled to be normotensive (normal blood pressure), what exactly does 116/72 mm Hg mean?

The blood pressure in the large arteries is caused by the heart's pumping activity. When the ventricles contract, blood is pumped out of the ventricle into the artery, thereby increasing pressure. The pressure in the arteries at the peak of ventricular contraction (systole) is called the **systolic pressure**; it is the top number (e.g., 116 mm Hg). The **diastolic pressure** is the pressure in the large arteries when the ventricles of the heart are relaxing (diastole). The diastolic reading is the bottom number (e.g., 72 mm Hg).

By measuring blood pressure, you can also calculate **pulse pressure**. The pulse pressure is the difference between the systolic and the diastolic pressure. For example, your blood pressure is 116/72 mm Hg. Your pulse pressure is 44 mm Hg (116 minus 72).

 Do You Know...

About the MABP?

A blood pressure is expressed as 120/80 mm Hg. What is the mean arterial blood pressure (MABP)? MABP is calculated as follows:

MABP = 2/3 diastolic pressure + 1/3 systolic pressure

or

MABP = diastolic pressure + 1/3 pulse pressure

For a blood pressure of 120/80 mm Hg, the MABP is 94 mm Hg. Why is the MABP important? It is important because the organs are perfused by or "feel" the MABP. Note that the MABP expresses more of the diastolic pressure than the systolic pressure. The dominance of the MABP by the diastolic pressure is the basis for the clinical concern for the diastolic reading.

NORMAL AND ABNORMAL

Blood pressure readings vary according to age, gender, and size (and don't discount your emotional state). For example, the normal blood pressure of a 2-year-old child is 95/65 mm Hg. The normal blood pressure for an adult is defined as a systolic pressure of less than 120 mm Hg and a diastolic pressure of less than 80 mm Hg. For many years, a blood pressure of 120/80 mm Hg was considered normal for an adult; today, it is classified as prehypertensive. The maintenance of normal blood pressure is extremely important. If blood pressure becomes too low (**hypotension**), blood flow to vital organs decreases, and the person is said to be in shock. Without immediate treatment, the person may die. If the blood pressure becomes elevated (**hypertension**), the blood vessels may burst, or rupture. A ruptured blood vessel in the brain, for example, is a major cause of stroke, resulting in loss of speech, paralysis, and possible death. Hypertension also puts added strain on the heart, damages the blood vessels in the kidneys, and damages the retina, causing loss of vision. Chronic hypertension is a major cause of heart failure. You will spend much time "taking" blood pressures and will be expected to interpret abnormal readings.

 Do You Know...

About "White Coat Hypertension"?

Often a patient's blood pressure elevates in response to a health care worker (wearing a white coat) recording his or her blood pressure, hence the term *white coat hypertension*. In fact, the person's blood pressure should be recorded a second time after he or she has relaxed. Emotions matter! Diagnosis and treatment are never based on a single blood pressure recording. There are other considerations in recording blood pressure, including proper cuff size and the patient's position (sitting with feet on the floor). The person should not be talking. One study has indicated that over 90% of blood pressure recordings in a single clinic violate proper procedure.

"TAKING" A BLOOD PRESSURE

Measurement of blood pressure provides valuable information regarding a person's general health. Blood pressure is most commonly measured over the brachial artery in the arm. Blood pressure is expressed in millimeters of mercury (mm Hg). Unless otherwise stated, the term *blood pressure* refers to the blood pressure in the large arteries.

The instrument used to take a blood pressure recording is the sphygmomanometer (sfig-moh-mah-NOM-eh-ter), which is a device with two basic components: a dial indicating the pressure and an inflatable cuff. The cuff is wrapped around the patient's arm and inflated with air until the brachial artery is compressed and the flow of blood through the artery is stopped. Then, with a stethoscope placed over the brachial artery distal to, or below, the cuff, the examiner listens for "tap tap tap" sounds. These sounds, called **Korotkoff (kor-ROT-koff) sounds**, are caused by the turbulent flow of blood through the brachial artery. The measurement of blood pressure is further explained in Figure 19-1.

? **Re-Think**

1. Your patient's blood pressure is 145/88 mm Hg. To what do the top and bottom numbers refer?
2. Your patient's initial blood pressure was 145/88 mm Hg. After 10 minutes, his blood pressure had declined to 122/76 mm Hg. What is a likely explanation for this spontaneous decline in blood pressure?

SYSTOLIC PRESSURE **DIASTOLIC PRESSURE**

Cuff pressure is inflated (no pulse sounds heard)

Pressure in cuff is lowered

Pressure in cuff is lowered more

Sounds first heard at 116 mm Hg

Sounds disappearing at 72 mm Hg

Brachial artery

no sound

Korotkoff sounds

Brachial artery closed by cuff, no blood flow

Blood spurts into constricted artery

Blood flows freely

A **B** **C** **D**

FIGURE 19-1 Taking a blood pressure. The measurement of blood pressure requires a sphygmomanometer and a stethoscope. Follow the panels for an explanation of the systolic (116 mm Hg) and diastolic (72 mm Hg) pressures. **A,** Identify the location of the brachial artery. **B,** Inflate the cuff, thereby squeezing the upper arm. At this point, the cuff pressure has become greater than the blood pressure in the brachial artery. The cuff pressure collapses the brachial artery, thereby stopping the flow of blood. No sound can be heard through the stethoscope. **C,** As the pressure in the cuff gradually diminishes, the artery opens slightly and blood spurts through the blood vessel in response to the pressure in the brachial artery. You can hear the spurting effect of the blood as soft tapping sounds. The number on the sphygmomanometer that corresponds to the tapping sounds is recorded as the systolic blood pressure (116 mm Hg). With further reduction in cuff pressure, the brachial artery opens wider and allows blood flow through the artery to increase. **D,** As cuff pressure declines even further, the brachial artery opens completely and normal blood flow through the artery resumes. At this point, the sounds heard through the stethoscope disappear or sound muffled. The pressure at which the sounds disappear is read as the diastolic blood pressure (72 mm Hg).

BLOOD PRESSURE IN DIFFERENT BLOOD VESSELS

Blood pressures vary from one type of blood vessel to the next (Figure 19-2). Note that the blood pressure is highest in the aorta because it is closest to the left ventricle; the left ventricle pumps blood with great force. The blood pressure gradually declines as the blood flows from the large arteries into the arterioles, into the capillaries, into the venules and, finally, into the veins. This difference in pressure causes blood to flow from the arterial side of the circulation to the venous side. Note that a blood pressure of 116/72 mm Hg is normal only for large blood vessels. Capillary pressure is generally much lower. Pressure within the large veins is around 0 mm Hg.

BLOOD PRESSURE AND VENOUS RETURN

Although blood pressure is very high in the arterial circulation, it decreases to almost 0 mm Hg in the veins. The blood pressure in the veins is so low, in fact, that it alone cannot return blood from the veins back to the heart. Three other mechanisms come to the rescue: skeletal muscle action, respiratory movements, and constriction of the veins.

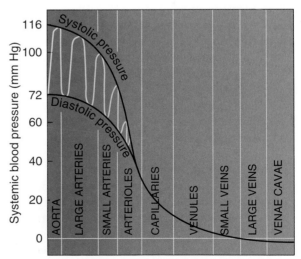

FIGURE 19-2 Blood pressure in the different blood vessels.

Skeletal Muscle Action

As Figure 19-3 shows, the large veins in the leg are surrounded by skeletal muscles. When the skeletal muscles are relaxed and blood flow slows, the valves close. As the skeletal muscles contract, they squeeze

To heart

Closed
valve

Open
valve

Vein

Muscle

FIGURE 19-3 Skeletal muscle pump.

the large veins, thereby opening the valves and forcing blood toward the heart. This mechanism is called the *skeletal muscle pump*. The pump explains the beneficial effects of exercise for your patients. Exercise improves venous return of blood to the heart and prevents stagnation of blood and thrombosis (blood clot formation).

Respiratory Movements

The act of breathing is performed by the contraction and relaxation of the skeletal muscles of the chest. These respiratory movements cause the pressures in the chest cavity to change. Inhalation decreases pressure within the thorax and increases pressure within the abdominal cavity. The respiratory-induced change in pressures forces blood toward the heart, thereby increasing venous return. This is called the *respiratory pump*. Encouraging your patient to "deep breathe" not only improves respiratory function, but also improves the circulation of blood.

Constriction of the Veins

Because most of the blood is located in the venous side of the circulation (capacitance vessels), constriction of the veins pushes additional blood out of the veins toward the heart. Both sympathetic nervous system stimulation and some hormones cause venoconstriction (VEE-noh-kahn-STRIK-shun), thereby increasing venous return of blood to the heart.

❓ Re-Think

1. List three mechanisms that improve venous return of blood to the heart.
2. Why does walking prevent stagnation of blood in the legs?

2+2 Sum It Up!

The blood vessels deliver blood to every organ in the body. The driving force for the movement of blood through the blood vessels is the blood pressure. Blood pressure is highest in the large arteries and lowest in the veins, accounting for the flow of blood from arteries to veins. However, venous pressure is so low in the venae cavae that venous blood flow needs help; it is aided by the skeletal muscle pump, respiratory pump, and venoconstriction.

WHAT DETERMINES BLOOD PRESSURE?

Blood pressure is determined by the heart (cardiac output) and the blood vessels (**systemic vascular resistance**).

> Blood Pressure = Cardiac Output × Systemic Vascular Resistance

HEART AND BLOOD PRESSURE

How does myocardial function affect blood pressure? You probably have watched enough television to know that when the heart stops beating, the blood pressure drops to 0 mm Hg and the person dies, indicating an obvious relationship between cardiac function and blood pressure.

What is the heart component of blood pressure? It is the cardiac output. Recall from Chapter 17 that cardiac output is determined by heart rate (HR) and stroke volume (SV). The stronger the force of contraction, the greater the stroke volume, the greater the cardiac output, and the higher the blood pressure. The faster the heart rate, the greater the cardiac output, and the higher the blood pressure. Conversely, a decline in heart rate and/or stroke volume decreases cardiac output and blood pressure.

BLOOD VESSELS AND BLOOD PRESSURE

How do the peripheral blood vessels affect blood pressure? A garden hose illustrates the blood vessels' effect on blood pressure. In Figure 19-4, *A*, the hose is hooked up to a faucet. When the faucet is turned on, water flows through the hose and falls to the ground in big droplets. In Figure 19-4, *B*, a nozzle has been attached to the end of the hose, thereby narrowing the end of the hose. The nozzle has increased the resistance to the flow of water. Because of the resistance of the nozzle, water does not fall out of the hose in big droplets, as in Figure 19-4, *A*; instead, water squirts out of the end of the hose. Notice how much further the squirted water travels. What is the reason for this difference? If you were to measure the pressures at point X, you would record a higher pressure in the hose with the nozzle on it. The nozzle increases resistance to the flow of water and causes the pressure behind the nozzle to

FIGURE 19-4 Effect of resistance on pressure. **A,** Low resistance and low pressure. **B,** High resistance and high pressure. **C,** Vasodilation, low resistance, and low pressure. **D,** Vasoconstriction, high resistance, and high pressure.

increase. The increased pressure in the nozzled hose simply pushes the water further.

How does the example of the hose apply to blood pressure? The large blood vessels are similar to the hose. The smaller vessels, especially the arterioles, act as nozzles. Because the arterioles are composed largely of smooth muscle, the contraction and relaxation of the muscle allow the arterioles to change their diameter and therefore their resistance to blood flow. *Systemic vascular resistance* (SVR) is the clinical term that refers to the resistance offered by all the peripheral blood vessels; it is the same as *total peripheral resistance* (TPR).

Arteriolar smooth muscle determines resistance. **Vasodilation** occurs when arteriolar smooth muscle relaxes and increases the diameter of the blood vessels. The process is comparable to removing the nozzle from the end of the hose (see Figure 19-4, *C*). Vasodilation decreases resistance in the blood vessels and decreases blood pressure. When the smooth muscle contracts, the diameter of the arteriole becomes smaller. This process is known as **vasoconstriction** and is comparable to adding a nozzle to the hose (see Figure 19-4, *D*). Vasoconstriction increases SVR and raises blood

pressure. Thus, the arterioles' ability to dilate and constrict helps determine blood pressure.

Do You Know...
About Obesity and the Miles and Miles of New Blood Vessels?

Blood pressure is determined by cardiac output and SVR. SVR is usually determined by changes in the diameter of the arterioles. Other resistance terms such as *blood vessel length* and *blood viscosity* are normally ignored. However, the accumulation of excess fat tissue not only adds pounds; it also contributes miles of additional new blood vessels, making blood vessel length a significant contributor to SVR. Fat tissue also secretes hormones that narrow or constrict blood vessels. Excess fat therefore elevates SVR, making the person hypertensive. What to do to lower that blood pressure? Lose weight!

? Re-Think

1. What are the two determinants of blood pressure?
2. Why would peripheral vasodilation cause dizziness and possibly syncope (fainting)?

Do You Know...

About Venodilation and This "Fainting" Balloon?

If a patient takes a drug that causes venodilation, the following events occur: blood "pools" in the veins; less blood returns to the heart (decreased venous return); myocardial contraction decreases (Starling effect); cardiac output decreases; and blood pressure decreases (hypotension). If the patient attempts to change position quickly, as in rising from a supine (lying down) to a standing position, insufficient blood is pumped to the brain, causing dizziness, fainting, and falling. This series of events is called *postural hypotension*, because it usually occurs when the patient assumes an upright posture. The water-filled balloon illustrates venodilation and pooling when the position of the balloon changes from a lying (horizontal) to standing (vertical) position. Lesson? Advise your patients to get up slowly from lying to sitting to upright. Other common causes of postural hypotension are blood volume depletion (dehydration), an aging cardiovascular system, and autonomic dysfunction. Elderly persons are especially prone to postural hypotension.

HOW BLOOD PRESSURE STAYS WITHIN NORMAL LIMITS

Under normal conditions, blood pressure remains relatively constant, at slightly less than 120/80 mm Hg. Regulation of blood pressure involves rapidly acting and slowly acting mechanisms.

RAPIDLY ACTING MECHANISMS

The most important of the rapidly acting mechanisms is a nervous mechanism called the **baroreceptor reflex**. This reflex consists of the following structures: receptors, sensory nerves, medulla oblongata, and motor nerves. (Follow the arrows in Figure 19-5 as you read about the components of the baroreceptor reflex.)

- *Receptors*. The special receptors, called *baroreceptors* (bar-oh-ree-SEP-tors), or pressure receptors, are located in the walls of the aortic arch and carotid sinus, located in the lower part of the internal carotid arteries. The baroreceptors sense sudden change in blood pressure.
- *Sensory nerves*. Once the baroreceptors have been activated, the sensory information travels along the nerves to the brain. The nerves that carry the sensory information are cranial nerves (CNs) IX (glossopharyngeal) and X (vagus).
- *Medulla oblongata*. The medulla oblongata of the brain stem interprets sensory information coming from the baroreceptors. The medulla oblongata then decides what to do. If the blood pressure is low, the medulla oblongata tells the heart and blood vessels to increase blood pressure. If the medulla oblongata receives information that the blood pressure is high, it tells the heart and blood vessels to decrease blood pressure.
- *Motor nerves*. Once the medulla oblongata has identified adjustments needed to restore blood pressure to normal, the motor nerves carry information to the heart and blood vessels. The motor nerves involved are the nerves of the autonomic nervous system (sympathetic and parasympathetic nervous systems).

What happens if a person's blood pressure suddenly declines as in hemorrhage? The decline in blood pressure is sensed by the baroreceptors and the information carried by sensory nerves (CNs IX and X) to the medulla oblongata. The medulla oblongata then fires the sympathetic nervous system. Stimulation of the sympathetic nerves causes the sinoatrial (SA) node to fire more quickly, thereby increasing heart rate. Sympathetic firing also causes the ventricular myocardium to contract more forcefully, increasing stroke volume. Both of these responses increase cardiac output and blood pressure. Firing of the sympathetic nerves also causes vasoconstriction of the arterioles, thereby increasing systemic vascular resistance and blood pressure.

The same series of events occurs in a person who suddenly experiences a sudden, drug-induced (e.g., nitroglycerin) decline in blood pressure. Activation of the baroreceptors causes an increase in heart rate, or reflex tachycardia. The tachycardia can overburden a damaged heart, causing angina (chest pain) and additional myocardial damage. The effect of drugs on baroreceptor responses is huge!

What happens if a person's blood pressure suddenly increases? Parasympathetic (vagal) stimulation decreases heart rate and therefore decreases cardiac output and blood pressure. Blood pressure also decreases because the blood vessels dilate, thereby decreasing resistance. If the blood vessels do not contain parasympathetic nerves, why do they dilate? The vasodilation is not caused by parasympathetic

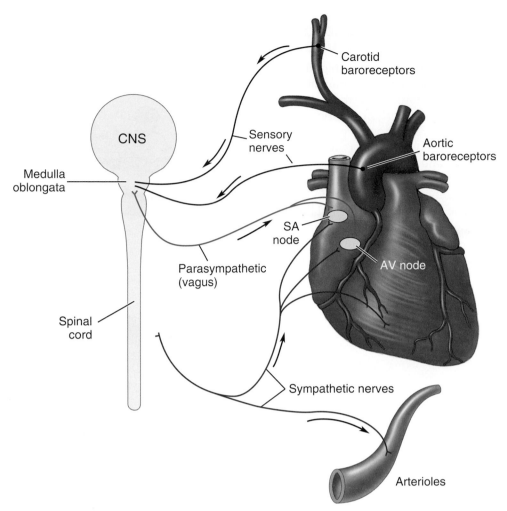

FIGURE 19-5 Baroreceptor reflex.

activity; it occurs because the sympathetic nerves become less active when the parasympathetic nerves fire.

Carotid sinus syncope also illustrates the baroreceptor response to a sudden increase in blood pressure. A tight collar exerts pressure over a hypersensitive carotid sinus, activating the baroreceptors. The medulla oblongata falsely interprets the blood pressure information as an elevation in blood pressure. Information sent from the brain to the heart and blood vessels lowers the blood pressure, so much so that the person faints (syncope). This response is called *carotid sinus syncope*. Other stimuli for carotid sinus syncope include shaving over the neck region, showering with strong spurts of water, and the use of shoulder strap seat belts.

 Re-Think

What is the baroreceptor response to excess vasodilation, as often occurs in the pharmacological treatment of hypertension?

A second, but less important, rapidly acting mechanism is the secretion of epinephrine and norepinephrine from the medulla of the adrenal gland. These hormones increase cardiac output and cause vasoconstriction, thus increasing blood pressure.

Do You Know...

About Val Salva's Most Embarrassing Medical Moment?

Val was constipated! Sounds like an insignificant problem, but in a person with a history of coronary artery disease (CAD), constipation can prove fatal. While "straining at stools," Val suffered a near-fatal heart attack. Straining at stools initiates the Valsalva maneuver, which occurs when a person tries to force an exhalation with the mouth and nose closed (as in having a bowel movement). The forced exhalation increases pressure in the chest, which in turn increases blood pressure. The sudden increase in blood pressure activates the baroreceptor reflex, causing a sudden burst of parasympathetic activity that not only slows heart rate, but triggers a fatal dysrhythmia, leading to cardiac arrest. Unfortunately, it is a rather common occurrence that someone with a history of CAD has a heart attack while on the "porcelain throne." How embarrassing—and to think it might have been prevented by a stool softener or laxative.

SLOWER ACTING MECHANISMS AND LONG-TERM REGULATION OF BLOOD PRESSURE

Several mechanisms act slowly to control blood pressure. These hormonally mediated mechanisms are more concerned with the long-term regulation of blood pressure. The most important of the slowly acting mechanisms is the renin-angiotensin-aldosterone mechanism. Activation of this mechanism increases blood volume and causes vasoconstriction. Both of these effects increase blood pressure (see Chapter 24). Other hormones that affect blood pressure include antidiuretic hormone (ADH). ADH is also called *vasopressin* because it exerts a **vasopressor** effect (increases blood pressure). Atrial natriuretic peptide (ANP) and brain natriuretic peptide (BNP), secreted by the distended walls of the heart, lower blood pressure by causing vasodilation and by decreasing blood volume through the renal (kidney) secretion of sodium and water.

2+2 Sum It Up!

Blood pressure is defined as the force that blood exerts against the walls of the blood vessels. Blood pressure is determined by the activity of the heart (cardiac output) and blood vessels, especially the arterioles (systemic vascular resistance). Remember: Blood pressure = cardiac output × systemic vascular resistance. Several mechanisms regulate blood pressure. The most important rapidly acting mechanism is the baroreceptor reflex; a sudden decline in blood pressure triggers a sympathetic discharge, whereas a sudden increase in blood pressure triggers parasympathetic or vagal discharge. The secretion of epinephrine and norepinephrine contributes to the rapid-response system. Long-term mechanisms are hormonal and include the renin-angiotensin-aldosterone system, antidiuretic hormone (ADH), and the natriuretic peptides.

BLOOD VESSELS ACT AS EXCHANGE VESSELS

The capillaries engage in the exchange of nutrients and waste between the blood and cells. Accordingly, the capillaries are called *exchange vessels*. The capillaries are the most numerous of the blood vessels. If all the capillaries in the body were lined up end to end, they would encircle the earth 2.5 times.

A

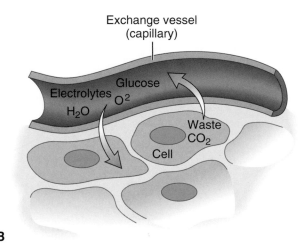

B

FIGURE 19-6 **Capillary exchange**: deliveries and pickup.
A, Waiters delivering food and picking up empty trays.
B, Capillary exchange.

WHAT IS AN EXCHANGE VESSEL?

An exchange vessel exchanges or swaps substances, much like a waiter (Figure 19-6, *A*). For example, a waiter delivers food to hungry guests. After some time has passed, the waiter picks up the waste—the empty trays, dirty dishes, and leftover food. Note the exchange part; food is dropped off and waste is picked up.

The capillaries work like the waiter (see Figure 19-6, *B*). As blood flows through the capillaries, substances move out of the capillary into the surrounding tissue spaces (interstitium). These substances include oxygen, water, electrolytes, and various nutrients such as glucose; they are the substances that the cell needs to live, work, and grow.

Oxygen and nutrients are taken up and used by the cells. As the cells carry on their work, they produce waste material such as carbon dioxide. The cellular waste diffuses out of the cell, into the interstitium, and then into the blood within the capillary. The blood carries the waste away from the capillary to the organs of excretion, such as the kidneys and the lungs.

WHY CAPILLARIES ARE GOOD EXCHANGE VESSELS

Three characteristics make the capillaries good exchange vessels: thin capillary walls, large numbers of capillaries, and slow blood flow through the capillaries.

THIN CAPILLARY WALLS

The capillary wall consists of a single layer of epithelium that sits on a delicate basement membrane. The epithelial layer has many holes, or pores, through which water and solute easily move.

MILLIONS OF CAPILLARIES

The millions of capillaries provide a huge surface for exchange; the larger the capillary surface, the greater the rate of exchange.

SLOW VELOCITY OF BLOOD FLOW

The large numbers of capillaries also affect the rate of blood flow. The greater the number of capillaries, the slower the flow of blood. The slow blood flow allows more time for exchange.

CAPILLARY FORCES: EXCHANGE

How do the nutrients and waste "know" where to go? There are forces that move water, nutrients, and waste in and out of the capillaries. These forces are diffusion and a filtration-osmosis balancing act.

EXCHANGE INVOLVING DIFFUSION

Diffusion is the primary process causing substances to move across the capillary wall. Diffusion means that a substance moves downhill from an area of high concentration to an area of low concentration. For example, the concentration of oxygen is higher in the capillary than in the tissue fluid. Thus, oxygen diffuses from the capillary into the interstitium and then into the cell. On the other hand, carbon dioxide concentration is higher in the interstitium than in the capillaries. Thus, carbon dioxide diffuses from the interstitium into the capillary.

EXCHANGE INVOLVING FILTRATION-OSMOSIS

A second process of exchange involves filtration-osmosis and is particularly important for water exchange. Filtration is illustrated in the syringe in Figure 19-7, A. A syringe is loaded with water. When the plunger is pushed, the pressure within the barrel of the syringe increases and water is forced out of the syringe through the needle. What would happen if you were to punch holes in the side of the syringe and push on the plunger? Not only would water flow through the needle end, it would also squirt out of the side of the syringe in response to the pressure.

The plunger and syringe are similar to the heart and capillaries (see Figure 19-7, B). The heart, like the plunger, creates a pressure that accomplishes two things. First, blood is pushed forward from the arterial end of the capillary to the venous end of the capillary. Second, because of the pores in the capillary wall, water and the smaller substances (electrolytes, glucose) squirt into the interstitium. Plasma proteins, such as albumin, are too large to fit through the capillary pores and therefore remain in the capillaries.

The pushing of the water and dissolved substances through the pores is filtration. Note that the cause of filtration is blood pressure. Note also the direction of filtration. In response to the pressure in the capillary, water and the dissolved substances are pushed out of the capillary into the interstitium.

What happens to all the substances pushed into the interstitium? The nutrients are used by the cells. What about the water that was filtered? The water is reabsorbed at the venous end of the capillary. The force that is responsible for the reabsorption of water is the oncotic pressure. The **oncotic pressure** is the plasma osmotic pressure that is due to the plasma proteins. Figure 19-7, C, shows that the oncotic pressure in the capillary is higher than in the interstitium. The capillary oncotic pressure is higher because of the plasma proteins trapped within the capillaries. The high oncotic pressure causes the water to diffuse from the interstitium into the capillary. Lymphatic drainage removes excess water from the interstitium (see Chapter 20).

What is the balancing act? The exact amount of water filtered at one end of the capillary is reabsorbed at the other end. The balancing act is important. If the amount of water filtered out of the capillary exceeds the amount reabsorbed from the tissue space, fluid collects in the tissue space. Excess fluid collection in the interstitium is called *edema*. If more water is reabsorbed from the tissue space than was filtered, the tissue space becomes depleted and the patient appears dehydrated. Fluid imbalances occur in many clinical conditions.

MECHANISMS OF EDEMA FORMATION

The forces that determine the movement of water across the capillary walls are disrupted in many clinical conditions. Some of the more common conditions are described here.

Heart Failure

A patient in heart failure retains water and develops excess blood volume (hypervolemia). The expanded blood volume, in turn, increases capillary filtration pressure, thereby increasing the amount of water filtered out of the capillaries into the interstitium. The excess filtration of water exceeds the ability of the capillaries to reabsorb water. Thus, the excess water remains in the interstitium, causing edema.

FIGURE 19-7 Filtration and osmosis. **A,** Syringe filled with water (H_2O). The plunger pushes the water out of the syringe. **B,** Capillary filled with blood. The heart pushes blood out of the capillary. **C,** Movement of water back into the capillary because of the oncotic pressure in the capillary.

Excess filtration of water into the lungs is called *pulmonary edema* and results in impaired oxygenation. Excess fluid accumulation in the feet is called *pedal edema*.

Severe Burn

A patient is admitted to the emergency room with severe burns on the lower extremities. In response to the thermal injury, the capillary pores dilate, thereby allowing the escape of excess water and plasma proteins into the interstitium. The "leaked" protein causes edema for two reasons. First, the reduction in plasma protein decreases oncotic pressure within the capillary; this decreases reabsorption of water. Second, the leaked protein "holds" the water in the interstitium by slowing its reabsorption.

Kidney Disease

A child is diagnosed with a kidney disease called *nephrotic syndrome*. The child's mother first noticed edema around his eyes (periorbital edema) and difficulty in fastening the waist of his pants. Nephrotic syndrome is characterized by the excretion of large amounts of the plasma protein, albumin, in the urine (albuminuria); this results in low plasma levels of albumin (hypoalbuminemia). The edema of nephrotic syndrome is caused in part by the hypoalbuminemia, resulting in a decreased plasma oncotic pressure.

Blocked Lymphatic Drainage

A woman goes to a clinic complaining of a grossly swollen leg and is eventually diagnosed with a large tumor in her lower pelvis. The tumor has compressed

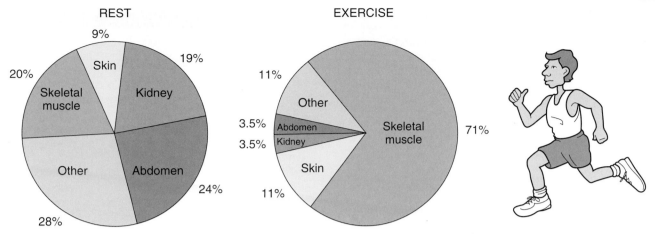

FIGURE 19-8 Distribution of blood flow at rest and during exercise.

the lymphatic vessels, thereby impairing the drainage of lymph; impaired lymph drainage causes the accumulation of fluid in the interstitium (edema). For this same reason, edema develops with the surgical removal of a breast (mastectomy) and lymph node dissection.

? Re-Think

1. Why are capillaries good exchange vessels?
2. Why is water filtered at the arterial end of the capillary? Why is water reabsorbed at the venous end of the capillary?
3. Explain how the body can "borrow" water from the interstitium in a dehydrated person?

2+2 Sum It Up!

The capillaries are well suited for exchange because of three characteristics: thin capillary wall, large surface area of capillaries, and slow velocity of capillary blood flow. Most solute exchanges by simple diffusion. Water (and some solute) exchange using the filtration-osmosis pressures (filtration at the arterial end and osmosis at the venous end of the capillary). Edema formation is due to an imbalance of the filtration-osmosis transport mechanisms at the capillary level.

BLOOD VESSELS DISTRIBUTE BLOOD

Blood vessels are also "in charge" of distributing blood according to changing body needs. As Figure 19-8 shows, blood flow to a particular area of the body can change. For example, in the resting state, the skeletal muscle receives 20% of the total blood flow, and the kidney and abdomen receive 19% and 24%, respectively. Note what happens during strenuous exercise. Blood flow is redirected; the percentage of blood flow pumped to skeletal muscle greatly increases (to 71% of total flow). Why? Exercising muscle needs more oxygen and nutrients. In addition, the increased blood flow carries heat and waste products away from the exercising muscles. At the same time, the percentage

of blood that flows through the kidney and abdomen decreases (3.5% of total flow). In other words, the blood is directed to sites where it is most needed, such as the skeletal muscle. Note also that the blood flow to the skin increases from 9% to 11% of total flow. The increased blood flow to the skin helps lose the excess heat, thereby helping regulate body temperature.

BLOOD VESSELS REGULATE BODY TEMPERATURE

The regulation of body temperature is described in Chapter 7. In essence, the blood vessels help dissipate (get rid of) or conserve heat. For example, with exercise and temperature elevation, the blood vessels dilate, thereby allowing more blood to flow to the skin. This activity transfers heat from the deeper tissues to the surface of the body. The heat radiates from the flushed skin, thereby lowering body temperature. Conversely, heat is conserved when the blood vessels of the skin constrict, diverting the warm blood from surface blood vessels into deeper parts of the body.

2+2 Sum It Up!

The circulatory system does more than run around in circles. It acts as a delivery system, regulates blood pressure, engages in the exchange of nutrients and waste, redistributes blood in response to changing body needs, and helps in the regulation of body temperature.

As You Age

1. The circulatory system is one of the body systems most affected by age. The walls of the arteries thicken and become less elastic and stiffer. Two major consequences occur: blood flow to vital organs (e.g., the brain) decreases, and blood pressure increases, thereby increasing the work of the heart.
2. Changes occur in both the walls and the valves of the veins. As a result, older persons are more prone to the development of varicose veins.
3. The inner surface of the blood vessels becomes roughened because of age-related changes in the vessel wall and the development of fatty plaques. As a result, older persons are more prone to thrombus formation.
4. The baroreceptors become less sensitive. Cardiovascular adjustments to changes in position are slowed, and the person may become dizzy and tend to fall.
5. Permeability of the capillary membrane increases with age, thereby increasing edema formation in older persons.

MEDICAL TERMINOLOGY AND DISORDERS — Disorders Involving the Peripheral Vasculature

Medical Term	Word Parts	Word Part Meaning or Derivation	Description
Words			
angioplasty	angi/o-	vessel	An **angioplasty** is *the surgical repair of a blood vessel, either by the insertion of a balloon-tipped catheter or reconstruction of the vessel.* The widened blood vessel improves blood flow to the myocardium.
	-plasty	surgical repair of or reconstruction	
intravenous	intra-	within	Refers to *the space within a vein.* Access is achieved by a venipuncture, or the insertion of a needle into a vein. Fluids and drugs are often administered intravenously.
	-ven/o-	vein	
	-ous	pertaining to	
phlebotomy	phleb/o-	vein	A **phlebotomy** is *the entrance into a vein for the purpose of obtaining blood for analysis or treatment.*
	-otomy	incision into	
vascular	vascul/o-	vessel	A term that *refers to blood vessels,* as in vascular disease or vascular resistance.
	-ar	pertaining to	
Disorders			
aneurysm		From a Greek word meaning "dilation" or "wide"	An **aneurysm** is *an abnormal bulging or ballooning of the walls of blood vessels, especially the arteries.* Aneurysms have two shapes: fusiform and saccular. The **fusiform aneurysm** is a weakness along an extended section of the aorta and involves the entire circumference of the aorta. A **saccular aneurysm** is a small bulge or sac on one side of the aorta. There are three types of aneurysms based on location: aortic, cerebral (or berry), or peripheral aneurysm. The **aortic aneurysms** are classified as thoracic and abdominal. **Cerebral (or berry) aneurysms** occur in an artery of the brain and are often berry sized. **Peripheral aneurysms** are those that occur in arteries other than the aorta and brain. An aortic aneurysm can also occur with dissection **(dissecting aneurysm),** in which a small tear in the aortic wall allows the blood to flow through the layers, thereby extending the tear and occluding blood vessels supplying other organs.
angioma	angi/o-	blood vessel	An **angioma** is *a benign tumor composed of blood vessels or lymph vessels that usually appear at the surface of skin.* There are many types of angiomas: a **hemangioma,** such as a **port-wine stain,** is a proliferation of endothelial cells lining a blood vessel. The angioma often looks like a stain created by spilled red wine.
	-oma	tumor	

MEDICAL TERMINOLOGY AND DISORDERS   Disorders Involving the Peripheral Vasculature—cont'd

Medical Term	Word Parts	Word Part Meaning or Derivation	Description
claudication		From a Latin word, *claudicare*, meaning "limping"	**Claudication** is *a condition that usually occurs in the legs*. **Vascular claudication** refers to discomfort caused by poor circulation to the extremities and is common in persons with diabetes. **Spinal or neurogenic claudication** is due to nerve root compression (e.g., herniated disk, bone spurs, scar tissue) or stenosis of the spinal canal. Claudication usually presents as pain, discomfort, or tiredness in calf muscles while walking; it is often described in terms of city blocks. A "one-block claudication" refers to the onset of claudication when the person experiences discomfort after walking one city block. There is also two-block or three-block claudication. Claudication may occur intermittently with exercise or occur at rest. **Rest claudication** is usually indicative of more serious underlying pathology.
hypertension	hyper-	excessive	*High blood pressure* (**hypertension**) is defined as a blood pressure >140/90 mm Hg. Hypertension can cause blood vessels to rupture with catastrophic results, such as a hemorrhage into brain tissue. Chronic hypertension increases the workload of the heart, gradually causing the heart to enlarge (ventricular hypertrophy) and fail. Hypertension also causes damage to other organs such as the kidneys, eyes, and brain.
	-tension	From a Latin word, *tendere*, meaning "to stretch"	
hypotension	hypo-	below	*Low blood pressure* (**hypotension**) is a blood pressure <90/60 mm Hg. Hypotension reduces blood flow to vital organs. Very low blood flow to the brain causes a loss of consciousness (syncope). Low blood flow to the heart may cause ischemic chest pain and necrosis (myocardial infarction).
	-tension	From a Latin word, *tendere*, meaning "to stretch"	
ischemia	isch/o-	blockage	**Ischemia** means *insufficient blood supply to a tissue or an organ*. The ischemic tissue is deprived of oxygen and nutrients. Examples include myocardial ischemia and an ischemic gut.
	-emia	blood condition	
peripheral arterial disease			**Peripheral arterial disease (PAD)** involves *an atherosclerotic narrowing and deterioration of the arteries of the neck, abdomen, and periphery*. The most significant risk factors are hypertension, elevated cholesterol, diabetes mellitus, and, chiefly, cigarette smoking. Although any artery can be affected, PAD most often involves the coronary, carotid, distal abdominal aorta, iliac, and femoral arteries.
Raynaud's phenomenon		Named for French physician Dr. Maurice Raynaud (1834–1881)	**Raynaud's phenomenon** is *an episodic vasospasm (involuntary contraction of the blood vessels), most often of the cutaneous blood vessels of the fingers and toes (also ears and nose)*. Vasospastic episodes cause the digits to change color: pallor (white) to cyanosis (bluish-purple) to rubor (red). Poor perfusion to the digits causes pain and tissue changes and damage, including gangrene.
shock			**Shock** is a general term used to characterize *a hypoperfusion of tissues and impairment of cellular metabolism. Shock is caused by low blood flow or maldistribution of blood flow*. Low blood flow is caused by poor cardiac function (**cardiogenic shock**) or low blood volume (**hypovolemic shock**). Hypovolemia is a consequence of hemorrhage, pooling of blood, and systemic vasodilation. Maldistribution of blood flow is caused by **neurogenic shock** (spinal cord injury), **septic shock** (infection), and **anaphylactic shock** (severe allergic response).

Continued

MEDICAL TERMINOLOGY AND DISORDERS   Disorders Involving the Peripheral Vasculature—cont'd

Medical Term	Word Parts	Word Part Meaning or Derivation	Description
thrombophlebitis	thromb/o-	From the Greek word *thrombos*, meaning "clot or curdled milk"	**Thrombophlebitis** is *the most common disorder of the veins; it is the formation of a thrombus (blood clot) in association with inflammation of the vein.* Classifications include **superficial thrombophlebitis** and the more clinically significant **deep vein thrombosis (DVT).** DVT is characterized by **Virchow's triad:** venous stasis, damage of the venous endothelium, and hypercoagulability. The thrombus most often forms in the deep veins of the legs; a piece of the thrombus may break off, becoming an embolus that lodges in the pulmonary circulation **(pulmonary embolus).** **Phlebothrombosis** refers to the development of a thrombus in the veins without the associated inflammation. It is usually caused by sluggish circulation in the legs, caused by prolonged bed rest, long car trips, or extended air travel.
	-phleb/o-	vein	
	-itis	inflammation	
varices		From a Latin word meaning "raised area," a reference to the bulging area of the legs associated with varicose veins	**Varices** are *abnormally dilated and lengthened arteries, veins, or lymph nodes.* In the lower extremities, varices are known as **varicose veins.** These are large, tortuous veins; they are of cosmetic concern and cause discomfort and a feeling of heaviness while standing. Other veins throughout the body can be affected. In the digestive system, esophageal varices develop in the lower esophagus in response to elevated portal pressure caused by cirrhosis of the liver. The concern is that the varices will rupture and bleed. In the rectal area, varices are called *hemorrhoids.* **Hemorrhoids** may be external or internal. **External hemorrhoids** are often painful, are accompanied by irritation and itching, and are prone to thrombosis. **Internal hemorrhoids** are generally not painful, but may bleed when irritated. A scrotal varicosity is called a **varicocele. Telangiectasia** is an enlargement of superficial cutaneous blood vessels that are most visible on the face and thighs.

Get Ready for Exams!

Summary Outline

The blood vessels perform five main functions.

I. Functions as a Delivery System
  A. The blood vessels deliver oxygen, nutrients, and hormones to the cells.
  B. The blood vessels pick up waste from the cells and deliver it to the organs of excretion.

II. Regulates Blood Pressure
  A. The blood vessels maintain a blood pressure to ensure an adequate flow of blood to the body.
  B. The normal blood pressure is slightly less than 120/80 mm Hg; 116/72 mm Hg is a normal blood pressure—116 is the systolic reading, and 72 is the diastolic reading.
  C. Blood pressure varies throughout the circulatory system; it is highest in the aorta and lowest in the venae cavae.
  D. Blood pressure in the veins is so low that help is needed—via skeletal muscle pump, respiratory pump, and venoconstriction—in order to return blood to the right heart.
  E. Blood pressure is determined by the action of the heart and blood vessels. The heart affects blood pressure by increasing or decreasing cardiac output. The blood vessels affect blood pressure by constricting or dilating the arterioles (systemic vascular resistance).
  F. Blood pressure is regulated on a daily basis by the baroreceptor reflex. A sudden decline in blood pressure causes the sympathetic nerves to fire. A sudden increase in blood pressure causes the parasympathetic (vagus) nerves to fire.
  G. Other mechanisms can correct blood pressure more slowly. The most important is the renin-angiotensin-aldosterone system.

III. Acts as Exchange Vessels
  A. The capillaries are the site of exchange of nutrients and waste between the blood and tissue fluid.
  B. Factors that make the capillaries ideal exchange vessels are the thin capillary walls with many pores, millions of capillaries, and a slow rate of blood flow through the capillaries.
  C. Most exchange occurs by diffusion.
  D. Water and dissolved substances exchange by filtration-osmosis. The capillary pressure pushes (filtration) water out of the capillary at its arterial end. Water and dissolved waste move from the

tissue fluid into the capillaries in response to plasma oncotic pressure.

IV. Distributes Blood According to Need
   A. Figure 19-8 compares the distribution of blood during rest and exercise.
   B. Note the change in skeletal muscle blood flow during rest (20%) and exercise (71%).

V. Regulates Body Temperature
   A. Vasodilation of the blood vessels of the skin encourages heat loss.
   B. Vasoconstriction of the blood vessels of the skin decreases heat loss.

Review Your Knowledge

Matching: Blood Pressure Terms
Directions: Match the following words with their descriptions below. Some of the words may be used more than once.
a. systolic pressure
b. diastolic pressure
c. pulse pressure
d. mean arterial blood pressure (MABP)
e. reflex tachycardia
f. Korotkoff sounds
g. brachial artery
h. baroreceptors

1. ____ ⅔ diastolic pressure + ⅓ systolic pressure
2. ____ Silent...tap...tap...tap...tap...muffle
3. ____ Pressure reading that reflects myocardial contraction
4. ____ Cells in the carotid sinus and aortic arch that detect changes in blood pressure
5. ____ Usual site of blood pressure recording
6. ____ The top number of a blood pressure recording
7. ____ The bottom number of a blood pressure recording
8. ____ The difference between the systolic and diastolic pressures
9. ____ Pressure reading that reflects myocardial relaxation
10. ____ A cardiac consequence of a sudden drop in blood pressure

Matching: Blood Pressure Readings
Directions: Match the following blood pressure readings with their descriptions below.
a. 116/72 mm Hg
b. 70/40 mm Hg
c. 220/120 mm Hg

1. ____ Normal blood pressure recorded in the aorta
2. ____ Normal blood pressure recorded in the brachial artery
3. ____ A "shocky" blood pressure
4. ____ A hypertensive blood pressure
5. ____ A hypotensive blood pressure
6. ____ Normotensive reading
7. ____ A postoperative blood pressure that may require a vasopressor drug
8. ____ A blood pressure that requires immediate treatment with an antihypertensive drug
9. ____ Has a pulse pressure of 44
10. ____ Blood pressure that is most likely to cause a reflex tachycardia

Matching: Changes in Blood Pressure
Directions: Indicate if the following (a) increases blood pressure or (b) decreases blood pressure.
1. ____ Sympathetic nerve stimulation
2. ____ Vagal discharge
3. ____ Effects of a vasopressor agent
4. ____ Effects of epinephrine and angiotensin II
5. ____ Increased systemic vascular resistance (SVR)
6. ____ Decreased cardiac output
7. ____ Arteriolar constriction
8. ____ Administration of an alpha$_1$-adrenergic blocker
9. ____ IV infusion of Levophed (norepinephrine)
10. ____ Administration of a beta$_1$-adrenergic agonist

Multiple Choice
1. The ability of the arterioles to contract and relax allows them to
   a. regulate heart rate.
   b. prevent the backflow of venous blood.
   c. function as resistance vessels.
   d. function as exchange vessels.
2. Which of the following is not a consequence of sympathetic nerve stimulation?
   a. Increased cardiac output
   b. Peripheral vasoconstriction
   c. Elevation of blood pressure
   d. Decreased systemic vascular resistance
3. A sudden decrease in blood pressure is most likely to cause
   a. edema.
   b. reflex tachycardia.
   c. increase in the synthesis of albumin.
   d. arteriolar dilation.
4. Which of the following is true of an increase in systemic vascular resistance?
   a. Increases blood pressure
   b. Is caused by vagal discharge
   c. Is caused by peripheral vasodilation
   d. Is due to relaxation of the aorta
5. In which of the following vessels is blood flow slowest?
   a. Aorta
   b. Arterioles
   c. Capillaries
   d. Veins
6. Which of the following is most apt to lower plasma oncotic pressure?
   a. Dehydration
   b. Hypoalbuminemia
   c. Hypertension
   d. Blood transfusion
7. The skeletal muscle pump
   a. increases systemic vascular resistance.
   b. lowers blood pressure.
   c. enhances venous return of blood to the right heart.
   d. closes the valves within the large veins during exercise.
8. Which of the following is most apt to cause edema?
   a. Decreased filtration pressure as in dehydration
   b. Increased plasma oncotic pressure
   c. Accumulation of albumin in the interstitium (tissue space)
   d. Hypotension

9. Which of the following occurs in the dehydrated state?
   a. The capillary oncotic pressure decreases and fluid accumulates in the tissue spaces.
   b. The capillary filtration pressure decreases and tissue fluid is absorbed into the capillaries.
   c. The capillary filtration rate increases, thereby increasing lymph formation.
   d. Plasma protein is filtered into the tissue spaces, thereby causing edema.

Go Figure

1. **According to Figure 19-2**
   a. Pressure within the capillaries is less than the pressure within the venae cavae.
   b. The pulse pressure within the capillaries is equal to the pulse pressure within the large arteries.
   c. Arteriolar pressure is greater than venous pressure.
   d. Pressure is lowest in the arterioles.

2. **According to Figure 19-1, *B*, neither the systolic pressure nor diastolic pressure can be heard because**
   a. The cuff has not been inflated sufficiently.
   b. The brachial artery is compressed, thereby blocking any flow of blood.
   c. The stethoscope is in the wrong place; it should be proximal to the cuff.
   d. Korotkoff sounds can only be heard when the cuff is inflated to more than 200 mm Hg.

3. **According to Figure 19-3**
   a. Valves in the deep veins of the leg remain open when the person is in a sitting position.
   b. Leg movement, as in exercise, induces stagnation of blood in the deep veins of the legs.
   c. Contraction of the muscles of the leg compresses the veins and enhances the flow of blood toward the heart.
   d. Blood returns to the heart because the valves in the veins of the leg contract and force blood in a forward direction.

4. **According to Figure 19-4**
   a. Resistance is greater in panel *A* than in panel *B*.
   b. The radius of the arterioles in panels *C* and *D* determine resistance to flow (of blood).
   c. Vasoconstriction decreases resistance to flow.
   d. Vasodilation increases resistance to flow.

5. **According to Figure 19-5**
   a. The baroreceptors are located in the SA and AV nodes.
   b. Sensory neurons of cranial nerves IX and X carry pressure information from the SA and AV nodes to the aortic arch and the carotid sinus.
   c. Motor information regarding the adjustment of blood pressure is transmitted to the heart and blood vessels.
   d. Motor information regarding the adjustment of blood pressure is transmitted to the carotid sinus and the aortic arch.

6. **According to Figure 19-7**
   a. In panel *B,* water is oncotically reabsorbed into the capillary.
   b. In panel *B,* the plasma proteins (albumin) are filtered into the interstitium.
   c. In panel *C,* water is oncotically reabsorbed from the interstitium into the capillary.
   d. Oncotic pressure is primarily caused by the plasma electrolytes and glucose.

7. **According to Figure 19-7**
   a. Albumin is filtered at the arterial end of the capillary.
   b. Water is reabsorbed by both the venous end of the capillary and the lymphatic vessels.
   c. The capillary membrane is impermeable to water, electrolytes, and plasma protein.
   d. The lymphatic vessel is impermeable to albumin, electrolytes, and water.

Lymphatic System

Key Terms

lymph (p. 373)
lymph nodes (p. 375)
lymphatic ducts (p. 374)

lymphatic vessels (p. 373)
spleen (p. 378)

thymus gland (p. 376)
tonsils (p. 376)

Objective

1. List three functions of the lymphatic system.
2. Describe the composition and flow of lymph.
3. Describe the lymph nodes, and state the location of the cervical nodes, axillary nodes, and inguinal nodes.

4. Describe the other lymphoid organs: tonsils, thymus gland, and spleen.

The woman in Figure 20-1 has a condition called *elephantiasis*. The name is an obvious reference to the size and shape of her leg. Elephantiasis is caused by the invasion and blockage of the lymphatic vessels by small worms called *filariae*. The amount of swelling illustrates the importance of the lymphatic system, which drains fluid from our tissue spaces.

The lymphatic system contains lymph, lymphatic vessels, lymphoid organs, and lymphoid tissue, which are widely scattered throughout the body. The three main functions of the lymphatic system are as follows:

• The lymphatic vessels return tissue fluid to the blood.

• Specialized lymphatic vessels play an important role in the intestinal absorption of fats and fat-soluble vitamins.
• Lymphoid tissue helps the body defend itself against disease.

THE LYMPHATIC SYSTEM

LYMPH: WHAT IT IS, WHERE IT COMES FROM

Lymph (limf) is a clear fluid that resembles plasma. Lymph is composed primarily of water, electrolytes, waste from metabolizing cells, and some protein that leaks out of the capillaries of the systemic circulation. Where does lymph come from? It is formed from the plasma during capillary exchange. About 20 L/day of lymph is filtered from the blood into the interstitium, or tissue spaces. It leaves the interstitium through the lymphatic vessels, which then carry the lymph toward the heart and eventually empty it into the blood.

Water and dissolved substances are continuously filtered out of the blood capillaries into the interstitium to form tissue fluid. Approximately 85% of this tissue fluid moves back into the blood capillaries and is carried away as part of the venous blood. What about the 15% of the tissue fluid that does not re-enter the blood capillaries? This fluid is drained by the lymphatic capillaries that surround the blood capillaries (Figure 20-2). The tissue fluid entering the lymphatic vessels is the lymph.

LYMPHATIC VESSELS

The lymphatic vessels include lymphatic capillaries and several larger lymphatic vessels. Like the blood

FIGURE 20-1 Elephantiasis, a form of lymphedema.

FIGURE 20-2 Lymph capillaries and blood capillaries.

vessels, the lymphatic vessels form an extensive network. The distribution of lymphatic vessels is similar to the distribution of veins. With the exception of the CNS, every organ in the body has a rich supply of lymphatic vessels. These pick up tissue fluid and transport it toward the heart. Figure 20-3 shows the relationship between the circulatory system and the lymphatic system. Note especially the close relationship of the lymphatic vessels with the veins.

The walls of the lymphatic capillaries are made up of a single layer of epithelium and have large pores. This large-pore structure allows the lymphatic capillaries to drain tissue fluid and proteins, thereby forming lymph. Once absorbed by the lymphatic capillaries, the lymph flows toward the heart through a series of larger and larger lymphatic vessels until it reaches the large lymphatic ducts.

For example, lymph from the right arm and right side of the head and thorax drains into the right lymphatic duct. Lymph from the rest of the body drains into the thoracic duct (Figure 20-4). Both ducts empty the lymph into the subclavian veins. The right lymphatic duct drains lymph into the right subclavian vein; the thoracic duct drains lymph into the left subclavian vein.

MOVEMENT THROUGH THE LYMPHATIC VESSELS

Whereas blood moves because it is pumped by the heart, lymph depends on other means for movement. Lymph moves in response to the following:
- The "milking" action of the skeletal muscles. As the skeletal muscles contract, they squeeze the surrounding lymphatic vessels, thereby pushing lymph toward the heart.
- The movement of the chest during respiration. Contraction and relaxation of the chest muscles cause changes in the pressure within the thorax. The

changes in intrathoracic pressure increase the flow of lymph.
- The rhythmic contraction of the smooth muscle in the lymphatic vessels. The alternating contraction and relaxation of the smooth muscle cause lymph to flow.
- The presence of valves. Like the veins, the lymphatic vessels contain valves. Valves prevent any backflow of lymph; if lymph moves at all, it must move toward the heart.

❓ Re-Think

1. A patient has had a radical mastectomy (removal of the breast) with lymph node dissection. Why might she develop edema in the affected arm?
2. What is the function of the right lymphatic and thoracic ducts?

2+2 Sum It Up!

Lymphatic vessels accompany venous blood vessels throughout the body. They drain fluid and protein from tissue spaces; the lymph drains into the main lymphatic ducts (right lymphatic duct and thoracic duct). The main lymphatic ducts drain into the general circulation through the subclavian veins. Lymph is not pumped by the heart; it moves in response to skeletal and smooth muscle activity.

LYMPHOID ORGANS

The lymphoid organs include the lymph nodes, tonsils, thymus gland, and spleen (Figure 20-5, A). Lymphoid tissue is also found scattered throughout the body in many other organs and particularly in mucous membranes, where it is referred to as *MALT* (*m*ucosal-*a*ssociated *l*ymphoid *t*issue). In general, the lymphoid organs and lymphoid tissue help defend the body

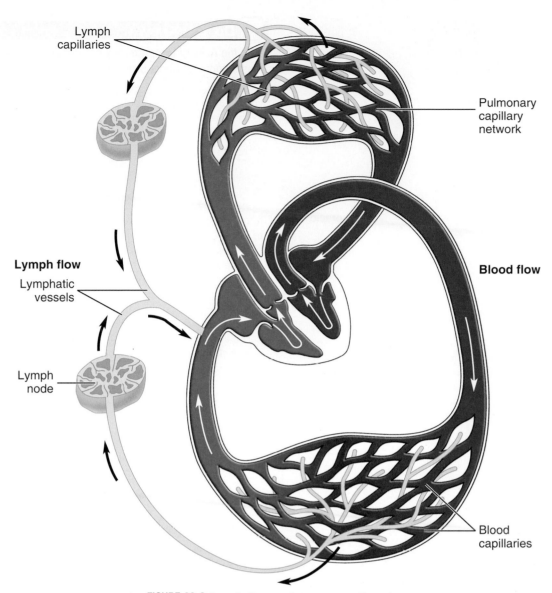

Lymph capillaries

Pulmonary capillary network

Lymph flow

Lymphatic vessels

Blood flow

Lymph node

Blood capillaries

FIGURE 20-3 Lymphatic vessels accompany the veins.

against disease by filtering particles such as pathogens and cancer cells from the lymph, tissue fluid, and blood and by supporting the activities of the lymphocytes, which provide immunity against disease.

LYMPH NODES

Lymph nodes are small pea-shaped patches of lymphatic tissue strategically located to filter the lymph as it flows through the lymphatic vessels. Lymph nodes tend to appear in clusters (see Figure 20-5, *B*). The larger clusters include the following:

- *Cervical lymph nodes* drain and cleanse lymph coming from the head and neck areas. Enlarged, tender cervical lymph nodes often accompany upper respiratory infections.

- *Axillary lymph nodes* are located in the axillary area, or armpit. These nodes drain and cleanse lymph coming from the upper extremities, shoulders, and breast area. Cancer cells that escape from the breast are often found in the axillary lymph nodes.
- *Inguinal lymph nodes* are located in the groin region. These nodes drain and cleanse lymph from the lower extremities and external genitalia.

What does a lymph node look like? A lymph node contains several compartments, called *lymph nodules,* that are separated by lymph sinuses (Figure 20-6). The lymph nodules are masses of lymphocytes and macrophages. These cells are defensive cells and are concerned with immunity and phagocytosis; they protect the body against disease. The lymph nodules are separated by lymph sinuses; these are lymph-filled spaces. Afferent lymphatic vessels carry lymph into the node

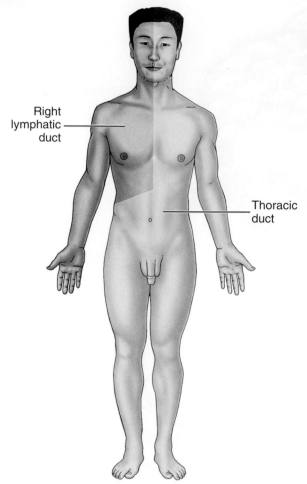

Right lymphatic duct

Thoracic duct

FIGURE 20-4 Main lymphatic ducts: right lymphatic duct and thoracic duct.

for cleansing. The lymph leaves the node through the efferent lymphatic vessels as it continues its journey toward the heart.

TONSILS

Tonsils are partially encapsulated lymph nodes in the throat area (see Figure 20-5, *A* and *C*). They filter tissue fluid contaminated by pathogens that enter the body through the nose, mouth, or both. The three sets of tonsils are as follows:

- *Palatine tonsils* are small masses of lymphoid tissue located at the opening of the oral cavity into the pharynx. A tonsillectomy is most often performed on this particular set of tonsils.
- *Pharyngeal tonsils* are also called the *adenoids.* They are located near the opening of the nasal cavity in the upper pharynx. The adenoids atrophy during adolescence. Enlargement of the adenoids may interfere with breathing and may require surgical removal, a procedure known as *adenoidectomy.*
- *Lingual tonsils* are located at the back of the tongue.

 Do You Know...

Why the Axillary Lymph Nodes Are Removed during a Mastectomy (Surgical Breast Removal)?

Many cancers metastasize, or spread, by way of the lymphatic vessels. Cancer of the breast commonly metastasizes to the axillary lymph nodes. In an attempt to rid the body of all cancer cells, the surgeon removes the breast and associated axillary lymph nodes. Each lymph node is then biopsied; further treatment often depends on how many of the lymph nodes are positive (i.e., are cancerous, or malignant). Removal of the axillary lymph nodes frequently impairs lymphatic drainage. Consequently, the woman may develop edema of the affected arm and shoulder. Because the edema develops in response to impaired drainage of lymph, it is called *lymphedema.*

A new technique is the sentinel node biopsy. The procedure was developed to determine if a cancer has spread without doing the traditional lymph node dissection. It is based on the following observation. Lymph ducts of the breast usually drain to one lymph node first and then to the others in the axillary region. The lymph node that receives the initial drainage is called the *sentinel lymph node* and is identified by the injection of dye. If the sentinel node biopsy is negative, it is assumed that the cancer has not spread to the axillary lymph nodes.

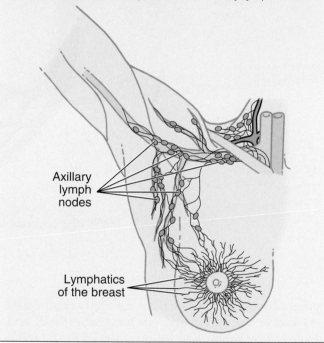

Axillary lymph nodes

Lymphatics of the breast

THYMUS GLAND

The **thymus gland** is located in the mediastinum of the thoracic cavity (see Figure 20-5, *A*). The thymus gland plays a crucial role in the development of the immune system before birth and in the first few months after birth. After puberty, the gland shrinks or involutes, but remains active throughout life.

The thymus gland secretes hormones called *thymosins.* Thymosins promote the proliferation and maturation of special lymphocytes (T cells) in lymphoid tissue throughout the body (see Chapter 21).

FIGURE 20-5 Location of lymphoid tissue. **A,** Lymphoid organs. **B,** Distribution of lymph nodes. **C,** Tonsils.

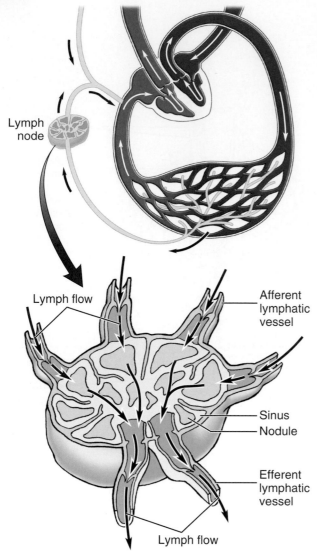

FIGURE 20-6 Cross-section of a lymph node.

Why "Lose That Spleen" Was a Slogan for Ancient Roman Marathoners?

In ancient Roman times, the rumor in marathon circles was that removal of the spleen would make a person a faster runner. The spleen was removed surgically or burnt out with a hot iron—ouch! Unfortunately, the rumor was based on a misreading of a biblical text, which does indeed say that the removal of the spleen made for a faster runner. The misreading? The shrinkage of the biblical spleen was achieved by an oral medicine concocted by the priests and not by surgery or a hot poker. Fortunately, the practice died out quickly...unfortunately, so did the victims of this "misreading."

In addition to its cleansing role, the spleen has other functions. The spleen stores blood, especially platelets. (As much as 30% of the platelets are stored in the spleen.) The spleen also destroys and phagocytoses old, worn-out red blood cells (RBCs). Therefore, the spleen is called the "graveyard" of the RBCs. Finally, the spleen plays a role in fetal erythropoiesis. After birth, the spleen stops producing RBCs but continues its lifelong production of lymphocytes.

Because of its location, the spleen is commonly injured. Because it is difficult to repair and prone to bleed, the spleen may be removed surgically. The splenectomized patient can live quite well without a spleen but may be more prone to infection.

SPLEEN

The spleen is the largest lymphoid organ in the body. It is located in the left upper quadrant of the abdominal cavity, just beneath the diaphragm, and is normally protected by the lower rib cage (Figure 20-7). Although the spleen is much larger, it resembles a lymph node.

The spleen filters blood rather than lymph. The spleen is composed of two types of tissue: white pulp and red pulp. The white pulp is lymphoid tissue consisting primarily of lymphocytes surrounding arteries. The red pulp contains venous sinuses filled with blood and disease-preventing cells such as lymphocytes and macrophages. Blood enters the spleen through the splenic artery. The blood is cleansed as it slowly flows through the spleen. Microorganisms trapped by the spleen are destroyed by the leukocytes in the spleen. The cleansed blood leaves the spleen through the splenic vein.

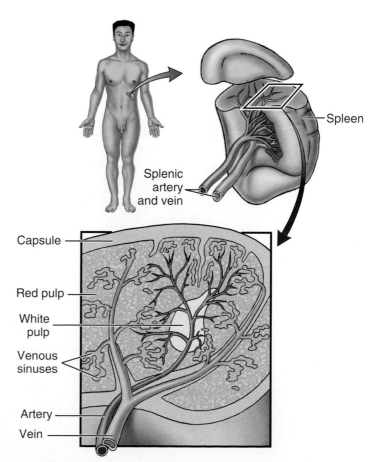

FIGURE 20-7 Spleen, composed of white pulp and red pulp.

Re-Think

1. List four lymphoid organs.
2. List three functions of the spleen.

2+2 Sum It Up!

Lymphocyte-containing organs, called *lymphoid organs,* include the lymph nodes, tonsils, thymus gland, and spleen. Lymph nodes are scattered throughout the body; some are clustered as the cervical, axillary, and inguinal lymph nodes. Three sets of tonsils (partially encapsulated lymph nodes) are the palatine, pharyngeal (adenoids), and lingual tonsils. Lymphoid tissue, in general, plays a crucial role in the prevention of disease. The spleen also acts as a storage site for RBCs and platelets.

As You Age

1. Lymphoid tissue reaches its peak development at puberty and then progressively shrinks with age.
2. After puberty, the thymus gland involutes, or shrivels up, and is replaced by connective tissue. This process involves a decrease in the amount of thymosins produced. Because of these changes, the defense mechanisms of the body diminish with age.

MEDICAL TERMINOLOGY AND DISORDERS   Disorders of the Lymphatic System

Medical Term	Word Parts	Word Part Meaning or Derivation	Description
Words			
hypersplenism	hyper-	excessive	**Hypersplenism** is *a disorder in which an overactive spleen prematurely destroys red blood cells, white blood cells, and platelets, thereby causing anemia, leukopenia, and thrombocytopenia.*
	-splen/o-	spleen	
	-ism	condition of	
lingual	lingul/o-	tongue	There are three pairs of tonsils: the palatine, the pharyngeal, and the **lingual,** located on the posterior tongue.
	-al	pertaining to	
splenomegaly	splen/o-	spleen	**Splenomegaly** is *an enlarged spleen; it usually accompanies hypersplenism and the excessive destruction of blood cells.*
	-megaly	enlargement	
tonsillectomy	tonsil/o-	tonsil	A **tonsillectomy** is *the removal of the tonsils,* usually the palatine tonsils.
	-ectomy	removal of	
Disorders			
lymphadenopathy	lymph/o-	lymph	Means *disease of the lymph nodes,* but is used synonymously with "swollen or enlarged lymph nodes." Lymph nodes swell in response to a number of conditions, both localized and systemic (infectious mononucleosis), autoimmune diseases and malignancies. Rarely is the distinction made between lymphadenopathy and **lymphadenitis,** *an inflammation of the lymph nodes.*
	-aden/o-	gland	
	-pathy	disease	
lymphedema	lymph/o-	lymph	Also called **lymphatic obstruction;** it is *a condition in which there is localized tissue swelling caused by damaged lymphatic vessels and poor drainage of tissue fluid.* The most common cause of lymphedema in the United States is related to the treatment of cancer: lymph node dissection, cancer surgery, and radiation therapy. In tropical regions of the world a common cause of severe lymphedema is filariasis, a parasitic infection.
	-edema	From a Greek word meaning a "swelling tumor"	
lymphoma	lymph/o-	lymph	*A solid malignant tumor of lymphoid cells, specifically the lymphocytes.* Abnormal lymphocytes collect and grow in lymph nodes or in lymphoid organs such as the spleen and tonsils, forming tumors that eventually metastasize throughout the body. There are two main categories of lymphomas: Hodgkin lymphoma (HL) and non-Hodgkin lymphoma (NHL).
	-oma	tumor	

Get Ready for Exams!

Summary Outline

The main functions of the lymphatic system are defense of the body against infection, return of fluid from the tissue spaces to the blood, and absorption of fat and fat-soluble vitamins from the digestive tract.

I. The Lymphatic System
  A. Lymph
   1. Lymph is a clear fluid containing water, electrolytes, waste, and some protein.
   2. Water and electrolytes are filtered from the plasma into the tissue spaces. Tissue fluid leaves the interstitium by way of the lymphatic vessels; in the lymphatic vessels, the fluid is known as *lymph*.
  B. Lymphatic vessels
   1. Lymphatic vessels are similar to the blood capillaries and the veins. The large holes in the lymphatic capillaries absorb fluid and protein from the tissue spaces.
   2. Lymph drains into the right lymphatic duct and thoracic duct; both ducts drain into the subclavian veins.
  C. Movement of lymph
   1. Lymph is not pumped by the heart like blood.
   2. Lymph moves in response to skeletal muscle contraction (through milking action), chest movement, and contraction of smooth muscle in the lymphatic vessels.

II. Lymphoid Organs
  A. Lymph nodes
   1. The major clusters of lymph nodes are the cervical, axillary, and inguinal nodes.
   2. Lymph nodes help protect the body against infection.
  B. Tonsils
   1. Tonsils are encapsulated lymph nodes.
   2. The tonsils are the palatine, pharyngeal (adenoids), and lingual tonsils.
  C. Thymus gland
   1. The thymus gland produces and helps differentiate T lymphocytes.
   2. The thymus gland secretes thymosins.
  D. Spleen
   1. It functions as a large lymph node.
   2. It has a store of WBCs that phagocytose microorganisms and participate in the immune process.
   3. It stores blood and removes worn-out red blood cells and platelets.
   4. It engages in fetal erythropoiesis.

Review Your Knowledge

Matching: Lymph Terms
Directions: Match the following words with their descriptions below.
a. lymph nodes
b. subclavian veins
c. thoracic duct
d. spleen
e. tonsils

1. ___ Pharyngeal, lingual, palatine
2. ___ Most of the lymph drains into this large duct.
3. ___ The large lymphatic ducts empty lymph into these blood vessels.
4. ___ Contains red pulp and white pulp; it is the largest lymphoid organ in the body
5. ___ Small, pea-shaped lymphoid structures that filter lymph as it flows through the lymphatic vessels

Multiple Choice
1. Which of the following is least characteristic of adenoids?
   a. They are considered lymphoid organs.
   b. They are tonsils.
   c. They cannot be surgically removed.
   d. They contain cells that fight infection.
2. The spleen
   a. is located in the right upper quadrant.
   b. cannot be removed without causing death.
   c. removes worn-out RBCs and platelets from the circulation.
   d. is avascular.
3. An overly active spleen may prematurely remove platelets from the circulation, thereby
   a. making the person hypertensive.
   b. predisposing the person to infection.
   c. predisposing the person to bleeding.
   d. causing hyperbilirubinemia and jaundice.
4. Which complication is most apt to develop in the patient who has had a breast removed (mastectomy) and lymph node dissection?
   a. Infectious mononucleosis
   b. Bleeding
   c. Lymphedema
   d. Jaundice
5. Which of the following statements is true about tonsils?
   a. Tonsils are nonlymphoid tissue.
   b. The pharyngeal tonsils are called *adenoids*.
   c. The lingual tonsils are the tonsils most often removed surgically.
   d. The pharyngeal tonsils may enlarge but never get infected.
6. The right lymphatic duct and the thoracic duct deliver
   a. blood to the lymphoid organs.
   b. venous blood to the right heart.
   c. lymph to the subclavian veins.
   d. lymph to the axillary lymph nodes.

7. The term MALT
   a. refers to lymphoid tissue in the mucosal membrane of many organs.
   b. is the medical term for lymph.
   c. is restricted to the spleen.
   d. is located exclusively in the mediastinum.
8. Which of the following is not true of lymph?
   a. It is formed from tissue or interstitial fluid.
   b. It is pumped into the main lymphatic ducts by the heart.
   c. It drains from the right lymphatic and thoracic ducts into the subclavian veins.
   d. It is cleansed by phagocytes as it flows through lymphoid organs.

Go Figure

1. **According to Figures 20-2, 20-3, and 20-4**
   a. The lymphatic vessels accompany the distribution of veins.
   b. Lymph nodes act as pumps to move the lymph from node to node.
   c. Most lymph drains into the right lymphatic duct.
   d. All lymph eventually drains into the thoracic duct.

2. **According to Figures 20-1 and 20-2**
   a. Water and protein are normally filtered by the lymphatic capillaries into the interstitium.
   b. Lymphatic capillaries normally reabsorb water from the interstitium.
   c. Lymphatic vessels surround and accompany the aorta.
   d. Lymphatic vessels are found exclusively in the upper torso.

3. **According to Figures 20-5 and 20-6**
   a. Lymphoid organs are restricted to the abdominopelvic cavity.
   b. Tonsils are considered cervical lymph nodes.
   c. *Adenoids* is another name for the spleen.
   d. The lymphatic system is widely dispersed throughout the body.

Key Terms

active immunity (p. 391)
allergens (p. 393)
antibodies (p. 389)
antibody-mediated immunity
    (AMI) (p. 387)
antigen (p. 386)
artificially acquired
    immunity (p. 391)

autoimmunity (p. 393)
B lymphocytes (B cells) (p. 387)
cell-mediated immunity
    (CMI) (p. 387)
clone (p. 388)
complement proteins (p. 385)
immunity (p. 382)
immunoglobulins (p. 389)

inflammation (p. 384)
interferons (p. 385)
macrophages (p. 384)
naturally acquired immunity (p. 391)
passive immunity (p. 391)
phagocytosis (p. 384)
T lymphocytes (T cells) (p. 387)
vaccine (p. 391)

Objective

1. Discuss nonspecific immunity, including:
   - Describe the process of phagocytosis.
   - Explain the causes of the signs of inflammation.
   - Explain the role of fever in fighting infection.
2. Discuss specific immunity, including:
   - Differentiate between specific and nonspecific immunity.
   - Explain the role of T cells in cell-mediated immunity.
   - Explain the role of B cells in antibody-mediated immunity.

3. Differentiate between genetic immunity and acquired immunity.
4. Describe naturally and artificially acquired active and passive immunity.
5. Describe other immune responses, including:
   - Identify the steps in the development of anaphylaxis.
   - Define _autoimmunity_.
   - Explain ways to prevent organ rejection.

Joey was born with an immunodeficiency disease; his immune system was not functioning well. This condition put Joey at high risk for life-threatening infections. As a result of this constant danger of infection, Joey spent most of his life in the sterile environment of a plastic bubble. The bubble protected him from a world of microorganisms. For persons with healthy immune systems, most microorganisms are harmless, but for Joey, the same microorganisms became dangerous pathogens. The use of bone marrow transplants has now eliminated the lifelong use of bubbles and has offered new hope for children with immunodeficiency diseases. Today we are more apt to encounter persons

who are immunosuppressed because of human immunodeficiency virus (HIV) infection or treatment for cancer in the form of chemotherapy or radiation.

The study of the immune system is called _immunology_. The human body has an elaborate defense system called immunity. In addition to protecting the body from pathogens, the immune system protects the body from other foreign agents, including pollens such as ragweed, toxins such as bee stings, and our own cells that have gone astray (cancer cells).

CLASSIFICATION OF THE IMMUNE SYSTEM

The defense mechanisms of the immune system are classified as nonspecific and specific immunity.

NONSPECIFIC IMMUNITY

Nonspecific immunity protects the body against many different types of foreign agents. With nonspecific immunity, the body need not recognize the specific foreign agent. A number of defense mechanisms are included in the category of nonspecific immunity (Figure 21-1). Nonspecific immunity can be divided into lines of defense. The first line of defense includes mechanical barriers, chemical barriers, and reflexes. The second line of defense includes phagocytosis, inflammation, fever, protective proteins (interferons and complement proteins), and natural killer (NK) cells. Remember that the nonspecific defense mechanisms work against all foreign agents; no recognition of a specific agent is necessary. Table 21-1 (later in this chapter) lists the many types of cells involved in the immune response.

FIRST LINE OF DEFENSE

The first line of defense includes mechanical barriers, chemical barriers, and reflexes. Intact skin and mucous membranes serve as mechanical barriers; pathogens cannot cross these structures and enter the body. Destruction of mechanical barriers is an invitation to microbial invasion and subsequent infection (see Figure 21-1). Assisting the skin and mucous membranes with their defensive functions are their secretions, the chemical barriers.

For example, tears, saliva, and perspiration provide chemical barriers that wash away microorganisms. They also establish a hostile environment, thereby killing the potential pathogens. The acid and digestive enzymes secreted by the cells of the stomach kill most of the microorganisms that are swallowed. Tears secrete a substance called *lysozyme,* which discourages the growth of pathogens on the surface of the eye.

Other secretions make the environment sticky and so provide another type of chemical barrier. The mucus secreted by the mucous membranes of the respiratory tract traps inhaled foreign material. Then the cilia, which line most of the respiratory structures, sweep the entrapped material toward the throat so that the material can eventually be coughed up or swallowed. In addition to the mechanical and chemical barriers, reflexes assist in the removal of pathogens. Sneezing and coughing help remove pathogens from the respiratory tract, whereas vomiting and diarrhea help remove pathogens from the digestive tract.

Mechanical barriers, chemical barriers, and reflexes are not an adequate defense against all pathogens, however. If a pathogen penetrates this first line of defense, it encounters processes that make up the second line of defense.

FIGURE 21-1 Nonspecific immunity. First line of defense: mechanical barriers, chemical barriers, and reflexes. Second line of defense: phagocytosis, inflammation, fever, protective proteins, and natural killer (NK) cells.

SECOND LINE OF DEFENSE

The second line of defense includes phagocytosis, inflammation, fever, protective proteins, and natural killer (NK) cells.

Phagocytosis

Some of the white blood cells (leukocytes) can ingest and destroy pathogens and other foreign substances by **phagocytosis**. Some phagocytes—the neutrophils and monocytes—are *motile*; they wander around the body through the blood and tissue fluid, doing their job. Other phagocytes are confined within a particular tissue and are *fixed*.

Traveling through the blood to the site of infection, the neutrophils and monocytes can squeeze through the tiny gaps between the endothelial cells of the capillary walls and enter the tissue spaces at the site of infection. The process of squeezing through the tiny gaps is called *diapedesis* (dye-ah-peh-DEE-sis). How do the neutrophils and monocytes know where to go? Chemicals released by injured cells attract them to the injured site. This signaling to attract phagocytes is called *chemotaxis* (kee-moh-TAK-sis). This process is similar to a bloodhound tracking a scent; the hound picks up the signal (odor), which identifies its source.

What Does a Phagocyte Do?

A phagocyte engulfs, or eats, particles or pathogens, much like an ameba does. The phagocyte's plasma membrane sends out pseudopods ("false feet") that surround the pathogen. The surfaces of the pseudopods then fuse, thereby enclosing the pathogen within the phagocyte. The trapped pathogen encounters a lysosome; the lysosomal membrane fuses with the pathogen, releasing potent enzymes that destroy the pathogen. The process of phagocytosis can be summarized as "ingested (eaten) and digested."

One group of phagocytic cells, the monocytes, deposit themselves in various organs and give rise to **macrophages**. As the name implies, the macrophages are big eaters. They become fixed within a particular organ and are thus nonmotile. They can, however, divide and produce new macrophages at their fixed site. The Kupffer (KOOP-fer) cells in the liver, for example, are fixed to the walls of the large capillaries called *sinusoids*. As blood flows through the sinusoids, pathogens and other foreign substances are removed from the blood and phagocytosed. The liver, spleen, lungs, and lymph nodes have a particularly rich supply of fixed phagocytes. Some fixed macrophages in the lungs are called "dust" cells because they phagocytose inhaled solid particles (better known as dust).

Inflammation

Inflammation refers to the responses the body makes when confronted by an irritant. The irritant can be almost anything; common irritants include pathogens, friction, excessive heat or cold, radiation, injuries, and chemicals. If the irritant is caused by a pathogen, the inflammation is called an *infection*.

Inflammation is characterized by redness, heat, swelling, and pain (see Figure 21-1). What are the causes of these symptoms? When the tissues are injured or irritated, injured cells release histamine and other chemicals. These chemicals cause the blood vessels in the injured tissue to dilate. The dilated blood vessels bring more blood to the area; the increased blood flow causes redness and heat. The histamine causes the blood vessel walls to leak fluid and dissolved substances into the tissue spaces, causing swelling. Fluid and irritating chemicals accumulating at the injured site also stimulate pain receptors; therefore, the person experiences pain. Redness, heat, swelling, and pain are the classic signs of inflammation.

The increased blood flow also carries an increased number of phagocytes (neutrophils and monocytes) to the injured site. As the phagocytes do their job, many are killed in the process. In a severe infection, the area becomes filled with dead leukocytes, pathogens, injured cells, and tissue fluid. This thick, yellowish accumulation of dead material is called *pus*. The presence of pus indicates that the phagocytes are doing their job.

Because of the leaky blood vessels, fluid collects in the tissue spaces. This tissue fluid contains some blood-clotting factors, such as fibrinogen, a protein present in plasma. Fibrinogen creates fibrin threads within the tissue spaces. Later, fibroblasts, the cells that form connective tissue, may also invade the injured area. The connective tissue helps contain, or restrict, the area of inflammation and thereby prevents the infection from spreading throughout the body. Fibroblastic activity is also involved in tissue repair.

 Do You Know...

How and Why the Body "Walls Off the Pus"?

When an area becomes infected, the cells involved in the inflammatory response do two things. First, they kill the pathogens. As the war continues, dead cells (including phagocytes, injured cells, and pathogens) and secretions accumulate in the area as pus. Second, the cells build a wall of tissue around the infected debris. This walled-off area is an abscess. An abscess performs a beneficial role in that it restricts the spread of the infection throughout the body. A large abscess may require a surgical procedure in which the abscess is lanced and drained.

 Re-Think

1. In what sense does a phagocyte act like an ameba?
2. List the four signs of inflammation and explain the physiological basis of each.

Fever

Fever, also known as *pyrexia* (pye-REK-see-ah), is an abnormal elevation in body temperature. As phagocytes perform their duty, they release fever-producing substances called *pyrogens* (from the Latin word for "fire"). The pyrogens stimulate the hypothalamus in the brain to reset the body's temperature, producing a fever. The elevation in temperature is thought to be beneficial in two ways: a fever stimulates phagocytosis and decreases the ability of certain pathogens to multiply. In fact, the elimination of mild fevers may do more harm than good.

What happens when the hypothalamus resets the body temperature? First, the person shivers in an attempt to generate heat; the heat is conserved as the blood vessels of the skin constrict. The person may have chills and feel cold and clammy, even though the body temperature is rising. The elevated temperature hovers around the new set point while the pathogen is active, but when the infection is contained and the secretion of pyrogens diminishes, the hypothalamus resets its thermostat back to normal. Heat-losing mechanisms are activated and the blood vessels of the skin dilate, thereby losing heat as the person sweats.

Evidence suggests that the reduction of fever prolongs an infection. Note, however, that a very high fever must be reduced because high body temperature may cause severe and irreversible brain damage. High fever, especially in children, is frequently accompanied by seizures. Seizures resulting from an elevated body temperature are called *febrile (fever) seizures*.

? **Re-Think**

Explain why pyrexia, but not hyperthermia, is considered a second line of defense. (Refer back to Chapter 7, if needed.)

Protective Proteins

Two groups of protective proteins, the interferons and complement proteins, act nonspecifically to protect the body (see Figure 21-1). **Interferons** (in-ter-FEER-ons) are a group of proteins secreted by cells infected by a virus. The interferons diffuse to surrounding cells where they prevent viral replication. Researchers first found interferons in cells infected by the influenza virus and named them accordingly because they interfered with viral replication. Interferons also activate NK cells and macrophages, thus boosting the immune system.

A second group of proteins that protect the body are the complement proteins. **Complement proteins** circulate in the blood in their inactive form. When the complement proteins are activated against a bacterium, they swarm over it. The complement attaches to

Interferons

Complement

Bacterium

the bacterium's outer membrane and punches holes in it. The holes in the membrane allow fluid and electrolytes to flow into the bacterium, causing it to burst and die. The activated complements perform other functions that enhance phagocytosis and the inflammatory response.

Natural Killer Cells

Natural killer (NK) cells are a special type of lymphocyte that acts nonspecifically to kill a variety of cells. NK cells are effective against many microbes and certain cancer cells. NK cells cooperate with the specific defense mechanisms to mount the most effective defense possible.

2+2 Sum It Up!

Figure 21-2 summarizes the functions of the nonspecific defense mechanisms. The wall of the fortress is the first line of defense. It protects the body from invaders such as bacteria, fungi, and viruses. The first line of defense includes mechanical barriers, chemical barriers, and reflexes. Behind the wall of the fortress is the second line of defense: phagocytosis, inflammation, fever, protective proteins, and NK cells. The third line of defense includes lymphocytes that are concerned with specific immunity, the topic of the next section.

SPECIFIC IMMUNITY: THIRD LINE OF DEFENSE

Specific immunity homes in on a foreign substance and provides protection against one specific substance but not others. It protects against a specific foreign agent such as the measles virus (a specific pathogen) or ragweed pollen. The two cells that play key roles in specific immunity are the lymphocytes (B lymphocytes and T lymphocytes) and the macrophages. Understanding the function of lymphocytes requires an understanding of antigens.

ANTIGENS

An **antigen** is a substance that stimulates the formation of antibodies. Antigens are generally large molecules; most are proteins, but a few are polysaccharides and lipids. Antigens are found on the surface of many substances, such as pathogens, red blood cells, pollens, foods, toxins, and cancer cells. Foreign substances that display antigens are described as antigenic. Antigenic substances are attacked by lymphocytes.

SELF AND NONSELF: IS THAT ME?

Before birth, your lymphocytes somehow get to know who belongs and who does not. In effect, your

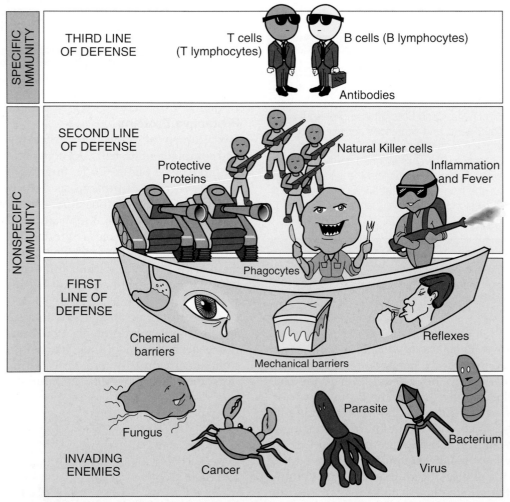

FIGURE 21-2 The immune system wages its battle with three lines of defense. (Read from bottom to top.)

Table 21-1	Cells Involved in Immunity	
CELL TYPE	**PRODUCTION SITE**	**FUNCTION**
Granular Leukocytes		
Neutrophils	Bone marrow	Phagocytosis
Basophils	Bone marrow	Secrete histamine and heparin
Eosinophils	Bone marrow	Destroy parasites
Nongranular Leukocytes		
Monocytes	Bone marrow	Phagocytosis; they enter tissues and are transformed into macrophages
Lymphocytes		
• B cells	Bone marrow	Antibody-mediated immunity; accounts for 20% to 30% of blood lymphocytes
Plasma cells		Secrete antibodies
Memory B cells		Remember the antigens
• T cells	Bone marrow and lymphoid tissue	Cell-mediated immunity; accounts for 70% to 80% of blood lymphocytes
Killer T cells		Kill cells
Helper T cells		Secrete lymphokines, which activate B cells and other cells
Suppressor T cells		Inhibit B-cell and T-cell activity (help control immune response)
Memory T cells		Remember the antigens
• Natural killer (NK) cells	Lymphoid tissue	Kill cells
Other Cells		
Macrophages	Almost all organs and tissues	Phagocytosis; present antigens to lymphocytes
Mast cells	Almost all organs and tissues, especially liver and lungs	Release histamine and other chemicals involved in inflammation

lymphocytes learn to recognize "you" (self) and take steps to eliminate "not you" (nonself, or foreign agent). Your body perceives your own cells and secretions as nonantigenic and other cells as antigenic. The antigenic cells are subsequently eliminated. Recognition of self is called *immunotolerance*. Sometimes, a person's immune system fails to identify self and mounts an immune attack against its own cells. This attack is the basis of autoimmune diseases, such as rheumatoid arthritis.

LYMPHOCYTES

The two types of lymphocytes are **T lymphocytes (T cells)** and **B lymphocytes (B cells)**. Although both come from the stem cells in the bone marrow, they differ in their development and functions (Table 21-1).

Why the Names "T" and "B" Cells?

During fetal development, stem cells in bone marrow produce lymphocytes. The blood carries lymphocytes throughout the body. About half of the lymphocytes travel to the thymus gland, where they mature and differentiate into T cells (the "T" is for *t*hymus-derived lymphocytes). Eventually, the blood carries T cells away from the thymus gland to various lymphoid tissues, particularly the lymph nodes and spleen. T cells live, work, and reproduce in the lymphoid tissue

as well as circulate in the blood, making up 70% to 80% of the blood's lymphocytes.

What about the B lymphocytes? B cells differentiate in the fetal liver and bone marrow (the "B" is for *b*one marrow). Like the T cells, the B cells take up residence in lymphoid tissue. B cells make up 20% to 30% of the circulating lymphocytes.

Both T cells and B cells attack antigens, but they do so in different ways. T cells attack antigens directly, through cell-to-cell contact. This immune response is called **cell-mediated immunity (CMI)**. B cells, on the other hand, interact with the antigen indirectly, through the secretion of antibodies. This response is called **antibody-mediated immunity (AMI)**. Because the antibodies are carried by the blood and other tissue fluid (the body "humors"), this type of immunity is also called *humoral immunity*.

Cell-Mediated Immunity: T-Cell Function

CMI is effective against many pathogens, tumor cells, and foreign tissue such as organ transplants. Refer to Figure 21-3 as you read about the following steps in CMI:

• *Step 1.* The antigen, on the surface of the pathogen, is phagocytosed by a macrophage. The macrophage digests the antigen and pushes the antigen to its surface. The macrophage's ability to push the antigen to its surface is called *antigen presentation*.

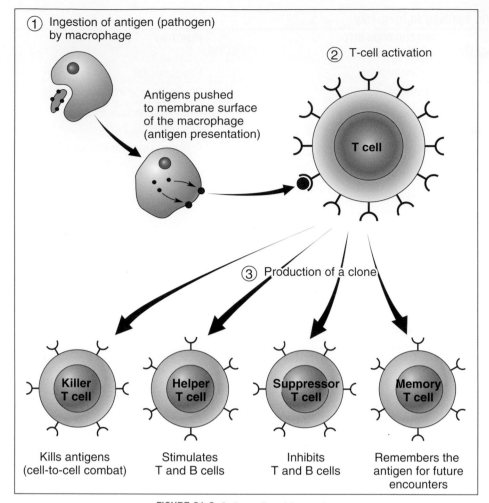

① Ingestion of antigen (pathogen) by macrophage

② T-cell activation

Antigens pushed to membrane surface of the macrophage (antigen presentation)

T cell

③ Production of a clone

Killer T cell	Helper T cell	Suppressor T cell	Memory T cell
Kills antigens (cell-to-cell combat)	Stimulates T and B cells	Inhibits T and B cells	Remembers the antigen for future encounters

FIGURE 21-3 Cell-mediated immunity.

- *Step 2.* T cells that have receptor sites bind to the antigen and become activated. This process is called *T-cell activation.* Activation of the T cell always requires an antigen-presenting cell, such as a macrophage.
- *Step 3.* The activated T cell divides repeatedly, resulting in large numbers of T cells. This group of T cells is called a **clone**, a group of identical cells formed from the same parent cell. Four subgroups are within the clone: killer T cells, helper T cells, suppressor T cells, and memory T cells.

The killer T cells destroy the antigen (pathogen) through the use of two mechanisms, punching holes in the pathogen's cell membrane and secreting substances called *lymphokines,* which enhance phagocytic activity. The killer T cells engage in cell-to-cell combat. The helper T cells also secrete a lymphokine that stimulates T cells and B cells and, in general, enhances the immune response. The suppressor T cells inhibit the immune response when the antigen has been destroyed. The suppressor T cells control B- and T-cell activity.

The memory T cells do not participate in the destruction of the antigen. These cells "remember" the initial

encounter with the antigen. If the antigen is presented at some future time, the memory cells quickly reproduce and thus allow a faster immune response to occur.

Antibody-Mediated Immunity: B-Cell Function

B cells engage in AMI. Activated B cells produce a clone of cells that secrete antibodies. The antibodies are carried by the blood and body fluids to the antigen-bearing pathogens. Individual B cells can produce over 10 million different antibodies, each of which reacts against a specific antigen. The large numbers of antibodies allow the body to develop immunity against many different diseases. Follow Figure 21-4 as you read about the following steps in AMI:

- *Step 1.* A macrophage engulfs and processes an antigen. The antigen is pushed to the surface of the macrophage and presented to the B cell and helper T cell.
- *Step 2.* The presented antigens bind to the B cell and helper T cell, activating both cells. Only those B cells and helper T cells with the proper receptors are activated.

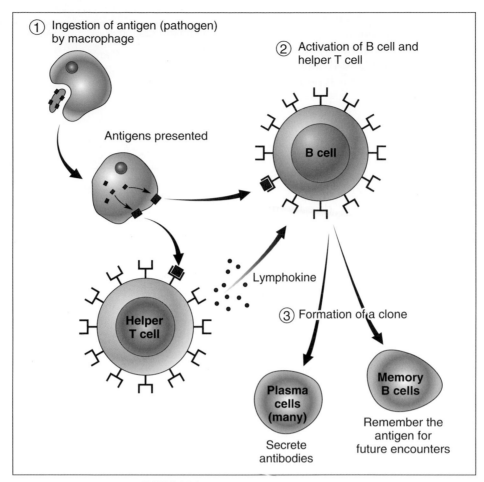

① Ingestion of antigen (pathogen) by macrophage

② Activation of B cell and helper T cell

Antigens presented

B cell

Lymphokine

Helper T cell

③ Formation of a clone

Plasma cells (many)

Secrete antibodies

Memory B cells

Remember the antigen for future encounters

FIGURE 21-4 Antibody-mediated immunity.

• *Step 3.* The activated helper T cells secrete a lymphokine that stimulates the B cells to reproduce, producing a clone. The two subgroups of the clone include plasma cells and memory B cells. Plasma cells produce large quantities of antibodies that travel through the blood to the antigens (pathogens). The memory B cells do not participate in the attack; they remember the specific antigen during future encounters and allow a quicker response to the invading antigen.

Note that B- and T-cell activation depends on helper T-cell activity. HIV attacks the helper T cells, thereby producing severe impairment of the immune system. This syndrome is called *acquired immunodeficiency syndrome* (AIDS). Because of the impairment of their immune system, persons with HIV infection and AIDS experience numerous bouts of infection, some of which may be lethal. The immune response of an AIDs patient may be so inadequate that even the common cold presents a life-threatening challenge.

The helper T cell is also called the CD4$^+$ T-cell (because of a surface protein called CD4). The CD4$^+$ T cell is a marker for immune function and the progression of HIV infection is monitored by the CD4$^+$ T-cell count. The CD4$^+$ T-cell count usually decreases as the infection progresses.

? Re-Think

1. List two lymphocytes that engage in specific immunity.
2. What is the consequence of the failure of the immune system to "recognize self"?
3. How does the action of the killer T cell differ from that of the plasma cell?

ANTIBODIES

What Antibodies Are

The **antibodies** secreted by the B cells are proteins called **immunoglobulins**. There are five major types of immunoglobulins. The three most abundant immunoglobulins are immunoglobulin G, immunoglobulin A, and immunoglobulin M. A fourth immunoglobulin, immunoglobulin D, is present in small amounts. A fifth immunoglobulin, immunoglobulin E, is involved in hypersensitivity reactions and is described later in this chapter.

• Immunoglobulin G (IgG) is an antibody found in plasma and body fluids. It is particularly effective against certain bacteria, viruses, and toxins.
• Immunoglobulin A (IgA) is an antibody found primarily in the secretions of exocrine glands. IgA in milk, tears, and gastric juice helps protect against

infection. Breast milk contains IgA antibodies and helps the infant ward off infection.

- Immunoglobulin M (IgM) is an antibody found in blood plasma. The anti-A and anti-B antibodies associated with red blood cells are a type of IgM antibody.

What Antibodies Do

Antibodies destroy antigens. They accomplish this task directly by attacking the membrane and indirectly by activating complement proteins that in turn facilitate the attack on the antigens.

When antibodies react with antigens directly, the antibodies bind to antigens in a process called an *antigen–antibody reaction*. By engaging in an antigen–antibody reaction, the antigen–antibody components clump together, or agglutinate (ah-GLOO-tin-ate). Agglutination makes it easier for the phagocytic cells to destroy the antigen. Under normal conditions, direct attack by the antibodies is not very helpful in protecting the body against invasion by pathogens.

A more effective way for antibodies to attack an antigen is through activation of the complement proteins. These activated complement proteins cause a variety of effects: they stimulate chemotaxis (attract more phagocytes), promote agglutination, make pathogens more susceptible to phagocytosis, and encourage lysis, or rupture of the pathogen's cell membrane. Direct and indirect attacks by antibodies provide an effective defense against foreign agents.

FIGURE 21-5 Primary and secondary responses to an antigen.

turn, induce the formation of many antibody-secreting plasma cells.

What does the secondary response mean for you? It means that you won't get the disease a second time; you are immune to that disease. For example, if you had measles as a child, you developed measles antibodies and many memory cells. If you are then exposed to the measles virus later in life, the memory cells "remember" the first exposure and produce antibody-secreting plasma cells very quickly. The measles antibodies, in turn, attack the measles virus and prevent you from becoming ill.

The level of antibodies in your blood is called an *antibody titer*. If you have had measles, for example, your measles antibody titer is higher than the titer of someone who has never had measles.

? Re-Think

1. CMI achieves cell death by cell-to-cell combat. How does AMI achieve the death of a pathogen?
2. How does agglutination help out the phagocytes?

Remember Me? Primary and Secondary Responses

Activated when exposed to an antigen, B cells produce many plasma cells and memory cells. The plasma cells secrete antibodies. This initial response to an antigen is called the *primary response* (Figure 21-5). The primary response develops slowly and produces a small number of antibodies. Note what happens when the immune system is challenged for a second time by the same antigen. The immune system responds quickly and produces a larger number of antibodies. This second challenge is called the *secondary response*. Compare the plasma levels of antibodies in the primary and secondary responses.

Why is the secondary response so much greater? The initial exposure to the antigen has stimulated the formation of antibody-secreting plasma cells and memory cells. The memory cells, which live for a long time in the plasma, are activated very quickly on the second exposure. The activated memory cells, in

---

? Re-Think

List two ways that the secondary response differs from the primary response.

2+2 Sum It Up!

Specific immunity forms the third line of defense of the immune response. It allows the immune system to recognize and destroy specific substances called *antigens*. The B and T lymphocytes and the macrophages are the most important cells associated with specific immunity. T cells engage in cell-to-cell combat (CMI), whereas B cells fight at a distance through the mediation of antibodies (AMI). Macrophages not only engage in phagocytosis, but also present the antigen to the lymphocytes. Antibodies are called *immunoglobulins* (IgG, IgA, IgM, IgD, and IgE); they engage antigens causing agglutination. Agglutination, in turn, facilitates phagocytosis. The primary and secondary responses refer to the secretion of antibodies by plasma cells in response to antigen stimulation.

TYPES OF IMMUNITY

The two main categories of immunity are genetic immunity and acquired immunity (Figure 21-6).

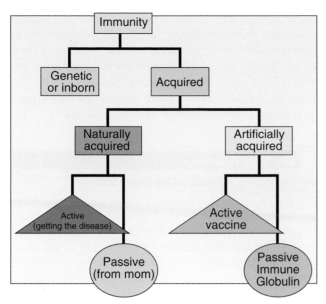

FIGURE 21-6 Types of immunity.

GENETIC IMMUNITY

Do you ever wonder why you have never gotten heart-worms from your dog or why your dog did not pick up chickenpox from you? As a human, you have inherited immunity to certain diseases such as canine heartworm; you are immunologically protected from your pet. Similarly, your dog will never contract chickenpox; Rover is immunologically protected from you. Another comforting thought is that neither you nor your dog is in danger of contracting Dutch elm disease from your tree. Each of you was born with genetic information that provides immunity to certain diseases. Genetic immunity is also called *inborn, innate,* or *species immunity.* As you can see, your species protects you from many diseases that afflict other species.

ACQUIRED IMMUNITY

Unlike genetic immunity, acquired immunity is received during a person's lifetime. Acquired immunity comes either naturally or artificially.

NATURALLY ACQUIRED IMMUNITY

You can acquire immunity naturally in two ways. The first is by getting the disease. As a child, you probably had one of the childhood diseases such as chickenpox. Your body responded to the specific pathogen by developing antibodies. After that first exposure, you never became ill with chickenpox again because your immune system had a ready supply of antibodies and memory cells with which to respond quickly to the second invasion of the chickenpox virus. Because your own body produced the antibodies, this type of **naturally acquired immunity** is called **active immunity**. Active immunity is generally long lasting.

The second way to acquire immunity naturally is by receiving antibodies from your mother. Some antibodies (IgG) crossed the placenta from your mother into you as a fetus. Your mother developed these antibodies in response to the pathogens that she encountered throughout her lifetime. Because your immune system did not produce these antibodies (you received them as a gift from your mother), this type of immunity is called **passive immunity**. Antibodies can also be transferred passively from mother to infant through breast milk. Breast milk contains IgA antibodies.

Unlike active immunity, which often lasts a lifetime, passive immunity is short lived. The antibodies that are acquired passively are broken down and eliminated from the baby's body. The mother's antibodies afford protection to the infant for about the first 6 months after birth. Breast-feeding may extend the length of immunoprotection.

ARTIFICIALLY ACQUIRED IMMUNITY

You can also acquire immunity artificially in two ways. The first is by a vaccine; the second is by injection of immune globulin. Both provide **artificially acquired immunity**.

A **vaccine** is an antigen-bearing substance, such as a pathogen, injected into a person in an attempt to stimulate antibody production. For example, the measles virus is first killed or weakened or attenuated (ay-TEN-yoo-ayt-ed). The attenuated virus cannot cause the disease (measles) when injected into the person, but it can still act as an antigen and stimulate the person's immune system to produce antibodies. The use of a dead or attenuated pathogen to stimulate antibody production is vaccination, or immunization. The solution of dead or attenuated pathogens is the vaccine. Because the use of a vaccine stimulates the body to produce its own antibodies, vaccines induce active immunity.

A vaccine can also be made from the toxin secreted by the pathogen. The toxin is altered to reduce its harmfulness, but it can still act as an antigen to induce immunity. The altered toxin is called a *toxoid.* Because a toxoid stimulates the production of antibodies, it causes active immunity.

The purpose of vaccination is to provide an initial exposure and stimulate the formation of memory cells (the primary response). The purpose of a booster shot is to stimulate the secondary response by administering another dose of the vaccine.

Vaccines have almost eradicated certain diseases. For example, infants routinely receive a series of DTP injections. DTP injections stimulate active immunity for *d*iphtheria (diphtheria toxoid), *t*etanus (tetanus toxoid), and *p*ertussis, or whooping cough (pertussis vaccine). MMR vaccine (*m*easles-rubeola, *m*umps, and *r*ubella) is also used preventively during early childhood.

Immune globulin differs from a vaccine. Immune globulin is obtained from a donor (human or animal) and contains antibodies (immune globulins). The antibodies are formed in the donor in response to a specific antigen. These preformed antibodies are taken from the donor and injected into a recipient, thereby conveying passive immunity.

 Do You Know...

Why Joey is Mooing?

Here's the story. Vaccination against smallpox was originally accomplished by injecting the cowpox virus, a cousin to the smallpox virus. Although Edward Jenner (circa 1850) had demonstrated some success with vaccination, many doctors opposed the procedure. His fellow doctors therefore spread a nasty rumor designed to scare the peasant population. The rumor claimed that the injection of the cowpox virus makes the child take on the characteristics of a cow...Moooooo! Pictures were widely distributed of Joey mooing, swatting flies with his tail, and clanging a cow bell hung around his neck.

Fortunately, the peasants weren't duped because they knew that milkmaids rarely came down with smallpox. Most attributed the immunity of the milkmaids to the cowpox lesions that developed when the milkmaid milked the cows infected with the cowpox virus. (Holy cow—this sounds like bull!) Just remember, the Latin word for cow is *vacca*, the root word for *vaccination*.

Why might this procedure be done? Assume for the moment that you are not immune to hepatitis B and so do not have antibodies against the hepatitis B virus. You are then exposed to the virus. Because you have no immunity to the virus, you may receive immune globulin (antibodies) in an attempt to provide immediate protection against the virus. Because this is a form of passive immunity, the immunity is short-lived. Immune globulins are available for rubella (German measles), hepatitis A and B, rabies, and tetanus. A comparison of the different types of acquired immunity appears in Table 21-2.

Other forms of passive immunity are commonly used to prevent the disease or the development of

severe symptoms of the disease. Antitoxins contain antibodies that neutralize the toxins secreted by the pathogens but have no effect on the pathogens themselves. Examples of antitoxins include tetanus antitoxin (TAT) and the antitoxins for diphtheria and botulism. Antivenoms contain antibodies that combat the effects of the poisonous venom of snakes.

 Do You Know...

Why the Ancient "Charmers" Ate Snake Venom?

Long ago, Indian snake charmers squeezed the venom from their cobras and drank it. Why? They realized that by eating the venom, they developed resistance to the bite of the family pet. This practice was observed by a number of physicians, and the concept eventually evolved into our modern-day immunology.

 Re-Think

1. Differentiate between active and passive immunity. Give an example of each.
2. Differentiate between naturally and artificially acquired immunity. Give an example of each.

OTHER IMMUNE RESPONSES

Normally the immune system protects the body from nonself; foreign agents are recognized and eliminated. Sometimes, however, the immune system goes awry: it attacks the self, causing autoimmune disease, or it overreacts, causing allergies.

ALLERGIC REACTIONS

The immune system sometimes forms antibodies to substances not usually recognized as foreign. This response forms the basis of allergic reactions. The two common allergic reactions are the delayed-reaction allergy and the immediate-reaction allergy.

Table 21-2   **Types of Acquired Immunity**

TYPE	STIMULUS	RESULT
Naturally Acquired		
Active immunity	Exposed to live pathogens (e.g., get the disease)	Long-term immunity; makes antibodies
Passive immunity	Antibodies are passed from mother to infant (across placenta and/or by breast-feeding)	Short-term immunity (lasts approximately for the first 6 months and for duration of breast-feeding); does not stimulate the production of antibodies
Artificially Acquired		
Active immunity	Vaccination	Long-term immunity; makes antibodies
Passive immunity	Injection with gamma globulin (antibodies)	Short-term immunity; does not stimulate the production of antibodies

The *delayed-reaction allergy* is so named because it usually takes about 48 hours to occur; its onset is delayed. This type of allergic response can occur in anyone. It usually results from the repeated exposure of the skin to chemicals such as household detergents. Repeated exposure to the chemical activates T cells, which eventually accumulate in the skin. Local tissue response to T-cell activity causes skin eruptions and other signs of inflammation. This skin response is called *contact dermatitis*. Other forms of contact dermatitis are associated with poison ivy, poison oak, certain cosmetics, and soaps.

The *immediate-reaction allergy*, as its name implies, occurs rapidly in response to its stimulus. It is more commonly called *immediate hypersensitivity reaction* and involves immunoglobulin E, the IgE antibodies. **Allergens** (antigens) are substances capable of inducing allergy. Allergens that are apt to be involved in this type of allergic response include pollens, such as ragweed, insect venom, drugs such as penicillin, and foods such as peanuts. See Figure 21-7, the steps involved in the development of an immediate hypersensitivity reaction.

- *Step 1.* An allergen activates a B cell.
- *Step 2.* The activated B cell forms a clone of antibody-secreting plasma cells.
- *Step 3.* The plasma cells secrete large amounts of IgE antibodies against the specific allergen.
- *Step 4.* The IgE antibodies bind to the mast cells in body tissues.
- *Step 5.* More of the allergen invades the body.

The allergen binds with the IgE antibodies on the mast cells. The mast cells release large amounts of histamine, leukotrienes, and other chemicals that cause systemic effects. The systemic effects can be severe; they include a massive vasodilation, which causes a sharp drop in blood pressure and severe constriction of the respiratory passages (bronchoconstriction), making breathing extremely difficult and, in some cases, impossible. This severe form of the immediate hypersensitivity reaction is called *anaphylaxis* or *anaphylactic shock*. Persons allergic to penicillin are at particular risk for anaphylaxis. As a result, always ask a person about allergies to medications before administering any type of drug, particularly antibiotics. (Some persons are even allergic to aspirin.)

 Re-Think

Describe the steps involved in the development of anaphylaxis.

AUTOIMMUNE DISEASE

Sometimes, a person's T cells attack his or her own body, causing extensive tissue damage and organ dysfunction. This process is **autoimmunity**. Diseases that

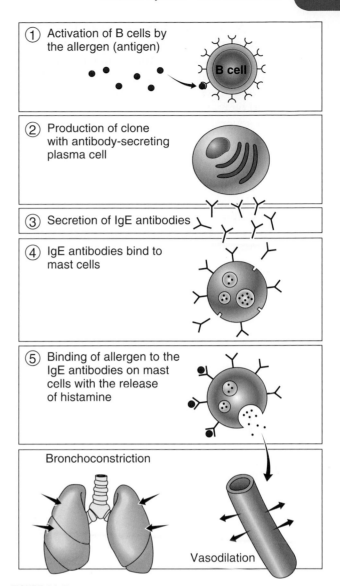

① Activation of B cells by the allergen (antigen)

B cell

② Production of clone with antibody-secreting plasma cell

③ Secretion of IgE antibodies

④ IgE antibodies bind to mast cells

⑤ Binding of allergen to the IgE antibodies on mast cells with the release of histamine

Bronchoconstriction

Vasodilation

FIGURE 21-7 Immediate hypersensitivity reaction.

develop in response to self-attack are called *autoimmune diseases*. A surprisingly large number of diseases are considered autoimmune.

Consider this. The immune system is affected by your endocrine system and your nervous system. Your endocrine and nervous systems are both affected by your emotional state (happy, sad, angry). What are the chances that your emotional state can affect your immune system and hence your physical well-being? In other words, does happiness promote health, whereas anger and depression cause disease? A branch of science called *psychoneuroimmunology* seeks to explore this relationship. In the meantime, be happy!

ORGAN REJECTION

Organ transplantation has become a common means of dealing with organ failure. A patient in kidney failure, for example, may receive a kidney transplant.

One of the greatest problems associated with this surgical technology is organ rejection. The recipient's immune system recognizes the donated kidney as foreign and mounts an immune attack against it. When the immune attack is successful, the organ is destroyed and is said to be rejected.

There are several ways to prevent organ rejection. The physician first selects a donor organ that is immunologically similar to the recipient's tissues. The physician then administers drugs that suppress the recipient's immune system. Cyclosporine is a commonly used immunosuppressant that inhibits the secretion of certain lymphokines, which, in turn, diminishes the immune attack against the donated organ. Unfortunately, these measures are not always successful, and the recipient may ultimately reject the organ.

 Do You Know...

Why This Bee Might Kill Auntie Bea?

Auntie Bea has become sensitized to bee venom (antigen). IgE antibodies to the bee venom attached to the surface of her mast cells. If Auntie is stung again, the bee venom antigen will bind to the IgE antibodies on the mast cells, causing a massive release of histamine. The histamine causes an anaphylactic reaction. Unless treated immediately, she is apt to die of anaphylactic shock. Treatment is usually an injection of epinephrine (Adrenalin), which opens breathing passages and elevates blood pressure. Steroids (cortisol) are also given to suppress the immune response.

 Do You Know...

About the Ultimate Rejection?

When dealing with transplant patients, we watch closely for signs of organ rejection by the host (recipient). However, some patients experience the opposite—the transplanted organ (or blood) rejects the host. This response is called *graft-versus-host disease* (GVHD); GVHD usually occurs in immunodeficient patients and is caused in part by transplanted T cells. The target organs for rejection are the skin, digestive tract, and liver. The biggest clinical problem is a variety of infections that gradually overwhelm the granulocytopenic patient. Imagine being rejected by an organ!

 Sum It Up!

Immunity is classified as genetic or acquired. Immunity may be acquired naturally or artificially. Immunity is also classified as active or passive. If a person makes antibodies in his or her own body, the immunity is active. If the person merely receives antibodies that were made by another person or animal, the immunity is passive. Active immunity is generally long lasting, whereas passive immunity is short lasting. Although the immune system normally works to protect the body, it can go awry, causing allergic reactions and autoimmune disease. Anaphylaxis is a serious IgE hypersensitivity reaction that is life threatening.

As You Age

1. T-cell and B-cell function are somewhat deficient in older adults. Depressed lymphocyte function is accompanied by a decrease in macrophage activity. Consequently, older adults are more prone to develop infections and they recover more slowly. Depressed lymphocyte function might also explain the higher incidence of cancer in older adults.
2. Older adults often have a reduced fever response to infection and may therefore have difficulty in combating infection.
3. Older adults have increased levels of circulating autoantibodies (antibodies directed against self). This increase explains, in part, why they are more prone to the development of autoimmune disease.
4. Older adults often take drugs or undergo treatment that depresses the immune system. For example, the use of steroids in the treatment of arthritis and the use of drugs and radiation in the treatment of cancer all cause immunosuppression.

MEDICAL TERMINOLOGY AND DISORDERS · Disorders of the Immune System

Medical Term	Word Parts	Word Part Meaning or Derivation	Description
Words			
anaphylaxis	ana-	up	**Anaphylaxis** is *a life-threatening hypersensitivity reaction mediated by IgE antibodies.*
	-phylaxis	From a Greek word meaning "watching or guarding"	
immune	immune/o-	From a Latin word meaning "exempt from"	To be **immune** is *to be exempt or protected from a particular disease.*
lymphocyte	lymph/o-	lymph	A **lymphocyte** is *a nongranular white blood cell.* There are T lymphocytes (T cells) and B lymphocytes (B cells).
	-cyte	cell	
macrophage	macro-	large	A **macrophage** (fixed or wandering) is *a type of white blood cell that digests foreign materials, including pathogens.*
	-phage	eat	
wheal and flare reaction			A **wheal and flare reaction** is *a skin reaction to an allergen or antigen.* The response is a circular (wheal) blanched area surrounded by an area of redness.
Disorders			
hypersensitivity reactions			A **hypersensitivity reaction** is *the immune system response to a foreign substance, or what is perceived as "foreign" in the case of autoimmune disease. Hypersensitivity reactions include allergies and autoimmune diseases.*
allergies			An **allergy** occurs when the immune system reacts to a foreign substance. Allergies are described in many ways: atopic, bacterial, contact, cold, drug, immediate, delayed, etc. The symptoms vary in intensity from mild to life threatening. An **atopic allergy** is genetic and refers to the development of a hypersensitivity reaction to an environmental allergen (e.g., pollen, bee venom, dander, food, environmental chemicals). Atopic reactions generally include eczema (atopic dermatitis), allergic rhinitis (hay fever), allergic conjunctivitis, or allergic asthma. A **latex allergy** is an allergic reaction to proteins found in natural rubber latex. Latex is found in many articles, such as shoes, balloons, condoms, medical equipment, drugs, paints, and adhesives, and for some is considered a major occupational hazard. About 50% of persons with latex allergy have allergic reactions to certain foods: avocado, banana, plum, strawberry, and tomato. **Anaphylaxis** is a severe and life-threatening hypersensitivity reaction, mediated by IgE antibodies.
autoimmune diseases	auto-	self	**Autoimmune system disorders** occur *when a person's immune system produces antibodies against its own cells; the immune system no longer recognizes self from nonself.* There are many **autoimmune diseases,** including rheumatoid arthritis, Hashimoto thyroiditis, diabetes mellitus (type 1), and rheumatic fever. **Rheumatic fever** is an immune disorder in which the antibodies produced in response to a streptococcal infection attack the heart muscle and its valves. Many of the autoimmune diseases are described in other chapters.
	-immun/o-	immunity	

Continued

MEDICAL TERMINOLOGY AND DISORDERS   Disorders of the Immune System—cont'd

Medical Term	Word Parts	Word Part Meaning or Derivation	Description
immunodeficiency disorders	immun/o-		*Disorders caused by an impaired immune response.* Immunodeficiency disorders are classified as primary or secondary. **Primary immunodeficiency disorders** are rare, an example being **severe combined immunodeficiency disease (SCID). Secondary immunodeficiency disorders** are common, the most common cause being a drug-induced immune deficiency such as the granulocytopenia resulting from cancer chemotherapy. Other causes include radiation therapy, steroid therapy, stress, malignancies, aging, and many diseases, especially infection with the human immunodeficiency virus (HIV). **HIV infection** is usually transmitted sexually. Because it is also transmitted through accidental or intended sharing of injection equipment, HIV is a serious threat to hospital workers and others who routinely handle blood or blood-related products or equipment. Initial infection with HIV causes **viremia** (virus in the blood), which persists for many years and which targets the immune system, particularly the CD4⁺ T cells (helper T cells). The late and severe manifestation of HIV infection is called **acquired immunodeficiency syndrome (AIDS).** At this stage all organ systems are adversely affected and death is most often caused by infection.
	-deficiency		
scleroderma	scler/o-	hard	*A chronic autoimmune disease characterized by a hardening of the skin or other organs.* The systemic form of the disease may be fatal because of heart, kidney, lung, and intestinal involvement. The limited form of the disease is called **CREST,** an acronym for the five main signs: *C*alcinosis, *R*aynaud's syndrome, *E*sophageal dysfunction, *S*clerodactyly (hardness of fingers or toes), *T*elangiectasia. CREST usually spares the lungs and kidneys.
	-derm/o	skin	
systemic lupus erythematosus (SLE)		From the Latin word meaning "wolf" (lupus)	**SLE** is a chronic autoimmune disorder. Symptoms are due to inflammation and are highly variable, but all persons experience joint pain (especially fingers, hands, wrist, and knees). A "butterfly" rash over the bridge of the nose and patchy skin color are characteristic of SLE. Persons who experience only the skin symptoms have **discoid erythematosus.** A **drug-induced lupus erythematosus (DIL)** can develop in response to certain medications; symptoms gradually disappear when the medication is stopped.

Get Ready for Exams!

Summary Outline

The immune system is a defense system that protects the body from foreign agents such as pathogens, pollens, toxins, and cancer cells.

I. Nonspecific Immunity
A. Nonspecific immune mechanisms protect the body against many different types of foreign agents and do not require recognition of the specific agent.
B. Lines of defense
1. The first line of defense includes mechanical barriers, chemical barriers, and reflexes.
2. The second line of defense includes phagocytosis, inflammation, fever, protective proteins, and natural killer (NK) cells.

II. Immunity
A. Specific immunity protects the body against specific foreign agents and requires recognition of the specific agent involved.
B. T cells, or T lymphocytes
1. The T cells make up 70% to 80% of the blood's lymphocytes.
2. T cells engage in cell-mediated immunity.
3. Activated T cells produce a clone (killer T cells, helper T cells, suppressor T cells, and memory T cells).
C. B cells, or B lymphocytes
1. B cells make up 20% to 30% of the blood's lymphocytes.
2. B cells engage in antibody-mediated immunity.

3. Activated B cells produce a clone (memory cells and plasma cells). The plasma cells secrete antibodies that travel through the blood to the antigens.
4. The antibodies are called *immunoglobulins*.

III. Types of Immunity
A. Genetic or acquired immunity
   1. With genetic immunity, a person is genetically immune to an antigen.
   2. A person can acquire immunity naturally or artificially.
   3. A person can acquire immunity naturally in two ways: by getting the disease or by receiving antibodies from the mother across the placenta and/or through breast milk.
   4. Immunity can be acquired artificially in two ways: by the use of a vaccine or by injection of immune globulin made by another person or animal.
B. Active or passive immunity
   1. Active immunity means that a person's body makes the antibodies (usually long-lasting).
   2. Passive immunity means that the antibodies are made by another animal and then injected into a patient's body (usually short-lasting).

IV. Other Immune Responses
A. Allergic reactions
   1. Allergic reactions are caused by the formation of antibodies to substances usually not recognized as foreign.
   2. There are two types of allergic reactions: delayed-onset allergy and immediate-reaction allergy.
   3. A delayed-onset allergy takes about 48 hours to develop. Contact dermatitis to a household chemical is a common example.
   4. An immediate-reaction allergy (also called an *immediate hypersensitivity reaction*) is often caused by exposure to pollens and drugs such as penicillin. The most severe form is anaphylaxis.
B. Autoimmunity and tissue or organ rejection
   1. Autoimmune disease develops when the immune system mounts an attack against self.
   2. Tissue or organ rejection occurs when the immune system recognizes the transplanted organ as foreign and attacks it.

Review Your Knowledge

Matching: Nonspecific Immunity
Directions: Match the following words with their descriptions below. Some words may be used more than once.
a. protective proteins
b. phagocytosis
c. inflammation
d. fever

1. ___ Caused by pyrogens
2. ___ Eats debris and pathogens
3. ___ Redness, heat, swelling, and pain
4. ___ Neutrophils and monocytes
5. ___ Complement and interferons

Matching: Specific Immunity
Directions: Match the following words with their descriptions below.
a. immunotolerance
b. cell-mediated immunity
c. antibody-mediated immunity
d. macrophage
e. plasma cells

1. ___ Subgroup of the B-cell clone that secretes antibodies
2. ___ Recognition of self
3. ___ The cell responsible for antigen presentation
4. ___ Also called *humoral immunity*
5. ___ T-cell immunity

Matching: Active and Passive Immunity
Directions: Indicate whether the following conveys active immunity (a) or passive immunity (b).
1. ___ Vaccine
2. ___ Antivenom
3. ___ Antitoxin
4. ___ Toxoid
5. ___ Gamma globulin
6. ___ Getting the disease

Multiple Choice
1. Complement and interferons are
   a. considered to be specific immunity.
   b. protective proteins engaged in nonspecific immunity.
   c. secreted by B cells and T cells.
   d. vaccines.
2. T and B cells
   a. engage in nonspecific immunity.
   b. refer to neutrophils.
   c. both engage in antibody-mediated immunity.
   d. are lymphocytes that are responsible for specific immunity.
3. Which of the following is not related to cell-mediated immunity?
   a. Cell-to-cell combat
   b. Killer T cells
   c. Immunoglobulins
   d. Antigen presentation by a macrophage
4. Which of the following best describes the killer T cell, helper T cell, memory T cell, and suppressor T cell?
   a. Immunoglobulins
   b. Macrophages
   c. Clone
   d. Agglutination
5. Pyrexia, pyrogens, and febrile seizures are most related to this nonspecific form of immunity?
   a. Inflammation
   b. Fever
   c. Anaphylaxis
   d. Diapedesis, chemotaxis, and phagocytosis
6. Plasma cells
   a. refer to T cells.
   b. are the same as NK cells.
   c. secrete antibodies.
   d. secrete interferons.

7. With which of the following is anaphylaxis most associated?
   a. Interferons
   b. Phagocytosis
   c. IgE
   d. Contact dermatitis

8. What is the primary concern regarding the care of a person experiencing an anaphylactic reaction?
   a. Inability to breathe
   b. Development of hives
   c. Development of febrile seizures
   d. Intense itching and discomfort

9. Which of the following is least characteristic of a vaccine?
   a. Artificially acquired immunity
   b. Active immunity
   c. Conveys long-lasting immunity
   d. Passive, immediate-onset, and short-lived immunity

10. Inflammation is
    a. specific immunity.
    b. characterized by redness, heat, swelling, and pain.
    c. known as *cell-mediated immunity*.
    d. synonymous with infection.

Go Figure

1. **According to Figures 21-1 and 21-2**
   a. The natural killer cell is a lymphocyte and is therefore considered a type of specific immunity.
   b. Phagocytosis, inflammation, and fever occur only in response to invasion by a pathogen.
   c. Interferons are lymphocytes.
   d. T and B cells are lymphocytes and are considered a form of specific immunity.

2. **According to Figures 21-3 and 21-4**
   a. Antigens are presented by macrophages in both cell-mediated immunity (CMI) and antibody-mediated immunity (AMI).
   b. Antibodies are secreted by plasma cells in AMI.
   c. Helper T cells enhance B-cell response.
   d. All of the above are true.

3. **According to Figures 21-3 and 21-4**
   a. Only T cells have memory cells in their clone.
   b. A deficiency of helper T cells, as in HIV infection, depresses B-cell activity.
   c. Suppressor T cells engage in cell-to-cell combat.
   d. Helper T cells secrete lymphokines, which in turn suppress B-cell activity.

4. **According to Figures 21-5 and 21-6**
   a. Antibody concentration is higher with the first exposure to a pathogen than the second.
   b. "Getting the disease" is a form of artificially acquired active immunity.
   c. Naturally acquired passive immunity describes the immunity of a breast-fed infant.
   d. A vaccine conveys long-lasting passive immunity.

5. **According to Figure 21-7**
   a. IgE antibodies are released by mast cells.
   b. IgE antibodies bind to mast cells, causing the release of histamine.
   c. Histamine causes peripheral vasoconstriction and anemia.
   d. Histamine binds to mast cells, causing the release of IgE antibodies.

6. **According to Figures 21-4 and 21-7**
   a. T cell activation produces plasma cells.
   b. Plasma cells secrete lymphokines which, in turn, activate helper T cells.
   c. Plasma cells secrete antibodies.
   d. Histamine binds to mast cells.

Respiratory System

Key Terms

alveolus (p. 406)
bronchioles (p. 406)
bronchus (p. 404)
compliance (p. 410)
epiglottis (p. 401)
exhalation (p. 411)

glottis (p. 401)
inhalation (p. 411)
intrapleural pressure (p. 409)
larynx (p. 401)
partial pressure (p. 415)
pharynx (p. 401)

pleurae (p. 407)
surfactants (p. 408)
tidal volume (p. 416)
trachea (p. 404)
ventilation (p. 411)
vital capacity (p. 417)

Objective

1. Describe the structure and functions of the organs of the respiratory system and trace the movement of air from the nostrils to the alveoli.
2. Describe why lungs collapse or expand and the role of pulmonary surfactants.
3. Discuss the three steps in respiration, including:
   • Describe the relationship of Boyle's law to ventilation.
   • Explain how respiratory muscles affect thoracic volume.

• List three conditions that make the alveoli well-suited for the exchange of oxygen and carbon dioxide.
4. List lung volumes and capacities.
5. Discuss the voluntary and involuntary control of breathing, including:
   • Explain the neural and chemical control of respiration.
   • Describe common variations and abnormalities of breathing.

Is he breathing? This is the first question asked about a person who has been seriously injured. The question indicates the importance of each breath. To breathe is to live; not to breathe is to die. Each breath is a breath of life.

Because of its close connection with life, ancient peoples attributed the act of breathing to the divine. Even the phases of breathing are called *inspiration* and *expiration,* references to a divine spirit moving into and out of our lungs. The creation story in Genesis, in which God breathes life into the little clay figure of Adam, vividly expresses an image of divine breath. Poetry also describes breathing as the life force. For example, the great Persian poet Sa'di echoed the sacredness of breath in a prayer: "Each respiration holds two blessings. Life is inhaled, and stale, foul air is exhaled. Therefore, thank God twice every breath you take."

STRUCTURE: ORGANS OF THE RESPIRATORY SYSTEM

UPPER AND LOWER RESPIRATORY TRACTS

The respiratory system contains the upper and lower respiratory tracts (Figure 22-1). The upper respiratory tract contains the respiratory organs located outside the chest cavity: the nose and nasal cavities, pharynx, larynx, and upper trachea. The lower respiratory tract consists of organs located in the chest cavity: the lower trachea, bronchi, bronchioles, and alveoli. The lower parts of the bronchi, bronchioles, and alveoli are located in the lungs. The pleural membranes and the muscles that form the chest cavity are also part of the lower respiratory tract.

Most of the respiratory organs are concerned with conduction, or movement, of air through the respiratory passages. The alveoli are the tiny air sacs located at the end of the respiratory passages. They are concerned with the exchange of oxygen and carbon dioxide between the air and the blood across the walls of the pulmonary capillaries. It is critical that the airway remains open; airway obstruction is life threatening!

NOSE AND NASAL CAVITIES

The nose includes an external portion that forms part of the face and an internal portion called the *nasal cavities.* The nasal cavities are separated into right and left halves by a partition called the *nasal septum,* which is made of bone and cartilage. Air enters the nasal cavities through two openings called the *nostrils,* or *nares.* Nasal hairs in the nostrils filter large particles of dust

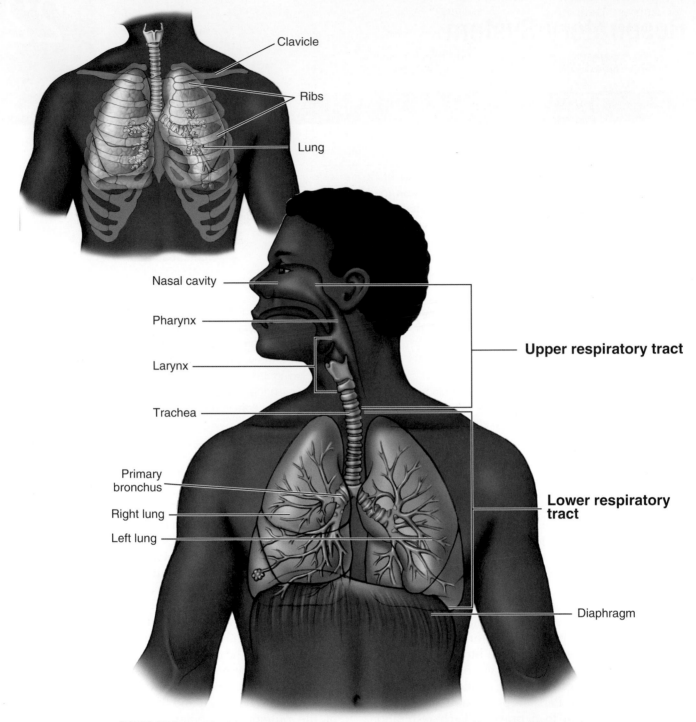

FIGURE 22-1 Organs of the respiratory system: upper respiratory tract and lower respiratory tract.

that might otherwise be inhaled. In addition to its respiratory function, the nasal cavity contains the receptor cells for the sense of smell. The olfactory receptors cover the mucous membrane of the upper parts of the nasal cavity and a part of the nasal septum.

Three bony projections called *nasal conchae* (KONCH-ay) appear on the lateral walls of the nasal cavities. The conchae increase the surface area of the nasal cavities and support the ciliated mucous membranes, which line the nasal cavities. Mucous

membranes contain many blood vessels and mucus-secreting cells. The rich supply of blood warms and moistens the air, and the sticky mucus traps dust, pollen, and other small particles, thereby cleansing the air as it is inhaled. Because the nose helps warm, moisten, and cleanse the air, breathing through the nose is better than mouth breathing.

The nasal cavities contain several drainage openings. Mucus from the paranasal sinuses (see Figure 8-8) drains into the nasal cavities. The paranasal sinuses include the maxillary, frontal, ethmoidal, and sphenoidal sinuses. Tears from the nasolacrimal ducts also drain into the nasal cavities. (Cry and your nose runs.)

Do You Know...

That Your Nose Is More Than Just a Smeller?

The nose does a few things real well; as you know, the nose knows smells. It also "nose" how to clean and humidify air. Equally important, the nose plays a big cosmetic role: it makes us look good and, if it doesn't, we simply rearrange it surgically until it is fashioned into a great-looking nose. Nose-related medical conditions or procedures are named after the rhino, who sports the mother of all noses. For instance, a *rhinoplasty* refers to the surgical reshaping, resizing, or realigning of the nose. *Rhinorrhea* refers to a runny nose, as in the common cold or the discharge of cerebrospinal fluid from the nose. *Rhinokyphosis* is a humpback nose, and, of course, you can have a pain in the nose—*rhinodynia*. It is interesting that the rhino has captured the nose words, since the rhino's nose is merely hardened hair; it doesn't sniff or drip, and it certainly doesn't check itself in for a nose job

In some persons, the nasal septum may bend toward one side or the other, thereby obstructing the flow of air and making breathing difficult. This abnormal positioning of the septum is called a *deviated septum*. Surgical repair of the deviated septum (septoplasty) corrects the problem.

And for the nose that snorts cocaine? Chronic exposure to the drug causes intense vasoconstriction of the blood vessels that supply the septum. The septal cartilage dies, thereby creating a hole in the septum and giving the nose a collapsed or "caved-in" appearance. Not a good look!

PHARYNX

The **pharynx** (FAIR-inks), or throat, is located behind the oral cavity and between the nasal cavities and the larynx (Figure 22-2). The pharynx includes three parts: the nasopharynx (upper section), the oropharynx (middle section), and the laryngopharynx (lower section). The oropharynx and the laryngopharynx are part of both the digestive and respiratory systems and function as a passageway for both food and air. The pharynx conducts food toward the esophagus (tube

for food to enter the stomach). The pharynx also conducts air to the larynx as it moves toward the lungs.

The pharynx contains two other structures: the openings from the eustachian tubes (auditory tubes) and the tonsils. The eustachian tube connects the nasopharynx with the middle ear.

Eustachian tube

LARYNX

WHERE AND WHAT IS YOUR VOICE BOX?

The **larynx** (LAIR-inks), also called the *voice box*, is located between the pharynx and trachea (see Figure 22-2, *A*). The larynx has three functions: it acts as a passageway for air during breathing, it produces sound (your voice), and it prevents food and other foreign objects from entering the distal respiratory structures. The larynx is a triangular structure made primarily of cartilage, muscles, and ligaments (see Figure 22-2, *C* and *D*).

The largest of the cartilaginous structures in the larynx is the thyroid cartilage. It is a tough hyaline cartilage and protrudes in the front of the neck. The thyroid cartilage is larger in men and is called the *Adam's apple* (see Figure 22-2, *B*).

The **epiglottis** (ep-i-GLOT-iss) is another cartilaginous structure, located at the top of the larynx (see Figure 22-2, *A* and *B*). The epiglottis acts as a flap, a very important flap. It covers the opening of the trachea during eating so food does not enter the lungs.

VOCAL CORDS

The larynx is called the *voice box* because it contains the vocal cords (see Figure 22-2, *A* and *C*). The vocal cords are folds of tissue composed of muscle and elastic ligaments and covered by mucous membrane. The cords stretch across the upper part of the larynx. The **glottis** is the space between the vocal cords.

TRUE OR FALSE

The two types of vocal cords are the false and true vocal cords. The false vocal cords are called "false" because they do not produce sounds. Instead, the muscles in this structure help to close the airway during swallowing. The true vocal cords produce

FIGURE 22-2 A, Organs of the upper respiratory tract. **B,** Larynx, showing the thyroid cartilage (Adam's apple). **C,** Vocal cords and glottis (closed). **D,** Vocal cords and glottis (open).

sound. Air flowing from the lungs through the glottis during exhalation causes the true vocal cords to vibrate, thereby producing sound.

The loudness of your voice depends on the force with which the air moves past the true vocal cords. The pitch of your voice depends on the tension exerted on the muscles of the true vocal cords. You form sound into words with your pharynx, oral cavity, tongue, and lip movement. The nasal cavities, sinuses, and pharynx act as resonating chambers, thereby altering the quality of your voice. Listen to the different voices of your friends. One voice may sound high and squeaky, whereas another may sound low and booming.

DOWN THE WRONG WAY

As shown in Figure 22-2, *A,* the pharynx acts as a passageway for food, water, and air. Food and water in the pharynx, however, should not enter the larynx. How is food and water normally kept out of the larynx? When you breathe in air, the glottis opens, and air moves through the glottis into tubes that carry it to the lungs.

When you swallow food, however, the epiglottis covers the glottis, thereby preventing food from entering the lower respiratory passages. Instead, the food enters the esophagus, the tube that empties into the stomach. How does this happen? During swallowing, the larynx moves upward and forward while the epiglottis moves downward. If you place your fingers on your larynx as you swallow, you can feel the larynx move upward and forward. In addition to the movement of the epiglottis, the glottis closes. Compare the size of the glottis in Figure 22-2, *C* and *D.*

Note that swallowing plays a key role in preventing the entrance of food or water into the respiratory tubes. Some patients develop difficulty in swallowing, particularly those who have suffered neurological damage such as a stroke. Any patient who experiences difficulty in swallowing is at risk for aspiration (entrance of food or water into the lungs). Aspiration is a large clinical problem.

FROM BOY TO YOUNG MAN

Why is Jack's voice lower than Jill's? At puberty, under the influence of testosterone, the male larynx enlarges and the vocal cords become longer and thicker. The larger vocal cords deepen the male voice. Changes in the larynx and vocal cords cause the boy's voice to "break" as he matures into a young man. In an earlier period in history, young choir boys with beautiful high voices were castrated. Castration, the surgical excision of the testes, removes the source of testosterone and prevents thickening of the vocal cords. These unfortunate castrated boys continued to sing beautifully as members of the castrati choir. For obvious reasons, this practice eventually disappeared.

? Re-Think

1. Trace the flow of air from the nose to the trachea.
2. Explain why food and water do not enter the respiratory structures during swallowing.

Do You Know...

Who Heimlich Is and What He Maneuvered?

Dr. Heimlich is a physician who developed a procedure designed to dislodge the obstructing object in a choking person. The Heimlich maneuver, or abdominal thrust, is a simple technique. The "bear hug" procedure is demonstrated on an adult below. Here are the steps for the adult:

1. Stand behind the choking person and wrap your arms around the person's waist.
2. Position your hands (fist position) between the person's navel and the bottom of the rib cage.
3. Press your fist into the abdomen with a quick upward movement.
4. Repeat several times as necessary.

Heimlich maneuver (adult)

Do You Know...

How "Dumb Plant" Was Used to Control Gossip (Without, of Course, Killing the Gossiper)?

A tea made from dieffenbachia ("dumb plant") was given to Roman slaves before they were sent to the market to shop. The tea caused the slave's tongue and mouth to swell and paralyzed the throat. The slave was therefore unable to speak and gossip about household affairs. It is still used by some African tribes as a punishment for gossip. An overdose of the poison causes excessive swelling, obstruction of the respiratory passageways, and death by suffocation. On an updated note, acute respiratory obstruction can be induced when a patient is given a drug or food to which she is allergic. "Dumb plant ingestion" may be dead, but the anaphylactic response (respiratory obstruction) is very much alive and well.

TRACHEA

WHERE IT SITS AND WHERE IT SPLITS

The trachea (TRAY-kee-ah), or windpipe, is a tube 4 to 5 inches (10 to 12.5 cm) long and 1 inch (2.5 cm) in diameter (Figure 22-3). The trachea extends from the larynx downward into the thoracic cavity, where it splits into the right and left bronchi (sing., bronchus). The trachea splits, or bifurcates, at a point called the *carina* (kah-RYE-nah) at the manubriosternal junction (where the manubrium of the sternum meets the sternal body). Why is the carina so important clinically? The carina is very sensitive; touching it during suctioning causes vigorous coughing. The purpose of the trachea? It conducts air to and from the lungs.

KEEPING IT OPEN

The trachea lies in front of the esophagus, the food tube. C-shaped rings of cartilage partially surround the trachea for its entire length and serve to keep it open. The rings are open on the back side of the trachea so that the esophagus can bulge forward as food moves along the esophagus to the stomach. You can feel the cartilaginous rings if you run your fingers along the front of your neck. Without this strong cartilaginous support, the trachea would collapse and shut off the flow of air through the respiratory passages. Because of the cartilaginous rings, a tight collar or necktie does not collapse the trachea. A severe blow to the anterior neck, however, can crush the trachea and cause an acute respiratory obstruction. The trachea must be kept open.

BRONCHIAL TREE: BRONCHI, BRONCHIOLES, AND ALVEOLI

The bronchial tree consists of the bronchi, the bronchioles, and the alveoli. It is called a *tree* because the bronchi and their many branches resemble an upside-down tree. Most of the bronchial tree is in the lungs.

Bronchial tree

BRONCHI

The right and left primary bronchi are formed as the lower part of the trachea divides into two tubes. The primary bronchi enter the lungs at a region called

 Do You Know...

What a Tracheostomy Is?

Sometimes a part of the upper respiratory tract becomes blocked, thereby obstructing the flow of air into the lungs. To restore air flow, an emergency tracheostomy may be performed. This procedure is the insertion of a tube through a surgical incision into the trachea below the level of the obstruction. The tracheostomy bypasses the obstruction and allows air to flow through the tube into the lungs.

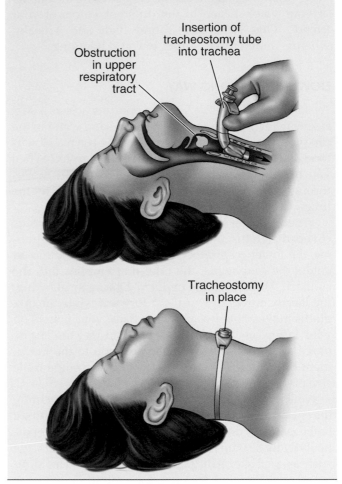

the *hilus*. The primary bronchi branch into secondary bronchi, which branch into smaller tertiary bronchi. Because the heart lies toward the left side of the chest, the left bronchus is narrower and positioned more horizontally than the right bronchus. The right bronchus is shorter and wider than the left bronchus and extends downward in a more vertical direction. Because of the differences in the size and positioning of the bronchi, food particles and small objects are more easily inhaled, or aspirated, into the right bronchus.

Why are tiny toys not good for tiny tots? Young children generally put toys in their mouths. The tiny toy may become lodged in the larynx or bronchus, causing an acute respiratory obstruction. Unless relieved immediately, the obstruction can be fatal. Tiny toys are responsible for many toy recalls.

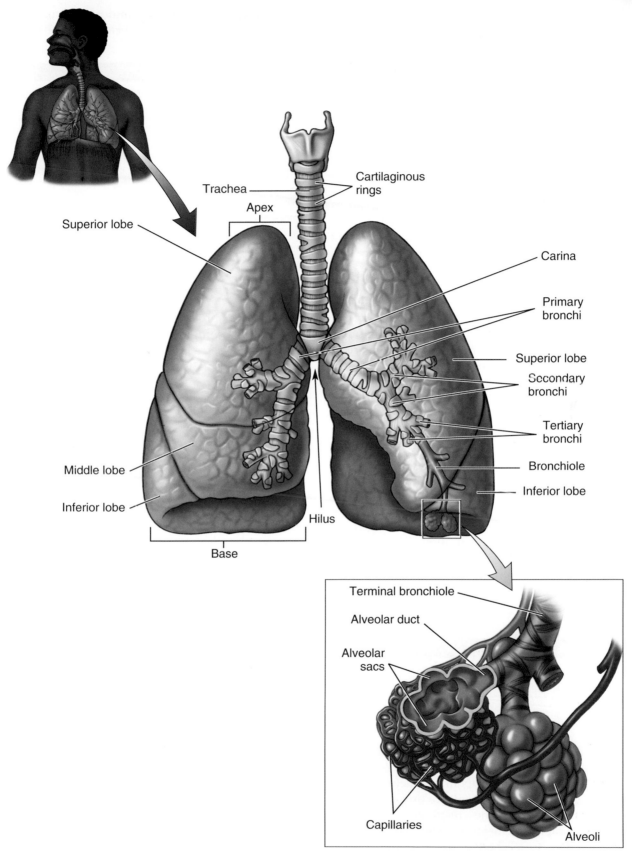

FIGURE 22-3 Trachea and bronchial tree (bronchi, bronchioles, and alveoli).

The upper segments of the bronchi have C-shaped cartilaginous rings, which help keep the bronchi open. As the bronchi extend into the lungs, however, the amount of cartilage decreases and finally disappears. The finer and more distal branches of the bronchi contain no cartilage.

BRONCHIOLES

The bronchi divide repeatedly into smaller tubes called **bronchioles** (BRON-kee-ohls). The walls of the bronchioles contain smooth muscle and no cartilage. The bronchioles regulate the flow of air to the alveoli. Contraction of the bronchiolar smooth muscle causes the bronchioles to constrict, thereby decreasing the bronchiolar lumen (opening) and thus decreasing the flow of air. Relaxation of the bronchioles causes the lumen to increase, thereby increasing the flow of air.

An asthma attack illustrates the effect of bronchiolar smooth muscle constriction. In a person with asthma, the bronchioles hyperrespond to a particular stimulus. The bronchiolar smooth muscle then constricts, decreasing the flow of air into the lungs. The person complains of a tight chest and expends much energy trying to force air through the constricted bronchioles into the lungs. Forced air causes a wheezing sound. Bronchiolar smooth muscle relaxants are medications that cause bronchodilation, thereby improving air flow and relieving the wheezing.

Let's translate this into autonomic pharmacology. The bronchioles contain beta$_2$-adrenergic receptors. Stimulation of these receptors causes relaxation of the bronchiolar smooth muscle, thus inducing bronchodilation and improved air flow. Albuterol, a beta$_2$-adrenergic agonist, is a bronchodilator drug. Conversely, a beta$_2$-adrenergic blocker, such as propranolol, causes bronchoconstriction and is therefore contraindicated in asthmatic patients.

? Re-Think

1. Explain why the trachea remains open.
2. What is the "problem" caused by bronchoconstriction?

ALVEOLI

The bronchioles continue to divide and give rise to many tubes called *alveolar ducts* (see Figure 22-3). These ducts end in very small, grapelike structures called *alveoli* (sing., **alveolus**). The alveoli are tiny air sacs that form at the ends of the respiratory passages. A pulmonary capillary surrounds each alveolus. The alveoli function to exchange oxygen and carbon dioxide across the alveolar-pulmonary capillary membrane. Oxygen diffuses from the alveoli into the blood; carbon dioxide diffuses from the blood into the alveoli. The term *atelectasis* refers to collapsed and airless alveoli. Atelectasis occurs commonly as a postoperative complication and as a result of conditions such as pneumonia and cancer of the lung.

 Do You Know...

Why You May Diagnose Cystic Fibrosis by Kissing Your Baby's Face?

Cystic fibrosis (CF) is a hereditary disease that is characterized by thickened secretions of most exocrine glands. Consequently CF affects many organs including the liver, pancreas, and especially the lungs. The production of thick bronchial secretions is of particular concern because the secretions block narrow breathing passages, causing atelectasis and pulmonary infections. Eventually lung tissue is destroyed; for this reason the clinical picture of CF is dominated by lung dysfunction. In addition, sweat glands and salivary glands produce a very salty secretion; mothers often notice the salty taste of their infants upon kissing them.

Certain respiratory diseases may destroy alveoli or cause a thickening of the alveolar wall. As a result, the exchange of gases is slowed. Oxygenation of the blood may decrease, causing hypoxemia and cyanosis, and the blood may retain carbon dioxide, causing a disturbance in acid–base balance (acidosis).

 Do You Know...

Why Your Fingers Go "Clubbing"?

Patients who experience chronic hypoxemia, such as those with impaired lung and heart function, often develop clubbing of the fingers and toes. Clubbing is characterized by enlarged fingertips and toes and changes in the thickness and shape of the nails. The enlargement is due to the formation of additional capillaries and tissue hypertrophy in an attempt to deliver oxygen to the oxygen-deprived cells.

LUNGS

RIGHT AND LEFT

The two lungs, located in the pleural cavities, extend from an area just above the clavicles to the diaphragm. The lungs are soft cone-shaped organs so large that they occupy most of the space in the thoracic cavity (see Figure 22-3). The lungs are subdivided into lobes. The right lung has three lobes: the superior, middle, and inferior lobes. Because of the location of the heart in the left side of the chest, the left lung has only two lobes: the superior lobe and the inferior lobe.

The upper rounded part of the lung is called the *apex*, and the lower portion is called the *base*. The base of the lung rests on the diaphragm. The amount of air the lungs can hold varies with a person's body build, age, and physical conditioning. For instance, a tall person has larger lungs than a short person. A swimmer generally has larger lungs than a "couch potato," and the trained singer has larger lungs than the typical "shower singer."

That Charles Dickens "Nailed It" in His Novel
The Pickwick Papers?

Yup, the creator of our beloved Tiny Tim in *A Christmas Carol* was the first to accurately describe (but not name) the syndrome of obesity-associated alveolar hypoventilation, or Pickwickian syndrome. In Dickens' description in *Pickwick Papers,* he refers to "a fat boy and red-faced boy in a state of somnolency" (extreme sleepiness). He subsequently addresses the boy as "Young Dropsy" (a reference to his obesity), Young Opium-eater (a reference to his somnolency), and Young Boa Constrictor (a reference to his excessive appetite). Physiologically, this is what Dickens meant to say: The boy's immense abdominal girth causes ventilatory insufficiency (periodic respirations and hypoventilation) and hypoxemia, explaining his extreme sleepiness (somnolence). The hypoxemia also stimulates RBC production and polycythemia (through erythropoietin) in an attempt to increase oxygen in the blood; this accounts for the boy's red appearance. Had Dickens known a little pathophysiology, he would have thrown into the mix a probable hematocrit of 65, expanded blood volume, hypercapnia with mild respiratory acidosis, alveolar hypoventilation, and an enlarged right heart. He would have explained that right heart failure, in turn, causes distention of the neck veins (JVD), hepatomegaly and pedal edema.

Although Dickens didn't throw around much medical terminology, Young Dropsy's appearance described the syndrome quite accurately. So why is Pickwickian syndrome of such concern today? Because of the prevalence of obesity in our society and the wide varieties of obesity-related health conditions! Our increasing girth continues to "expand" upward. The short-term solution may be to increase the size of clothes, chairs, and caskets, but the real solution is to waste the waist. The good news? Weight loss appears to reverse the signs and symptoms of Pickwickian syndrome, including the "obesity heart disease."

? **Re-Think**

1. What is the primary function of the alveoli?
2. Reviewing the structures of the respiratory tract, identify at least three ways that a patient can develop an acute respiratory obstruction.

PLEURAL MEMBRANES

PLEURA

The outside of each lung and the inner chest wall are lined with a continuous serous membrane called the **pleurae** (Figure 22-4). The pleurae are named according to their location. The membrane on the outer surface of each lung is called the *visceral pleura;* the membrane lining the chest wall is called the *parietal pleura.* The visceral pleura and the parietal pleura are attracted to each other like two flat plates of glass whose surfaces are wet. The plates of glass can slide past one another but offer some resistance when you try to pull them apart.

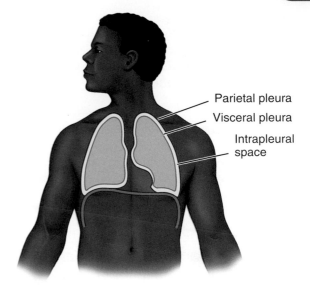

FIGURE 22-4 Lungs, pleural membranes, and the intrapleural space.

PLEURAL CAVITY: A POTENTIAL SPACE

Between the visceral pleura and the parietal pleura is a space called the *intrapleural space.* The pleural membranes secrete a small amount of serous fluid (approximately 25 mL). The fluid lubricates the pleural membranes and allows them to slide past one another with little friction or discomfort. Under abnormal conditions, the intrapleural space has the potential to accumulate excess fluid, blood, and air. An excess secretion of pleural fluid is called *pleural effusion.* Purulent (pus) pleural effusion is called *empyema.*

2+2 **Sum It Up!**

Air moves through the following structures—from the nasal cavities, to the pharynx, to the larynx, to the trachea, to the bronchi, to the bronchioles, and finally to the alveoli. When the air reaches the alveoli (the tiny air sacs at the end of the bronchial tree), the respiratory gases oxygen and carbon dioxide diffuse across the alveolar–pulmonary capillary membrane. Most of the respiratory structures conduct air to and from the lungs. Only the alveoli function in the exchange of the respiratory gases between the outside air and the blood. The lungs contain the structures of the lower respiratory tract. Pleural membranes surround the lungs and line the thoracic cavity, creating the intrapleural space or pleural cavity.

COLLAPSED AND EXPANDED LUNGS

Figure 22-1 shows that the lungs occupy most of the thoracic cage, but this statement must be qualified: the *expanded* lungs occupy most of the thoracic cage. Under normal conditions, the lungs expand like inflated balloons. Under abnormal conditions, however, a lung may collapse. What determines whether or not the lungs collapse or expand?

WHY LUNGS COLLAPSE

If the thoracic cavity is entered surgically, the lungs collapse. There are two reasons why the lungs collapse: elastic recoil and surface tension.

ELASTIC RECOIL

Consider a balloon and a lung (Figure 22-5, *A*). If you blow up a balloon but fail to tie off the open end, the air rushes out and the balloon collapses. It collapses because of the arrangement of its elastic fibers. When these fibers stretch, they remain stretched only when tension is applied (the air blown into the balloon stretches the balloon). If the end of the balloon is not tied off, the elastic fibers recoil, forcing air out and collapsing the balloon. The same can be said of the lung. The arrangement of the lung's elastic tissue is similar to the arrangement of the elastic fibers in the balloon. The elastic tissue of the lung can stretch, but it recoils and returns to its unstretched position if tension is released (see Figure 22-5, *B*). This is called *elastic recoil*.

SURFACE TENSION

The lung also collapses for a second reason, a force called *surface tension*. The single alveolus in Figure 22-5, *C*, illustrates surface tension. A thin layer of water lines the inside of the alveolus. Water is a polar molecule; one end of the water molecule has a positive (+) charge, whereas the other end of the molecule has a negative (−) charge. Note how the water molecules line up. The positive (+) end of one water molecule is attracted to the negative (−) charge on the second water molecule. Each water molecule pulls on the other and on the water molecules beneath them. The electrical attraction of the water molecules is the surface tension. As the water molecules pull on one another, they tend to make the alveolus smaller; in other words, they tend to collapse the alveoli.

NOTE: The surface tension of pure water is normally very high. In the mature normal lung, special alveolar cells secrete pulmonary surfactants. **Surfactants** (sur-FAK-tants) are detergent-like lipoproteins that decrease surface tension by interfering with the electrical attraction between the water molecules on the inner surface of the alveolus (see Figure 22-5, *C*). The secretion of surfactant is stimulated by a sigh. After every five or six breaths, a person takes a larger than normal breath (a sigh); the sigh stretches the alveoli, promoting the secretion of surfactant. Surfactants lower surface tension but do not eliminate it. Surface tension remains a force that acts to collapse the alveoli.

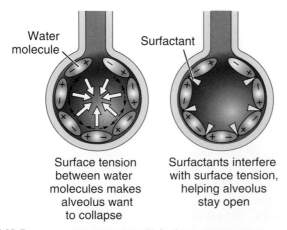

Elastic tissue

Elastic tissue is stretched

Elastic tissue recoils to unstretched position

B

Water molecule

Surfactant

Surface tension between water molecules makes alveolus want to collapse

Surfactants interfere with surface tension, helping alveolus stay open

C

FIGURE 22-5 **A** and **B,** Elastic recoil. **C,** Surface tension: water and the effect of surfactants.

🧠 Do You Know...

Why a Premature Infant Is More Apt Than a Full-Term Infant to Develop Respiratory Distress Syndrome?

Surfactant-secreting cells appear only during the later stages of fetal development. An infant born 2 to 3 months prematurely generally has insufficient surfactant-secreting cells. As a result, surface tension within the alveoli is excessively high, the alveoli collapse, and the infant experiences respiratory distress. The infant may die in respiratory failure. This condition is commonly called *respiratory distress syndrome*. Before delivery the mother may be given steroids to hasten the development of surfactant-secreting cells. In addition, a premature infant is given surfactants through inhalation in an attempt to prevent this life-threatening condition.

WHY LUNGS EXPAND

If elastic recoil and surface tension collapse the lungs, why do they remain expanded in the normal closed thorax? Lung expansion depends on pressure within the intrapleural space. A series of diagrams in Figure 22-6 illustrates this point. In Figure 22-6, *A*, the three pressures are labeled P1, P2, and P3. P1 is the pressure outside the chest (the pressure in the room), also called the *atmospheric pressure*. P2 is the pressure in the lung, also called the *intrapulmonic pressure*. P3 is the pressure in the intrapleural space, also called the **intrapleural pressure**. Note in Figure 22-6, *A*, that the lungs are normally expanded.

Figure 22-6, *B* and *C*, shows why the lungs expand. To illustrate this point, a hole is created in the right chest wall so that the right lung collapses. Note the pressures. Because of the hole in the chest wall, all the pressures are equal. In other words, P1 = P2 = P3. In Figure 22-6, *C*, a tube is inserted through the hole of the right chest wall into the intrapleural space. The tube is attached to a pump, which removes air from the intrapleural space. As air moves from the intrapleural space, the intrapleural pressure (P3) decreases and becomes negative. This negative intrapleural pressure (P3) merely means that it is lower than the atmospheric pressure (P1) or the intrapulmonic pressure (P2).

What is the effect of a negative intrapleural pressure? Because P2 (intrapulmonic pressure) is greater than P3 (intrapleural pressure), the lung is pushed toward the chest wall, causing the lung to expand. Also, because P1 (atmospheric pressure) is higher than P3, the chest wall is pushed inward toward the lung. When the chest wall and the lungs meet, the lung is

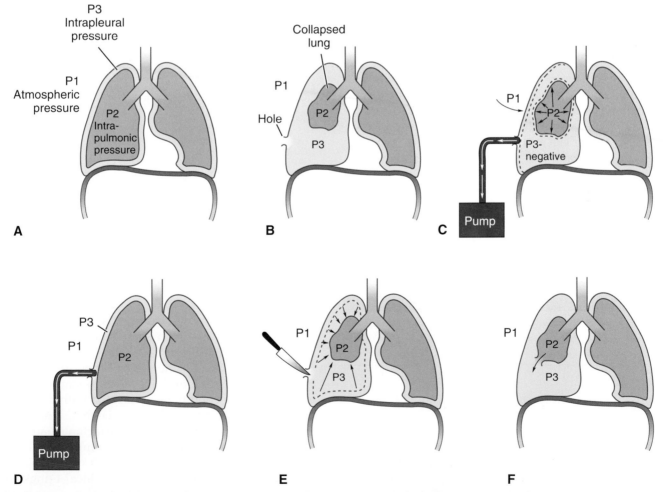

FIGURE 22-6 Lung expansion and collapse. **A,** The lungs expand. **B,** The right lung collapses because of the hole in the chest wall. **C,** Air is pumped out of the intrapleural space, creating a negative intrapleural pressure. **D,** The lung expands because of the negative intrapleural pressure. **E,** The lung collapses because of the hole (knife wound) in the chest wall. **F,** The lung collapses because of a hole in the lung.

expanded (see Figure 22-6, *C* and *D*). The important point is that the lung expands and remains expanded because the intrapleural pressure is negative.

What happens if the pump is removed, thereby recreating the hole in the chest wall? Because P1 is higher than P3, air rushes into the intrapleural space through the hole and eliminates the negative intrapleural pressure. As a result, the lung collapses. Remember that the lung expands only when the intrapleural pressure is negative.

Figure 22-6, *E,* illustrates the effects of a stab wound to the chest. The hole created by the knife allows the air to rush into the intrapleural space and eliminate the negative intrapleural pressure. The introduction of air into the intrapleural space and subsequent collapse of the lung is called a *pneumothorax* (*pneumo-* means air; *thorax* means chest). Air in the intrapleural space is also why the lungs collapse when a surgical incision is made into the chest wall.

Figure 22-6, *F,* shows the effect of a hole in the lung. Because the intrapulmonic pressure (P2) is higher than the intrapleural pressure (P3), air rushes into the intrapleural space through the hole in the lung, thereby eliminating the negative intrapleural pressure and collapsing the lung. Sometimes, people with emphysema develop blebs, or blisters, on the outer surface of their lungs. The blebs rupture and create a hole between the intrapulmonic and intrapleural spaces, causing air to rush into the intrapleural space and collapsing the lung.

What can be done for a collapsed lung? The physician inserts a tube through the chest wall into the intrapleural space and pulls air out of the intrapleural space. As the air leaves the intrapleural space, negative pressure is reestablished, and the lung expands. Sometimes, the physician inserts a large needle into the intrapleural space to aspirate, or withdraw, air, blood, and pus in a procedure called a *thoracentesis*. It facilitates lung expansion.

NOTE: The intrapleural pressure remains negative only when no hole exists in the chest wall or the lungs.

Do You Know...

Why This Person's Chest Looks Like a Barrel?

This person has emphysema, a condition characterized by damaged tissue in the lower respiratory structures and overinflated alveoli. As a result, the lungs cannot exhale the proper amount of air, and the air remains trapped in the alveoli. (*Emphysema* means "puffed up" alveoli.) Consequently, the alveoli and lungs become overinflated and cause the chest to be shaped like a barrel, so a person with severe emphysema is described as barrel-chested.

Normal adult

Barrel-chest

? Re-Think

Explain why the lungs remain expanded. Use the terms *atmospheric pressure*, *intrapleural pressure*, and *intrapulmonic pressure* in your explanation.

SAYING IT ANOTHER WAY: COMPLIANCE

Compliance is the measure of elastic recoil and can be illustrated by two balloons. One balloon has never been inflated and is stiff. A second balloon has been inflated many times and has lost some of its elasticity (elastic recoil); it appears baggy. Which balloon is easier to inflate? The baggy balloon is easier to inflate because it has lost some of its elasticity and is less stiff.

Translation: The baggy balloon is more compliant (stretchy). The new balloon is less compliant (stiff) and is therefore more difficult to inflate.

The same is true for the lungs. When lung compliance decreases (stiff lungs), the lungs are more difficult to inflate. Some conditions associated with decreased lung compliance are pulmonary edema, respiratory distress syndrome (deficiency of surfactants), and pulmonary fibrosis. Decreased lung compliance is not good!

What about increased lung compliance? Lungs that are too stretchy also cause problems. For example, the patient with emphysema has damaged lung structure and reduced elastic recoil. Lung compliance has increased too much; there is not enough elastic recoil to completely expel air on exhalation. The increased compliance also contributes to the formation of the barrel chest appearance that characterizes a person with chronic lung disease.

 Re-Think

Explain compliance using the example of two springs: a heavy duty spring used on garage doors and the tiny springs found in ball-point pens.

2+2 **Sum It Up!**

The expanded lungs normally fill the thoracic cavity. Unless pressure conditions in the pleural cavity are correct, the lungs collapse. The tendency of the lungs to collapse is due to the result of two factors: elastic recoil and alveolar surface tension. The expansion of the lungs is caused by a negative intrapleural pressure within the intrapleural space. If the negative intrapleural pressure is eliminated, the lungs collapse.

RESPIRATORY FUNCTION

THREE STEPS IN RESPIRATION

Most of us equate breathing with respiration. Respiration includes breathing, but it is more than breathing; it involves the entire process of gas exchange between the atmosphere and the body's cells. Respiration includes the following three steps:
- Ventilation, or breathing
- Exchange of oxygen and carbon dioxide
- Transport of oxygen and carbon dioxide by the blood

STEP 1: VENTILATION OR BREATHING
What It Is
Movement of air into and out of the lungs is called **ventilation**; it is more commonly called *breathing*. The two phases of ventilation are inhalation and exhalation. **Inhalation**, also called *inspiration*, is the breathing-in phase. During inhalation, oxygen-rich air moves into tiny air sacs in the lungs. **Exhalation**, also called *expiration*, is the breathing-out phase. During exhalation, air rich in carbon dioxide is moved out of the lungs. One inhalation and one exhalation make up one respiratory cycle.

Boyle's Law: Pressure and Volume
To understand ventilation, you need some background information. You need to know the relationship between pressure and volume, a relationship called *Boyle's law*. Note the two tubes in Figure 22-7. Tube A is a small tube that fits into a bicycle tire. When filled, the tube can hold 1 liter (L) of air. Tube B is larger and fits into a truck tire. When filled, it can hold 10 L of air.

Thus, the volume of the truck tube (B) is 10 times greater than the volume of the bicycle tube.

In the upper panel of Figure 22-7, both tubes are empty. Let's add 1 L of air to each tube and measure the pressure in each tube. By touching the surfaces of the tubes, you can get a rough estimate of the pressures. Tube A feels firm, whereas tube B feels soft. In other words, the pressure in tube A is higher than the pressure in tube B. Both tubes received the same amount of air, so why are the pressures different? The different volumes of the tubes cause the different pressures. The pressure is higher in tube A because the volume of tube A is small; 1 L of air completely fills the tube. The pressure in tube B is lower because its volume is large (10 L). One L of air only partially fills the truck tube. The smaller the volume, the higher the pressure; the greater the volume, the lower the pressure. If volume changes, the pressure changes. This is Boyle's law, the principle on which ventilation is based.

 Do You Know...

About the Pink Puffers and Blue Bloaters?

Both Pink Puffers and Blue Bloaters suffer from breathing difficulties, such as asthma, emphysema, or chronic obstructive pulmonary disease (COPD). Pink Puffers gasp for breath and, in doing so, turn red in the face. Blue Bloaters, having suffered from poor pulmonary function for a longer time, are accustomed to struggling for air and so don't gasp and struggle like the Pink Puffers. The Blue Bloaters, with weakened respiratory muscles, don't have the energy to puff away and turn red; rather, they tend to inhale a large volume of air, hold it, and become bloated. This type of respiratory activity causes their oxygen levels to decline, thereby causing hypoxemia and cyanosis (blueness). Complicating the hypoxemia is an accumulation of carbon dioxide in the blood, which in turn causes respiratory acidosis. Of the two, Blue Bloaters are generally the most seriously ill and in need of treatment. Furthermore, their already depleted oxygen levels decline quickly if they develop an acute complication such as pneumonia.

Boyle's Law and Breathing
What does Boyle's law have to do with ventilation? On inhalation (breathing in), air flows into the lungs. What is the force that causes the air to flow in? Place your hands on your rib cage. Inhale. Notice that the thoracic cage moves up and out on inhalation (Figure 22-8, *A* and *C*). This movement increases the volume of the thoracic cavity and lungs. As the volume in the lung increases, the pressure in the lung (P2) decreases (satisfying Boyle's law). As a result, P2 becomes less than P1 (atmospheric pressure, the air you breathe). Air flows from higher pressure to lower pressure, through the nose into the lungs.

What happens on exhalation? Another change in lung volume. Place your hands on your rib cage and exhale. The thoracic and lung volumes decrease as the rib cage returns to its resting position (see Figure 22-8,

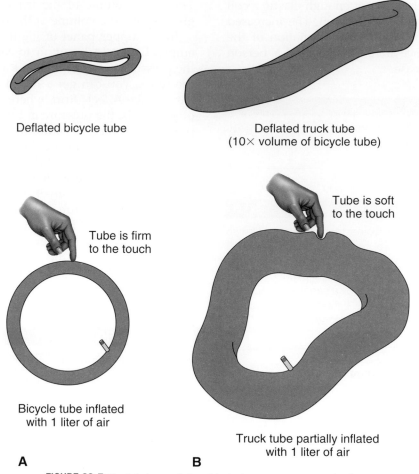

Deflated bicycle tube

Deflated truck tube
(10× volume of bicycle tube)

Tube is firm
to the touch

Tube is soft
to the touch

Bicycle tube inflated
with 1 liter of air

Truck tube partially inflated
with 1 liter of air

A   **B**

FIGURE 22-7 Boyle's law: relationship between pressure and volume.

B and *D*). The decreased lung volume causes the pressure within the lungs (P2) to increase. Now P2 is higher than P1, and air flows out of the lungs through the nose. Let us clarify the relationship between Boyle's law and ventilation:

- Air flows in response to changes in pressure. As the lung volume increases on inhalation, the intrapulmonic pressure (P2) decreases, and air flows into the lungs.
- On exhalation, lung volume decreases, intrapulmonic pressure (P2) increases, and air flows out of the lungs.
- Air flows in response to pressure changes. Pressure changes occur in response to changes in volume. Inhalation is associated with an increase in thoracic volume; exhalation is associated with a decrease in thoracic volume.

? Re-Think

Explain ventilation in terms of Boyle's law.

The Muscles of Respiration

What causes the thoracic volume to change? The change in thoracic volume is caused by the contraction and relaxation of the respiratory muscles. On inhalation, the respiratory muscles, diaphragm, and intercostal muscles contract (see Figure 22-8, *A* and *C*). The diaphragm is a dome-shaped muscle that forms the floor of the thoracic cavity and separates the thoracic cavity from the abdominal cavity. The diaphragm is the chief muscle of inhalation. Contraction of the diaphragm flattens the muscle and pulls it downward, toward the abdomen. This movement increases the length of the thoracic cavity. During quiet breathing, the diaphragm accounts for most of the increase in the thoracic volume.

The two intercostal muscles, the external and internal intercostals, are located between the ribs. When the external intercostal muscles contract, the rib cage moves up and out, thereby increasing the width of the thoracic cavity. Note that the size of the thoracic cavity increases in three directions: from front to back, from side to side, and lengthwise. Why is this increase in thoracic volume so important? As the thoracic volume increases, so does the volume of the lungs. According to Boyle's law, the increase in volume decreases the pressure in the lungs and, as a result, air flows into the lungs. Some of the accessory muscles of respiration, located in

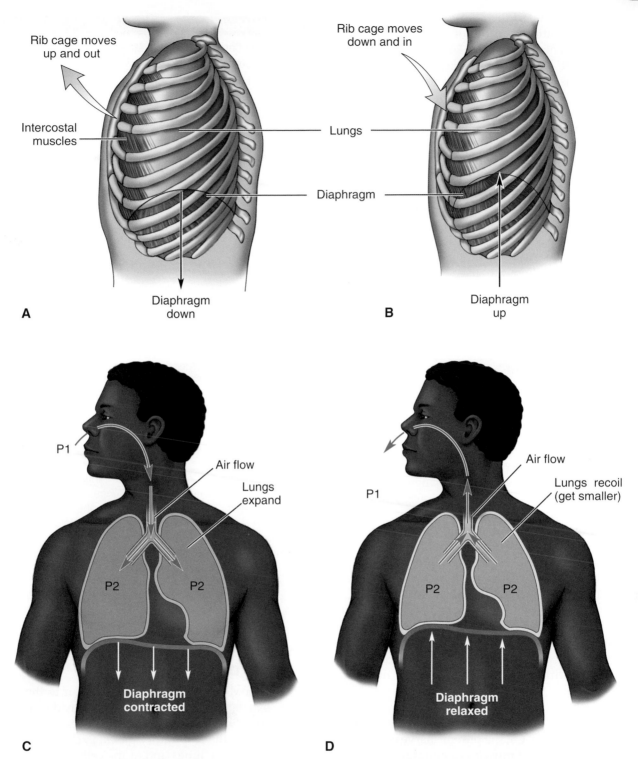

FIGURE 22-8 Inhalation and exhalation. The thoracic volume increases, and air rushes into the lungs **(A and C).** The thoracic volume decreases, and air rushes out of the lungs **(B and D).**

the neck and chest, can move the rib cage even farther during exertion.

On exhalation, the muscles of respiration relax and allow the ribs and diaphragm to return to their original positions (see Figure 22-8, *B* and *D*). This movement decreases thoracic and lung volume and increases pressure in the lungs. Consequently, air flows out of

the lungs. Elastic recoil of lung tissue and surface tension within the alveoli aid with exhalation. Forced exhalation uses the accessory muscles of respiration. These include the muscles of the abdominal wall and the internal intercostal muscles. Contraction of the accessory muscles of respiration pulls the bottom of the rib cage down and in, and it forces the abdominal viscera upward toward the relaxed diaphragm. These actions force additional air out of the lungs.

How much energy does it take to breathe? Inhalation is a result of the contraction of the respiratory muscles, so it is an active process. The muscles use up energy (ATP) as they contract. Exhalation associated with normal quiet breathing is passive. Exhalation is caused by muscle relaxation; no energy is required for muscle relaxation. Thus, in normal quiet breathing, we use up energy during half of the respiratory cycle (inhalation). We rest on exhalation. During forced exhalation (as in exercise), however, the accessory muscles of respiration must contract, and exhalation becomes energy using, or active.

With certain lung diseases such as emphysema, exhalation can be achieved only when the accessory muscles of respiration are used. The patient with emphysema therefore uses energy during both inhalation and exhalation. This process is physically exhausting, and these patients usually complain of being very tired.

 Re-Think

1. What muscles are used for inhalation?
2. Explain why different muscles are used in exhalation and forced exhalation. Why might a person force exhale?

Nerves That Supply the Respiratory Muscles

Ventilation occurs in response to changes in the thoracic volume, and the changes in thoracic volume are caused by muscle contraction and relaxation. The respiratory muscles, being skeletal muscles, must be stimulated by motor nerves to contract. The motor nerves supplying the respiratory muscles are the phrenic nerve and intercostal nerves. The phrenic nerve exits from the spinal cord at the level of C4, travels within the cervical plexus, and is distributed to the diaphragm. Firing of the phrenic nerve stimulates the diaphragm to contract. The intercostal nerves supply the intercostal muscles. Thus, inhalation is initiated by the firing of the phrenic and intercostal nerves.

You will be caring for patients whose nerve and muscle function is impaired. For example, if the spinal cord is severed above C4, the phrenic nerve cannot fire. As a result, the skeletal muscles (diaphragm and intercostals) cannot contract. The person not only is quadriplegic, but also can breathe only with the assistance of a ventilator. Other patients experience difficulty in breathing because of the effects of certain drugs. Curare, for example, is a drug commonly used during surgery to cause muscle relaxation. It is a neuromuscular blocking agent that interferes with the transmission of the electrical signal from nerve to muscle. The block occurs within the neuromuscular junction. The patient is not only unable to move the body voluntarily, but also is unable to breathe.

 Do You Know...

That a Boa Constrictor Knows More about Boyle's Law Than the Early Corset Makers?

The boa knows that by wrapping itself around an animal's chest, it can suffocate the victim by preventing chest expansion and inhalation (Boyle's law). Early corset makers, however, ignored this basic information. Corsets were designed to constrict the waist—the tighter the corset, the smaller the waist. A successfully corseted young lady might boast of a 12-inch–diameter waist! Problem was, the upper part of the corset included the lower part of the rib cage. What was the result of this constant binding? The corset prevented adequate ventilation and caused a permanent deformity of the rib cage, to say nothing of the displaced abdominal organs. The corseted young lovely couldn't breathe and often fainted. Herein lies the physiological basis of the swoon and delicate weakness that characterized wealthy young women. They were not weak because of their female X chromosomes; they were merely hypoxemic—no oxygen going to the brain. Fortunately, only the wealthiest could make a fashion statement by fainting.

 Re-Think

What is the respiratory consequence of an injured or severed phrenic nerve?

 Sum It Up!

The three steps in respiration are ventilation, exchange of oxygen and carbon dioxide in the lungs and cells, and transport of oxygen and carbon dioxide by the blood. Ventilation occurs in response to changes in thoracic volumes, which in turn cause changes in intrapulmonic pressures. Inhalation occurs when the respiratory muscles contract and enlarge the thoracic cage. Exhalation occurs when the respiratory muscles relax, allowing the thorax to return to its smaller, resting thoracic volume. The muscles of respiration contract in response to stimulation of the phrenic and intercostal nerves.

STEP 2: EXCHANGE OF OXYGEN AND CARBON DIOXIDE

Inhalation delivers fresh oxygen-rich air to the alveoli and exhalation removes carbon dioxide–laden air from the alveoli. The second step of respiration is the exchange of the respiratory gases. Exchange occurs at two sites: in the lungs and at the cells (Figure 22-9).

Why the Lungs Are Good Gas Exchangers

Gas exchange occurs in the lungs, specifically across the membranes of the alveoli and pulmonary capillaries. Three conditions make the alveoli well suited for the exchange of oxygen and carbon dioxide: a large surface area, thin alveolar and pulmonary capillary walls, and a short distance between the alveoli and pulmonary capillaries.

- *Large surface area.* Millions of alveoli, approximately 350 million per lung, create a total surface area

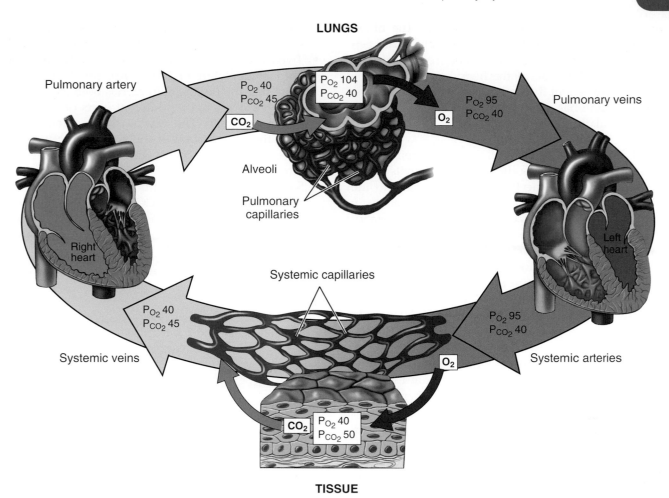

LUNGS

Pulmonary artery

P_{O_2} 40
P_{CO_2} 45

P_{O_2} 104
P_{CO_2} 40

CO_2

P_{O_2} 95
P_{CO_2} 40

O_2

Pulmonary veins

Alveoli

Pulmonary
capillaries

Right
heart

Left
heart

Systemic capillaries

P_{O_2} 40
P_{CO_2} 45

P_{O_2} 95
P_{CO_2} 40

O_2

Systemic veins

Systemic arteries

CO_2

P_{O_2} 40
P_{CO_2} 50

TISSUE

FIGURE 22-9 Partial pressures of oxygen (pO_2) and carbon dioxide (pCO_2) within the lungs and at the cellular level (in mm Hg).

about half the size of a tennis court. The large surface increases the amount of oxygen and carbon dioxide exchanged across the alveolar membranes.

• *Thin alveolar and pulmonary capillary walls.* The thin walls favor diffusion because they do not offer much resistance to the movement of oxygen and carbon dioxide across the membranes.

• *Closeness of the alveoli to the pulmonary capillaries.* Each alveolus is very close to a pulmonary capillary. For diffusion, closeness ensures a high rate of diffusion.

Partial Pressures and the Diffusion of Gases
What Causes the Respiratory Gases to Diffuse? Chapter 3 describes how molecules diffuse from an area of higher concentration to an area of lower concentration. For gases such as oxygen and carbon dioxide, however, concentration is related to pressure. When the molecules of a gas are highly concentrated, the gas creates a high pressure. Consequently, we can talk about diffusion from areas of higher pressure to areas of lower pressure.

Ordinary room air is a gas composed of 78% nitrogen, 21% oxygen, and 0.04% carbon dioxide. Each part of the gas contributes to the total pressure. The amount

of pressure each gas contributes is called the **partial pressure**. The symbol for the partial pressure of oxygen is pO_2; the symbol for the partial pressure of carbon dioxide is pCO_2. (Because the body does not use nitrogen gas, we can ignore it.)

Partial Pressures within the Lungs. Let us analyze the partial pressures of the respiratory gases in the alveoli and pulmonary capillaries (see Figure 22-9). The pO_2 of air in the alveoli is 104 mm Hg, whereas the pO_2 of venous blood (the blue end of the pulmonary capillary) is 40 mm Hg. Oxygen diffuses from the area of higher pressure (the alveolus) to the area of lower pressure (the pulmonary capillary). Note that the pO_2 in the blood goes from 40 mm Hg (blue) to 95 mm Hg (red). The partial pressure of oxygen increases because the blood has been oxygenated.

As for the waste, the carbon dioxide, the pCO_2 in the blood (blue capillary) is 45 mm Hg, whereas the pCO_2 in the alveolus is only 40 mm Hg. Carbon dioxide diffuses from the capillary, the area of higher pressure, to the alveolus, the area of lower pressure. Because of the diffusion of carbon dioxide out of the blood, the pCO_2 of the blood goes from 45 mm Hg at the blue end of the capillary to 40 mm Hg at the red end of the capillary. What has been accomplished? The blood coming from the right side of the heart (blue) has been oxygenated and the oxygenated blood (red) eventually returns to the left side of the heart so that it can be pumped throughout the body. As oxygenation occurs, carbon dioxide has been removed; it leaves the lungs during exhalation.

Partial Pressure at the Cells. What happens to the gases at the tissues, or body cells? Two events occur. First, oxygen leaves the blood and diffuses into the cells, where it can be used during cell metabolism. Second, carbon dioxide, a consequence of cell metabolism, diffuses into the blood.

What partial pressures cause these events to happen? The pO_2 of the arterial blood is 95 mm Hg, whereas the cellular pO_2 is only 40 mm Hg. During gas exchange, oxygen diffuses from the blood into the space surrounding the cells. The pCO_2 of the cells is 50 mm Hg and the arterial pCO_2 is only 40 mm Hg. Carbon dioxide therefore diffuses from the cells into the blood. The blood then carries the carbon dioxide to the lungs for excretion. Thus, oxygenated blood from the lungs carries the oxygen to the cells; the oxygen then diffuses from the blood into the cells. The carbon dioxide, or the waste produced by the metabolizing cells, diffuses into the blood, which carries it to the lungs for excretion. Note the venous blood leaving the cells. The pO_2 is 40 mm Hg because the oxygen has been used up by the cells. The pCO_2 is 45 mm Hg because the waste was removed from the cells.

STEP 3: TRANSPORT OF OXYGEN AND CARBON DIOXIDE

The third step in respiration is the blood's mechanism for transporting oxygen and carbon dioxide between the lungs and body cells. Although the blood transports both oxygen and carbon dioxide, the way in which blood transports each gas differs.

Oxygen Transport

Almost all the oxygen (98%) is transported by the hemoglobin in the red blood cells. The remaining 2% of the oxygen is dissolved in the plasma. As soon as oxygen enters the blood in the pulmonary capillaries, it immediately forms a loose bond with the iron portion of the hemoglobin molecule. This new molecule is oxyhemoglobin. As the oxygenated blood travels to the cells throughout the body, the oxygen unloads from the hemoglobin molecule and diffuses across the capillary walls to the cells. The oxygen is eventually used up by the metabolizing cells.

Carbon Dioxide Transport

Blood carries carbon dioxide from the metabolizing cells to the lungs, where it is exhaled. Blood carries carbon dioxide in the following three forms:

- Ten percent of the carbon dioxide is dissolved in plasma.
- Twenty percent of the carbon dioxide combines with hemoglobin to form carbaminohemoglobin. Note that the hemoglobin carries both oxygen and carbon dioxide but by different parts of the hemoglobin molecule. The oxygen forms a loose bond with the iron portion of the hemoglobin, whereas the carbon dioxide bonds with the globin, or protein (amino acids) portion, of the hemoglobin.
- Seventy percent of the carbon dioxide is converted to the bicarbonate ion (HCO_3^-). Note that the blood carries most of the carbon dioxide in the form of bicarbonate.

? Re-Think

1. What is the pO_2 in the alveoli, pulmonary veins, tissue, and vena cava?
2. What is the driving force for oxygen to move from the alveoli into the blood? From the blood into the tissues?
3. How does the blood transport oxygen? Carbon dioxide?

2+2 Sum It Up!

The exchange of the respiratory gases occurs at two sites: the lungs and the cells. Oxygen diffuses from the alveoli into the pulmonary capillaries. Carbon dioxide diffuses from the pulmonary capillaries into the alveoli. At the cellular sites, oxygen diffuses from the capillaries into the cells; carbon dioxide diffuses from the cells into the capillaries. Blood transports oxygen and carbon dioxide. Hemoglobin carries most of the oxygen as oxyhemoglobin. The blood carries most of the carbon dioxide in the form of a bicarbonate ion (HCO_3^-).

AMOUNTS OF AIR

LUNG VOLUMES

Think about all the ways that you can vary the amount of air you breathe. For example, you can inhale a small amount of air or you can take a deep breath. How are you breathing now? Probably slowly and effortlessly. With strenuous exercise, you would breathe more rapidly and deeply. If you become anxious, your breathing pattern becomes more rapid and shallow. With certain diseases, your respirations might increase or decrease. In other words, the amount, or volume, of air you breathe can vary significantly.

The different volumes of air you breathe have names. The four pulmonary volumes are *tidal volume, inspiratory reserve volume, expiratory reserve volume,* and *residual volume.* A spirometer (spih-ROM-eh-ter) is a device that measures pulmonary volumes. The patient blows into the spirometer, which measures the amount of air and prints the results on graph paper. A recording of the volumes appears in Figure 22-10 and is summarized in Table 22-1:

- *Tidal volume.* Breathe in and out. The amount of air moved into or out of the lungs with each breath is called the **tidal volume**. The average tidal volume

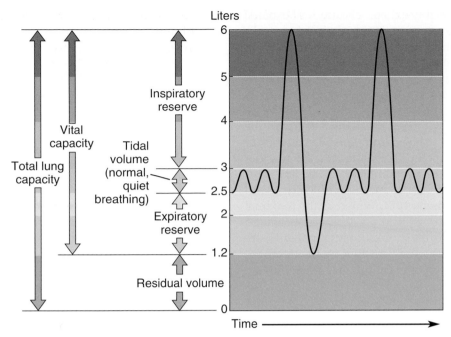

FIGURE 22-10   Pulmonary volumes and capacities.

during normal quiet breathing is about 500 mL. Tidal volume increases with exercise.

- *Inspiratory reserve volume.* Inhale a normal volume of air. Now, in addition to this normal amount of air, inhale as much as you possibly can. The additional volume of air is called the *inspiratory reserve volume*. This extra volume is approximately 3000 mL.
- *Expiratory reserve volume.* Exhale a normal amount of air. Now, in addition to this normal amount of air, exhale as much as you possibly can. The extra volume of exhaled air is called the *expiratory reserve volume*. It is about 1100 mL.
- *Residual volume.* Even after a forced exhalation, about 1200 mL of air remains in the lungs. This remaining air is the *residual volume*. Residual air remains in the lungs at all times, even between

breaths. Note in Figure 22-10 that the four pulmonary volumes add up to the total lung capacity.

LUNG CAPACITIES

In addition to four pulmonary volumes, there are four pulmonary capacities (two described here). A pulmonary capacity is a combination of pulmonary volumes. For example, **vital capacity** (4600 mL) refers to the combination of tidal volume (500 mL), inspiratory reserve volume (3000 mL), and expiratory reserve volume (1100 mL). The measurement of vital capacity is a commonly used pulmonary function test.

You can measure vital capacity as follows. Take the deepest breath possible. Exhale all the air you possibly can into a spirometer. The spirometer measures the

Table **22-1**	Lung Volumes and Capacities	
NAME	**DESCRIPTION**	**AMOUNT (mL)**
Volumes		
Tidal volume	The volume of air moved into or out of the lungs during one respiratory cycle	500
Residual volume	The volume of air that remains in the lungs after a forceful exhalation	1200
Inspiratory reserve volume	The volume of air that can be forcefully inhaled after normal inhalation	3000
Expiratory reserve volume	The volume of air that can be forcefully exhaled after normal exhalation	1100
Capacities		
Vital capacity	The maximum volume of air that can be exhaled following maximal inhalation	4600
Functional residual capacity	The volume of air remaining in the lungs following exhalation during quiet breathing	2300
Total lung capacity	The volume of air in the lungs following a maximal inhalation	5800

amount of air you forcibly exhale. The amount exhaled should be approximately 4600 mL. In other words, vital capacity is the maximal amount of air exhaled after a maximal inhalation. Vital capacity measures pulmonary function in patients with lung diseases such as emphysema and asthma. A more commonly used clinical term for forced vital capacity is the *forced expiratory volume* (FEV). The FEV is the fraction of the forced vital capacity exhaled in a specific number of seconds. The subscript in FEV_1 indicates the number of seconds that the measurement lasted. The term *peak expiratory flow rate* (PEFR) is another clinically useful respiratory measurement. It is defined as the maximal rate of air flow during expiration. PEFR is measured by a handheld flow meter. Asthmatic patients are taught to measure FEV_1 and/or PEFR in an attempt to manage their asthma. (Other pulmonary capacities are listed in Table 22-1.)

DEAD SPACE

Some of the air you inhale never reaches the alveoli. It stays in the conducting passageways of the trachea, bronchi, and bronchioles. Because this air does not reach the alveoli, it is not available for gas exchange and is said to occupy anatomical dead space. The dead space holds about 150 mL of air. Breathing slowly and deeply increases the amount of well-oxygenated air that reaches the alveoli. Conversely, rapid panting delivers a poorer quality of air to the alveoli because a greater percentage of the inhaled volume of air remains in the anatomical dead space. Therefore, when you encourage your patients to take deep breaths, you are also helping supply the alveoli with well-oxygenated air.

? Re-Think

1. Differentiate between tidal volume and vital capacity.
2. Explain to your patient in two to three sentences what to do in order to measure vital capacity.

CONTROL OF BREATHING

Normal breathing is rhythmic and involuntary. For example, as you read, you are breathing effortlessly, about 16 times/min. (The normal respiratory rate ranges from 12 to 20 breaths/min in an adult and from 20 to 40 breaths/min in a child, depending on the age and size of the child.) You do not have to remember to breathe in and out, nor do you have to calculate how deeply to breathe. Fortunately, breathing occurs automatically.

You can voluntarily control breathing up to a point. Hold your breath for 5 seconds. Now try to hold your breath for 3 minutes. You can't do it; you must breathe. The need to breathe means that Sammy should not hold you hostage with his temper tantrums. No matter how good his performance and how long he holds

his breath, he will eventually take a really deep breath and live.

NEURAL CONTROL OF RESPIRATION

How does the body control breathing? The two means of controlling breathing are nervous and chemical mechanisms. The nervous mechanism involves several areas of the brain, the most important being the brain stem. Special groups of neurons are widely scattered throughout the brain stem, particularly in the medulla oblongata and the pons (Figure 22-11). The main control center for breathing, in the medulla oblongata, is called the *medullary respiratory control center*. It sets the basic breathing rhythm.

Inhalation occurs when the inspiratory neurons in the medulla oblongata fire, giving rise to nerve impulses. The nerve impulses travel from the medulla oblongata along the phrenic and intercostal nerves to the muscles of respiration. Contraction of the respiratory muscles causes inhalation. Exhalation occurs when the expiratory neurons in the medulla oblongata fire and shut down the inspiratory neurons. This process inhibits the formation of nerve impulses and causes the respiratory muscles to relax. Thus, breathing is the result of the alternate firing of the inspiratory and expiratory neurons.

Although the medulla oblongata is the main control center for breathing, the pons also plays an important role. The pons contains the pneumotaxic center and the apneustic center. These areas in the pons modify and help control breathing patterns.

The medullary respiratory center is very sensitive to the effects of narcotics. Narcotics (opioids), such as morphine, depress the medulla oblongata and slow respirations. If the narcotic overdose is large enough, respirations may even cease, causing respiratory arrest and death. Because of the profound effect of narcotics on respirations, you must check a patient's respiratory rate before administering narcotics.

? Re-Think

1. What part of the brain stem exerts the greatest control of respiration?
2. Why will a downward herniation of the brain stem through the foramen magnum cause respiratory arrest?

Although the brain stem normally determines the basic rate and depth of breathing, other areas of the brain, including the hypothalamus and cerebral cortex, can also affect breathing patterns. For example, the hypothalamus processes our emotional responses, such as anxiety and fear. The hypothalamus, in turn,

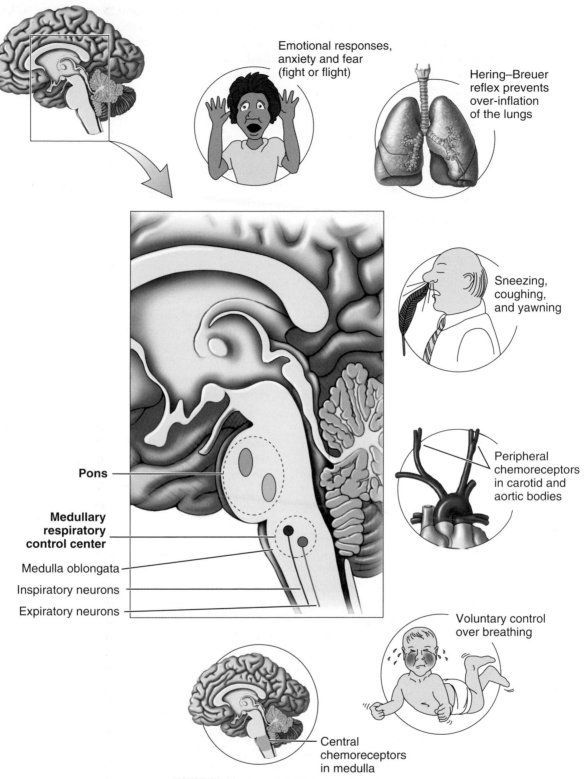

Emotional responses, anxiety and fear (fight or flight)

Hering–Breuer reflex prevents over-inflation of the lungs

Sneezing, coughing, and yawning

Peripheral chemoreceptors in carotid and aortic bodies

Pons

Medullary respiratory control center

Medulla oblongata

Inspiratory neurons

Expiratory neurons

Voluntary control over breathing

Central chemoreceptors in medulla

FIGURE 22-11 Factors that influence breathing.

stimulates the brain stem and changes the breathing pattern. Rapid breathing, a response to anxiety or fear, is part of the fight-or-flight response. The cerebral cortex can also affect respiration; cortical activity allows us to control the depth and rate of breathing voluntarily.

Several other nervous pathways affect the respiratory system. For example, the vagus nerve carries nerve impulses from the lungs to the brain stem. When the lungs become inflated, nerve impulses travel to the brain stem, inhibiting the inspiratory neurons. This response is called the *Hering-Breuer reflex*. It prevents overinflation of the lungs. The nervous structures not only control breathing patterns, but also affect several reflexes associated with the respiratory system. These include coughing, sneezing, and yawning.

CHEMICAL CONTROL OF RESPIRATION

Chemicals dissolved in the blood also affect breathing (see Figure 22-11), including carbon dioxide, hydrogen ion (which determines the pH), and oxygen. These chemicals are detected by chemosensitive cells called *chemoreceptors*. When activated, the chemoreceptors stimulate the areas of the brain stem concerned with respiration. The two types of chemoreceptors are central chemoreceptors, located in the central nervous system (CNS), and peripheral chemoreceptors, located outside the CNS.

The central chemoreceptors in the medulla oblongata detect changes in the blood concentrations of carbon dioxide and hydrogen ions. If carbon dioxide or hydrogen ion concentration increases, the central chemoreceptors signal the respiratory center to increase its activity. This response causes an increase in the rate and depth of breathing. As a result of the increase in breathing, carbon dioxide is exhaled and the blood levels of carbon dioxide decrease. Conversely, if the blood levels of carbon dioxide and hydrogen ions decrease, breathing decreases, thereby allowing concentrations of both carbon dioxide and hydrogen ions to increase. Breathing is controlled primarily by blood concentrations of carbon dioxide and hydrogen ions, which trigger the central chemoreceptors.

The peripheral chemoreceptors are in the walls of the carotid arteries and the walls of the aorta in the neck and chest region. They are called the *carotid* and *aortic bodies*. (Do not confuse the chemoreceptors with the baroreceptors, which are located in the same general area.) The peripheral chemoreceptors are sensitive primarily to low concentrations of oxygen and increased hydrogen ion concentration. Blood concentrations of oxygen, however, must be very low to trigger the peripheral chemoreceptors. Thus, oxygen plays only a minor role in the regulation of breathing. *Remember: pCO_2 is the major regulator of respirations.*

Respiratory patterns change, most often in response to changing body needs and sometimes in response to underlying pathology. Table 22-2 includes respiratory terms commonly used to describe altered respiratory activity.

Table 22-2	Common Respiratory Terms
TERM	**DESCRIPTION**
Apnea	Temporary cessation of breathing
Cheyne-Stokes respirations	An irregular breathing pattern characterized by a series of shallow breaths that gradually increase in depth and rate; the series of increased respirations is followed by breaths that gradually decrease in depth and rate. A period of apnea lasting 10 to 60 seconds follows; the cycle then repeats.
Cyanosis	A bluish color of the skin or mucous membrane caused by a low concentration of oxygen in the blood
Dyspnea	Difficult or labored breathing
Eupnea	Normal, quiet breathing
Hypoxia	An abnormally low concentration of oxygen in the tissues
Hypoxemia	An abnormally low concentration of oxygen in the blood
Hypercapnia	An abnormally high concentration of carbon dioxide in the blood
Hypocapnia	An abnormally low concentration of carbon dioxide in the blood
Hyperventilation	An increase in the rate and depth of respiration. Hyperventilation causes an excess exhalation of carbon dioxide and alkalosis.
Hypoventilation	A decrease in the rate and depth of respiration. Hypoventilation causes a retention of carbon dioxide and acidosis.
Kussmaul breathing	An increase in rate and depth of respiration stimulated by metabolic acidosis
Orthopnea	Difficulty in breathing that is relieved by a sitting-up position
Rales	Crackles (as in snap, *crackle*, and pop) are small clicking sounds in the lungs that resemble rubbing hair together next to the ear. They are typically inspiratory and are believed to occur when air opens closed air spaces. Rales or crackles can be further described as moist, dry, fine, and coarse.

Table 22-2	Common Respiratory Terms—cont'd
TERM	**DESCRIPTION**
Rhonchi	Snoring-like sounds that generally occur with obstruction of air in the large airways (trachea and bronchi)
Stridor	High-pitched, wheezelike sound that can be heard on both inhalation and/or exhalation. It is caused by an obstruction of air flow in the upper airway, such as the trachea, or in the back of the throat.
Tachypnea	Rapid breathing
Wheezes	High-pitched sounds typically on exhalation. Wheezing and other abnormal sounds can sometimes be heard without a stethoscope. Wheezing occurs when air is forced through narrow airways. Although commonly associated with asthma, wheezing may also be caused by other obstructing conditions (e.g., tumors, swelling, foreign bodies).

? Re-Think

Explain how pCO_2 affects respiratory rate.

2+2 Sum It Up!

Normal breathing is rhythmic and involuntary. Nervous and chemical mechanisms control breathing. The nervous mechanism involves several areas of the brain, the most important of which is the brain stem. The inspiratory and expiratory neurons in the medulla oblongata determine the basic breathing pattern, which can be modified by the apneustic center and pneumotaxic center in the pons. Chemicals in the blood help control respirations. The central chemoreceptors in the brain are sensitive to carbon dioxide and hydrogen ions, and the peripheral chemoreceptors are sensitive to low blood levels of oxygen and an increase in the hydrogen ion concentration. pCO_2 is the major regulator of respirations.

❧ As You Age

1. As a person ages, lung capacity decreases. The decrease in lung capacity is caused by the loss of elasticity of the lung tissue and diminished efficiency of the respiratory muscles. By the age of 70 years, vital capacity has decreased 33%.
2. With aging, many of the protective mechanisms of the respiratory system decline. The ciliary activity of the mucosa decreases, for example, and the phagocytes in the lungs become less effective. As a result, older adults are at greater risk for respiratory infections, especially pneumonia and bronchitis.
3. With age-related structural changes, the number of alveoli diminishes. The resulting decrease in oxygenation ultimately diminishes the capacity for physical activity.
4. Respiratory control is altered; consequently, the pO_2 drops to a lower level whereas the pCO_2 increases to a higher level.
5. Having breathed a lifetime's worth of various harmful substances (e.g., cigarette smoke, pollutants, pollens, pathogens), the lungs of an older person often show evidence of wear and tear, leading to emphysema and other respiratory disorders.

🖳 MEDICAL TERMINOLOGY AND DISORDERS   Disorders of the Respiratory System

Medical Term	Word Parts	Word Part Meaning or Derivation	Description
Words			
epistaxis		From a Greek word meaning "to drip"	**Epistaxis** is *a nosebleed.*
eupnea (and other "-pnea" words)	eu-	normal	**Eupnea** means *normal breathing.* To contrast, **bradypnea** (brady- = slow) is slow breathing, whereas **tachypnea** (tachy- = rapid) means rapid breathing. **Apnea** (a- = without) refers to the temporary cessation of breathing, **dyspnea** (dys- = difficult) is difficulty in breathing, and **orthopnea** (ortho- = straight) is the inability to breathe unless in an upright position.
	-pnea	breathing	
inspiration	in-	in	**Inspiration** refers to *breathing in or inhalation;* **expiration** (ex- = out) refers to *breathing out or exhalation.*
	-spir/o	breathing	
oximeter	-ox/i-	oxygen	A pulse **oximeter** is *a mechanical device used to measure oxygen levels in the blood.*
	-meter	measure	

Continued

MEDICAL TERMINOLOGY AND DISORDERS   Disorders of the Respiratory System—cont'd

Medical Term	Word Parts	Word Part Meaning or Derivation	Description
thoracentesis	thorac/o-	chest	A **thoracentesis** is *the incision through the chest wall in order to aspirate fluid or air for therapeutic or diagnostic purposes.*
	-centesis	surgical puncture	
Disorders			
influenza		From an Italian word meaning "influence of the cold"	*A respiratory infection (also known as* **the flu***) that can be caused by several influenza viruses.*
pharyngitis	pharyng/o-	pharynx or throat	*Also called a sore throat; refers to an inflammation of the pharynx or throat.* Approximately 70% of the cases are virally induced. Infection by beta-hemolytic streptococcus is called *strep throat.*
	-itis	inflammation of	
rhinitis	rhin/o-	nose	Refers to the inflammation of the nasal mucosa. **Allergic rhinitis** refers to the response of the nasal mucosa to an allergen. **Seasonal allergic rhinitis** is triggered by high pollen counts. **Perennial allergic rhinitis** is present constantly throughout the year and is triggered by pet dander, cockroaches, and dust mites. **Acute viral rhinitis** is the **common cold** or **acute coryza.**
	-itis	inflammation of	
sinusitis (acute)	sinus/o-	sinus	*Refers to inflammation of the sinuses and is most often due to a swelling and narrowing of passages that drain the sinuses.*
	-itis	inflammation of	
Lower Respiratory Disorders			
asthma		From a Greek word meaning "to breathe hard" or "to pant"	*A chronic immune-mediated airway inflammation, characterized by breathlessness, tightness of the chest, dyspnea, wheezing, and coughing.* The inflammatory process produces **bronchial hyperreactivity,** so that milder stimuli, such as exercise, act as triggers.
bronchiectasis	bronch/o-	bronchus	*Refers to the permanent and abnormal dilation of the bronchi.* The characteristic sign of bronchiectasis is a persistent or recurrent cough and the production of purulent sputum.
	-ectasis	stretching or dilation	
bronchocarcinoma	bronch/o-	bronchus	A common cause of cancer-related deaths in the United States. It is especially common in persons >50 years with a long history of cigarette smoking. More than 90% of lung cancers are bronchogenic and arise from the bronchial epithelium.
	-carcin/o-	cancer	
	-oma	tumor	
tuberculosis	tubercul/o-	tubercle	Commonly called TB. It is known historically as "consumption" and was responsible for the "white plague." Globally TB is responsible for more deaths than any other infectious disease. TB is caused by *Mycobacterium tuberculosis,* or the "acid-fast" bacillus, and is generally spread by droplet infection through inhalation of the pathogen. It usually affects the upper lobes of the lungs, but can infect many other organs and spread or seed throughout the body (miliary TB). Following inhalation, the mycobacteria continue to multiply without any resistance from the host. In about 10 to 20 days a cellular immune response limits the growth and spread of the infection by the formation of a granuloma. The inner core of the granuloma is called the *Ghon tubercle;* it undergoes caseous necrosis, thereby forming a cheesy mass of dead cells and debris. The lesion may also liquefy and drain into surrounding bronchi, causing cavitation. The primary lesion often becomes fibrotic and calcifies. The infection enters a latent period during which mycobacteria become dormant. The activation of the dormant mycobacteria can occur at any time, particularly in an immunosuppressed person and in patients taking steroids.
	-osis	condition of	

MEDICAL TERMINOLOGY AND DISORDERS   Disorders of the Respiratory System—cont'd

Medical Term	Word Parts	Word Part Meaning or Derivation	Description
Restrictive Lung Disorders			
Disorders characterized by decreased "stretchiness" of the lungs and/or chest wall. They are classified as extrapulmonary and intrapulmonary disorders. Extrapulmonary causes of restrictive disorders include disorders of the CNS, the neuromuscular junction, and the chest wall. The intrapulmonary disorders are described as follows.			
pleuritis	pleur/o-	pleura	*Also called* **pleurisy** *and refers to an inflammation of the pleura.* Pleurisy is classified as **dry pleurisy** (fibrinous) and **wet pleurisy** (serofibrinous, with an increased secretion of pleural fluid).
	-itis	inflammation	
pleural effusion	pleur/o-	pleura	*Refers to the accumulation of excess fluid between the two pleural membranes.* (An effusion is an escape of a fluid into a body cavity.) The two types of pleural effusion are the transudative and the exudative.
	-al	pertaining to	
	effusion	From a Latin word meaning "to pour out"	
pneumothorax	pneum/o-	air or lung	*Refers to the accumulation of air within the pleural space, causing the lung to collapse.* A pneumothorax can be opened or closed. An open pneumothorax occurs when the chest wall is penetrated, as in stabbing or gunshot wounds. A **closed pneumothorax** is not caused by an external wound; its cause originates within, as in a ruptured bleb (air bubble or blister) in a person with emphysema, ventilator-induced lung injury, and lung injury from broken ribs. A **tension pneumothorax** is due to a rapid accumulation of air in the pleural space. In addition to air, the lung may also collapse in response to the accumulation of blood in the pleural space (**hemothorax;** hem/o- = blood) or lymph (**chylothorax;** chyl/o- = lymph).
	-thorac/o-	chest	
interstitial lung diseases (ILDs)			*A general term that includes many disorders characterized by inflammation and fibrosis.* The largest group of disorders appears in occupations and environments where there is significant inhalation of dust, gas, or fumes. ILDs also occur in response to infections and as a result of connective tissue disorders such as rheumatoid arthritis and scleroderma. **Sarcoidosis** and **idiopathic pulmonary fibrosis** are the two most common ILDs with an unknown etiology.
pneumonia	pneum/o-	air or lung	*Refers to an inflammation of lung tissue.* Pneumonia is the leading cause of death by infectious disease in the United States and has the highest mortality rate of all nosocomial (hospital-acquired) infections. There are many types of pneumonia. Pneumonia may be classified according to its cause: bacterium, virus, fungus, *Mycoplasma,* parasite, and chemical. Pneumonia is also classified according to whether it is community-acquired pneumonia or hospital-acquired pneumonia. **Community-acquired pneumonia (CAP)** is most commonly caused by *Streptococcus pneumoniae* and has its onset in the community or during the first 48 hours of hospitalization. **Hospital-acquired pneumonia (HAP)** occurs after 48 hours of admission to a hospital. The causative organisms of HAP are primarily bacterial, and differ from those involved with CAP. **Aspiration pneumonia** refers to the response of lung tissue to the entry of a foreign substance from the mouth or stomach. It usually occurs in persons with a diminished gag or cough reflex as occurs with loss of consciousness. **Opportunistic pneumonia** refers to pneumonia that develops in immunosuppressed persons. Immunosuppression is common in persons receiving cancer chemotherapy and radiation therapy.
	-ia	condition of	

Continued

MEDICAL TERMINOLOGY AND DISORDERS | Disorders of the Respiratory System—cont'd

Medical Term	Word Parts	Word Part Meaning or Derivation	Description
acute respiratory distress syndrome (ARDS)			**Adult respiratory distress syndrome,** or ARDS, is *a syndrome that leads to multiple organ failure and death.* **Infant respiratory distress syndrome (IRDS)** occurs in the premature infant and is due to the lack of pulmonary surfactants. (IRDS was formerly called **hyaline membrane disease.**)

Chronic Obstructive Pulmonary Diseases

Called COPD and includes diseases (chronic bronchitis and emphysema) characterized by increased air flow obstruction. The major risk factor is cigarette smoking.

emphysema		From a Greek word meaning "puffed up or bloated"	*Characterized by hyperinflation and destruction of the alveoli, obstruction of the small airways, and loss of elasticity of the lung tissue.*
chronic bronchitis	bronch/o-	bronchus	*The excessive production of mucus in the bronchi and the development of a recurrent and productive cough.* Chronic bronchitis is characterized by hyperplasia of the mucus-secreting cells in the trachea and bronchi; this causes narrowing of the airways and alters the functioning of the macrophages.
	-itis	inflammation of	

Vascular Lung Disorders

pulmonary edema			*A collection of fluid within the alveolar and interstitial spaces of the lungs.* The presence of fluid impairs the diffusion of respiratory gases causing dyspnea, hypoxemia, CO_2 retention, and respiratory acidosis.
pulmonary embolism			*The lodging of an embolus or emboli in the pulmonary arterial circulation.* The affected part of the lung is therefore ventilated, but not perfused (with blood). The most common causes of pulmonary embolus are a blood clot arising from a thrombus in the deep veins of the legs or a clot originating in the right side of the heart in a person with atrial fibrillation.
pulmonary artery hypertension			*An elevation in pulmonary artery pressure.* Pulmonary hypertension increases the workload of the right ventricle causing ventricular hypertrophy and cor pulmonale.

Get Ready for Exams!

Summary Outline

The respiratory system is primarily concerned with the delivery of oxygen to every cell in the body and the elimination of carbon dioxide.

I. Structures: Organs of the Respiratory System

A. Consists of the upper and lower respiratory tracts

B. Nose and nasal cavities
1. The nose and nasal cavities warm and humidify inhaled air.
2. Olfactory receptors are located in the nose.
3. The nasal cavities receive drainage from the paranasal sinuses and tear ducts.

C. Pharynx (throat)
1. The nasopharynx forms a passage for air only.
2. The oropharynx and laryngopharynx form passageways for both air and food.

D. Larynx (voice box)
1. The larynx is a passage for air.
2. The epiglottis is the uppermost cartilage and covers the larynx during swallowing.

E. Trachea (windpipe)
1. It bifurcates into the right and left bronchi.
2. C-shaped rings of cartilage keep the trachea open.

F. Bronchial tree
1. The bronchial tree contains the bronchi, bronchioles, and alveoli.
2. The bronchioles determine the radius of the respiratory air passages and therefore affect the amount of air that can enter the alveoli.
3. The alveoli are tiny grapelike air sacs surrounded by pulmonary capillaries.
4. Gas exchange occurs across the thin walls of the alveoli.

G. Lungs
1. The right lung has three lobes and the left lung has only two lobes.
2. The lungs contain the structures of the lower respiratory tract.
H. Pleural membranes
1. The serous membranes in the chest cavity are the parietal pleura and the visceral pleura.
2. Serous fluid between the pleural membranes prevents friction.
3. For the lungs to remain expanded, pressure in the intrapleural space must be negative.

II. Respiratory Function
A. Respiration includes three steps: ventilation, exchange of respiratory gases, and transport of respiratory gases in the blood.
1. Ventilation (breathing)
   a. The two phases of ventilation are inhalation and exhalation.
   b. Ventilation occurs in response to changes in the thoracic volume (Boyle's law).
   c. Thoracic volume changes because of the contraction and relaxation of the respiratory muscles.
   d. The phrenic and intercostal nerves are motor nerves that supply the diaphragm and the intercostal muscles.
   e. Inhalation is an active process (ATP is used during muscle contraction). Unforced exhalation is passive (no ATP used).
2. Exchange of gases
   a. Exchange of respiratory gases occurs by diffusion across the alveoli and pulmonary capillaries.
   b. Oxygen diffuses from the air in the alveoli into the blood while carbon dioxide diffuses from the blood into the alveoli.
   c. At the cellular layer, oxygen diffuses from the capillaries to the cells. Carbon dioxide diffuses from the cells into the capillaries, where it is transported to the lungs for excretion.
3. Transport of gases in the blood
   a. Most of the oxygen is transported by the red blood cell (oxyhemoglobin).
   b. The blood transports most carbon dioxide in the form of bicarbonate ion (HCO_3^-).
B. Amounts of air
1. Pulmonary volumes
   a. Refers to the amounts of air moved into and out of the lungs
   b. Pulmonary volumes are illustrated in Figure 22-10 and summarized in Table 22-1.
2. Vital capacity and anatomical dead space
   a. Lung capacities are combinations of pulmonary volumes.
   b. Vital capacity is the amount of air that can be exhaled after a maximal inhalation.
   c. Anatomical dead space refers to air remaining in the large conducting passageways that is unavailable for gas exchange, approximately 150 mL of air.

C. Control of breathing
1. Neural control of breathing
   a. The respiratory center is located in the brain stem.
   b. The medullary respiratory center contains inspiratory and expiratory neurons. Nerve impulses travel along the phrenic and intercostal nerves to the muscles of respiration.
   c. The pneumotaxic center and apneustic center are in the pons. These centers help control the medullary respiratory center to produce a normal breathing pattern.
   d. Two other areas of the brain can affect respirations: the hypothalamus and cerebral cortex.
2. Chemical control of respiration
   a. Central chemoreceptors are stimulated by carbon dioxide (pCO_2) and [H^+].
   b. Peripheral chemoreceptors are sensitive to low concentrations of oxygen and increased hydrogen ion concentration in the blood.

Review Your Knowledge

Matching: Structures of the Respiratory Tract
Directions: Match the following words with their descriptions below. Some words may be used more than once.

a. pharynx
b. trachea
c. larynx
d. bronchus
e. paranasal sinuses
f. bronchioles
g. carina
h. alveoli

1. ____ The trachea branches into a right and left _____
2. ____ Called the *voice box* because it contains the vocal cords
3. ____ Mucus drains from these mucous membrane-lined structures into the nasal passages.
4. ____ The respiratory structure connected to the middle ear by the eustachian tube
5. ____ Large tube supported by rings of cartilage; called the *windpipe*
6. ____ The respiratory structure(s) concerned with the exchange of the respiratory gases
7. ____ Structure closest to the pulmonary capillaries
8. ____ Tiny respiratory passages that deliver air to the alveoli
9. ____ Respiratory passage that delivers air to the bronchioles
10. ____ The point at which the trachea splits; causes intense coughing when stimulated by a suction catheter

Matching: Thoracic Cavity and Ventilation

Directions: Match the following words with their descriptions below. Some words may be used more than once.

a. parietal pleura
b. thoracic cavity
c. intrapleural space
d. visceral pleura
e. phrenic
f. diaphragm

1. ___ Membrane on the outer surface of each lung
2. ___ Contains the pleural cavity, pericardial cavity, and mediastinum
3. ___ The lung collapses when air or fluid collects in this space.
4. ___ The motor neuron that innervates the diaphragm
5. ___ Dome-shaped muscle that is the chief muscle of inhalation
6. ___ Membrane that lines the walls of the pleural cavity
7. ___ Must have a negative pressure here

Multiple Choice

1. Inhalation and exhalation are
   a. caused by contraction of the diaphragm and intercostal muscles.
   b. caused by contraction and relaxation of the bronchiolar smooth muscle.
   c. referred to as *ventilation*.
   d. caused by the relaxation of the diaphragm and intercostal muscles.
2. The bronchi, bronchioles, and alveoli are
   a. concerned with the exchange of respiratory gases.
   b. upper respiratory structures.
   c. collectively referred to as the *bronchial tree*.
   d. surrounded by rings of cartilage.
3. The diameter of the bronchioles determines the
   a. amount of mucus secreted by the respiratory membranes.
   b. rate of surfactant secretion.
   c. air flow to the alveoli.
   d. ventilatory rate.
4. Which of the following best describes the visceral and parietal pleura?
   a. They line the inner wall of the trachea and bronchi.
   b. They line the mediastinum.
   c. They are serous membranes.
   d. They are surfactant-secreting membranes.
5. If intrapleural pressure equals or exceeds intrapulmonic pressure,
   a. surfactant secretion ceases.
   b. the lung collapses.
   c. the larynx can no longer generate sound.
   d. pulmonary edema develops.
6. Which of the following does not occur on inhalation?
   a. Air moves into the lungs.
   b. Thoracic volume increases.
   c. The diaphragm contracts.
   d. Pressure within the intrapleural space becomes positive.

7. Which of the following describes Boyle's law?
   a. An increase in thoracic volume causes an increase in intrapleural pressure.
   b. There is no relationship between intrapulmonic pressure and thoracic volume.
   c. An increase in thoracic volume decreases intrapulmonic pressure.
   d. An increase in thoracic volume forces air out of the lungs.

Go Figure

1. **According to Figure 22-1**
   a. All respiratory structures distal to the larynx are located within the lung.
   b. The alveoli are the most distal of all structures of the bronchial tree.
   c. The bronchioles have cartilaginous rings similar to the trachea.
   d. Gas exchange occurs across all respiratory structures located in the lung.

2. **According to Figure 22-2**
   a. The glottis is also called the *true vocal cords*.
   b. The epiglottis prevents the entrance of food and water into the respiratory structures.
   c. The esophagus is "covered" by the epiglottis during swallowing.
   d. The larynx is part of both the respiratory system and the digestive system.

3. **According to Figure 22-3**
   a. The carina is located within the larynx.
   b. Alveoli are composed of a single layer of cells held open by cartilaginous rings.
   c. The alveoli are proximal to the bronchioles.
   d. The left lung has two lobes whereas the right lung has three lobes.

4. **Which statement is not true about Figure 22-5?**
   a. Elastic recoil wants to collapse the lungs.
   b. The surface tension of water wants to collapse the lungs.
   c. Surfactants want to collapse the lungs.
   d. Surfactants decrease the surface tension of water.

5. **According to Figures 22-4 and 22-6**
   a. The lung collapses when the intrapulmonic pressure exceeds intrapleural pressure.
   b. The lung collapses when intrapulmonic pressure exceeds atmospheric pressure.
   c. The lung collapses when intrapleural pressure is lower than intrapulmonic pressure.
   d. Pressure is normally negative in the space between the visceral and parietal pleurae.

6. **According to Figure 22-7 and Boyle's Law**
   a. When volume increases, pressure increases.
   b. When volume decreases, pressure decreases.
   c. There is no relationship between volume and pressure.
   d. When volume increases, pressure decreases.

7. **According to Figure 22-8**
   a. Air moves into the lungs when thoracic volume decreases.
   b. Air moves out of the lungs when thoracic volume increases.
   c. Air moves out of the lungs when the diaphragm and intercostal muscles contract.
   d. Intrapulmonic pressure decreases when the diaphragm contracts.

8. **According to Figure 22-9**
   a. Tissue pO_2 is 95 mm Hg.
   b. Venous pO_2 is 95 mm Hg whereas pCO_2 is 45 mm Hg.
   c. Aortic blood pO_2 and pCO_2 are both 95 mm Hg.
   d. Arterial pO_2 is higher than tissue pO_2.

9. **According to Figure 22-10**
   a. Tidal volume and vital capacity equals the total lung capacity.
   b. Vital capacity is equal to the sum of the resting tidal volume and expiratory reserve volume.
   c. Vital capacity is equal to the tidal volume, inspiratory reserve volume, and expiratory reserve volume.
   d. Expiratory reserve volume is the same as residual volume.

10. **According to Figure 22-11**
    a. Inspiratory and expiratory neurons are located within the respiratory control center of the medulla oblongata.
    b. All respiratory control is located within the brain stem.
    c. All respiratory control is voluntary.
    d. The medulla oblongata is the only brain stem structure that affects respirations.

Key Terms

absorption (p. 429)
amylase (p. 448)
appendix (p. 438)
bile (p. 443)
biliary tree (p. 445)
cecum (p. 438)
chyle (p. 438)
chyme (p. 434)
colon (p. 438)

common bile duct (p. 445)
digestion (p. 429)
duodenum (p. 437)
emulsification (p. 449)
esophagus (p. 434)
gallbladder (p. 445)
ileum (p. 438)
jejunum (p. 438)
lipase (p. 449)

liver lobule (p. 443)
minerals (p. 452)
pancreas (p. 445)
peristalsis (p. 430)
protease (p. 449)
stomach (p. 434)
villus (p. 438)
vitamins (p. 451)

Objectives

1. Discuss the basic anatomy and physiology of the digestive system, including:
   - List four functions of the digestive system.
   - Explain the processes of digestion and absorption.
   - Describe the four layers, nerves, and membranes of the digestive tract.
2. Describe the structure and functions of the organs and accessory organs of the digestive tract.

3. Explain the physiology of digestion and absorption, including:
   - Describe the effects of amylases, proteases, and lipases.
   - Describe the role of bile in the digestion of fats.
4. Discuss nutrition concepts, including:
   - Describe five categories of nutrients.
   - Discuss the importance of a balanced diet.
   - Explain how energy is measured, balanced, and expended in the body.

Most of us have no difficulty in eating our way through the Thanksgiving holiday turkey dinner, although the hours after the feeding frenzy can be a digestive challenge. Our digestive systems work very efficiently to digest and absorb as much of the food as possible. Before the holiday is over, the turkey dinner will be a part of every cell in your body.

Before dinner

After dinner

Cells require a constant supply of nutrients and energy. Food is their source. The purpose of the digestive system is to break down or digest the food into particles that are small and simple enough to be absorbed. Thus, the digestive system ingests food, digests it, absorbs the end products of digestion, and eliminates the waste. The study of the digestive tract is called *gastroenterology*.

OVERVIEW OF THE DIGESTIVE SYSTEM

The digestive tract and the accessory organs of digestion make up the digestive system. The digestive tract, also called the *alimentary canal* or the *gastrointestinal (GI) tract,* is a hollow tube extending from the mouth to the anus (Figure 23-1). The structures of the digestive or GI tract include the mouth, pharynx, esophagus, stomach, small intestine, large intestine, rectum, and anus.

The accessory organs of digestion include the salivary glands, teeth, liver, gallbladder, and pancreas. The salivary glands empty their secretions into the mouth; the liver, gallbladder, and pancreas empty their secretions into the small intestine.

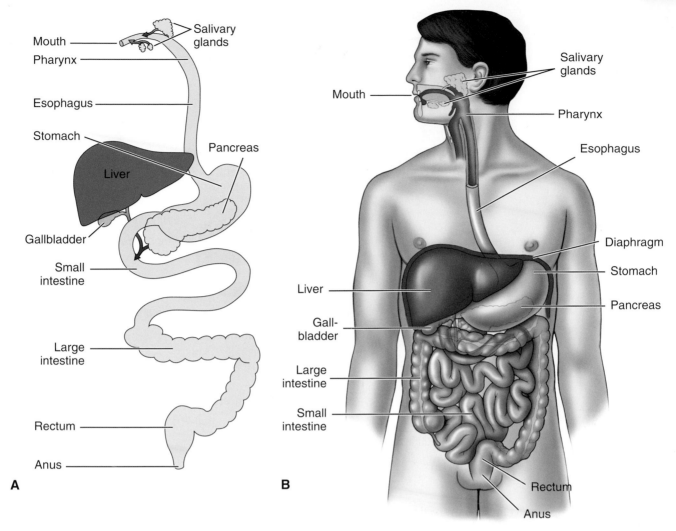

FIGURE 23-1 The digestive system. **A,** Hollow tube. **B,** Anatomical arrangement.

DIGESTION AND ABSORPTION

Digestion is the process by which food is broken down into smaller particles suitable for absorption. Digestion takes place within the digestive tract. **Absorption** is the process whereby the end products of digestion move across the walls of the digestive tract into the blood for distribution throughout the body.

The two forms of digestion are mechanical and chemical. Mechanical digestion is the breakdown of large food particles into smaller pieces by physical means. This process is usually achieved by chewing and by the mashing, or squishing, actions of the muscles in the digestive tract. Chemical digestion is the chemical alteration of food. For example, a protein changes chemically into amino acids. Chemical substances such as digestive enzymes, acid, and bile accomplish chemical digestion.

The end products of digestion are absorbed by moving across the lining of the digestive tract into the blood. Digested nutrients eventually reach every

cell in the body. The food that cannot be digested and absorbed is eliminated from the body as feces. Elimination of waste products is the last stage of the digestive process.

? **Re-Think**

1. Differentiate between digestion and absorption.
2. Differentiate between mechanical and chemical digestion.

LAYERS, NERVES, AND MEMBRANES

Although modified for specific functions in different organs, the wall of the digestive tract has a similar structure throughout its length (Figure 23-2). The wall of the digestive tract has four layers: the mucosa, the submucosa, the muscle layer, and the serosa.

MUCOSA

The innermost layer of the digestive tract, the mucosa, consists of the mucous membrane. Glands secrete mucus, digestive enzymes, and hormones. Ducts from

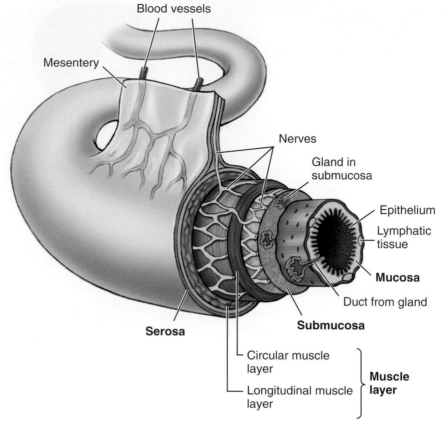

FIGURE 23-2 Layers of the digestive tract.

exocrine glands empty into the lumen of the digestive tract.

SUBMUCOSA

A thick layer of loose connective tissue, the submucosa, lies beneath the mucosa. The submucosa contains blood vessels, nerves, glands, and lymphatic vessels.

MUSCLE LAYER

The third layer of the digestive tract is the muscle layer. Two layers of smooth muscles are an inner circular layer and an outer longitudinal layer. The muscle layer is responsible for several types of movements in the digestive tract. Repeated contraction and relaxation of the stomach muscles digest the food mechanically and mix the particles with digestive juices.

A second type of muscle movement is peristalsis (pair-i-STAL-sis), a rhythmic alternating contraction and relaxation of the muscles. Peristalsis pushes the food in a forward direction through the digestive tract. It's a gutsy move! Peristalsis moves food in the same way that toothpaste squirts from a tube, as illustrated here by G.I. Joe. The toothpaste squirts in a forward direction because the bottom of the tube is squeezed. Peristaltic waves squeeze the food from behind and push it forward. Peristaltic waves are stimulated by the presence of food.

What happens if peristalsis stops? After surgery, intestinal peristalsis is often sluggish and may actually cease. This condition is called *paralytic ileus*. When this happens, food, gas, and liquid accumulate within the digestive tract, creating a life-threatening situation that demands immediate intervention.

Muscle activity is also responsible for other types of movement, such as swallowing and defecation (the elimination of waste from the digestive tract).

SEROSA

The outermost lining of the digestive tract is the serosa. The serosa extends as peritoneal membranes.

INNERVATION

The digestive tract has a unique nervous network called the *enteric nervous system* (ENS). The ENS regulates gastrointestinal (gut) motility and secretion; its activity is modulated by autonomic nerves, especially the parasympathetic (vagal) fibers. Some refer to the gut as a second brain. Why? Because so many of the neurotransmitters that affect the brain also affect the gut. Ever have a "gut" feeling that something is wrong? Your gut might be telling you something!

PERITONEAL MEMBRANES

The peritoneal membranes in the abdominal cavity are extensions of the serosa. These form large flat and folded structures that perform several important functions. They help anchor the digestive organs in place; carry blood vessels, lymph vessels, and nerves to the abdominal organs; and help restrict the spread of infection in the abdominal cavity.

The peritoneal membranes, located behind the digestive organs, are called the *mesentery* and *mesocolon*. When located in front of the organs, they are called the *greater* and *lesser omentum*. The greater omentum is a double layer of peritoneum that contains a considerable amount of fat and resembles an apron draped over the abdominal organs.

2+2 Sum It Up!

The digestive system is made up of a hollow tube that extends from the mouth to the anus and the accessory organs of digestion. The digestive system has four functions: ingestion, digestion, absorption, and elimination. The wall of the digestive tract has four layers: mucosa, submucosa, muscle layer, and serosa. The muscle layer enables the digestive tract to mix, mash, and move food through the tract; the forward movement of food is caused by peristalsis. The enteric nervous system regulates gastrointestinal (gut) motility and secretion; its activity is modulated by autonomic nerves, especially the parasympathetic (vagal) fibers. Large, flat peritoneal membranes in the abdominal cavity help anchor the digestive organs in place.

STRUCTURES AND ORGANS

MOUTH

The digestive tract begins with the mouth, also known as the *oral cavity*. The mouth contains structures that assist in the digestive process. These include the teeth, tongue, salivary glands, and several other structures. The buccal cavity, as part of the oral cavity, refers to the area between the gums and the cheek or lips.

TEETH

The purpose of the teeth is to chew food and to begin mechanical digestion. During the process of chewing, or mastication (mass-ti-KAY-shun), the teeth break down large pieces of food into smaller pieces. Once moistened by the secretions in the mouth, the small pieces of food are easily swallowed.

During a lifetime, a person will have two sets of teeth: deciduous and permanent. The deciduous (deh-SID-yoo-us) teeth are also called *baby teeth* or *milk teeth*. There are 20 deciduous teeth. They begin to appear at the age of 6 months and are generally in place by the age of 2½ years. Between the ages of 6 and 12 years, these teeth are pushed out and replaced by the permanent teeth. There are 32 permanent teeth (Figure 23-3, *A*).

Note the positions and names of the teeth: the incisors, cuspids (canines), premolars (bicuspids), and molars, including wisdom teeth. The shape and location of each tooth determines its function. For example, the sharp, chisel-shaped incisors and cone-shaped cuspids are front teeth used to tear or grasp food. The larger flatter molars, the back teeth, are more suited for grinding food.

A tooth has three parts: the crown, the neck, and the root (see Figure 23-3, *B*). The crown of the tooth is above the level of the gum, or gingiva (JIN-ji-vah), and is covered with hard brittle enamel. The neck connects the crown with the root of the tooth. The root is that part of the tooth embedded in the jawbone. The outer surface of the root is anchored to the periodontal membrane by cementum. The bulk of the tooth consists of a bonelike material called *dentin*. Nerves, blood vessels, and connective tissue, called *pulp*, penetrate the dentin through the pulp cavity and supply the tooth with sensation and nutrients. As the pulp cavity extends into the root, it is called the *root canal*. The *periodontium* is the name given to the tissues that surround the teeth and include the gums, soft tissue, and bone. Gingivitis and stomatitis are mouth conditions that are often drug induced. Both cause considerable discomfort and interfere with nutrition. Gingivitis is inflammation of the gums. Stomatitis refers to inflammation or ulcers of the oral mucosa of the mouth area.

Do You Know...

The Meaning of These Tooth Words?

Four back molars can appear later in life (at 17 to 25 years of age, when you have "become wiser") and are therefore called *wisdom teeth*. In many individuals, the wisdom teeth remain embedded in the jawbone and are said to be impacted. Because impacted teeth serve no function and are often a source of infection, they are frequently removed.

Lacking some naming creativity, the canine teeth are commonly called *eyeteeth* because they are positioned under the eyes. To be "long in the tooth" is a not-too-flattering reference to advanced age; the gums recede with aging, thereby exposing more of the tooth.

TONGUE

The tongue is a muscular organ that occupies the floor of the mouth and serves two major roles in the digestive process. First, it facilitates chewing and swallowing by continuously repositioning the food in the mouth. As swallowing begins, the tongue pushes the food, which it has molded into a ball-like mass called a *bolus*, toward the pharynx. Second, the tongue contains the taste buds and allows us to taste food.

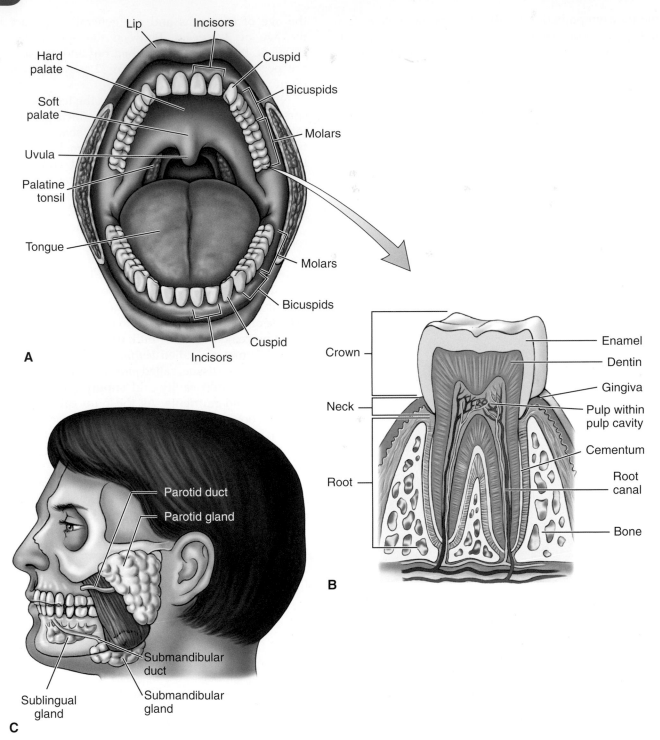

FIGURE 23-3 Oral cavity. **A,** Structures in the mouth. **B,** Longitudinal view of a tooth. **C,** Location of the salivary glands.

If you look under your tongue in the mirror, you will notice two structures. One is a small piece of mucous membrane called the *frenulum*, which anchors the tongue to the floor of the mouth. The second structure is an extensive capillary network that provides the sublingual (under the tongue) area with a rich supply of blood. Because the blood supply is so good, medications are absorbed rapidly when administered sublingually.

? Re-Think

1. What is peristalsis? What causes it? What does it do?
2. A patient is taking three medications: one by the oral route, the second by the buccal route, and the third to be administered sublingually. Explain the difference between the three routes of administration.

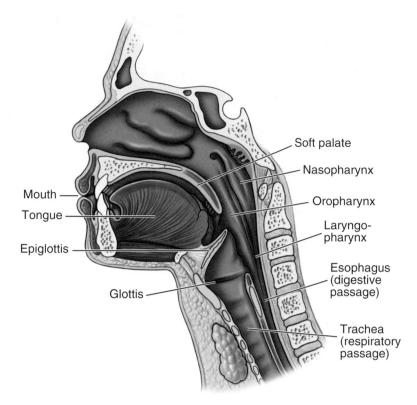

FIGURE 23-4 Eating and swallowing structures: from mouth to pharynx to esophagus.

SALIVARY GLANDS

Three pairs of salivary glands secrete their contents into the mouth: the parotid glands, the submandibular glands, and the sublingual glands (see Figure 23-3, C). The parotid glands are the largest of the three glands and lie below and anterior to the ears. These are the glands infected by the mumps virus, which results in a chipmunk-like appearance. The submandibular glands are located on the floor of the mouth. The sublingual glands are located under the tongue and are the smallest of the salivary glands. The salivary glands are exocrine glands that secrete saliva (from a Greek word meaning "spittle"), a watery fluid that contains mucus and one digestive enzyme called *salivary amylase,* or *ptyalin.* Approximately 1 L of saliva is secreted each day. Saliva reaches the mouth by way of tiny ducts. The most important function of saliva is to soften and moisten food and thereby facilitate swallowing.

What does one do with 1 L of saliva? Normally, the saliva is swallowed. If someone is unable to swallow, however, the saliva must be suctioned so that it is not aspirated into the lungs. This problem occurs in patients who experience inflammation, tumors, or surgery of structures of the upper digestive tract.

Occasionally, one of the salivary ducts becomes obstructed by a stone. The condition is called *sialolithiasis* (si-ah-lo-li-THI-ah-sis) and is characterized by intense pain on eating when the salivary juices start to flow.

OTHER STRUCTURES WITHIN THE MOUTH

The hard and soft palates form the roof of the mouth (see Figure 23-3, *A*). The anterior hard palate separates the oral cavity from the nasal passages, and the posterior soft palate separates the oral cavity from the nasopharynx. The soft palate extends toward the back of the oral cavity as the uvula (YOO-vyoo-lah), the V-shaped piece of soft tissue that hangs down from the upper back region of the mouth. The uvula plays a role in swallowing. The palatine tonsils are masses of lymphoid tissue located along the sides of the posterior oral cavity. These play a role in the body's defense against infection (further explained in Chapter 21).

PHARYNX

The tongue pushes the food from the mouth into the pharynx (throat). The pharynx is involved in swallowing (deglutition). The three parts of the pharynx are the nasopharynx, the oropharynx, and the laryngopharynx (Figure 23-4). Only the oropharynx and laryngopharynx are part of the digestive system.

The pharynx communicates with the nasal, respiratory, and digestive passages. The act of swallowing normally directs food from the throat into the esophagus, a long tube that empties into the stomach. Food does not normally enter the nasal or respiratory passages because swallowing temporarily closes off the openings to both. For example, during swallowing, the soft palate moves toward the opening to the nasopharynx. Similarly, the laryngeal opening is closed when the trachea moves upward and allows the epiglottis to cover the entrance to the respiratory passages. You can see this process as the up-and-down movement of the Adam's apple, part of the larynx or voice box.

> ### ? Re-Think
> 1. List the three salivary glands.
> 2. Explain how food or water can be aspirated into the respiratory tract.

ESOPHAGUS

The esophagus (eh-SOF-ah-gus) is the food tube that carries food from the pharynx to the stomach (see Figure 23-1). The esophagus, which is approximately 10 inches (25 cm) in length, descends through the chest cavity and penetrates the diaphragm. The act of swallowing pushes the bolus of food into the esophagus. The presence of food in the esophagus stimulates peristaltic activity and causes the food to move through the esophagus into the stomach. Glands within the mucosa of the esophagus secrete mucus, which lubricates the bolus and facilitates its passage along the esophagus.

The two esophageal sphincters are the pharyngoesophageal sphincter located at the top of the esophagus, and the gastroesophageal, or lower esophageal sphincter (LES), located at the base of the esophagus (Figure 23-5). Swallowing pushes food past the pharyngoesophageal sphincter into the esophagus. Relaxation of the LES keeps the base of the esophagus open, thereby allowing the passage of food into the stomach. When contracted, however, the LES closes the base of the esophagus, thereby preventing reflux, or regurgitation, of acidic stomach contents back into the esophagus.

In some persons a poorly functioning LES allows for reflux of stomach contents into the esophagus. The condition is called *gastroesophageal reflux disease* (GERD) and is characterized by a burning sensation called *heartburn* or *pyrosis*. The burning sensation is a result of the high acidity of stomach contents. (Note that the word *pyrosis* is related to the word *pyromaniac*, a person who loves to set fires, and to the word *pyretic*, referring to fever.)

STOMACH

WHAT IT DOES

The stomach is a pouchlike organ that lies in the upper part of the abdominal cavity under the diaphragm (see Figure 23-1). It performs five important digestive functions:

- Secretion of gastric (stomach) juice, which includes digestive enzymes, hydrochloric acid, and intrinsic factor.
- Secretion of gastric hormones.
- Regulation of the rate at which the partially digested food is delivered to the small intestine. This is the most important function of the stomach.
- Digestion of food. The stomach plays an important role in the mechanical digestion (mixing and mashing) of food. Chemical digestion is limited.
- Absorption of small quantities of water and dissolved substances. The stomach is not well suited for an absorptive role. It can, however, absorb alcohol efficiently. Therefore, the consumption of alcoholic beverages on an empty stomach can quickly increase blood levels of alcohol.

REGIONS OF THE STOMACH

The major regions of the stomach include the fundus, the body, and the pylorus (see Figure 23-5, *A*). The pylorus, which literally means "gatekeeper," continues as the pyloric canal. A pyloric sphincter is located at the end of the pyloric canal and helps regulate the rate at which gastric contents are delivered to the small intestine. Other landmarks of the stomach include the greater curvature and the lesser curvature.

How big can your stomach get? The empty stomach lies in thick accordion-like folds called *rugae* (ROO-gay). The rugae allow the stomach to expand. For example, when the stomach is empty, it is the size and shape of a sausage. Following a large meal, however, the stomach may expand to approximately 1 L. Think of your turkey dinner sitting in your very expanded stomach—it feels like you are going to pop! Sadly, the stomach can keep stretching in response to continued overeating.

MUSCLES OF THE STOMACH

The stomach has three layers of muscles that lie in three directions: longitudinal, oblique, and circular (see Figure 23-5, *B*). This arrangement allows the stomach to churn and mix the food with gastric juice to create a thick, pastelike mixture called chyme (kime). The stomach is your personal organ grinder. The muscles of the stomach also generate peristaltic waves that squeeze the food toward the pylorus.

GLANDS OF THE STOMACH

The mucous membranes of the stomach contain gastric glands (see Figure 23-5, *C*). These glands contain three types of secretory cells: (1) the mucous cells, which secrete mucus; (2) the chief cells, which secrete digestive enzymes; and (3) the parietal cells, which secrete hydrochloric acid (HCl) and intrinsic factor. The secretions of the gastric glands are called *gastric juice*. An interesting note: the HCl in gastric juice is strong enough to eat the varnish off furniture. In addition to the gastric juice, other cells secrete thicker mucus and bicarbonate that adheres closely to the stomach lining. This secretion forms a protective coating for the stomach lining and prevents the acidic gastric juices from digesting the stomach itself.

FIGURE 23-5 Stomach. **A,** Regions of the stomach: fundus, body, and pylorus. **B,** Three muscle layers of the stomach. **C,** Mucosa of the stomach, showing the mucus, parietal, and chief cells.

? Re-Think

1. Locate the following structures: LES, fundus of the stomach, pyloric sphincter, and the greater and lesser curvatures.
2. What is the most important function of the stomach?
3. What "burns" the base of the esophagus in patients with GERD?

VOMITING

Vomiting, or emesis, is and is not a stomach event. It is a stomach event in that the stomach is emptied on vomiting. However, vomiting is not a stomach event in terms of mechanism. Vomiting is part of the emetic reflex controlled by the medulla oblongata. In response to stimuli sent to the medullary vomiting center, the

LES relaxes and the diaphragm and abdominal muscles contract, thereby compressing the stomach and ejecting its contents. You should become a keen observer of vomited stomach contents and its surrounding events. For example, you will want to know if the vomiting was preceded by nausea or vertigo (dizziness), or related to food or drug intake. Record the frequency—is it an isolated event or more frequent? Record the amount and contents, including drugs, and note the color and any evidence of blood (blood that is changed because of the stomach acid can have a bright red or coffee grounds–like appearance). A lot of clinically valuable information can be obtained through your observations. Don't rush to flush!

WHEN THE STOMACH IS NOT WORKING RIGHT

The stomach gets a lot of attention clinically. Note how it is shown in Figure 23-6:

- *Ulcer* (see Figure 23-6, *A*). A healthy digestive tract has an intact inner mucous membrane. The stomach lining may erode, or break down, thereby creating a lesion called an *ulcer*. Some ulcers are caused by the *Helicobacter pylori* microorganism and are painful and prone to bleeding. An antiulcer drug plan for this type of ulcer includes an antibiotic in addition to drugs that decrease or neutralize acid.
- *Hiatal hernia* (see Figure 23-6, *B*). The stomach is located in the upper abdominal cavity immediately

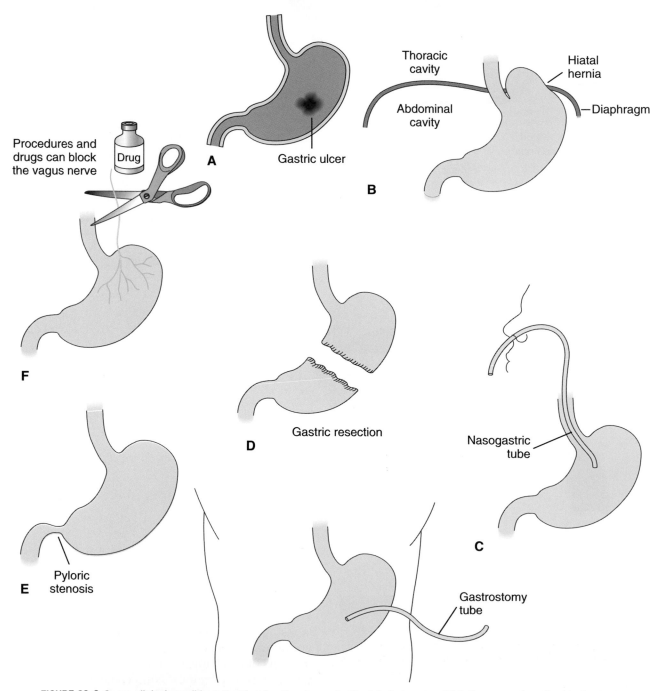

FIGURE 23-6 Some clinical conditions that involve the stomach. The labeled parts of this figure are described in the text.

below the diaphragm. The esophagus enters the abdominal cavity through an opening in the diaphragm. If that opening is weakened or enlarged, the stomach may protrude, or herniate, from the abdominal cavity into the thoracic cavity. This condition is called a *hiatal hernia*.

- *Nasogastric tube* (see Figure 23-6, *C*). Many conditions require that a nasogastric (NG) tube be inserted through the nasal passages into the stomach. Usually, the NG tube is used to empty the stomach to prevent vomiting. When a person cannot eat normally, a tube may be surgically inserted through the abdominal wall into the stomach. Food is introduced directly into the stomach through this tube. This procedure is called a *gastrostomy*.

- *Gastric resection* (see Figure 23-6, *D*). An important function of the stomach is to regulate the rate at which chyme is delivered to the duodenum. A person with cancer of the stomach may require a surgical procedure that removes the stomach, or part of it. The procedure is called a *gastric resection*, or *gastrectomy*. A serious consequence of gastric resection is the inability to regulate the rate at which chyme is delivered to the duodenum. Because food (chyme) is literally dumped into the duodenum, since there is no stomach, a condition called *dumping syndrome* develops. The person experiencing dumping syndrome looks and acts "shocky," with severe nausea, perspiration, dizziness, and tachycardia.

- *Pyloric stenosis* (see Figure 23-6, *E*). The digestive tract is a hollow tube that must remain open. Occasionally, during infancy, the pylorus is too narrow and impedes the movement of food out of the stomach. This condition is pyloric stenosis (narrowing). Pyloric stenosis is characterized by projectile vomiting immediately after feeding. Interestingly, pyloric stenosis is more common in male infants than in female infants. Fortunately, a simple surgical procedure corrects the defect.

- *Gastric hyperactivity* (see Figure 23-6, *F*). Stimulation of the vagus nerve increases gastric secretion and motility. Certain drugs block the effects of the vagus nerve, thereby decreasing gastric secretion and motility. The administration of a vagolytic drug is like cutting the vagus nerve (vagotomy).

- Autonomic translation. Stimulation of the vagus nerve activates muscarinic receptors. Drugs that activate muscarinic receptors stimulate gut motility and secretion and are used to treat "slow" gut conditions such as gastroparesis. Anticholinergic or antimuscarinic (atropine) drugs block muscarinic receptors, thus slowing gut motility and decreasing gastric secretions.

? Re-Think

What functions are lost in the patient who has a total gastrectomy?

2+2 Sum It Up!

The mouth begins the process of mechanical and chemical digestion. The bolus of food is swallowed and moves from the mouth, through the pharynx and esophagus, and into the stomach. The stomach continues the digestive process by mashing the food into chyme. Gastric juice minimally helps to break down food chemically. The stomach delivers chyme to the duodenum (small intestine) at the proper rate.

SMALL INTESTINE

LOCATION AND PARTS

An acidic chyme is ejected by the stomach into the small intestine (see Figure 23-1). The small intestine is called "small" because its diameter is smaller than the diameter of the large intestine. However, the word "small" does not refer to the length of the small intestine; it is considerably longer (about 20 feet [6 m]) than the large intestine (5 feet [1.5 m]). The small intestine is located in the central and lower abdominal cavity and is held in place by the mesentery. The small intestine is concerned primarily with chemical digestion and the absorption of digested food. It consists of three parts: the duodenum, the jejunum, and the ileum. Although the stock market can make your guts churn, it can also help you remember the parts of the small intestine:

Dow	Duodenum
Jones	Jejunum
Industrials	Ileum

SEGMENTS OF THE SMALL INTESTINE

The **duodenum** (doo-oh-DEE-num) is the first segment of the small intestine. The word *duodenum* literally means "twelve" (*duo* means "two"; *denum* means "ten"). In this case, the reference is to the width of 12 fingers. Thus, the length of the duodenum is 12 fingerbreadths or approximately 10 inches (25 cm).

12 fingers

Why is the duodenum considered the meeting point for digestion? In addition to receiving chyme from the stomach, the duodenum also receives secretions from several accessory organs of digestion such as the liver, gallbladder, and pancreas (see Figure 23-1). These secretions, in addition to those from the mouth, stomach, and duodenum, are responsible for the digestion of all food. Most digestion and absorption occur in the duodenum and the first third of the jejunum, the next segment. *To repeat: Most digestion and absorption occur in the duodenum and first third of the jejunum.*

The jejunum (jeh-JOO-num) is the second segment of the small intestine. It is approximately 8 feet (2.4 m) in length. Digestion and absorption of food occurs in the first third of the jejunum.

 Do You Know...

What Borborygmus Is?

"Gurgle, gurgle," growls your guts. How embarrassing is this as you look around the room! This gurgling sound that eminently emanates from your intestines is caused by the rapid movement of gas and liquid through the intestines. The sounds are louder and more noticeable when you are hungry because you tend to salivate more and swallow more air. "Gurgle, gurgle" is called *borborygmus* (bor-bor-IG-mus) and comes from the Greek word meaning "to rumble." Despite this long and ugly name, borborygmus is normal. Its only purpose? To embarrass you.

The ileum (IL-ee-um) is the third segment of the small intestine and is approximately 12 feet (3.6 m) in length. It extends from the jejunum to the ileocecal valve. The ileocecal valve prevents the reflux of contents from the cecum (first part of the large intestine) back into the ileum. The function of the ileum is to complete the process of absorption of digestive end products, vitamin B_{12}, and bile salts. The lining of the ileum contains numerous patches of lymphoid tissue called *Peyer's patches*. Peyer's patches diminish the bacterial content in the digestive system. The ileum performs another important role as an "ileal brake." Through a reflex mechanism, the presence of fatty acids in the ileum slows gut motility. What you eat affects gut motility and secretions.

FUNCTIONS OF THE SMALL INTESTINE

What is so special about the wall of the small intestine? The wall of the small intestine forms circular folds with fingerlike projections called *villi* (sing., villus) (Figure 23-7). The epithelial cells of each villus form extensions called *microvilli*. The large number of villi and microvilli increases the amount of digested food that can be absorbed.

What is a villus? Each villus consists of a layer of epithelial tissue that surrounds a network of blood capillaries and a lymphatic capillary called a *lacteal* (see Figure 23-7, *B*). The villus absorbs the end products of digestion from the duodenum into the blood capillaries or the lacteal. The capillary blood within the villus drains into the hepatic portal system and then into the liver. Thus, the end products of carbohydrate and protein digestion first go to the liver for processing before being distributed throughout the body. The

end products of fat digestion enter the lacteal, forming a milky-white lymph called chyle (kile). The chyle empties directly into the lymphatic system. (Do not confuse the words *chyle* and *chyme*.)

In addition to forming a site for absorption, the cells of the intestinal wall also secrete several digestive enzymes and two important hormones: secretin and cholecystokinin (CCK). Table 23-1 lists the major intestinal enzymes and hormones.

Peristalsis and Absorption in the Small Intestine

Like other parts of the digestive tract, peristalsis moves its digestive contents through the small intestines. The peristalsis in the small intestine, however, is unique. Instead of merely pushing the digestive contents forward, the peristalsis also generates a swishing and swaying motion. This motion continually washes the nutrient-rich digestive contents across the villi, thereby increasing absorption. That which is not absorbed is moved forward by peristaltic waves toward the large intestine.

 Re-Think

1. List the three segments of the small intestine.
2. Where does most digestion and absorption take place?

LARGE INTESTINE

The large intestine is approximately 5 feet (1.5 m) long and extends from the ileocecal valve to the anus (Figure 23-8). The cecum, colon, rectum, and anal canal are parts of the large intestine.

SEGMENTS OF THE LARGE INTESTINE

The first part of the large intestine is the cecum. The cecum is located in the right lower quadrant and ascends on the right side as the ascending colon. Attached to the cecum is the appendix, a wormlike structure that contains lymphocytes and is a source of immune cells.

Occasionally, the appendix becomes inflamed, causing appendicitis, and must be surgically removed through an appendectomy. Failure to remove an inflamed appendix causes it to rupture. The discharge of fecal material into the peritoneal cavity causes a life-threatening infection called *peritonitis*. RLQ pain? Think appendicitis and get thee to a doctor.

The ascending colon ascends on the right side and curves acutely near the liver at the hepatic flexure. As it crosses the upper abdomen, it is known as the *transverse colon*. The colon then bends near the spleen at the splenic flexure to become the descending colon. The descending colon descends on the left side of the abdomen into an S-shaped segment called the *sigmoid colon*. Structures distal to the sigmoid colon include the rectum, anal canal, and anus. The anal canal ends at the anus, a structure composed primarily of two sphincter muscles (an involuntary internal sphincter

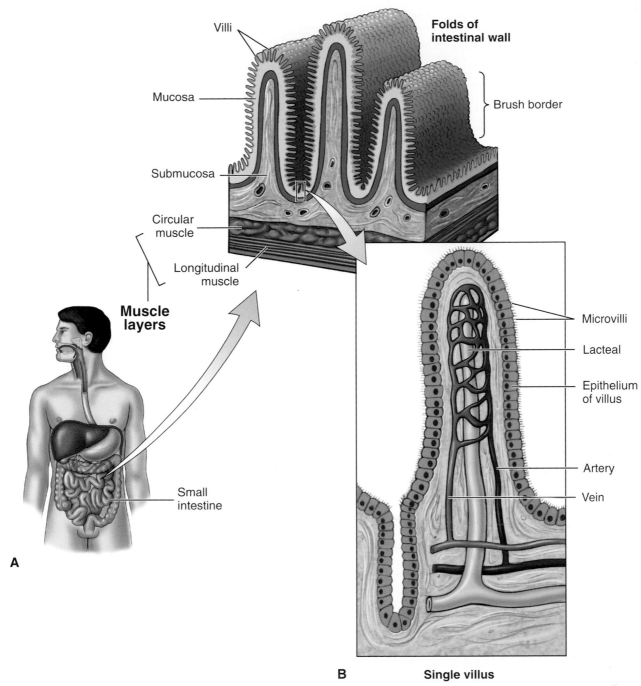

FIGURE 23-7 Small intestine. **A,** Folds of the intestinal wall. **B,** Single villus showing the blood capillaries and the lacteal.

and a voluntary external sphincter). The sphincters are closed except during the expulsion of the feces. Feces (FEE-seez) is waste composed primarily of nondigestible food residue; it forms the stool, or bowel movement (BM). Expulsion of feces is called *defecation*.

FUNCTIONS OF THE LARGE INTESTINE

The four functions of the large intestine are as follows:
- Absorption of water and electrolytes
- Synthesis of certain vitamins by the intestinal bacteria (especially vitamin K and some B vitamins)
- Temporary storage site of waste (feces)
- Elimination of waste from the body (defecation)

Peristalsis and Absorption

Intermittent and well-spaced peristaltic waves move the fecal material from the cecum through the colon. As the fecal material moves through the colon, water is continuously reabsorbed from the feces, across the intestinal wall, into the capillaries. Consequently, as the feces enter the rectum, it has changed from a watery consistency to a semisolid mass. Feces that remain in the large intestine for an extended period lose excess water, and the person experiences constipation. Rapid movement through the intestine allows insufficient time for water reabsorption, causing diarrhea.

Table 23-1 Major Secretions of the Digestive System

NAME	SOURCE	DIGESTIVE FUNCTION
Enzymes		
Salivary Enzyme		
• Amylase (ptyalin)	Salivary glands	Begins carbohydrate digestion to disaccharides
Gastric Enzyme		
• Pepsin	Gastric glands	Begins digestion of protein
Pancreatic Enzymes		
• Amylase	Pancreas	Digests polysaccharides to disaccharides
• Lipase	Pancreas	Digests fats to fatty acids and glycerol
• Proteases	Pancreas	Digests proteins to peptides and amino acids
Trypsin		
Chymotrypsin		
Intestinal Enzymes		
• Peptidases	Intestine	Digests peptides to amino acids
• Disaccharidases	Intestine	Digests disaccharides to monosaccharides
Sucrase		
Lactase		
Maltase		
• Lipase	Intestine	Digests fats to fatty acids and glycerol
• Enterokinase	Intestine	Activates trypsinogen to trypsin
Digestive Aids		
Hydrochloric acid	Stomach	Helps unravel proteins; kills microorganisms that are ingested in food
Intrinsic factor	Stomach	Assists in the absorption of vitamin B_{12}
Bile	Liver	Emulsifies fats; aids in the absorption of fatty acids and the fat-soluble vitamins (A, D, E, K)
Mucus	Entire digestive tract	Softens food; lubricates food and eases its passage through the digestive tract
Hormones		
Gastrin	Stomach	Stimulates gastric glands to secrete gastric juice
Cholecystokinin	Duodenum	Stimulates the gallbladder to contract and release bile; stimulates release of pancreatic digestive enzymes; slows gastric emptying
Secretin	Duodenum	Stimulates the pancreas to secrete sodium bicarbonate; called "nature's own antacid"; makes chyme alkaline

 Do You Know...

Why Hirschsprung's Disease Is Also Called Megacolon?

Hirschsprung's disease is a congenital disorder characterized by a lack of the enteric nerve network (no ganglia) in the distal colon near the rectum. The aganglionic colon "feels" no urge to defecate and enlarges in response to accumulated feces (earning its alternative name, *megacolon*, or *congenital aganglionosis*). When the megacolon finally produces a stool, it is huge and noteworthy! This condition attests to the role of the enteric nerves in "moving things along."

Drugs may be administered to increase or decrease the motility of the large intestine. For example, a person with diarrhea may take a drug that slows motility. Slower motility allows for more water reabsorption and the formation of a drier stool. In contrast, a person with constipation requires an increase in motility, so as to prevent additional water reabsorption. Thus, a laxative, which increases motility, is often prescribed to relieve constipation.

Bacterial Action

What do bacteria do in the large intestine? The bacterial content in the feces is normally high, accounting for an impressive 30% of the fecal content. (The presence of bacteria in the intestinal tract is normal and is called the *normal flora*.) Some of these bacteria, *Escherichia coli* for example, synthesize vitamins. Although *E. coli* is normal and beneficial in the intestinal tract, it can cause serious medical conditions in urine and blood. Bacteria are also responsible for the formation of malodorous molecules that provide stools with their characteristic aroma.

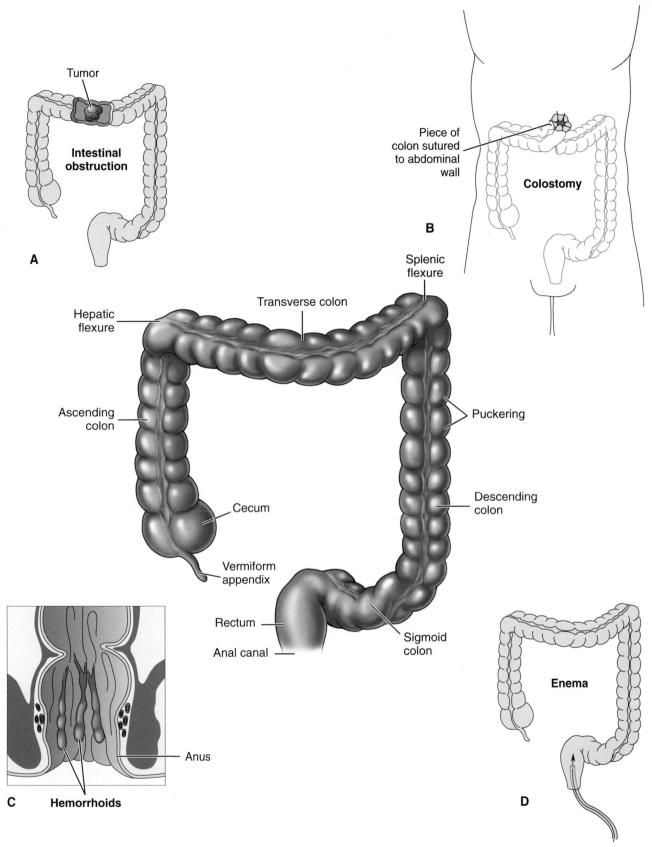

FIGURE 23-8 Large intestine *(center)* and some clinical conditions that affect the large intestine. The labeled parts of this figure are described in the text.

About the Clinical Concern for *Clostridium Difficile*?

Clostridium difficile, a gram-positive bacillus, is a part of the intestinal normal flora; it normally causes no problems. If the intestinal flora is disrupted, as may occur with antibiotic therapy, the number of *C. difficile* increases, causing a serious antibiotic-associated colitis. The combination of antibiotic therapy and severe diarrhea should send up a red flag: the possibility of superinfection with *C. difficile*. How did *C. difficile* get its name? From its uncooperative nature; it is difficult to grow in the lab.

Intestinal Gas

We have our own natural gas line! The average person expels about 500 mL of gas/day (always a crowd pleaser). The expelled gas is called *flatus* (FLAY-tus), and the process is called *flatulence* (FLATCH-yoo-lints). From a Ms. Manners perspective, most episodes of flatulence can be controlled, a much appreciated act of kindness. Gas is normally produced from air that is swallowed and as a byproduct of digestion, especially of gassy foods. Conditions such as lactose intolerance produce excess gas, causing severe cramping and discomfort. You will often hear surgeons ask patients if they have been "passing gas." A barely audible and embarrassed "yes" indicates that peristaltic activity, which often diminishes during surgery, has resumed. Passing gas after surgery is very good. The intestinal gases include methane and hydrogen gas, both of which are flammable. This is a concern in the operating room, where the use of electrical equipment (cautery) can cause the intestinal gas to explode. Not good. This just in—dinosaurs may have done themselves in through the expulsion of ginormous amounts of gas; the gas produced a toxic environment unsuitable for baby dinos.

 Re-Think

1. List the parts of the large intestine.
2. Why is it important to assess your patient's bowel sounds postoperatively?

WHEN THE LARGE INTESTINE IS NOT WORKING RIGHT

The large intestine is a common site of clinical disorders and discomfort. Some clinical conditions and procedures involving the large intestine are illustrated in Figure 23-8.

Because the digestive tract is a hollow tube that extends from the mouth to the anus, it occasionally becomes blocked, or occluded (see Figure 23-8, *A*). For example, a tumor may grow large enough to block a segment of the large intestine completely. Or, the bowel may become twisted on itself, causing a volvulus, and may occlude the lumen of the bowel. Both conditions result in intestinal obstruction, whereby the movement of feces is impaired.

In case of an intestinal obstruction, a surgical procedure may be performed to relieve the obstruction (see Figure 23-8, *B*). An incision into the colon and the rerouting of the colon onto the surface of the abdomen (colostomy) allows the feces to bypass the obstruction. Because of insufficient water reabsorption, a colostomy performed on the ascending colon is characterized by the drainage of liquid feces. Because of adequate water reabsorption along the length of the large intestine, however, a colostomy performed on the sigmoid colon is characterized by a well-formed stool.

All organs receive a supply of oxygen-rich blood from the arteries and are drained by veins. The walls of the veins are thin and may become damaged by excessive pressure. Sometimes, the veins that drain the anal region become stretched and distorted, causing varicosities. These varicosities are called *hemorrhoids* (see Figure 23-8, *C*).

For several reasons (e.g., constipation, preparation for x-ray examination), cleansing of the rectum or colon may be necessary. This procedure is accomplished by an enema, which infuses water through a tube inserted into the rectum (see Figure 23-8, *D*). The water stimulates the contraction of the muscle of the bowel, causing evacuation of its contents. Once the bowel is cleansed of fecal material, barium may be infused into the lower bowel (a procedure called a *barium enema*). The white translucent barium appears on the x-ray and outlines any tumor or other abnormality.

 Do You Know...

That the "Shepherd of the Anus" Was a High-Profile "Ca-rear"?

Ancient Egyptian medicine was divided into many specialties. Each area of the body had its own physician, or shepherd. The physician of the rectal area, comparable to today's proctologist, was called the "shepherd of the anus." Given the ancients' preoccupation with bowel irregularity and the popularity of emetics and purges, this shepherd was a very busy person—not too different from today if you note the staggering numbers of over-the-counter gastrointestinal drugs.

2+2 Sum It Up!

Chyme is discharged from the stomach into the small intestine: duodenum, jejunum, and ileum. Most digestion and absorption occur in the duodenum and first third of the jejunum. The end products of digestion are absorbed across the duodenal and jejunal walls into the villi of the small intestine. Glucose and amino acids are absorbed into the capillaries of the villi. The fats and fat-soluble vitamins are absorbed into the lacteals. Water and electrolytes are absorbed as the contents move through the small and large intestines (cecum, colon, and rectum). Digestive waste is eliminated as feces.

 Re-Think

List the structures through which food would pass on a mouth-to-anus travelogue.

ACCESSORY DIGESTIVE ORGANS

Three important organs—the liver, the gallbladder, and the pancreas—empty their secretions into the duodenum (Figure 23-9). These secretions are necessary for the digestion of food.

LIVER

The liver is a large reddish-brown organ located in the mid and right upper abdominal cavity (see Figure 23-9, *A*). It lies immediately below the diaphragm; much of the liver is tucked up under the right rib cage. The liver is the largest gland in the body and has two main lobes: a larger right lobe and a smaller left lobe separated by a ligament. This ligament secures the liver to surrounding structures. The liver is surrounded by a fibrous membrane called a *capsule*. The word *hepatic* refers to liver.

WHAT THE LIVER DOES

The liver is essential for life and performs many vital functions:

- *Synthesis of bile salts and secretion of bile.* Bile salts play an important role in fat digestion and in the absorption of fat-soluble vitamins. Bile secretion is the main digestive function of the liver.
- *Synthesis of plasma proteins.* The plasma proteins play an important role in maintaining blood volume and controlling blood coagulation.
- *Storage.* The liver stores many substances: glucose in the form of glycogen, the fat-soluble vitamins (A, D, E, and K), and vitamin B_{12}.
- *Detoxification.* The liver plays an important role in the detoxification of drugs and other harmful substances. The liver changes these toxic substances into substances that can be more easily eliminated from the body by the kidneys. The liver is the most important organ in the biotransformation of drugs!
- *Excretion.* The liver excretes many substances, including bilirubin, cholesterol, and drugs.
- *Metabolism of carbohydrates.* The liver plays an important role in the regulation of blood glucose levels. If blood glucose levels rise above normal, the liver removes glucose from the blood, converts it to glycogen, and then stores it for future use. If the blood glucose levels decline below normal, the liver makes glucose from glycogen and nonglucose substances (gluconeogenesis) and releases it into the blood.
- *Metabolism of protein.* The liver can make a variety of different amino acids. Also, because only the liver contains the urea cycle enzymes, nitrogen (from ammonia) is converted to urea in the liver for eventual excretion by the kidneys. Free ammonia in the blood is toxic to humans.
- *Metabolism of fats.* The liver can break down fatty acids, synthesize cholesterol and phospholipids, and convert excess dietary protein and carbohydrates to fat.
- *Phagocytosis.* The Kupffer cells are hepatic macrophages and can phagocytose bacteria and other substances.

? Re-Think

1. Explain how the liver helps to regulate blood glucose.
2. Explain why a person with poor hepatic function requires a smaller dose of a drug.
3. Explain the role of Kupffer cells.

BLOOD SUPPLY TO THE LIVER

Blood Supply and the Hepatic Portal System

The liver has a unique arrangement of blood vessels called the *hepatic portal system* (see Figure 18-7). The liver receives a lot of blood, approximately 1.5 L/min, from two sources: the portal vein, which provides most of the blood, and the hepatic artery. The portal vein drains blood from all of the organs of digestion and brings blood rich in digestive end products to the liver. The hepatic artery delivers oxygen-rich blood from the aorta to the liver. Blood leaves the liver through the hepatic veins and empties into the inferior vena cava, where it is returned to the heart for recirculation.

? Re-Think

1. Why does the liver require a blood supply from both the hepatic artery and the portal vein?
2. Why is portal blood flow to the liver much greater than the arterial flow?
3. Identify the blood vessels that carry the blood from the liver to the vena cava.

LIVER LOBULES

The liver contains thousands of liver lobules, the functional unit of the liver (see Figure 23-9, *B*). The liver lobules consist of a special arrangement of blood vessels and hepatic cells (hepatocytes). Note the central vein and the rows of hepatic cells that radiate away from the central vein. These cells are bathed by blood that enters the lobule from both the hepatic artery and the portal vein.

Blood from these two blood vessels mixes in the liver in spaces called *sinusoids* (SINE-u-soids), or large pore capillaries. The hepatic cells extract water and dissolved substances from the sinusoidal blood. Hepatic cells then secrete a greenish-yellow substance called *bile* into tiny canals called *canaliculi* (kan-ah-LIK-yoo-lye). These tiny bile canals merge with canals from other lobules to form larger hepatic bile ducts. Bile exits from the liver through two hepatic bile ducts.

BILE

Bile is a greenish-yellow secretion produced by the liver and stored in the gallbladder. Bile is composed

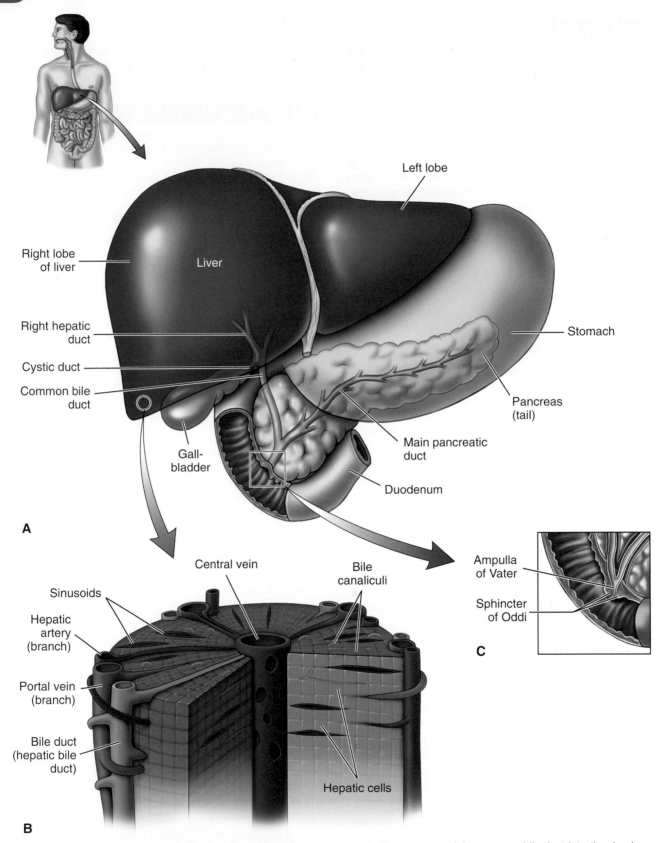

FIGURE 23-9 **A,** Liver, gallbladder, bile ducts, and pancreas. **B,** Liver lobule. **C,** The entrance of the common bile duct into the duodenum.

primarily of water, electrolytes, cholesterol, bile pigments, and bile salts. The bile pigments bilirubin and biliverdin are formed from the hemoglobin of worn-out red blood cells. The bile salts are the most abundant constituents of the bile. Only the bile salts have a digestive function; they play an important role in fat digestion and in the absorption of fat-soluble vitamins. Between 800 and 1000 mL of bile is secreted per day.

Bile pigments, especially urobilinogen (yoo-roh-bil-IN-oh-jen) (a breakdown product of bilirubin), also give the stool a brownish color. With gallbladder disease, a gallstone sometimes becomes lodged in the common bile duct, blocks the flow of bile into the duodenum, and deprives the stools of brown pigments. Common bile duct obstruction is therefore characterized by colorless, gray, or clay-colored stools.

Bile salts are made from cholesterol by the liver. If the liver is stimulated to make additional bile salts, more cholesterol is used up, thereby lowering the amount of cholesterol in the blood. The statins, popular cholesterol-lowering drugs, stimulate the hepatic synthesis of bile salts and are therefore useful in lowering cholesterol and preventing coronary artery disease.

BILIARY TREE

The ducts that connect the liver, gallbladder, and duodenum are called the biliary tree (see Figure 23-9, A). This network of ducts, the "bile aisle," includes the hepatic bile ducts, cystic duct, and common bile duct. The hepatic bile ducts receive bile from the canaliculi in the liver lobules. The hepatic ducts merge with the cystic duct to form the common bile duct, which carries bile from the hepatic ducts (liver) and the cystic duct (gallbladder) to the duodenum.

The base of the common bile duct swells to form the hepatopancreatic ampulla (ampulla of Vater; see Figure 23-9, C). The main pancreatic duct joins the common bile duct at this point. The hepatopancreatic sphincter (sphincter of Oddi) encircles the base of the ampulla, where it enters the duodenum. This sphincter helps regulate the delivery of bile to the duodenum and is sensitive to nervous, hormonal, and pharmacological control. (Do not confuse the ducts of the biliary tree with the hepatic blood vessels.)

Do You Know...

With No Hepatic Cells—Everything Swells?

The liver is a very busy organ. One of its functions is to make plasma proteins such as albumin. Plasma proteins help hold water in the blood vessels. In severe liver disease, insufficient protein is made, causing water to leak out of the blood vessels into the surrounding tissue. The waterlogged tissue is called *edema.* "Take care of that liver," says Sir Osis, who has cirrhosis. "And remember, too many drinks, liver shrinks. Too much nog, 'ammonia fog.' No hepatic cells, everything swells." Need those hepatic cells!

GALLBLADDER

The gallbladder is a pear-shaped sac attached to the underside of the liver (see Figure 23-9, A). The cystic duct connects the gallbladder with the common bile duct. Bile, produced in the liver, flows through the hepatic ducts and into the cystic duct and gallbladder. The function of the gallbladder is to concentrate and store bile. The gallbladder concentrates about 1200 mL of bile/day.

The presence of dietary fat in the duodenum stimulates the release of a hormone, cholecystokinin (koh-lee-sis-toh-KYE-nin) (CCK). This hormone enters the bloodstream and circulates to the gallbladder, where it causes the smooth muscle of the gallbladder to contract. When the gallbladder contracts, the bile is ejected into the cystic duct and then into the common bile duct and duodenum.

For unknown reasons, bile components often form stones. The larger stones remain in the gallbladder. However, the smaller stones can be pushed out of the gallbladder when bile is ejected. The stones then lodge in the common bile duct. Bile that backs up behind the stones causes jaundice and impairs hepatic function. The stagnant bile can also be forced into the main pancreatic duct, causing a life-threatening pancreatitis. The presence of stones in the gallbladder often causes an inflammation called *cholecystitis.* The presence of stones in the common bile duct is called *choledocholithiasis.* Both conditions may cause biliary colic (midepigastric pain that often radiates to the right subscapular area) and other digestive symptoms, such as nausea, vomiting, and pain.

How can a fatty meal trigger biliary colic in a person with cholecystitis? When the fat enters the duodenum, it causes the release of CCK. The CCK travels via the blood to the gallbladder and stimulates the inflamed gallbladder to contract. Ouch!

? Re-Think

1. Trace the flow of bile from its source to its point of excretion.
2. Explain the difference in function between the hepatic portal system and the hepatobiliary system.

PANCREAS

The pancreas is an accessory organ of digestion located just below the stomach (see Figure 23-9, A). The head of the pancreas rests in the curve of the duodenum, and the tail lies near the spleen in the left upper quadrant of the abdominal cavity. The main pancreatic duct, which travels the length of the pancreas, joins with the common bile duct at the ampulla of Vater. The pancreatic duct carries digestive enzymes from the pancreas to the duodenum—the meeting point for digestion.

The pancreas secretes both endocrine and exocrine substances. The exocrine secretions include the digestive enzymes and an alkaline secretion. These secretions form the pancreatic juice; the pancreas secretes about 1400 mL/day. *Note: The pancreatic enzymes are the most important of all the digestive enzymes.* Acinar cells secrete the pancreatic enzymes in their inactive form. The enzymes travel through the main pancreatic duct to the duodenum and are activated in the duodenum.

In addition to the digestive enzymes, the pancreas also secretes an alkaline juice rich in bicarbonate. The bicarbonate neutralizes the highly acidic chyme coming from the stomach into the duodenum. This neutralization is important because the digestive enzymes in the duodenum work best in an alkaline environment.

The secretion of the digestive enzymes and bicarbonate is under nervous (vagus) and hormonal control. The presence of food in the stomach and duodenum is the stimulus for the nervous and hormonal responses. For example, the presence of chyme in the duodenum stimulates the release of the hormone CCK from the duodenal walls. CCK travels by way of the blood to the pancreas, stimulating the release of pancreatic digestive enzymes. Note that CCK affects both the gallbladder and pancreas (see Table 23-1). The acid in the duodenum stimulates the release of a second hormone, secretin, from the duodenal walls. Secretin travels by way of the blood to the pancreas, stimulating release of the bicarbonate-rich juice. Bicarbonate neutralizes the gastric acid.

? Re-Think

1. What are the stimuli for the release of CCK and secretin? What are the effects of CCK and secretin?
2. How does the gallbladder "know" when to release bile into the common bile duct?

WHEN ACCESSORY DIGESTIVE ORGANS ARE NOT WORKING RIGHT

Disorders involving the liver, gallbladder, biliary tree, and pancreas are common. Some clinical conditions are shown in Figure 23-10.

- *Jaundice* (see Figure 23-10, *A*). The liver secretes bile, which is stored in the gallbladder for future use in the duodenum. When needed, bile travels through bile ducts to the duodenum. If the common bile duct becomes blocked with stones, the flow of bile stops. The bile backs up into the liver. The bile pigments, especially bilirubin, accumulate in the blood and are eventually carried throughout the body, where they are deposited in the skin. The skin turns yellow, and the person is described as being jaundiced. Because

the jaundice is caused by an obstruction, it is called *obstructive jaundice* (in contrast to hemolytic jaundice, which is caused by the rapid breakdown of red blood cells; see Chapter 15). Jaundice can also occur in response to liver disease (hepatitis). A person with hepatitis may become jaundiced because the inflamed hepatic tissue causes the bile canaliculi to swell and close. This closure diminishes the excretion of bile from the liver and causes backup of bilirubin in the blood. In addition, the hepatocytes are too damaged to metabolize bilirubin.

- *Bleeding* (see Figure 23-10, *B*). The liver synthesizes clotting factors such as prothrombin. What can make a person hypoprothrombinemic? A gallstone lodged in the common bile duct may cause hypoprothrombinemia. Because bile is necessary for the absorption of fat-soluble vitamins, bile duct obstruction causes diminished absorption of vitamin K. Vitamin K is necessary for the hepatic synthesis of a number of clotting factors, including prothrombin. Thus, common bile duct obstruction diminishes the hepatic synthesis of prothrombin, causing hypoprothrombinemia, a prolonged prothrombin time, and bleeding. Damaged hepatocytes are another hepatic cause of hypoprothrombinemia; they are simply too damaged to make prothrombin.

- *Portal hypertension and hemorrhage* (see Figure 23-10, *C*). The liver receives a large flow of blood from the portal vein. Normally, the blood passes through the liver quickly and easily. In alcoholic cirrhosis, however, the liver is so damaged that the flow of portal blood through the liver is greatly impeded. The blood backs up in the portal vein, elevating the pressure in the vein and causing portal hypertension. The increased portal pressure is felt not only by the portal vein, but also by all the veins that drain into the portal vein, including the small veins at the base of the esophagus. Over time, the small veins become stretched and damaged (varicose veins). If the portal pressure becomes too great, the weak varicose veins (esophageal varices) at the base of the esophagus may rupture, causing a massive hemorrhage (ruptured esophageal varices). The elevated portal pressure also causes some portal blood to bypass the liver, thereby allowing toxic amounts of ammonia (nitrogen) to enter the general circulation. This causes a type of disorientation called "ammonia fog"; the toxic effects of ammonia eventually causes hepatic encephalopathy (en-sef-ah-LOP-ath-ee).

- *Portal hypertension and ascites* (see Figure 23-10, *D*). In alcoholic cirrhosis, the portal hypertension may also cause fluid to seep across the blood vessels into the peritoneal cavity. The collection of fluid in the peritoneal cavity is called *ascites* (ah-SYE-tees). The ascites may be so severe that the accumulated fluid pushes up on the diaphragm and interferes with breathing. The fluid may be siphoned off by

Jaundice

A

Gallstones

B **Bleeding**

Acute pancreatitis

E

Ascites

Esophagus

Stomach

Bleeding
varices

C

**Portal hypertension
and bleeding
esophageal varices**

D **Paracentesis**

FIGURE 23-10 Some clinical conditions that affect the liver, gallbladder, and pancreas. The labeled parts of this figure are described in the text.

the insertion of a tube into the peritoneal cavity. This procedure is called *paracentesis* (pair-ah-sin-TEE-siss).

- *Pancreatitis* (see Figure 23-10, *E*). The pancreas secretes potent proteolytic enzymes in their inactive forms. These inactive enzymes normally flow through the main pancreatic duct into the duodenum, where the enzymes are activated. Sometimes, the enzymes become activated within the pancreas and digest the pancreatic tissue, causing severe inflammation in the form of acute pancreatitis.

2+2 Sum It Up!

The accessory digestive organs include the liver, gallbladder, and pancreas. These organs secrete substances that are eventually emptied into the duodenum, the meeting place for digestion. The liver performs many functions. The liver's primary digestive role is the secretion of bile. Bile is concentrated and stored in the gallbladder; it is released into the bile ducts in response to cholecystokinin. The pancreatic acinar cells secrete the most potent digestive enzymes (amylase, lipase, proteases). The pancreatic enzymes empty into the duodenum. In addition to the digestive enzymes, bicarbonate-rich pancreatic secretions assist the digestive process.

DIGESTION AND ABSORPTION

The primary purpose of the digestive system is to break down large pieces of food into small particles suitable for absorption. Food is digested mechanically and chemically. Mechanical digestion is the physical breakdown of food into small pieces. It is achieved by the chewing activity of the mouth and by the mixing and churning activities of the muscles of the digestive organs. Chemical digestion is the chemical change occurring primarily in response to the digestive enzymes. Whereas mechanical digestion refers to a breakdown in the size of the piece of food, chemical digestion refers to a change in the chemical composition of the food molecule.

Food is made up of carbohydrates, proteins, and fats. Digestive enzymes and several digestive agents (mucus, hydrochloric acid, and bile) play key roles in chemical digestion. Specific enzymes digest each type of food (see Table 23-1). (Review the structures of carbohydrates, protein, and fat in Chapter 4.)

CARBOHYDRATES AND CARBOHYDRATE-SPLITTING ENZYMES

Carbohydrates are classified according to size (see Figure 4-2). Monosaccharides are single (mono) sugars (saccharides). The three monosaccharides are glucose, fructose, and galactose. Glucose is the most important of the three monosaccharides. Disaccharides are double (di) sugars. The three disaccharides are sucrose (table sugar), lactose, and maltose. Polysaccharides are many (poly) glucose molecules linked together. The shorter monosaccharides and disaccharides are called *sugars*; the longer-chain polysaccharides are *starches*.

A polysaccharide is digested in two stages (Figure 23-11, *A*). First, enzymes called **amylases** (AM-eh-lays-ez) break the polysaccharide into disaccharides. The two amylases are salivary amylase (ptyalin) and pancreatic amylase. Second, disaccharidases break disaccharides into monosaccharides. The three disaccharidases are sucrase, lactase, and maltase. (The ending *-ase* indicates an enzyme.) The cells of the

FIGURE 23-11 Chemical digestion. **A,** Carbohydrate digestion. **B,** Protein digestion. **C,** Fat emulsification and digestion.

intestinal villi contain disaccharidases. Disaccharides therefore are split into monosaccharides in the duodenum at the surface of the villi. They are immediately absorbed across the villus into the blood capillaries.

Certain carbohydrates, such as cellulose, cannot be digested and therefore remain in the lumen of the digestive system. Although providing no direct nourishment, dietary cellulose is beneficial in that it provides fiber and bulk to the stool.

Many persons suffer from a deficiency of the enzyme lactase. They are unable to digest the sugar found in milk (lactose) and are said to be lactose intolerant. This enzyme deficiency prevents lactose-intolerant people from digesting milk and many milk products. An interesting note: Most people worldwide are lactose intolerant!

PROTEINS AND PROTEIN-SPLITTING ENZYMES

The building blocks of proteins are amino acids. Several amino acids linked together form a peptide. Many amino acids linked together form a polypeptide. Proteins are very long polypeptide chains; some proteins contain more than one polypeptide chain (see Figure 23-11, B). To be absorbed across the wall of the digestive tract, these chains must be uncoiled and broken down into small peptides and amino acids.

Enzymes called **proteases**, or proteolytic enzymes, digest proteins. Proteases are secreted by three organs: the stomach secretes pepsin, the intestinal cells secrete enterokinase, and the pancreas secretes several proteases, including trypsin and chymotrypsin. The pancreatic proteases are the most potent proteases. Proteins are broken down into small peptides and amino acids and are absorbed across the intestinal villi into the blood capillaries. (Interesting fact: Because it was thought to aid digestion, Pepsi was named after the enzyme pepsin.)

Although not an enzyme, HCl aids protein digestion. First, the HCl unravels the strands of protein, making the protein fragments more sensitive to the proteases. Second, the HCl activates a gastric proteolytic enzyme, pepsinogen, into pepsin. Pepsin then facilitates breaking protein into small peptides.

FATS, BILE, AND FAT-SPLITTING ENZYMES

Fats are long-chain molecules. Enzymes called **lipases** (LYE-pays-ez) digest fats. The most important is pancreatic lipase (see Figure 23-11, C). The end products of fat digestion are fatty acids and glycerol; fat is absorbed into the lacteals of the villi.

Why is bile necessary for fat digestion (see Figure 23-11, C)? Fats, unlike carbohydrates or proteins, are not soluble in water; they tend to clump together into large fat globules when added to water. If, for example, oil and water are placed in a test tube, the oil and water separate; the oil rises to the surface, and the water

settles at the bottom. Oil and water simply do not mix. The same separation occurs in the digestive tract. Dietary fat tends to form large fat globules. The lipase cannot readily digest the fat; it can attack only the outside surface of the fat globule.

Bile solves the large fat globule problem. Bile can split the large fat globule into thousands of tiny fat globules. This process is **emulsification** (ee-MULL-seh-feh-KAY-shun). Because of emulsification, the lipases can work on the surfaces of all the tiny fat globules, thereby digesting more fat. Bile performs two other important roles. Bile salts prevent the fatty acids (end products of fat digestion) from reforming large fat globules in the intestine before they can be absorbed across the intestinal villi. Bile salts also help the absorption of the fat-soluble vitamins A, D, E, and K.

? Re-Think

1. List the enzymes needed for carbohydrate, protein, and fat digestion.
2. Why does fat digestion require bile whereas carbohydrate and protein digestion do not?
3. Why may a high-fat meal "bother" a person with cholecystitis (inflammation of the gallbladder)?

2+2 Sum It Up!

How is a turkey dinner digested and absorbed (Figure 23-12)?
1. In the mouth, food is chewed into tiny pieces and mixed with saliva.
2. The smaller pieces of food are transported through the esophagus to the stomach, where they are mixed, mashed, and churned into chyme.
3. The partially digested food (chyme) squirts into the duodenum, where it mixes with bile and the pancreatic and intestinal enzymes. Pancreatic amylase and the disaccharidases digest the polysaccharides to monosaccharides. The pancreatic proteases (trypsin and chymotrypsin) and the intestinal proteases digest the proteins to amino acids. A pendulum-like peristaltic motion washes the digested food across each villus, thereby enhancing absorption.
4. The simple sugars and the amino acids are absorbed into the blood capillaries of the villi. These capillaries eventually empty into the portal vein for transport to the liver. Bile emulsifies the fats, and the pancreatic and intestinal lipases digest them. The end products of fat digestion are fatty acids and glycerol. The fat products are absorbed into the lacteals of the villi. Most of the digestion and absorption occurs in the duodenum and the proximal jejunum.
5. The unabsorbed food material continues along the jejunum and ileum and into the large intestine.
6. A large volume of water and certain electrolytes are absorbed along this route, and a semisolid stool is formed.
7. The presence of the fecal material in the rectum gives rise to an urge to defecate.

NUTRITION: CONCEPTS TO KNOW

Nutrition is the science that studies the relationship of food to the functioning of the body. Food consists of

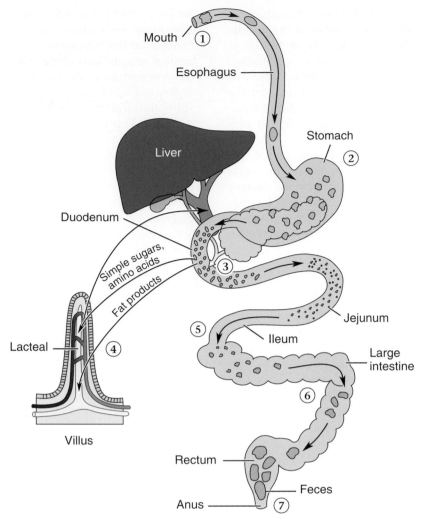

Mouth ①
Esophagus
Stomach ②
Liver
Duodenum
Simple sugars, amino acids
Fat products
③
Jejunum
Lacteal ④
⑤
Ileum
Large intestine
Villus
⑥
Rectum
Feces
Anus ⑦

FIGURE 23-12 Summary: digestion and absorption of the turkey meal.

nutrients, substances the body uses to promote normal growth, maintenance, and repair. The five categories of nutrients are carbohydrates, proteins, lipids, vitamins, and minerals.

CARBOHYDRATES

Dietary carbohydrates are classified as simple sugars and complex carbohydrates. A simple sugar is composed of monosaccharides and disaccharides. Glucose, the simplest carbohydrate, is the major fuel used to make ATP in most body cells. Most of the carbohydrates come from plants. The sugars are derived primarily from fruit, sugar cane, and milk.

The complex carbohydrates are larger sugar molecules (polysaccharides) and consist primarily of starch and fiber. Starch is found in cereal grains (wheat, oats, corn, barley), legumes (peas, beans), and root vegetables, such as potatoes. Fiber, or cellulose, is found primarily in vegetables.

Most dietary carbohydrate should be in the form of complex carbohydrates for two reasons. First, complex carbohydrates usually provide other nutrients, whereas simple sugars provide "empty calories" (nothing but

calories). Second, complex carbohydrates are absorbed at a slower rate than sugars, thereby preventing a sudden spike in blood glucose. The spiking of blood glucose has been linked to an oversecretion of insulin, impaired cellular uptake of glucose, and hypertension. Our excessive intake of corn syrup is fattening us up and raising our blood pressures. Is it also creating a nation of diabetics?

PROTEINS

Dietary proteins supply the body with amino acids. Because the body cannot store amino acids, a daily supply is necessary. Amino acids are classified as essential and nonessential. An essential amino acid cannot be synthesized by the body and must therefore be consumed in the diet. A nonessential amino acid can be synthesized by the body. It is not essential that these amino acids be consumed in the diet. Of the 20 amino acids, 9 are essential.

Proteins are classified as complete or incomplete. A complete protein contains all essential amino acids. Complete proteins are found in animal sources such as meat, eggs, and dairy products. Incomplete proteins do not contain all of the essential amino acids, and these proteins include vegetable proteins such as nuts, grains, and legumes. Vegetable proteins, if eaten in combinations, can supply a complete complement of amino acids. For example, a favorite Mexican dish containing rice and beans is complete in that it supplies all the essential amino acids, even though both the rice and the beans are incomplete proteins.

FATS (LIPIDS)

Most dietary lipids are triglycerides, or molecules that contain glycerol and fatty acids. Fatty acids are classified as saturated or unsaturated. A saturated fatty acid (e.g., butter, lard), which come primarily from animal sources, is solid at room temperature. Also included in this group are artificially hardened, or hydrogenated, fats such as vegetable shortening and margarine. An unsaturated fat is liquid at room temperature and is called an *oil*.

The body can synthesize all fatty acids, with one exception: linoleic acid, an important component of cell membranes. Because the body cannot synthesize it, linoleic acid is an essential fatty acid and therefore must be included in the diet.

Foods high in fat come from both animal and plant sources. Animal sources, however, tend to contain more saturated fat. They include meat, eggs, butter, and whole-milk products such as cheese. Plant sources include coconut oil and palm oil. Hydrogenated vegetable oils in shortening and margarine are also high in saturated fat. In addition to the fat content, these foods also tend to be high in cholesterol.

? Re-Think

1. What is the difference between an essential amino acid and a nonessential amino acid?
2. What is the difference between a complete and incomplete protein?

VITAMINS

Vitamins are small organic molecules that help regulate cell metabolism (Table 23-2). Vitamins are parts of enzymes or other organic substances essential for normal cell function and are classified as fat soluble or water soluble. The fat-soluble vitamins include vitamins A, D, E, and K. Because the body stores fat-soluble vitamins, excess intake may result in symptoms of toxicity (hypervitaminosis).

The water-soluble vitamins include vitamins B and C. These vitamins, for the most part, are not stored by the body. Excess water-soluble vitamins are generally excreted in the urine. Excretion, however, does not rule out the possibility of toxicity in response to megadosing with water-soluble vitamins.

Table 23-2 Selected Vitamins

VITAMIN	FUNCTION	DEFICIENCY
Fat-Soluble Vitamins		
Vitamin A	Necessary for skin, mucous membranes, and night vision	Night blindness; dry, scaly skin; disorders of mucous membranes
Vitamin D (calciferol)	Necessary for the absorption of calcium and phosphorus	Rickets in children; osteomalacia in adults
Vitamin E	Necessary for health of cell membrane	None defined
Vitamin K	Needed for the synthesis of prothrombin and other clotting factors	Bleeding
Water-Soluble Vitamins		
Thiamine (vitamin B_1)	Helps release energy from carbohydrates and amino acids; needed for growth	Beriberi; alcohol-induced Wernicke's syndrome
Riboflavin (vitamin B_2)	Essential for growth	Skin and tongue disorders; dermatitis
Niacin (vitamin B_3)	Helps release energy from nutrients	Pellagra with dermatitis, diarrhea, mental disorders
Pyridoxine (vitamin B_6)	Participates in the metabolism of amino acids and proteins	Nervous system and skin disorders
Vitamin B_{12}	Helps form red blood cells and deoxyribonucleic acid (DNA)	Anemias, particularly pernicious anemia
Folic acid	Participates in the formation of hemoglobin and DNA	Anemia; neural tube defects in embryo
Ascorbic acid (vitamin C)	Necessary for synthesis of collagen; helps maintain capillaries; aids in the absorption of iron	Scurvy; poor bone and wound healing

You can best appreciate the roles vitamins play by observing the effects of specific vitamin deficiencies. For example, vitamin A is necessary for healthy skin and night vision. Vitamin A deficiency is characterized by various skin lesions and by night blindness, or the inability to see in a darkened room. Vitamin D is necessary for the absorption of calcium and the development and formation of strong bones. Vitamin D deficiency causes rickets in children, a condition in which the bones are soft and often bow in response to weight bearing. Because the skin can synthesize vitamin D in response to exposure to ultraviolet radiation, the incidence of rickets is higher in places with little sunlight. Vitamin D deficiency in adults results in a bone-softening condition called *osteomalacia*.

Vitamin K plays a crucial role in hemostasis. It is necessary for the synthesis of prothrombin and several other hepatic clotting factors. A deficiency of vitamin K causes hypoprothrombinemia and a tendency to bleed excessively.

Finally, vitamin C is necessary for the integrity of the skin and mucous membranes. A deficiency of vitamin C causes scurvy, a condition involving skin lesions and inability of the tissues to heal. Historically, scurvy was common on ships that were at sea for months at a time. Having determined that limes prevented scurvy, the British sailors traveled around the world sipping lime juice. In response to this habit, they were dubbed "limeys." Other vitamin deficiencies are included in Table 23-2.

MINERALS

Minerals are inorganic substances necessary for normal body function (Table 23-3). Minerals have numerous functions, ranging from regulation of plasma volume (sodium, chloride) to bone growth (calcium) to oxygen transport (iron) to the regulation of metabolic rate (iodine).

Mineral deficiencies can cause serious health problems. For example, because iodine is necessary for the synthesis of the thyroid hormone thyroxine, iodine deficiency can cause an enlarged thyroid gland (goiter) and hypothyroidism. Because iron is necessary for the synthesis of hemoglobin, iron deficiency can cause anemia. This anemic state is characterized by fatigue and, depending on its severity, a diminished ability to transport oxygen around the body.

HEALTH AND A BALANCED DIET

A BALANCED DIET

A balanced diet contains all the essential nutrients and includes a variety of foods. The balanced diet is often displayed in the form of a food pyramid. The newest food pyramid "personalizes" food intake because it

Table 23-3	Selected Minerals	
MINERAL	**FUNCTION**	**DEFICIENCY**
Potassium (K)	Nerve and muscle activity	Nerve and muscle disorders
Sodium (Na)	Water balance; nerve impulse conduction	Weakness, cramps, diarrhea, dehydration, confusion
Calcium (Ca)	Component of bones and teeth, nerve conduction, muscle contraction, blood clotting	Rickets, tetany, bone softening
Phosphorus (P)	Component of bones and teeth; component of ATP, nucleic acids, and cell membranes	Bone demineralization
Iron (Fe)	Component of hemoglobin (red blood cells)	Anemia, dry skin
Iodine (I)	Necessary for synthesis of thyroid hormones	Hypothyroidism; iodine-deficient goiter
Magnesium (Mg)	Component of some enzymes; important in carbohydrate metabolism	Muscle spasm, dysrhythmias, vasodilation
Fluorine (F)	Component of bones and teeth	Dental caries
Trace minerals	Small amounts required for certain specific functions	Nerve and muscle disorders
• Zinc (Zn)	Nerve and muscle activity	Weakness, cramps, diarrhea, dehydration, confusion
• Copper (Cu)	Activates many enzymes	Loss of structural support resulting from a deficiency of connective tissues in many organs and blood vessels
• Manganese (Mn)	Component of bones and teeth; nerve conduction, muscle contraction, blood clotting	Bone demineralization
• Selenium (Se)	Not determined, plays a significant role in many enzymes, thereby affecting metabolism	Cardiomyopathy; other conditions not yet identified

also considers body build and level of activity. Exercise is a crucial part of the newest pyramid.

POORLY BALANCED DIET AND DISEASE

Many health problems are thought to originate in poor dietary choices. For example, a diet high in cholesterol or fat, or both, has been implicated in coronary artery disease, stroke, diabetes, and cancer.

Although overeating and obesity have been linked with health problems, a number of health problems are also related to a deficiency of certain foods. For example, infants who are fed fat-poor diets (skim milk) may become deficient in fats essential for the development of nervous tissue. Fat deficiency may cause nerve damage and developmental delay. In poverty-stricken areas of the world, protein deficiency diseases are common. Kwashiorkor, for example, is a protein-deficient state in which protein intake is inadequate to synthesize plasma proteins, muscle protein, and proteins necessary for healthy skin.

 Do You Know...

That Kwashiorkor Refers to a "Displaced" Child?

Kwashiorkor is a condition of severe protein deficiency resulting in emaciation, edema formation, and ascites. The African word *kwashiorkor* (displaced or deposed) indicates the cause of the condition. A breast-fed infant is prematurely weaned from breast milk and placed on a protein-poor cereal diet. Why the premature weaning? To make room for baby brother. The 9-month-old infant is displaced or deposed by the newborn.

Malnutrition usually refers to starvation or a profound weight loss caused by a calorie deficiency. Although malnutrition certainly takes this form in countries with limited food supplies, in the United States malnutrition appears most often in the overfed. The American diet and sedentary lifestyle have contributed to obesity, a national health problem. The magnitude of the problem is evident in the numbers of weight-reduction diets. The problem is so common that we now have a common term, *couch potato*, to describe a snack-prone sedentary person, someone who may well be obese.

One form of extreme wasting common in the United States is called *cachexia* (kah-KEK-see-ah). It is most often seen in patients who are terminally ill with cancer and other chronic diseases. The severe anorexia

and altered metabolism cause depletion of fat and protein stores, resulting in dramatic weight loss and starvation.

APPETITE CONTROL AND THE COUCH POTATO

What makes us eat and stop eating? Don't know. We know that the hypothalamus plays an important role. There is an area of the lateral hypothalamus called the *feeding center*. When destroyed, it leads to anorexia and starvation. Another hypothalamic area is called the *satiety center;* damage to it causes overeating and morbid obesity. There are numerous theories about what satisfies (satiety) and therefore suppresses appetite. The glucostat hypothesis states that the satiety center contains neurons called *glucostats* that absorb glucose and send inhibitory information to the feeding center. In response, appetite diminishes. The lipostat hypothesis states that adipocytes (fat cells) secrete an appetite-suppressing hormone called *leptin*. Alas! Couch Potato keeps eating, apparently ignoring the "stop eating" signals from his blitzed hypothalamus.

 Re-Think

List four fat-soluble vitamins and provide a function of each.

BODY ENERGY

Energy is essential for two reasons: (1) it provides the body with the power to do its work, and (2) it maintains body temperature.

MEASUREMENT OF ENERGY

Energy is measured in units called *kilocalories* (kcal), meaning "the large calorie." (A capital **"C"** means a large calorie.) One Calorie is the amount of energy required to raise the temperature of 1 kilogram (kg) of water by 1° Celsius (C). The energy yield of the three food groups—carbohydrates, proteins, and fats—is expressed in calories.

Carbohydrate, 1 g, yields 4 Cal/g
Protein, 1 g, yields 4 Cal/g
Fat, 1 g, yields 9 Cal/g

NOTE: The metabolism of 1 g of fat yields about twice as many calories as the metabolism of 1 g of carbohydrate or protein.

ENERGY BALANCE

Energy balance occurs when the input of energy (food) equals the output of energy (energy expenditure). Energy balance is not always achieved. If food intake exceeds energy expenditure, the excess energy is converted to and stored as fat, causing weight gain. Conversely, if food intake is less than the energy expended, weight loss occurs. Weight management programs therefore encourage both dietary restriction and exercise regimens.

ENERGY EXPENDITURE

Energy expenditure differs depending on whether the body is in a resting or nonresting state. The amount of energy the body requires per unit of time to perform essential activities at rest is the basal metabolic rate (BMR). These activities include breathing, kidney function, cardiac muscle contraction, and whatever minimal functions the body must perform to remain alive.

Several factors affect BMR. These include gender, age, body surface area, emotional state, overall health status, and several hormones. Men have a higher BMR than women. An adolescent has a higher BMR than an older person. A tiny bird has a higher BMR than an elephant. A person livid with rage has a higher metabolism than a peaceful person. A patient with an infection has a higher BMR than an infection-free person. The thyroid hormone thyroxine exerts the most profound effect on BMR. The hyperthyroid patient has a higher BMR than a euthyroid (normal thyroid) person. The metabolism of a hyperthyroid patient can be so high that the patient can consume in excess of 6000 Cal/day and still lose weight. In contrast, the hypothyroid patient has a lower than normal BMR and often consults a physician because of loss of energy and weight gain.

The body needs a certain amount of energy to maintain minimal function but requires additional energy when the person engages in activity above and beyond the resting state. In general, the more active the person is, the higher the metabolic rate and the greater the expenditure of energy.

2+2 Sum It Up!

The body uses food for energy, repair, and maintenance. A balanced diet contains specific amounts and types of nutrients: carbohydrates, proteins, fats, vitamins, and minerals. Failure to ingest certain nutrients causes malnutrition, deficiency states, and illness.

As You Age

1. The muscular wall of the digestive tract loses tone, causing constipation because of a slowing of peristalsis.
2. Secretion of saliva and digestive enzymes decreases, thereby decreasing digestion. The decrease in secretions also impairs the absorption of vitamins (vitamin B_{12}) and minerals (iron and calcium).
3. The sensations of taste and smell diminish with age. Consequently, food tastes different, and appetite may be affected.
4. The loss of teeth and an inability to chew food effectively makes eating difficult. The loss of teeth may also affect the choice of food, causing the older person to select a less nutritious diet such as tea and toast.
5. Peristalsis in the esophagus is no longer triggered with each swallow, and the lower esophageal sphincter relaxes more slowly. These changes hamper swallowing and cause an early feeling of fullness.
6. A weakened gag reflex increases the risk of aspiration.
7. The liver shrinks and receives a smaller supply of blood. The rate of drug detoxification by the liver declines, thereby prolonging the effects of drugs and predisposing the person to a drug overdose. (Remember that the liver is the chief organ of drug inactivation or biotransformation.)

MEDICAL TERMINOLOGY AND DISORDERS | Disorders of the Digestive System

Medical Term	Word Parts	Word Part Meaning or Derivation	Description
Words			
amylase	amyl/o-	starch	An **amylase** is *an enzyme that digests starch, a carbohydrate.* A **lipase** (lip/o- = fat) is *an enzyme that digests fat.* A **protease** is *an enzyme that digests protein.*
	-ase	enzyme	
buccal	bucc/o-	cheek	The **buccal** cavity is located between the teeth and cheeks.
	-al	pertaining to	
colonoscopy	colon/o-	colon, large intestine	A **colonoscopy** is *the visual examination of the colon using a scope.*
	-scopy	examination	
dyspepsia	dys-	difficult or faulty	**Dyspepsia** is *difficult or disturbed digestion.*
	-pepsia	digestion	
gastroenterology	gastr/o-	stomach	**Gastroenterology** is *the study of the digestive tract, made up largely of the stomach and intestines.*
	-enter/o-	intestines	
	-logy	study	
hematemesis	hemat/o-	blood	**Hematemesis** means *the vomiting of blood.*
	-emesis	vomiting	
melena	melan/o-	black	**Melena** *refers to dark-colored stools and is an indication of bleeding within the gastrointestinal tract.*
oral	or/o-	mouth	The **oral** cavity is the mouth. Many drugs are administered orally.
	-al	pertaining to	

MEDICAL TERMINOLOGY AND DISORDERS   Disorders of the Digestive System—cont'd

Medical Term	Word Parts	Word Part Meaning or Derivation	Description
postprandial	post-	after	**Postprandial** means *after a meal*, whereas **preprandial** means *before a meal*.
	-prand(ium)-	From a Latin word meaning "meal"	
	-al	pertaining to	
stomatitis	stomat/o-	mouth	**Stomatitis** means *inflammation of the oral mucosa (mouth).*
	-itis	inflammation	
sublingual	sub-	underneath	*Means underneath the tongue or hypoglossal.* Some drugs are administered **sublingually.**
	-lingul/o-	tongue	
Disorders			
diverticulitis	diverticul/o-	diverticulum	A **diverticulum** is *a sac formed by mucous membrane that herniates through a weakened muscular wall of the colon, especially the sigmoid colon.* **Diverticulitis** refers to *inflammation of the diverticula and surrounding tissue.* **Diverticulosis** refers to *the condition of having diverticula in the colon.*
	-itis	inflammation	
dysentery	dys-	difficult or abnormal	**Dysentery** is *a group of disorders characterized by inflammation of the intestines, especially the large intestine; it is characterized by cramping and the passage of bloody diarrhea.*
	-enter/o-	intestine	
	-ery	pertaining to	
gastroenteritis	gastr/o-	stomach	*Inflammation of the stomach and the intestine.* It can be caused by a variety of pathogens, including viruses, bacteria, and parasites.
	-enter/o-	intestine	
	-itis	inflammation	
gastroparesis	gastr/o-	stomach	**Gastroparesis** is *paralysis of the stomach causing slow gastric emptying and esophageal reflux.*
	-paresis	paralysis	
gastroesophageal reflux disease (GERD)	gastr/o-	stomach	**GERD** *refers to the backflow (reflux) of stomach contents into the esophagus.* Relaxation of the lower esophageal sphincter (LES) commonly occurs with GERD and is thought to be the chief cause of the reflux and heartburn, also known as **pyrosis** (pyr/o- = fire, burning).
	-esophagi/o-	esophagus	
gingivitis	gingiv/o-	gums	*Inflammation of the gums surrounding the teeth.* Gingivitis is a **periodontal disease.**
	-itis	inflammation	
hernia	hernia	Related to two Latin words meaning "rupture" and "intestine"	*A protrusion of an organ or part of an organ out of the cavity in which it is normally contained.* A hernia may be described as **incarcerated** (*the herniated intestine swells and becomes trapped*), **strangulated** (*the herniated intestine is trapped, swollen, and necrotic because its blood supply has been cut off*), **reducible** (*the herniated intestine can be pushed back into its proper cavity*), or **irreducible** (*the herniated intestine is not able to be pushed back into place*). Hernias develop in many different locations. An **inguinal hernia** refers to *the herniation of the intestine in the groin area.* A **femoral hernia** is *the herniation of intestine along a path used by the femoral artery as it leaves the abdomen and enters the thigh.* An **umbilical hernia** is *a herniation of intestine through the abdominal wall surrounding the umbilicus (belly button).* An **incisional hernia** is *the herniation of intestine through a surgically induced weakened abdominal wall.* Organs other than the intestine can herniate. A **hiatal hernia** refers to *the herniation of a part of the stomach into the thoracic cavity. Surgical repair of a hernia is called a* **herniorrhaphy.**

Continued

MEDICAL TERMINOLOGY AND DISORDERS — Disorders of the Digestive System—cont'd

Medical Term	Word Parts	Word Part Meaning or Derivation	Description
inflammatory bowel disease			Abbreviated as **IBD,** but also known as **ileitis** and **enteritis.** The two most common types of IBD are Crohn's disease and ulcerative colitis. **Crohn's disease** is *an inflammatory condition that can affect any part of the GI tract, most commonly the ileum.* **Ulcerative colitis** is *a chronic inflammatory condition that usually affects the inner lining of the colon and rectum.* **Irritable bowel syndrome (IBS)** *refers to periodic episodes of altered bowel function, diarrhea or constipation, and abdominal pain.*
intestinal obstruction			Also called a **bowel obstruction.** It is *a partial or complete blockage of the intestines that prevents the passage of food or fluid.* The obstruction may be mechanical, meaning that something is in the way. The obstruction may also be due to **paralytic ileus,** whereby *the intestinal or bowel muscles do not contract effectively to propel its contents forward.* There are many causes of intestinal obstruction: tumors, twisting, telescoping, hernias, and adhesions. Other conditions include **volvulus,** *a twisted intestine (like a twisted garden hose);* an **intussusception,** *a telescoped intestine;* **hernias,** *"trapped" intestines;* and **adhesions,** *bands of connective tissue that wrap around intestinal organs, such as the intestines, causing occlusion.*
peptic ulcer disease (PUD)			**Peptic ulcer disease (PUD)** *refers to a mucosal erosion (ulcer) in an area of the gastrointestinal tract that has acidic contents.* Most often the cause of PUD is due to *Helicobacter pylori;* the ulcers develop within the duodenum (duodenal ulcer) and/or stomach (gastric ulcer).
Liver, Gallbladder, Pancreas			
cholecystitis	chol/e- -cyst/o- -itis	bile bladder inflammation	*Inflammation of the gallbladder; characterized by nausea, vomiting, and severe RUQ pain that radiates to the right subscapular region.* The pain is called **biliary colic. Cholecystitis** is most often caused by gallstones in the gallbladder, a condition called **cholelithiasis** (chol/e- = bile; -lith/o- = stone). Sometimes the small gallstones escape from the gallbladder and become lodged in the common bile duct, called **choledocholithiasis** (chol/e- = bile; -doch/o- = duct; -lith/o- = stone), causing inflammation of the bile ducts, or **cholangitis** (chol/e- = bile; -angio- = vessel; -itis = inflammation), biliary obstruction, hyperbilirubinemia, and jaundice.
cirrhosis of the liver	cirrh- -osis	From the Greek word *kirrhos,* meaning "tawny" condition	*Scarring of the liver in response to repeated destruction and regeneration of the liver cells.* Despite hepatic regeneration, the architecture of the liver is altered so as to impair hepatic function and blood flow. Because of the obstruction of blood flow, blood bypasses the liver, eventually causing **hepatic encephalopathy.** Obstruction of blood flow also increases portal vein pressure, causing **portal vein hypertension,** which in turn causes ascites and esophageal varices.
hepatitis	hepat/o- -itis	liver inflammation	*An inflammation of the liver, usually caused by viral infection.* (There are nonviral causes of hepatitis.) There are five main types: A, B, C, D, and E. Hepatitis X is hepatitis caused by an unidentified virus. Hepatitis A and E are commonly transmitted by contaminated food or water. Hepatitis B and D are transmitted by contact with body fluids. Hepatitis C is transmitted by contact with contaminated blood and increases the patient's risk for cancer of the liver.
pancreatitis	pancreat/o- -itis	pancreas inflammation	**Pancreatitis** is *inflammation of the pancreas.* Approximately 70% of cases are caused by excess alcohol ingestion. **Acute pancreatitis** is *an emergency condition with severe abdominal pain as the most common symptom.* **Chronic pancreatitis** may persist for many years.

Get Ready for Exams!

Summary Outline

I. Overview of the Digestive System
A. Functions of the digestive system
1. Ingestion (eating)
2. Digestion
3. Absorption
4. Elimination
B. The wall of the digestive tract and membranes
1. Four layers: mucosa, submucosa, muscle, and serosa
2. Peritoneal membranes: mesentery, mesocolon, and greater and lesser omentum

II. Structures and Organs of the Digestive System
A. Mouth
1. Teeth and tongue
2. Salivary glands
   a. Parotid, submandibular, and sublingual glands
   b. Secretes saliva
B. Pharynx (oropharynx and laryngopharynx)
C. Esophagus
1. The esophagus is a long tube that connects the pharynx to the stomach.
2. There are two sphincters: pharyngoesophageal and LES.
D. Stomach
1. The three parts of the stomach are the fundus, body, and pylorus.
2. The stomach functions in digestion; its most important role is to regulate the rate at which chyme is delivered to the small intestine.
3. It secretes hormones, few digestive enzymes, HCl, and intrinsic factor.
E. Small intestine
1. The three segments of the small intestine are the duodenum, jejunum, and ileum.
2. Most of the digestion and absorption occurs within the duodenum and first third of the jejunum.
3. The end products of digestion are absorbed into villi (capillaries and lacteal).
4. The common bile duct enters the small intestine at the duodenum.
F. Large intestine
1. The large intestine consists of the cecum, ascending colon, transverse colon, descending colon, sigmoid colon, rectum, and anus.
2. The large intestine functions in absorption of water and electrolytes.

III. Accessory Digestive Organs
A. Liver
1. The liver has many functions; its most important digestive function is the secretion of bile.
2. The liver receives most of its blood from the portal vein; portal blood is rich in digestive end products.
3. The arterial blood is delivered by the hepatic artery (from the celiac trunk).
B. Biliary tree
1. The biliary tree is composed of the bile ducts that connect the liver, gallbladder, and duodenum.
2. The bile ducts are the hepatic ducts, cystic duct, and common bile duct.
3. The common bile duct empties into the duodenum.
C. Gallbladder
1. The gallbladder functions to store and concentrate bile.
2. The gallbladder contracts and releases bile into the bile ducts in response to the hormone cholecystokinin (CCK).
D. Pancreas
1. The pancreas secretes the most important digestive enzymes.
2. The pancreatic enzymes empty into the base of the common bile duct and then into the duodenum.
3. The pancreas is responsive to both cholecystokinin and secretin.

IV. Digestion and Absorption
A. Carbohydrate digestion
1. To be absorbed, carbohydrates must be broken down into monosaccharides, especially glucose.
2. Carbohydrates are digested by enzymes called *amylases* and *disaccharidases*.
B. Protein digestion
1. To be absorbed, proteins must be broken down into small peptides and amino acids.
2. Proteins are broken down by proteolytic enzymes or proteases.
C. Fat digestion
1. To be absorbed, fats must be broken down into fatty acids and glycerol.
2. Fats are emulsified by bile and then digested by enzymes called *lipases*.

V. Nutrition and Body Energy
A. Carbohydrates
1. Carbohydrates are simple or complex.
2. Glucose, the simplest carbohydrate, is the major fuel used by the body for energy.
B. Protein
1. The body needs essential amino acids, which it cannot synthesize, and nonessential amino acids, which it can synthesize.
2. Dietary proteins are complete or incomplete.
C. Fats (lipids)
1. Most dietary lipids are triglycerides.
2. Fats are saturated fats (like butter) or unsaturated fats (like oils).
D. Vitamins
1. Vitamins are small organic molecules that help regulate cell metabolism. Dietary vitamin deficiencies give rise to many diseases (see Table 23-2).
2. Vitamins are water soluble (vitamins B and C) or fat soluble (vitamins A, D, E, and K).
E. Minerals
1. Minerals are inorganic substances necessary for normal body function.
2. Mineral deficiencies can cause serious health problems (see Table 23-3).

F. Body Energy
   1. The body needs energy to do its work and maintain body temperature.
   2. The basal metabolic rate (BMR) is the amount of energy the body requires per unit of time to perform essential activities at rest.
   3. Metabolism is determined by many factors, including age, gender, surface area, emotional state, overall health status, and hormones, especially thyroxine.

Review Your Knowledge

Matching: Structures: Making the Connections

Directions: Match the following words with their description below.

a. ileum
b. sigmoid colon
c. jejunum
d. common bile duct
e. transverse colon
f. duodenum
g. esophagus
h. stomach

1. ___ Connects the duodenum to the ileum
2. ___ Connects the cystic and hepatic ducts to the duodenum
3. ___ Connects the rectum to the descending colon
4. ___ Connects the ascending colon to the descending colon
5. ___ Connects the esophagus to the duodenum
6. ___ Connects the pharynx to the stomach
7. ___ Connects the stomach to the jejunum
8. ___ Connects the jejunum to the cecum

Matching: Enzymes, Hormones, and Digestive Aids

Directions: Match the following words with their description below. Some words may be used more than once.

a. amylases
b. hydrochloric acid
c. disaccharidases
d. secretin
e. bile
f. proteases
g. cholecystokinin (CCK)
h. intrinsic factor
i. lipase

1. ___ Classification of trypsin and chymotrypsin
2. ___ Secreted by the parietal cells of the stomach; lowers gastric pH
3. ___ Digests sucrose, maltose, and lactose
4. ___ An emulsifying agent
5. ___ Digests fats to fatty acids and glycerol
6. ___ Hormone secreted by the duodenum in response to the presence of fat
7. ___ Digest starch and polysaccharides to disaccharides
8. ___ Hormone that stimulates the pancreas to secrete a bicarbonate-rich secretion
9. ___ Hormone that stimulates the gallbladder to contract
10. ___ Digests protein to small peptides and amino acids
11. ___ Secreted by the liver and stored in the gallbladder
12. ___ Necessary for the absorption of vitamin B_{12}
13. ___ Classification of sucrase, maltase, and lactase

Multiple Choice

1. The esophagus
   a. secretes potent proteolytic enzymes.
   b. secretes intrinsic factor that is necessary for the absorption of vitamin B_{12}.
   c. is a hollow tube that carries food from the pharynx to the stomach.
   d. is the primary site of digestion and absorption.

2. Which of the following is true regarding the stomach?
   a. Its most important function is the digestion of fat.
   b. It is lined with microvilli to maximize absorption.
   c. It is attached distally to the jejunum and proximally to the esophagus.
   d. Its most important function is to deliver chyme to the duodenum at the proper rate.

3. Which of the following is not descriptive of bile?
   a. Aids in fat digestion
   b. Is an emulsifying agent
   c. Is classified as a lipase
   d. Is stored by the gallbladder

4. Lipases, proteases, and amylases are
   a. gastric hormones.
   b. synthesized by the liver and stored in the gallbladder.
   c. digestive enzymes.
   d. bile-dependent digestive enzymes.

5. Which of the following is not a function of the liver?
   a. Makes blood-clotting factors such as prothrombin
   b. Makes bile
   c. Secretes cholecystokinin and secretin
   d. Stores fat-soluble vitamins

6. Which of the following best describes emulsification?
   a. A fat is chemically digested to fatty acids and glycerol.
   b. The fatty acids are absorbed into the lacteal, becoming chyle.
   c. A large fat globule is mechanically broken into smaller fat globules.
   d. A large protein forms ammonia.

7. The pancreas
   a. secretes the most potent digestive enzymes.
   b. secretes CCK and secretin.
   c. is only important because of its endocrine (insulin) function.
   d. empties its digestive enzymes into the appendix.

8. The duodenum is most concerned with
   a. the secretion of intrinsic factor and the absorption of vitamin B_{12}.
   b. digestion and absorption.
   c. the synthesis of clotting factors and plasma proteins.
   d. the synthesis of bile and emulsification.

9. Which of the following is true of trypsinogen, chymotrypsinogen, and pepsinogen?
   a. They are secreted by the gastric lining.
   b. They are inactive proteases.
   c. They are pancreatic lipases.
   d. They are emulsifying agents.
10. Gastrin, cholecystokinin (CCK), and secretin are
   a. secretions of the salivary glands.
   b. digestive enzymes.
   c. emulsifying agents.
   d. gastrointestinal hormones.

Go Figure

1. **According to Figure 23-1**
   a. All GI structures are located in the abdominopelvic cavity.
   b. The esophagus descends through the thoracic cavity.
   c. The small intestine is distal to the large intestine.
   d. The liver and pancreas empty their contents into the digestive tract at a point that is proximal to the stomach.

2. **According to Figure 23-2**
   a. The inner lining of the GI tract is composed of smooth muscle.
   b. GI smooth muscle is well innervated.
   c. The mesentery forms the inner lining of the GI tract.
   d. The nervous innervation of the GI is referred to as the *mesentery*.

3. **According to Figure 23-3**
   a. The salivary glands are endocrine glands.
   b. The secretions of the parotid, submandibular, and sublingual glands are carried to the mouth by salivary ducts.
   c. In a healthy tooth, enamel, gingiva, and dentin are visible.
   d. The uvula is the same as the adenoids (pharyngeal tonsils).

4. **According to Figure 23-5**
   a. The LES is distal to both the cardiac and the pyloric sphincters.
   b. The pyloric valve is distal to both the duodenum and the LES.
   c. Gastric contents can reflux from the stomach through the LES and into the base of the esophagus.
   d. With the exception of the sphincters, the stomach wall has no muscle.

5. **According to Figure 23-5**
   a. Parietal cells are located in the stomach lining.
   b. Chief cells secrete HCl and intrinsic factor.
   c. Rugae are found only within the pylorus.
   d. The greater curvature is a gastric structure and the lesser curvature is a duodenal structure.

6. **According to Figure 23-6**
   a. A hiatal hernia is located in the same general area as an inguinal hernia.
   b. Some drugs block vagal stimulation of the stomach.
   c. A pyloric valve stenosis impairs delivery of food from the duodenum to the stomach.
   d. Insertion of a nasogastric tube involves the surgical insertion of a tube through the abdominal wall into the stomach (for feeding purposes).

7. **According to Figure 23-7**
   a. Each villus contains capillaries that all empty into a lacteal.
   b. Villi are widely spread throughout the entire GI tract.
   c. Villi are found only in the stomach.
   d. Villi form the brush border of the small intestine.

8. **According to Figure 23-9**
   a. Both the common bile duct and the main pancreatic duct drain into the duodenum.
   b. The gallbladder ejects bile into the hepatic ducts where it is returned to the liver.
   c. The tail of the pancreas is closer to the ampulla of Vater than is the head of the pancreas.
   d. The green vessels in Figure 23-9, *B,* carry blood from the portal vein to the hepatic veins.

9. **According to Figure 23-11**
   a. Amylases digest disaccharides into monosaccharides.
   b. Lipases digest sucrose, lactose, and maltose into glucose, fructose, and galactose.
   c. Lipases emulsify fats.
   d. Bile breaks down large fat globules into smaller fat globules.

Key Terms

Objectives

1. List four organs of excretion.
2. Describe the major organs of the urinary system.
3. Describe the location, structure, blood supply, nerve supply, and functions of the kidneys.
4. Explain the role of the nephron unit in the formation of urine.
5. Explain the three processes involved in the formation of urine: filtration, reabsorption, and secretion.

6. Describe the hormonal control of water and electrolytes by the kidneys.
7. List the normal constituents of urine.
8. Describe the structure and function of the ureters, urinary bladder, and urethra.

Sammy with his soggy diaper is a friendly reminder of our hard-working urinary system. Sammy may be a bundle of joy, but he is generally a wet bundle. What makes Sammy wet? Like a round-the-clock factory, Sammy's body burns fuel and produces waste products. To remain healthy, his kidneys must remove the waste and constantly adjust the amount of water and the concentration of electrolytes in his body. The kidneys work hard to do this; a wet Sammy is a healthy Sammy.

EXCRETION

ORGANS OF EXCRETION

The kidneys are the most important excretory organs. They eliminate nitrogenous waste, water, electrolytes, toxins, and drugs. Other organs perform excretory functions; the sweat glands secrete small amounts of nitrogen compounds, water, and electrolytes; the lungs eliminate carbon dioxide and water; and the intestines excrete digestive wastes, bile pigments, and other minerals (Table 24-1). Whereas the skin, lungs, and intestines eliminate waste, only the kidneys can fine-tune the excretion of water and electrolytes to maintain the normal volume and composition of body fluids.

URINARY SYSTEM ORGANS

The urinary system, shown in Figure 24-1, makes urine, temporarily stores it, and finally eliminates it from the body. The major organs of the urinary system include the following:

- *Two kidneys.* The kidneys form urine from the blood.
- *Two ureters.* The ureters (YOOR-eh-ters) are tubes that conduct urine from the kidneys to the urinary bladder.

Table **24-1**	Organs of Excretion
ORGAN	**SUBSTANCES EXCRETED**
Kidneys	Water Electrolytes Nitrogenous waste
Skin (sweat glands)	Water Electrolytes Nitrogenous waste
Lungs	Carbon dioxide Water
Intestines	Digestive waste (feces) Bile pigments

- *One urinary bladder.* The **urinary bladder** acts as a temporary reservoir; it receives urine from the ureters and stores the urine until it can be eliminated.
- *One urethra.* The **urethra** (yoo-REE-thrah) is a tube that conducts urine from the bladder to the outside for elimination. (Do not confuse the ureters with the urethra.)

URINARY SYSTEM TERMS

There are several words that refer to the urinary system and specifically to the kidneys. The word *renal* refers to the kidney. Thus, *renal physiology* refers to the study of kidney function. *Nephrology* also refers to the study of kidney function. The term comes from the nephron unit—the unit in the kidney that makes urine. *Urology* is the study of the urinary system.

KIDNEYS

LOCATION

The kidneys are located high on the posterior wall of the abdominal cavity, behind the parietal peritoneum (retroperitoneal; see Figure 24-1, *A*). The kidneys are cushioned and protected by the renal fascia, adipose tissue pads, and lower rib cage.

 Do You Know...

What a Floating Kidney Is?

The kidney is normally held in position by connective and adipose tissue. A very thin person has little adipose tissue, so the kidney is more loosely attached to surrounding structures and may move about, or float. As you might expect, the floating kidney has a fancy medical name: nephroptosis. The downward displacement of the kidney causes the ureter to kink, thereby restricting the flow of urine.

STRUCTURE

The kidney is a reddish-brown, beanlike structure enclosed in a tough fibrous capsule. Each kidney is about 4 inches (10 cm) long, 2 inches (5 cm) wide, and 1 inch (2.5 cm) thick. The indentation of the bean-shaped kidney is called the *hilus.* It is the point at which the blood vessels, ureter, and nerves enter and exit the kidney.

What do you see when you cut open a kidney? As shown in Figure 24-1, *B,* a kidney has three distinct regions: the renal cortex, the renal medulla, and the renal pelvis. The lighter, outer region is the renal cortex. The darker triangular structure, the renal medulla, is located deeper within the kidney. The renal medulla forms striped, cone-shaped regions called *renal pyramids.* Each pyramid is separated by a renal column, an extension of the outer renal cortex. The lower ends of the pyramids point toward the renal pelvis, a basin that collects the urine made by the kidney and helps form the upper end of the ureter. The cuplike edges of the renal pelvis, closest to the pyramids, are calyces. Calyces (KAY-liss-ees) (sing., calyx) collect the urine formed in the kidney.

BLOOD SUPPLY

Blood is brought to the kidney by the **renal artery,** which arises from the abdominal aorta (see Figure 24-1, *B*). The renal arteries deliver a large amount of blood (about 20% to 25% of the cardiac output) to the kidneys. After entering the kidney, the renal artery branches into a series of smaller and smaller arteries, which deliver blood to the nephron units, the urine-making structures of the kidney. Blood leaves the kidney through a series of veins that finally merge to form the **renal vein.** The renal vein empties into the inferior vena cava.

NERVE SUPPLY

The renal nerves travel with the renal blood vessels to the kidney. The nerves are primarily sympathetic nerves that help control blood flow to the kidney and regulate the release of a blood pressure–regulating enzyme.

? **Re-Think**

1. List the major organs of the urinary system.
2. Explain why a physician may thump a patient in the upper left and right lumbar areas when assessing for evidence of a kidney infection.

FUNCTIONS OF THE KIDNEYS

In general, the kidneys cleanse the blood of waste products, help regulate the volume and composition

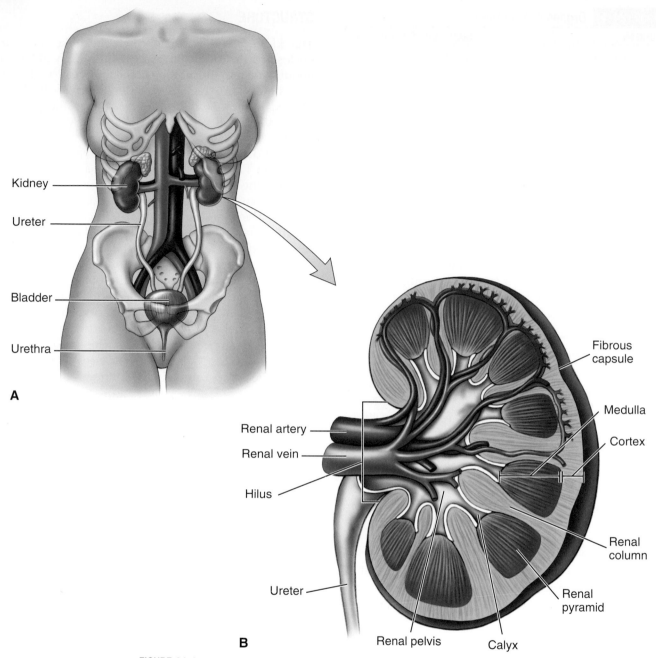

Kidney

Ureter

Bladder

Urethra

A

Renal artery

Renal vein

Hilus

Ureter

B

Fibrous capsule

Medulla

Cortex

Renal column

Renal pyramid

Renal pelvis

Calyx

FIGURE 24-1 **A,** Organs of the urinary system. **B,** Internal structure of a kidney.

of body fluids, and help regulate the pH of body fluids. Specifically, the kidneys perform the following tasks:

- Excrete nitrogenous waste such as urea, uric acid, ammonia, and creatinine
- Regulate blood volume by determining the amount of water excreted
- Help regulate the electrolyte content of the blood
- Play a major role in the regulation of acid–base balance (blood pH) by controlling the excretion of hydrogen ions (H^+). (See Chapter 25 for the renal regulation of acid–base balance.)
- Play a role in the long-term regulation of blood pressure

- Play a role in the regulation of red blood cell production through the secretion of erythropoietin

URINE MAKING: THE NEPHRON UNIT

STRUCTURES

The **nephron unit** is the functional unit, or urine-making unit, of the kidney. Each kidney contains about 1 million nephron units. The number of nephron units does not increase after birth, and they cannot be replaced if damaged. Each nephron unit has two parts: a tubular component (renal tubules) and a vascular component (blood vessels).

RENAL TUBULES

The renal tubules consist of a number of tubular structures. The glomerular capsule, called *Bowman's capsule,* is a C-shaped structure that partially surrounds a cluster of filtering capillaries called a glomerulus (gloh-MAIR-yoo-lus). Note that Figure 24-2 shows two views of a nephron unit: an anatomical view and a schematic view. You should become familiar with both.

Bowman's capsule extends from the glomerulus as a highly coiled tubule called the *proximal convoluted tubule.* The proximal convoluted tubule dips toward the renal pelvis to form a hairpin-shaped structure called the *loop of Henle.* The loop of Henle (HEN-lee) contains a descending and ascending limb. The ascending limb becomes the distal convoluted tubule. The distal convoluted tubules of several nephron units empty into a collecting duct. The collecting ducts run through the renal medulla to the calyx of the renal pelvis. Urine is formed in these tubules.

RENAL BLOOD VESSELS (VASCULAR STRUCTURES)

The kidney receives blood from the renal artery. The renal artery branches into smaller blood vessels that eventually form the afferent arteriole. The afferent arteriole branches into a cluster, or tuft, of capillaries called a *glomerulus* (as described in the previous section). The glomerulus sits in Bowman's capsule and exits from Bowman's capsule as the efferent arteriole. The efferent arteriole then forms a second capillary network called the peritubular capillaries. The peritubular capillaries surround the renal tubule and empty into the venules, larger veins and, finally, into the renal vein. (You need to understand the relationships of the vascular structures to the tubular structures. Become thoroughly familiar with Figure 24-2.)

? Re-Think

1. List all tubular structures as you trace a drop of urine from Bowman's capsule to the renal pelvis.
2. List all vascular structures as you trace a drop of blood from the renal artery to the renal vein.

URINE FORMATION

Urine is formed in the nephron units as water and dissolved substances move between the vascular and tubular structures. Identify all structures in Figure 24-2 as urine formation is described. Three processes are involved in the formation of urine: glomerular filtration, tubular reabsorption, and tubular secretion.

GLOMERULAR FILTRATION

Urine formation begins in the glomerulus and Bowman's capsule. Glomerular filtration causes water and dissolved substances to move from the glomerulus into Bowman's capsule. Understanding filtration means answering two questions: Why does filtration occur, and what substances are filtered across the glomerular membrane?

Why Filtration Occurs

Filtration occurs when the pressure on one side of a membrane is greater than the pressure on the opposite side. Blood pressure in the glomerulus is higher than the pressure in Bowman's capsule. This pressure difference provides the driving force for filtration. This pressure difference is called the *glomerular filtration pressure.* If blood pressure suddenly declines, as in shock, glomerular filtration pressure decreases, thereby reducing urinary output.

What Substances Are Filtered

The wall of the glomerulus contains pores and acts like a sieve or a strainer. The size of the pores determines which substances can move across the wall from the glomerulus into Bowman's capsule. Small substances such as water, sodium, potassium, chloride, glucose, uric acid, and creatinine move through the pores very easily. These substances are filtered in proportion to their plasma concentration. In other words, if the concentration of a particular substance in the plasma is high, much of that substance is filtered. Large molecules such as red blood cells and large proteins cannot fit through the pores and therefore remain within the glomerulus. The water and the dissolved substances filtered into Bowman's capsule are called the *glomerular filtrate.* Note that the glomerular filtrate is protein-free (called an *ultrafiltrate*); the presence of protein (proteinuria) in the urine indicates abnormally large holes in the glomerulus. The protein that is most often found in the urine is albumin (albuminuria).

The rate at which glomerular filtration occurs is called the *glomerular filtration rate* (GFR). Here is the amazing thing about GFR—the amount of filtrate formed is 125 mL/min, or 180 L (45 gallons) in 24 hours. Imagine 180 1-L bottles of cola. This is the amount of filtrate formed by your kidneys in 1 day. Obviously, you do not excrete 180 L of urine every day; otherwise, you would do little more than drink and urinate, and you would literally wash away within a few hours. You excrete only about 1.5 L each day, so the big question is what happens to the 178.5 L that are filtered into the tubules but not excreted as urine?

? Re-Think

1. Why does filtration occur across the glomerular membrane?
2. Why isn't protein (albumin) normally filtered across the glomerular membrane?
3. What happens to GFR if blood pressure declines to shock levels (70/40 mm Hg)? Explain why a patient in shock is usually oliguric.

FIGURE 24-2 The nephron unit: tubular and vascular structures.

TUBULAR REABSORPTION

Most of the filtrate, approximately 178.5 L, is reabsorbed in the kidney and returned to the circulation. Tubular reabsorption is the process whereby water and dissolved substances (glomerular filtrate) move from the tubules into the blood of the peritubular capillaries. Although reabsorption occurs throughout the entire length of the renal tubule, most occurs across the proximal convoluted tubule.

What is reabsorbed into the blood, and what is excreted into the urine? The kidney chooses the type and quantity of substances it reabsorbs. Some substances, such as glucose, are completely reabsorbed. For example, the amount of glucose filtered is the same as the amount reabsorbed, so glucose normally does not appear in the urine. In hyperglycemic conditions, however, excess glucose is filtered; the amount of filtered glucose exceeds the reabsorptive capacity of the tubules. The excess glucose therefore appears in the urine (glucosuria). Some substances are incompletely reabsorbed. For example, over 99% of water and sodium is reabsorbed, whereas only 50% of urea is reabsorbed. Some waste products such as **creatinine** (kree-AT-i-nin) are not reabsorbed at all. Those substances that are not reabsorbed remain in the tubules and become part of the urine.

 Do You Know...

Why Serum Creatinine Is a Measure of Kidney Function?

Creatinine is a waste product removed from the blood by the kidneys and eliminated in the urine. If kidney function declines, creatinine accumulates in the plasma. An increase in serum creatinine indicates that the kidneys are not able to excrete it. Thus, serum creatinine levels are used to monitor kidney function.

The reabsorption of substances by the kidney also varies with the mechanism of reabsorption. Absorption occurs through active or passive transport. For example, sodium is actively transported from the tubules into the peritubular capillaries. Water and chloride passively follow the movement of sodium. In general, when sodium is pumped from one location to another, water and chloride follow passively. This sequence is the basis for the action of most diuretics, drugs that increase the production of urine. Most diuretics block the tubular reabsorption of sodium and therefore also block the reabsorption of water. The excess sodium and water remain in the tubules and are eliminated as urine. The excess secretion of urine is called **diuresis** (dye-yoo-REE-sis). Hormones regulate the reabsorption of some substances; these hormones are described later in this chapter.

TUBULAR SECRETION

Although most of the water and dissolved substances enter the tubules because of filtration across the glomerulus, a second process moves very small amounts of select substances from the blood into the tubules. This process is tubular secretion. It involves the active transport of potassium ions (K^+), hydrogen ions (H^+), uric acid, ammonium ions (NH_4^+), and drugs from the peritubular capillaries into the tubules.

2+2 Sum It Up!

The urinary system is composed of the urine-making kidneys and the structures that transport, store, and eliminate urine from the body. The urine is made by the nephron units, the functional units of the kidney. Urine is formed by three processes: filtration, reabsorption, and secretion. Filtration causes water and dissolved substances to move from the glomeruli into the tubules. Reabsorption causes water and selected substances to move from the tubules into the peritubular capillaries. Secretion causes small amounts of specific substances to move from the peritubular capillaries into the tubules.

? Re-Think

Identify the specific vascular and tubular structures involved in filtration, reabsorption, and secretion.

HORMONES THAT WORK ON THE KIDNEYS

Several hormones act on the kidney to regulate water and electrolyte excretion. Thus, these hormones play an important role in the regulation of blood volume, blood pressure, and electrolyte composition of body fluids (Table 24-2).

ALDOSTERONE

Aldosterone is a hormone secreted by the adrenal cortex. Aldosterone acts primarily on the distal tubule and upper collecting duct of the nephron unit. It stimulates the reabsorption of sodium and water and the excretion of potassium. Because of its effect on Na^+, aldosterone is called the "salt-retaining" (NaCl) hormone. Because aldosterone increases Na^+ and water reabsorption, it expands or increases blood volume. The expanded blood volume, in turn, increases blood pressure. A deficiency of aldosterone causes severely diminished blood volume, decline in blood pressure, and shock.

What causes the release of aldosterone? One of the most important stimuli for the release of aldosterone is **renin**. Renin is an enzyme that activates the renin-angiotensin-aldosterone system. Renin is secreted by a specialized collection of cells called the **juxtaglomerular apparatus**, located in the afferent arterioles of the kidney. The renin-secreting cells are stimulated when blood pressure or blood volume declines. As Figure 24-3 shows, renin sets off the following series of events:

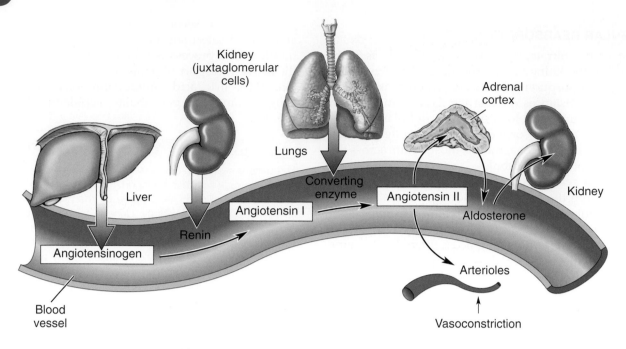

FIGURE 24-3 The renin-angiotensin-aldosterone system.

- Renin activates angiotensinogen (an-jee-oh-ten-SIN-oh-jen) to form angiotensin I. Angiotensinogen is secreted by the liver and circulates within the blood; angiotensinogen is inactive.
- An enzyme called *converting enzyme* changes angiotensin I to angiotensin II. (Converting enzyme is found in the blood throughout the body but is in particularly high concentration in the lungs.)
- Angiotensin II stimulates the adrenal cortex to release aldosterone. The aldosterone, in turn, stimulates the distal tubule to reabsorb sodium and water and to excrete potassium. The increased blood volume increases blood pressure.
- In addition to stimulating the release of aldosterone, angiotensin II is also a potent vasopressor (a blood pressure–elevating agent). Thus, the activation of the renin-angiotensin-aldosterone system regulates blood volume and blood pressure. A class of drugs called *angiotensin-converting enzyme* (ACE) *inhibitors* is used to lower blood pressure. They prevent the production of angiotensin II and aldosterone, both of which increase blood pressure. ACE inhibitors include the *-pril* drugs, such as lisinopril and captopril.

 Re-Think

If a patient takes a drug that blocks the production of aldosterone, why must he or she be monitored for hydration status, serum Na⁺ (hyponatremia), and serum K⁺ (hyperkalemia)?

ANTIDIURETIC HORMONE

A second hormone affecting water reabsorption is **antidiuretic hormone (ADH)**. The action of ADH allows the kidneys to concentrate urine. (Think of the term *antidiuretic hormone*. It literally means "against diuresis.") The posterior pituitary gland (neurohypophysis) secretes ADH.

Antidiuretic hormone works primarily on the collecting duct of the nephron unit by determining its permeability to water. In the presence of ADH, the collecting duct becomes permeable to water. Water is reabsorbed from the collecting duct into the peritubular capillaries. In other words, ADH decreases the excretion of water and causes excretion of a concentrated urine. In the absence of ADH, the membrane permeability of the collecting duct decreases and water cannot be reabsorbed; the result is excretion of a dilute urine. Because ADH affects the amount of water excreted by the kidneys, it plays an important role in the determination of blood volume and blood pressure. Excess ADH expands blood volume, whereas a deficiency of ADH diminishes blood volume.

Do You Know...

Why Both Diabetes Mellitus and Diabetes Insipidus Cause Polyuria?

Diabetes mellitus is a disease of insulin deficiency that results in hyperglycemia. The hyperglycemia, in turn, leads to excess filtration of glucose by the kidneys. Because all the filtered glucose cannot be reabsorbed, glucosuria develops. The excess glucose in the tubules requires the excretion of large amounts of water. Thus, the person with diabetes mellitus experiences polyuria (*poly-* means much; *-uria* means urine). Diabetes insipidus is a disease of ADH deficiency. ADH is necessary for the reabsorption of water from the collecting duct. In the absence of ADH, the person may excrete up to 25 L of a pale dilute urine. Note that both diabetes mellitus and diabetes insipidus are characterized by polyuria. The word *diabetes* refers to diuresis.

Table 24-2	Effects of Hormones on the Kidney	
HORMONE	**SECRETED BY**	**FUNCTION(S)**
Aldosterone	Adrenal cortex	Stimulates the reabsorption of sodium and water; stimulates the excretion of potassium; acts primarily on the distal tubule
Atrial natriuretic peptide (ANP)	Atria of the heart	Decreases the reabsorption of sodium; causes greater excretion of sodium and water by the kidney
Brain natriuretic peptide (BNP)	Ventricles of the heart	Decreases the reabsorption of sodium; causes greater excretion of sodium and water by the kidney; acts as a biological marker for heart failure
Antidiuretic hormone (ADH)	Neurohypophysis (posterior pituitary)	Stimulates the reabsorption of water, primarily by the collecting ducts
Parathyroid hormone (PTH)	Parathyroid gland	Stimulates the reabsorption of calcium and excretion of phosphate

The stimulus for the release of ADH is decreased blood volume and a concentrated plasma. Consider a person who becomes dehydrated by vomiting. The person loses large amounts of water and electrolytes. When the volume of blood decreases and the concentration of the blood increases, ADH is released. The ADH increases the reabsorption of water by the kidneys, expanding blood volume and diluting the blood. The increased blood volume eventually stops the stimulus for the release of ADH.

Disturbances of ADH secretion are common. The hypersecretion of ADH is associated with many clinical conditions. Head injuries are a common cause of the syndrome of inappropriate ADH release. Excess ADH increases the reabsorption of water and an expansion of the blood volume. Diluted blood can cause serious CNS effects such as seizures. Hyposecretion of ADH causes diabetes insipidus, a condition characterized by the excretion of a large volume of pale dilute urine.

? Re-Think

Give two reasons for the secretion of ADH in the dehydrated state.

NATRIURETIC PEPTIDES

Atrial natriuretic (nay-tree-yoo-RET-ik) peptide (ANP) and brain natriuretic peptide (BNP) cause excretion of sodium (Na^+), a process called **natriuresis** (nat-ree-yoo-REE-sis). ANP is secreted by the walls of the atria of the heart in response to an increase in the volume of blood. BNP is secreted by the walls of the ventricles in response to elevated ventricular volume. ANP and BNP decrease the secretion of aldosterone by the adrenal cortex. The effect is decreased sodium and water reabsorption. The effects of the **natriuretic peptides** are opposite of the effects of aldosterone and ADH. Since ventricular blood volume increases in the failing heart, BNP is used diagnostically in the assessment of heart failure.

PARATHYROID HORMONE

Parathyroid hormone (PTH) is secreted by the parathyroid glands. It does not affect water balance but plays an important role in the regulation of two electrolytes: calcium and phosphate. PTH stimulates the renal tubules to reabsorb calcium and excrete phosphate. The excretion of phosphate is called the *phosphaturic effect* of PTH. The primary stimulus for the release of PTH is a low plasma level of calcium (review Chapter 14 for a detailed description of PTH).

COMPOSITION OF URINE

Finally, we can answer this question. What is in urine? Urine is a sterile fluid composed mostly of water (95%), nitrogen-containing waste, and electrolytes. Important nitrogenous waste includes urea, uric acid, ammonia, and creatinine. The light yellow color of urine is caused by a pigment called *urochrome*, formed from the breakdown of hemoglobin in the liver. The average output of urine is 1500 mL/day. The term *oliguria* (*oligo-* means "scanty") refers to a urine output of less than 400 mL/day. Table 24-3 summarizes the composition of urine along with the significance of some abnormal constituents.

What is meant by the specific gravity of urine? **Specific gravity** is the ratio of the amount of solute to volume. The specific gravity of urine ranges from 1.001 to 1.035, depending on the amount of solute (substances such as Na^+ and creatinine) in the urine. The more solute, the higher is the specific gravity. If a patient is dehydrated, the kidneys filter less water; as a result, the volume of urine decreases. The ratio of solute to volume in the urine therefore increases. Thus, dehydration is characterized by an increase in **urinary specific gravity**. Very dilute urine, as in blood volume expansion, has a low specific gravity.

Regarding odor—it's not too bad if fresh. However, over time, bacteria degrade the urea to ammonia. That explains the "diaper pail" odor. Similarly, a bladder

Table 24-3 **Characteristics of Urine**

CHARACTERISTIC	DESCRIPTION
Amount (volume)	Average 1500 mL/day
pH	Average 6.0
Specific gravity	Slightly heavier than water (1.001–1.035)
Color	Yellow (amber, straw-colored, deep yellow in dehydration, pale yellow with overhydration)
Some Abnormal Constituents of Urine	
Albumin (protein)	Albuminuria—indicates an increased permeability of the glomerulus (e.g., nephrotic syndrome, glomerulonephritis, hypertension); sometimes exercise or pregnancy will result in albuminuria.
Glucose	Glycosuria (glucosuria)—usually indicates diabetes mellitus
Red blood cells	Hematuria—bleeding in the urinary tract; indicates inflammation, trauma, or disease
Hemoglobin	Hemoglobinuria—indicates hemolysis (transfusion reactions, hemolytic anemia)
White blood cells	Pyuria (pus)—indicates infection within the kidney or urinary tract
Ketone bodies	Ketonuria—usually indicates uncontrolled diabetes mellitus (fats are rapidly and incompletely metabolized)
Bilirubin	Bilirubinuria—usually indicates disease involving the liver and/or biliary tree

infection can often be detected by the rotten odor of the urine. Your sense of smell can help you in your medical sleuthing. Use it!

 Do You Know...

What Happens when Griz Doesn't Whiz?

As you know, Griz hibernates during the long winter months. Ever think about why he doesn't get ammonia-toxic and have to get up to whiz (urinate)? Griz has the ability to recycle his nitrogenous waste, such as urea, metabolically. In other words, the water and waste is converted into metabolic fuel and reused all winter until Mr. Lazy awakens. If Griz would give up his biochemical secret to scientists, perhaps persons with impaired renal function could do the recycle thing. "No-Whiz Griz" is just fine. He awakens in the spring … to have his fling … then off to sleep, without a peep. Ol' Griz … no whiz.

 Do You Know...

About Urine as a First-Aid Wash?

A scene from the old war stories journal! A soldier is seriously wounded in battle. He is propped up against a charred tree stump as the battle rages on. As his fellow soldiers pass by, they note a large gaping wound in his thigh. Each soldier stops and urinates on the wounded area. Seems rather hostile! However, urine is sterile and acidic. Given the unsanitary wartime conditions, the "cleansing" of the wounded area with urine helped prevent lethal wound infections. A urine wash—not recommended today, but it was better than nothing in the good ol' days.

 Re-Think

1. Why does dehydration cause an increase in urinary specific gravity?
2. What is the normal urinary pH, glucose concentration, and 24-hour output?

 Sum It Up!

Figure 24-4 summarizes the steps in urine formation. Water and dissolved solute (180 L/day) are filtered across the glomerulus into Bowman's capsule. Whereas reabsorption occurs throughout the entire length of the tubule, most occurs in the proximal tubule. Approximately 1.5 L of urine is excreted from the body in 24 hours. Water (178.5 L/day) moves from the tubules into the blood (peritubular capillaries). The kidneys respond to several hormones in regulating the composition of blood: aldosterone ("salt-retaining" hormone), ADH, ANP, BNP, and PTH.

 Do You Know...

Why a Patient with Poor Renal Function May Have to Take the Drug Epoetin?

The kidneys normally produce erythropoietin, a hormone that stimulates the bone marrow to make red blood cells. A patient in renal failure does not produce erythropoietin and therefore develops anemia ("the anemia of chronic renal failure"). The drug epoetin is erythropoietin; it stimulates the bone marrow to produce red blood cells (RBCs).

UREMIA AND DIALYSIS

There are many reasons why the kidneys fail. Nephrotoxic drugs, such as the aminoglycosides, and poisons such as antifreeze (ethylene glycol) destroy the kidneys. Infections, such as those caused by *E. coli*, found in

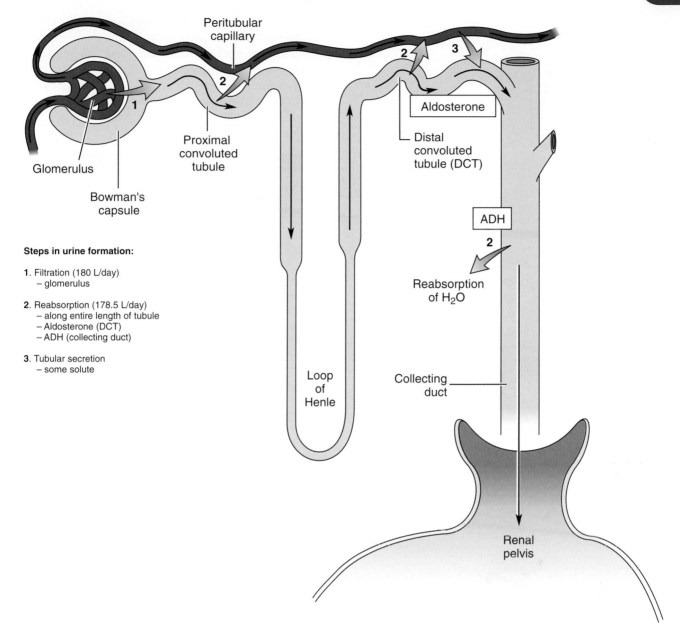

FIGURE 24-4 Steps in urine formation—filtration, reabsorption, and secretion—and the effects of aldosterone and ADH.

contaminated beef, can destroy the kidneys and are capable of causing a lethal hemolytic uremic syndrome (HUS). Finally, chronic diseases such as hypertension, diabetes mellitus, and gout are capable of destroying the kidneys.

Kidney failure is called *renal suppression*. The kidneys no longer make urine. The blood is not cleansed of its waste, and substances that should have been excreted in the urine remain in the blood. This condition is called *uremia* (yoo-REE-mee-ah), which literally means urine in the blood. Uremia may be prevented with the use of an artificial kidney, a form of **dialysis** (Figure 24-5). The artificial kidney consists of a cylinder filled with a plasma-like solution called the *dialysate*. The patient's blood is passed through a series of tiny tubes immersed in the dialysate. Waste products in the blood, such as potassium, creatinine, uric acid, and excess water, diffuse out of the tubules into the

dialysate. The blood is thereby cleansed of these waste products and returned to the patient. Because this procedure cleanses blood like a kidney, it is called an *artificial kidney*.

A second form of dialysis is peritoneal dialysis. With this procedure, the peritoneal cavity of the patient is used as the cylinder of an artificial kidney, and dialysate is infused into the peritoneal cavity. Waste products diffuse from the patient's blood into the dialysate. The dialysate eventually drains out of the peritoneal cavity and is discarded.

YOUR PLUMBING

Whereas the kidneys form urine, the remaining structures of the urinary system (ureters, urinary bladder, and urethra) function as plumbing and form the urinary tract (Figure 24-6). They do not alter the urine

FIGURE 24-5 Types of dialysis. **A,** Artificial kidney. **B,** Peritoneal dialysis.

in any way; instead, they store and conduct urine to the outside of the body for elimination. The urinary tract has an outer layer of connective tissue and a middle layer of smooth muscle. The tract is lined with mucous membrane.

URETERS

Two ureters connect the kidneys with the bladder. The ureters originate in the renal pelvis of the kidneys and terminate in the bladder. The ureters are long (10 to 13 inches [25 to 33 cm]), slender, muscular tubes capable of peristalsis. Urine moves along the ureters from the kidneys to the bladder in response to gravity and peristalsis.

Sometimes, a kidney stone (renal calculus or neph-rolithiasis) lodges in the slender ureter, and the urine backs up behind the stone, increasing pressure within the renal pelvis (hydronephrosis). The increased

pressure causes severe pain and renal colic and can adversely affect the kidney, causing a severe decline in GFR and irreversible kidney damage. The stone must be removed. Most stones simply wash out with the urine. Some must be extracted with an instrument inserted into the ureters via the bladder. Other methods include lithotripsy (crushing by ultrasound) and surgical removal.

Do You Know...

What Ka-plunk and Gush Have to Do with the Lithotomy Position?

"Ka-plunk!" echoed the giant stone as it flew out of the bladder into a bucket. So went the very first lithotomy, a crude and desperate surgical procedure used to extract stones (from the Greek word *lithos*) from the urinary bladder. A stone in the bladder acted like a plug, preventing the outflow of urine and causing the urine to accumulate in the bladder. Imagine the discomfort of not being able to urinate for days on end. Generally, the patient was in such excruciating pain that he or she agreed to have a sharp and dirty instrument pushed through the perineum into the bladder. Out popped the stones, followed by a major gush of urine and blessed relief of pressure. Because this position was used to perform the surgical procedure (removal of *lithos*, or stones), the position itself was named the *lithotomy position*, a term (and position) still in use today in gynecological practice.

URINARY BLADDER

The urinary bladder functions as a temporary reservoir for the storage of urine. When empty, the bladder is located below the peritoneal membrane and behind the symphysis pubis. When full, the bladder rises into the abdominal cavity. You can feel a distended bladder if you place your hand over your lower abdomen.

Four layers make up the wall of the bladder. The innermost layer is the mucous membrane and contains several thicknesses of transitional epithelium. The mucous membrane is continuous with the mucous membrane of the ureters and urethra. The second layer is the submucosa and consists of connective tissue and contains many elastic fibers. The third layer is composed of muscle. This involuntary smooth muscle is the **detrusor** (dee-TROO-sor) **muscle.** The outermost layer of the upper part of the bladder is the serosa.

How much can you hold? The bladder wall is arranged in folds called *rugae* that allow the bladder to stretch as it fills. The urge to urinate usually begins when it has accumulated about 200 mL of urine. As the volume of urine increases to 300 mL, the urge to urinate becomes more intense. A moderately full bladder contains about 500 mL, or 1 pint of urine. An overdistended bladder may contain more than 1 L of urine. With overdistention, the urge to urinate may be lost.

One specific area of the floor of the bladder is the trigone (TRY-gohn). It is a triangular area formed by three points: the entrance points of the two ureters and

Ureter

Bladder

Detrusor
muscle

Rugae

Ureteral
opening

Trigone

Internal
sphincter

External
sphincter

Urethra

FIGURE 24-6 Organs of the urinary tract: ureters, bladder, and urethra (your "plumbing").

the exit point of the urethra. The exit of the urinary bladder contains a sphincter muscle, called the *internal sphincter*. The internal sphincter is composed of smooth muscle that contracts involuntarily to prevent emptying. Below the internal sphincter, surrounding the upper region of the urethra, is the external sphincter. This sphincter is composed of skeletal muscle and is controlled voluntarily. Contraction of the external sphincter allows you to resist the urge to urinate.

 Do You Know...

That an Infection Can "Ascend"?

The urinary bladder, especially in the female, is a frequent site of infection. An infection of the urinary bladder is called *cystitis*. If cystitis is not treated promptly, pathogens can travel from the bladder up the ureter into the kidney, causing a kidney infection (pyelonephritis). Because the pathogens travel to the kidney from the bladder, a kidney infection is often called an *ascending infection*. In the female, the offending pathogen is usually *E. coli*, a resident of the large intestine. Because the female urethra is short, *E. coli* has a short journey from the meatus to the bladder.

URINATION

Urination, also called **micturition** (mik-too-RISH-un) or *voiding,* is the process of expelling urine from the bladder. What causes micturition? As the bladder fills with urine, stimulated stretch receptors send nerve impulses along sensory nerves to the spinal cord. The spinal cord reflexively sends motor nerve impulses back to the bladder, causing the bladder wall to contract rhythmically and the internal sphincter muscle to relax. This response is called the *micturition reflex*. This reflex gives rise to a sense of urgency. Contraction of the external sphincter prevents involuntary urination. In an infant, the micturition reflex causes the bladder to empty involuntarily. This is what caused baby Sammy to be a wet bundle of joy. As he matures, he will learn to override this reflex by voluntarily controlling the external sphincter. Only then can Sammy move from diapers to training pants.

A patient may experience urinary retention, or the inability to void or to empty the bladder. Urinary retention is usually caused by the effects of drugs used perioperatively. Note the difference between renal suppression and urinary retention. Renal suppression means that the kidneys do not make urine; urinary retention means that the bladder does not expel urine.

Many patients experience urinary incontinence, or the involuntary leakage of urine from the bladder. There are many causes of incontinence, such as an incompetent bladder sphincter, bladder infection, and excess external pressure as occurs during pregnancy. A chronically full bladder may cause an overflow incontinence. The patient does not urinate and empty the bladder; the excess dribbles out in small amounts. Finally, a sudden rise in bladder pressure as occurs in coughing or laughing causes incontinence; this is called *stress incontinence* and is the source of much embarrassment.

URETHRA

The urethra is a tube that carries urine from the bladder to the outside. It is lined with mucous membrane that contains numerous mucus-secreting glands. The muscular layer of the urethra contracts and helps expel urine during micturition.

The male and female urethras differ in several ways. In the female, the urethra is short (1.5 inches [3.8 cm]); it opens to the outside at the urethral meatus. The female urethral meatus is located in front of the vagina and between the labia minora.

In the male, the urethra is part of the urinary and the reproductive systems. The male urethra (8 inches [20 cm]) is much longer than the female urethra. As the male urethra leaves the bladder, it passes through the prostate gland and extends the length of the penis.

 Re-Think

1. List the urinary structures as you trace a drop of urine from the renal pelvis to the urethral meatus.
2. List the urinary structures as you trace the movement of *E. coli* from the urethral meatus to the renal pelvis of the kidney.

 Do You Know...

Why an Enlarged Prostate Gland "Slows the Stream" ... or Even Worse?

The male urethra is surrounded by the doughnut-shaped prostate gland. When the prostate gland enlarges, pressure is exerted on the outside of the urethra, constricting the lumen of the urethra and impeding the flow or "stream" of urine from the bladder. Urination becomes difficult (dysuria), and the incomplete emptying of the bladder sets the stage for repeated bladder infections. The incomplete emptying also causes nocturia (the need to urinate at night, thereby interfering with sleep), a bothersome symptom that may cause men to seek medical help.

AN AUTONOMIC MOMENT

The detrusor muscle of the urinary bladder and the internal sphincter have muscarinic receptors. Activation of the muscarinic receptors causes the detrusor muscle to contract and the sphincter to relax; this action causes the bladder to expel the urine. This can lead to two pharmacology issues. First, if a patient is experiencing urinary retention, she or he may be given a muscarinic agonist such as bethanechol (Urecholine). The muscarinic agonist causes contraction of the detrusor muscle and relaxation of the urinary sphincter. Second, if a person has been taking medications that have antimuscarinic side effects, he or she may experience difficulty in urinating. This often happens to persons who take preoperative drugs such as atropine and those who take anticholinergic antidepressants.

2+2 Sum It Up!

The kidneys make urine. The urine is stored and transported by the structures that make up the urinary tract: two ureters, bladder, and urethra. The accumulation of urine in the bladder is the stimulus for the micturition reflex and creates the urge to void. Voluntary control of the external sphincter allows you to void at a particular time. Urine exits the body through the urethral meatus.

As You Age

1. The number of nephron units progressively decreases so that by the age of 70 to 80 years, there has been a 50% reduction. Clinically, this decrease in nephron function causes a diminished ability to concentrate urine.
2. The glomerular filtration rate (GFR) declines with age. As a result, the older person excretes drugs more slowly and is at risk for drug overdose. The decrease in GFR also makes it difficult for the older person to excrete excess blood volume, so any intravenous fluids must be administered slowly and carefully. Overhydration is a common cause of heart failure in older adults.
3. The aging urinary bladder shrinks and becomes less able to contract and relax. As a result, the older person must void more frequently. Because of less effective bladder contraction and residual urine, the incidence of bladder infection increases. The weakening of the external sphincter and a decreased ability to sense a distended bladder increase the incidence of bladder incontinence. Frequent urination in men may be caused by an enlarged prostate gland, a common age-related disorder.

MEDICAL TERMINOLOGY AND DISORDERS | Disorders of the Urinary System

Medical Term	Word Parts	Word Part Meaning or Derivation	Description
azotemia	azote-	From a French word, *azote*, meaning "nitrogen"	**Azotemia** refers to *the presence of nitrogenous waste in the blood*; it develops in persons with renal failure who do not undergo dialysis.
	-emia	blood condition	
cystoscopy	cyst/o-	bladder	**Cystoscopy** is *a visual examination of the bladder.*
	-scopy	examination	
diuresis		From a Greek word meaning "prompting urine"	**Diuresis** refers to *an increase in urine production.* A diuretic drug is one that increases urine production.
polydipsia	poly-	much or many	Refers to *excessive thirst, most often experienced by an uncontrolled diabetic person.*
	-dips/o-	thirst	
glucosuria; other substances in the urine	gluc/o-	glucose	**Glucosuria** refers to *the presence of glucose in the urine;* also called **glycosuria** (glyc/o- = glucose). **Ketonuria** (keton/o- = ketone bodies) refers to *ketone bodies in the urine.* **Albuminuria,** a type of proteinuria, refers to *the presence of albumin in the urine and is usually indicative of glomerular dysfunction.* **Hematuria** is *the presence of blood in the urine;* the blood may come from the kidneys or other urinary tract structures such as the bladder and ureters. **Pyuria** is *pus in the urine and is indicative of an infection.*
	-uria	urine	
kaliuresis	kaliur-	From the Greek word *kalium,* meaning "potassium"	Kaliuresis is *the excretion of potassium in the urine;* aldosterone stimulates the renal excretion of potassium.
	-uresis	From the Greek word *ouresis,* meaning "urination"	

Continued

MEDICAL TERMINOLOGY AND DISORDERS Disorders of the Urinary System—cont'd

Medical Term	Word Parts	Word Part Meaning or Derivation	Description
lithotripsy	lith/o-	stone or calculus	**Lithotripsy** is *a medical procedure that crushes stones so that they can be expelled without surgical intervention.*
	-tripsis	Greek word meaning "to crush"	
oliguria and other "urias"	olig/o-	scanty	**Oliguria** refers to *scanty or insufficient urine production as occurs in response to protracted hypotension.* **Nocturia** (noct/i- = night) refers to *the necessity of needing to urinate at night.* **Polyuria** is *the excessive production of urine.*
	-uria	urine	
natriuresis	natri-	From two words meaning "salt" (Latin, *natrium*) and "urination" (Greek, *ouresis*)	**Natriuresis** is *the excretion of sodium in the urine.* Most diuretic drugs cause natriuresis, resulting in the excretion of sodium and water.
	-uresis		
Disorders			
acute tubular necrosis	necr/o-	death	*Also called* **ATN,** *it is a consequence of renal tubular damage.* A common cause of ATN is a prolonged period of hypotension (as in shock), in which the tubules are deprived of blood and the tubular cells die. The injured tubular cells cannot reabsorb tubular fluids and electrolytes properly.
	-osis	condition of	
enuresis	enuresis	From a Greek word meaning "to make water"	*The involuntary discharge of urine in a person old enough to be expected to have bladder control.* Commonly called bedwetting, or **nocturnal enuresis.**
glomerulonephritis	glomus-	From a Latin word meaning "ball of thread"	**Glomerulonephritis (GN)** is *an acute or chronic inflammation of the glomeruli; filtration by inflamed glomeruli is impaired so that the composition of urine is altered.* If GN occurs on its own, it is called **primary GN. Secondary GN** develops in response to another disorder, such as autoimmune disorders (lupus) or diabetes mellitus. GN occurs in many forms. One type is called **postinfectious GN;** it is an immune response to a pathogen (*Streptococcus pyogenes*) and classically occurs 10-14 days after a skin or pharyngeal (throat) infection.
	-nephr/o-	kidney	
	-itis	inflammation	
hydronephrosis	hydr/o-	water	*Literally means "water in the kidney."* **Hydronephrosis** refers to *the dilation of the renal pelvis and calyces caused by obstruction to the flow of urine out of the kidney.* The obstruction is usually a kidney stone in one of the ureters; other causes of obstruction include ureteral strictures, nephroptosis (dropped kidney, "floating kidney"), and abdominal adhesions.
	-nephr/o-	kidney	
	-osis	condition of	
nephrosis	nephr/o-	kidney	*Also called* **nephrotic syndrome,** *a group of symptoms that include proteinuria, hypercholesterolemia, elevated serum triglycerides, and edema.* Protein is filtered across the damaged glomeruli, causing albuminuria, hypoalbuminemia, and edema.
	-osis	condition of	
pyelonephritis	pyel/o-	From a Greek word meaning "tub-shaped vessel"	*Also called a* **kidney infection.** It generally begins in the urinary bladder and travels up to the kidney. This UTI is most often caused by *E. coli.*
	-nephr/o-	kidney	
	-itis	inflammation	
renal calculi	ren/o-	kidney	Urinary stones are classified by location: **nephrolithiasis** (kidney stones, renal calculi); **ureterolithiasis** (stones in the ureter); and **cystolithiasis** (stones in the bladder). Most stones are composed of calcium; this explains the increased risk of kidney stones in patients who are bedridden.
	-calcul/o-	stone	

MEDICAL TERMINOLOGY AND DISORDERS | Disorders of the Urinary System—cont'd

Medical Term	Word Parts	Word Part Meaning or Derivation	Description
renal failure			*Also called* **kidney failure.** *The kidneys fail to remove waste, concentrate urine, and maintain electrolyte balance.* There are many causes, including infection, hypovolemia, shock, blood clots in the renal blood vessels, and chronic diseases such as diabetes mellitus. Long-term diabetes mellitus causes **glomerulosclerosis,** *or scarring of the glomeruli.* Renal failure causes uremia, the presence of "urine" in the blood.
urinary incontinence	in-	not	*The inability to control the bladder with an involuntary leakage of urine.* Stress incontinence refers to involuntary discharge of urine when coughing, sneezing, or exercise. Urge incontinence, also called overactive bladder, bladder spasm, and detrusor hyperreflexia, is the sudden urge to urinate as a result of bladder muscle contractions.
	-continent	From a Latin word meaning "to hold in"	

Get Ready for Exams!

Summary Outline

The urinary system consists of organs that make urine, temporarily store it, and then eliminate it from the body. The kidneys contain the nephron units that make urine, thereby eliminating waste from the body and regulating water and electrolyte balance.

I. Excretion
   A. There are several organs of excretion: the kidneys, skin, lungs, and intestines.
   B. The urinary system organs include the kidneys, ureters, urinary bladder, and urethra.

II. Kidneys
   A. The kidney has three distinct regions: the cortex, medulla, and pelvis.
   B. The kidneys have many functions: excrete nitrogenous waste, regulate blood volume, regulate electrolyte concentration, regulate pH and blood pressure, and stimulate red blood cell production.

III. Urine Making: Nephron Unit
   A. The nephron unit is the functional (urine-making) unit of the kidney.
   B. The nephron unit is composed of tubular structures and vascular structures.
   C. There are three processes in urine formation:
      1. Glomerular filtration filters 180 L of filtrate in 24 hours.
      2. Tubular reabsorption causes the reabsorption of 178.5 L of filtrate.
         a. A substance is either completely or incompletely reabsorbed.
         b. A substance is reabsorbed actively or passively.
      3. Tubular secretion causes the secretion of small amounts of specific substances from the peritubular capillaries into the tubules.

IV. Hormones That Work on the Kidneys
   A. Aldosterone
      1. Aldosterone stimulates the distal tubule and upper collecting duct to reabsorb Na^+ and water and to excrete K^+.
      2. The secretion of aldosterone is regulated primarily by the renin-angiotensin-aldosterone system.
   B. Antidiuretic hormone (ADH)
      1. ADH stimulates the collecting duct to reabsorb water.
      2. ADH is released from the posterior pituitary gland in response to low blood volume and increased concentration of solute in the plasma.
   C. Natriuretic peptides (ANP, BNP) inhibit the reabsorption of Na^+ and water, thereby causing natriuresis and the excretion of water.
   D. Parathyroid hormone (PTH) stimulates the renal reabsorption of calcium and the excretion of phosphate.

V. Composition of Urine
(The characteristics of urine are summarized in Table 24-3.)
   A. Amount
   B. pH
   C. Specific gravity
   D. Color
   E. Abnormal constituents

VI. Uremia
   A. Kidney failure causes a syndrome called *uremia.*
   B. Dialysis can prevent uremia.

VII. Your Plumbing
   A. The two ureters are long slender tubes that carry urine from the renal pelvis to the bladder.

B. Urinary bladder
1. The urinary bladder is a temporary reservoir that holds the urine.
2. The detrusor muscle is a smooth muscle responsible for bladder contraction and the elimination of urine.
3. There are two sphincters: internal (involuntary) and external (voluntary).
4. The voluntary elimination of urine is called *urination* (micturition).
C. The urethra is a tube that carries urine from the bladder to the outside of the body.

Review Your Knowledge

Matching: Plumbing ... More or Less
Directions: Match the following words with their descriptions below. Some words may be used more than once.
a. urethra
b. kidneys
c. ureters
d. urinary bladder

1. ___ These two long tubes empty urine into the urinary bladder.
2. ___ The urine-making organs
3. ___ Urine leaves the bladder through this structure.
4. ___ The external urinary sphincter is located at the distal end of this structure.
5. ___ Its walls contain the detrusor muscle.
6. ___ Tubes that receive urine from the renal pelvis
7. ___ An enlarged prostate gland prevents the emptying of this structure.
8. ___ Cystitis is an inflammation of this urinary structure.
9. ___ Renal suppression is most associated with these structures.
10. ___ Urinary retention is most associated with this structure.

Matching: Nephron Unit
Directions: Match the following words with their descriptions below. Some words may be used more than once.
a. loop of Henle
b. glomerulus
c. afferent arterioles
d. collecting duct
e. proximal convoluted tubule
f. calyx
g. peritubular capillaries

1. ___ This structure receives urine from the distal convoluted tubule.
2. ___ The tuft of capillaries that sits within Bowman's capsule
3. ___ Urine flows from the proximal tubule into this structure.
4. ___ These capillaries surround the tubules and reabsorb huge amounts of water and solute.
5. ___ Filtration occurs across the membrane of this vascular structure.
6. ___ Most reabsorption occurs across this tubular structure.
7. ___ These tiny blood vessels deliver blood to the glomeruli.

8. ___ Hairpin tubular structure between the proximal and distal tubules
9. ___ A cuplike structure that receives urine from the collecting duct
10. ___ The tubular site that is most responsive to ADH

Matching: Hormones and Enzymes
Directions: Match the following words with their descriptions below. Some words may be used more than once.
a. aldosterone
b. renin
c. parathyroid hormone (PTH)
d. converting enzyme
e. antidiuretic hormone (ADH)
f. brain natriuretic peptide (BNP)
g. angiotensin II

1. ___ Secreted by the juxtaglomerular apparatus cells; activates angiotensinogen
2. ___ Stimulates the distal tubule to reabsorb Na^+ and excrete K^+
3. ___ Determines the membrane permeability of the collecting duct to water
4. ___ Mineralocorticoid secreted by the adrenal cortex
5. ___ Secreted by the walls of the heart; causes the renal excretion of Na^+ and water
6. ___ Called the "salt-retaining" hormone
7. ___ Deficiency of this hormone causes diabetes insipidus
8. ___ Stimulates the tubules to reabsorb calcium and excrete phosphate
9. ___ Secreted by the lungs; changes angiotensin I to angiotensin II
10. ___ A potent vasopressor that is generated by the action of converting enzyme

Multiple Choice
1. Micturition
   a. occurs in Bowman's capsule.
   b. refers to the filtration of 180 L of water.
   c. refers to the storage of urine by the bladder.
   d. refers to urination.
2. The filtration of 180 L/day of water
   a. is a micturition event.
   b. moves water from the renal tubules into the peritubular capillaries.
   c. is the rate at which urine flows into the urinary bladder.
   d. occurs across the glomerular membrane.
3. Which of the following is the first tubular structure to receive the glomerular ultrafiltrate?
   a. Collecting duct
   b. Renal pelvis
   c. Loop of Henle
   d. Bowman's capsule
4. The active pumping of Na^+ from the proximal convoluted tubule into the peritubular capillaries
   a. stimulates the micturition reflex.
   b. causes diuresis.
   c. is responsible for the passive reabsorption of water.
   d. can only occur in response to aldosterone.

5. Which of the following is least true of aldosterone?
   a. It is a mineralocorticoid.
   b. It is the "salt-retaining" hormone.
   c. It determines the membrane permeability of the collecting duct to water.
   d. It causes the tubular reabsorption of sodium and water.

6. ADH
   a. is released in response to excess blood volume and a dilute plasma.
   b. determines the membrane permeability of the collecting duct to water.
   c. makes the collecting duct impermeable to water.
   d. determines the pore size of the glomeruli.

7. A drug that blocks the renal reabsorption of Na$^+$ causes
   a. defecation.
   b. diuresis.
   c. oliguria.
   d. hypernatremia.

8. Why is glucose normally not excreted in the urine?
   a. No glucose is filtered.
   b. All filtered glucose is reabsorbed.
   c. Glucose is used up by the metabolizing nephron units.
   d. Glucose is converted to ammonia in the distal tubule and excreted as urea.

9. A drug that blocks the effects of aldosterone
   a. increases the reabsorption of Na$^+$ and water.
   b. is kaliuretic.
   c. may cause an increase in plasma K$^+$.
   d. causes oliguria.

10. Oliguria
    a. refers to a lowered serum potassium.
    b. develops in response to hypotension.
    c. is a response to a diuretic drug.
    d. most often accompanies a decline in serum creatinine.

Go Figure

1. **According to Figure 24-1**
   a. The kidneys are located in the pelvic cavity.
   b. The calyx is the opening through which the renal artery and renal vein enter and leave the kidney.
   c. The renal column is the same as the renal pyramid.
   d. The kidneys are connected to the urinary bladder by two ureters.

2. **According to Figure 24-2**
   a. The glomerulus sits within the renal pelvis.
   b. The glomeruli are attached to both the afferent and efferent arterioles.
   c. The peritubular capillaries sit within Bowman's capsule.
   d. The collecting duct empties urine into the loop of Henle.

3. **According to Figure 24-2**
   a. Blood from the afferent arterioles drain into the collecting duct.
   b. The loop of Henle is a hairpin-like tubular structure between the proximal and distal tubules.
   c. The proximal convoluted tubule is closer to the collecting duct than is the distal convoluted tubule.
   d. Blood from the peritubular capillaries drains into the renal artery and abdominal aorta.

4. **According to Table 24-2**
   a. ADH is a neurohypophyseal hormone whose target cells are in the collecting duct.
   b. Aldosterone, like ADH, is a salt-retaining steroid.
   c. An excess of aldosterone or ADH causes diuresis.
   d. Both ANP and BNP are secreted by the renal cortex.

5. **According to Figure 24-3**
   a. Renin converts angiotensin I to angiotensinogen.
   b. Converting enzyme changes angiotensin I to angiotensin II.
   c. Aldosterone changes angiotensin II to converting enzyme.
   d. Inhibition of converting enzyme expands blood volume and elevates blood pressure.

6. **According to Figure 24-4**
   a. Aldosterone exerts its effect primarily on the proximal convoluted tubule.
   b. Filtration occurs across the glomerulus into Bowman's capsule.
   c. ADH exerts its effect primarily on the descending limb of the loop of Henle.
   d. Most tubular secretion occurs across the glomeruli.

7. **According to Figure 24-6**
   a. The detrusor muscle forms the wall of the urinary bladder.
   b. The urinary bladder wall has rugae for expansion.
   c. The urinary bladder is drained by a urethra.
   d. All of the above are true.

Water, Electrolyte, and Acid–Base Balance

evolve

http://evolve.elsevier.com/Herlihy

Key Terms

acidosis (p. 483)
alkalosis (p. 483)
buffer (p. 483)
dehydration (p. 479)
electrolyte balance (p. 481)
extracellular fluid (p. 478)
hyperkalemia (p. 482)
hyperventilation (p. 485)

hypokalemia (p. 482)
hypoventilation (p. 485)
intake (p. 479)
interstitial fluid (p. 478)
intracellular fluid (p. 478)
kaliuretic (p. 482)
Kussmaul respirations (p. 485)
metabolic acidosis (p. 485)

metabolic alkalosis (p. 486)
output (p. 479)
respiratory acidosis (p. 485)
respiratory alkalosis (p. 485)
skin turgor (p. 480)
transcellular fluid (p. 478)

Objectives

1. Describe the two main fluid compartments and the composition of body fluids.
2. Define *intake* and *output*.
3. Explain the effects of water imbalances, fluid shift, and fluid spacing.

4. List factors that affect electrolyte balance.
5. Describe the most common ions found in the intracellular and extracellular compartments.
6. List three mechanisms that regulate pH in the body.
7. Discuss acid–base imbalances: acidosis and alkalosis.

The old saying "you're all wet" has some truth to it. Between 50% and 70% of a person's weight is water. In the average man, water makes up 60% of the weight (about 40 L); in the average woman, water makes up about 50%. An infant is composed of even more water—up to 75%. Because adipose tissue contains less water than muscle tissue, obese persons have less water than thin persons.

BODY FLUIDS: DISTRIBUTION AND COMPOSITION

FLUID COMPARTMENTS

Water and its dissolved electrolytes are distributed into two major compartments: an intracellular compartment

and an extracellular compartment (Figure 25-1). The intracellular compartment includes the water located in all the cells of the body. Most water, about 63%, is located in the intracellular compartment.

The extracellular compartment includes the fluid located outside all the cells and represents about 37% of the total body water. The extracellular compartment includes the water located between cells, called **interstitial fluid**, water within blood vessels (plasma), and water within lymphatic vessels (lymph). **Transcellular fluid** is extracellular fluid and includes cerebrospinal fluid, the aqueous and vitreous humors in the eyes, the synovial fluids of joints, the serous fluids in body cavities, and the glandular secretions. Interstitial fluid and plasma are the largest extracellular compartments.

COMPOSITION OF BODY FLUIDS

Intracellular and extracellular fluids vary in their concentrations of various electrolytes. **Extracellular fluids** contain high concentrations of sodium (Na^+), chloride (Cl^-), and bicarbonate (HCO_3^-) ions. The plasma portion (extracellular) contains more protein than do other extracellular fluids. **Intracellular fluid** contains high concentrations of potassium (K^+), phosphate (PO_4^{3-}), and magnesium (Mg^{2+}) ions. The concentration of an ion is indicated when it appears in brackets; thus, $[H^+]$ means the concentration of the hydrogen ion.

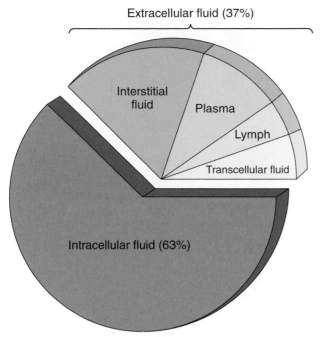

Extracellular fluid (37%)

Interstitial fluid

Plasma

Lymph

Transcellular fluid

Intracellular fluid (63%)

FIGURE 25-1 Fluid compartments: extracellular and intracellular.

Smaller concentrations of other ions are present in both intracellular and extracellular fluids. Although distributed across the fluid compartments, water and electrolytes can move from one compartment to another. The movement of fluid and electrolytes between compartments is well regulated.

 Do You Know...

What Is So "Normal" about Normal Saline and Why It Is Normally Given?

Some patients become deficient in body fluids. These may be surgical patients who are not permitted to drink, patients who have been vomiting, or those who are unconscious and unable to eat or drink. These patients often receive intravenous infusions of solutions that resemble plasma in ionic composition. Normal saline, for example, contains 0.9% sodium chloride, a concentration equal to that of plasma. Because the concentration of "salt" in normal saline resembles that of plasma, it is considered normal.

WATER BALANCE

Normally, the quantity of water taken in, which is **intake**, equals the amount of water eliminated from the body, which is **output**. Water balance exists when intake equals output (Figure 25-2). As part of your clinical responsibilities, you will be measuring intake and output.

WATER INTAKE

Although water intake can vary considerably, the average adult takes in about 2500 mL every day. About 60% comes from drinking liquids; an additional 30% comes from water in foods, while 10% comes from the

breakdown of foods. This latter portion is called the *water of metabolism*.

Thirst is the primary regulator of water intake. The thirst center is in the hypothalamus of the brain. As the body loses water, the thirst center in the hypothalamus is stimulated, thus causing you to drink. Drinking restores the water content of the body, so both your thirst and your hypothalamus are satisfied. Older adults have a diminished thirst mechanism and are therefore prone to dehydration.

WATER OUTPUT

In a healthy person, 24-hour intake and output are approximately equal; the individual who takes in 2500 mL of water should therefore eliminate 2500 mL. Water can leave the body through several routes: kidneys, skin, lungs, and digestive tract. The kidneys eliminate about 60% of the water as urine. About 28% is lost from the skin and lungs; 6% is eliminated in the feces, and another 6% is lost as sweat. The amount lost by sweat can vary considerably, depending on the level of exercise and environmental temperatures. Water loss through the skin and lungs increases in a hot, dry environment.

The kidneys are the primary regulator of water output. Water regulation occurs mainly through the action of antidiuretic hormone (ADH) on the collecting duct. When body water content is low, the posterior pituitary gland releases ADH. It stimulates the collecting duct to reabsorb water, thereby decreasing water in the urine and increasing blood volume. When body water content is high, the secretion of ADH decreases. As a result, less water is reabsorbed from the collecting duct, and the excess water is eliminated in the urine. Water balance is also regulated by aldosterone, discussed later in the chapter.

 Do You Know...

What a Prune and a Dehydrated Person Have in Common?

A prune is a dehydrated plum. As water is removed from the plum, its skin assumes a shriveled appearance. The same process occurs in a person who is dehydrated. As fluid is lost from the body, water moves from the interstitium (tissue spaces) into the blood vessels in an attempt to maintain adequate blood volume and blood pressure. As water is lost from the interstitium, the overlying skin appears shriveled, much like a prune. Both the dehydrated patient and prune are said to have poor skin turgor.

WATER IMBALANCES

DEHYDRATION

A deficiency of body water is called **dehydration**. Dehydration develops when water output exceeds water intake and commonly occurs in conditions such as excessive sweating, vomiting, diarrhea, and use of diuretics. A dehydrated person usually has poor skin

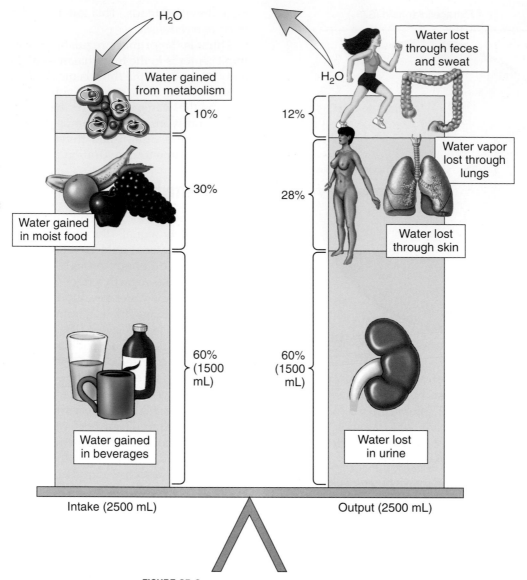

FIGURE 25-2 Water balance: intake equals output.

turgor. **Skin turgor** is assessed by pinching the skin and then observing how quickly the skin flattens, or returns to its normal position. If a person is well hydrated, the pinched skin quickly flattens out. The skin of a dehydrated person, however, flattens out more slowly, giving the skin the appearance of a tent—hence the term *tenting*. Tenting is caused by the depletion of fluid in the interstitial space. If untreated blood volume and blood pressure continue to decline, the person develops a low-volume (hypovolemic) shock.

EDEMA

The body can retain excess water and deposit it in various compartments, especially the interstitial space. Fluid retention is called *edema*. Edema can be intracellular or extracellular. Generally, we are concerned with interstitial edema. Excess body water can accumulate in various parts of the body. For example, water accumulation in the lungs is called *pulmonary edema*; it causes hypoxemia and cyanosis. Cerebral edema is the

accumulation of water in the brain; it causes a life-threatening increase in intracranial pressure and evidence of neurological dysfunction. Water accumulation in the ankle region is called *pedal edema*. As you can see, the consequences can be mild (pedal edema) or life threatening (pulmonary edema and cerebral edema). The goal of therapy is to remove excess fluid, relieve the symptoms, and treat the underlying cause of the edema.

? Re-Think

1. List four extracellular compartments.
2. Compare the volume of the interstitial space during dehydration and edema.

WHY DOES FLUID SHIFT?

The fluid shifts because of a change in the "pushing and pulling" forces affecting the capillaries. (See Chapter 19 for a discussion of capillary exchange and the mechanisms of edema formation.) The forces include the capillary filtration pressure, plasma oncotic pressure, effect of lymphatic drainage, and effects of plasma protein that becomes trapped in the tissue space. Alteration of any of these factors affects water movement.

DAILY WEIGHTS AND FLUID BALANCE

The daily measurement of body weight provides a reliable estimate of fluid balance. For example, if a person with heart failure suddenly gains 4.4 lb, you should suspect fluid retention. How is the amount estimated? One liter of water weighs 2.2 lb (1 kg). If a person has a sudden weight gain of 4.4 lb, you can assume that that person has retained 2 L of fluid. Another example is when a patient is given a diuretic and loses 2.2 lb overnight. You can assume that the patient excreted 1 L of fluid.

? Re-Think

A 210-lb edematous man was given a powerful diuretic; he lost 2 kg in 12 hours. How much does he weigh after losing that water weight?

FLUID SPACING—IN OTHER WORDS

Fluid spacing is a clinical term that refers to the distribution of body water. First spacing refers to the normal distribution of water as described previously. Second spacing refers to the accumulation of water in the interstitial spaces (interstitial edema). Generally, with adequate treatment, this water can be reabsorbed and excreted. Third spacing refers to the accumulation of water in spaces from which it is not easily absorbed. For example, the water that accumulates in the abdominal cavity as ascites is not easily reabsorbed. Similarly, the excess water that accumulates within the digestive tract as a result of a paralytic ileus is unavailable for easy reabsorption. The amount of water in "third spaces" can be large and life threatening. Monitoring of water distribution is a common clinical concern.

ELECTROLYTE BALANCE

Electrolyte balance exists when the amounts of the various electrolytes gained by the body equal the amounts lost. *Electrolyte imbalances* are common, serious clinical challenges. Electrolytes are important components of the body fluids. The kidneys control the composition of body fluids by regulating the renal excretion of electrolytes. Table 25-1 includes the major electrolytes and their normal levels and functions.

QUICK REFERENCE: ELECTROLYTES

Chapter 2 describes the chemical characteristics of electrolytes. You will want to review several of the terms listed here for quick reference:

- *Ion:* An element or compound that carries an electrical charge. Common ions are Na^+, Cl^-, K^+, Ca^{2+}, and Mg^{2+}.
- *Cation:* A positively charged ion, such as Na^+, K^+, and Ca^{2+}
- *Anion:* A negatively charged ion, such as Cl^- and HCO_3^- (bicarbonate). Most proteins (such as albumin) carry a negative charge.
- *Electrolyte:* Substances that form ions when they dissolve in water, such as NaCl (salt):

$$NaCl \rightarrow Na^+ \text{ (cation)} + Cl^- \text{ (anion)}$$

- *Ionization:* The chemical reaction caused when an electrolyte splits into two ions

MOST IMPORTANT IONS

SODIUM (Na⁺)

Sodium is the chief extracellular cation, accounting for almost 90% of the positively charged ions in the extracellular fluid. Sodium plays a key role in the regulation of water balance. The primary mechanism regulating sodium concentration is aldosterone. Aldosterone stimulates the distal tubule and upper collecting duct of the nephron unit to reabsorb sodium. Usually, "when sodium moves, water moves"; this

Table 25-1	Major Ions and Their Functions	
ELECTROLYTE	**PLASMA LEVEL (mEq/L)**	**FUNCTIONS**
Sodium (Na⁺)	136–145	Chief extracellular cation Regulates extracellular volume Participates in nerve–muscle function
Potassium (K⁺)	3.5–5.0	Chief intracellular cation Participates in nerve–muscle function
Calcium (Ca²⁺)	4.5–5.8	Strengthens bone and teeth Participates in muscle contraction Helps in blood clotting
Magnesium (Mg²⁺)	1.5–2.5	Strengthens bone Participates in nerve–muscle function
Chloride (Cl⁻)	95–108	Chief extracellular anion Involved in extracellular volume control
Bicarbonate (HCO₃⁻)	22–26	Part of bicarbonate buffer system Participates in acid–base balance
Phosphate (PO₄³⁻)	2.5–4.5	Strengthens bone Participates in acid–base balance

means that aldosterone causes the reabsorption of both Na^+ and water.

Hypernatremia (hye-per-nah-TREE-mee-ah) refers to excess Na^+ in the blood and is the result of excess water loss or increased Na^+ intake. Note the types of patients who develop hypernatremia:

- Older persons following surgery or fever. They are apt to have a low blood volume and diminished thirst mechanism.
- Patients who have been on prolonged diuretic therapy because of the loss of excessive water as urine.
- Uncontrolled diabetic patients with hyperglycemia. The glucosuria requires the excretion of large amounts of water (polyuria) leading to dehydration and hypernatremia.

Hyponatremia refers to a decrease in the concentration of plasma Na^+. Normal plasma Na^+ levels are essential for normal brain function. Often, a patient becomes hyponatremic because of excess water in the blood. The blood literally is diluted out with water, causing a dilutional hyponatremia, a condition that is serious because it can result in delirium and seizures. For example, a person with heart failure often has an expanded blood volume and a dilutional hyponatremia. Sometimes, runners drink too much water during a marathon, causing a dilutional hyponatremia. Psychiatric patients sometimes "water binge"; they too are at risk for dilutional hyponatremia.

POTASSIUM (K^+)

Potassium (K^+) is the chief intracellular cation. The primary hormone regulating K^+ concentration is aldosterone. Aldosterone stimulates the distal tubule and upper collecting duct of the nephron unit to excrete K^+ into the urine. The kidney is the primary organ responsible for the excretion of excess K^+. The monitoring of serum K^+ levels is an important clinical responsibility. Whereas only 2% of the K^+ is located in the extracellular space, plasma K^+ is important for normal muscle function, especially cardiac function. Changes in plasma levels of K^+ cause serious cardiac dysrhythmias.

Hyperkalemia (hye-per-kah-LEE-mee-ah) refers to excess K^+ (>5.5 mEq/L) in the blood. The primary cause of hyperkalemia is kidney disease, because the kidneys play a major role in the elimination of K^+. Hyperkalemia is an emergency situation and is treated in several ways, including dialysis or the IV administration of an insulin-glucose solution. Dialysis removes K^+ from the blood. The IV insulin drives the glucose and K^+ into the cells, lowering plasma levels of K^+.

Hypokalemia refers to a lower than normal amount of K^+ (<3.5 mEq/L) in the blood. Hypokalemia usually presents as muscle fatigue, leg cramps, abdominal distention, and cardiac rhythm disturbances. The most common cause of hypokalemia is the prolonged use of K^+-losing diuretics, known as **kaliuretics**

(cal-ee-yoo-RET-iks). Some diuretics, such as spironolactone, are not kaliuretic and cause the kidney to reabsorb potassium. These diuretics are called "potassium sparers"; they can cause hyperkalemia. Maintaining normal K^+ levels in a patient who requires diuretic therapy is a major clinical concern. You must know which diuretics excrete K^+ and which diuretics reabsorb or "spare" potassium. Large amounts of K^+ can also be lost through vomiting (or nasogastric tubes) and diarrhea. Hypokalemia is a serious condition and is treated by the administration of K^+.

 Do You Know...

Why Acidosis Can Cause Hypokalemia?

As acidosis develops, the body attempts to decrease the plasma $[H^+]$ by moving it from the blood into the cells. As H^+ enters the cells, it kicks K^+ out of the cells into the blood, where it is filtered by the kidneys and excreted in the urine. When the acidosis is corrected, the H^+ leaves the cells and goes back into the blood. The K^+ then re-enters the cells, thereby making the person hypokalemic.

CALCIUM (Ca^{2+})

Calcium is necessary for bone and teeth formation, muscle contraction, nerve impulse transmission, and blood clotting. Of the body's calcium, 99% is in the bones and teeth. Parathyroid hormone is the primary regulator of plasma levels of calcium. Hypercalcemia and hypocalcemia are described in Chapter 14. (Do not confuse the terms *hypercalcemia* and *hyperkalemia*.)

MAGNESIUM (Mg^{2+})

Next to K^+, magnesium is the most abundant cation in the intracellular fluid. Magnesium is important in the function of the heart, muscles, and nerves. Kidney disease is the major cause of hypermagnesemia. Other causes include overuse of magnesium-containing antacids. (Did you think that over-the-counter drugs couldn't kill you?) Hypomagnesemia is often seen in critically ill persons. It can be caused by aggressive diuretic therapy and is also seen in patients with chronic alcoholism, as well as in pregnant women with preeclampsia (high blood pressure of pregnancy).

CHLORIDE (Cl^-)

Chloride is the chief extracellular anion, and it usually follows sodium. That is, when sodium is actively pumped from the tubules into the peritubular capillaries, chloride follows the sodium passively. Changes in the plasma levels of chloride affect acid–base balance through its effect on bicarbonate. For example, when the plasma chloride level decreases (hypochloremia), the plasma bicarbonate level increases and causes alkalosis. Hyperchloremia, on the other hand, causes a decrease in the plasma bicarbonate level and a state of acidosis. Like sodium, chloride is greatly affected by diuretic therapy.

BICARBONATE (HCO_3^-)

Bicarbonate is an important anion in acid–base balance. Bicarbonate is an alkaline (basic) substance that helps remove excess acid (H^+) from the body. It is also the form in which carbon dioxide (CO_2) is transported in the blood. Bicarbonate excretion is controlled by the kidneys. Bicarbonate can be either reabsorbed or excreted, depending on the body's needs.

OTHER IONS

The plasma contains other ions, such as sulfate (SO_4^{2-}) and phosphate (PO_4^{3-}). The normal laboratory values for the major ions are summarized in Table 25-1.

2+2 Sum It Up!

The volume and composition of body fluids are closely regulated. Body fluids are found in two main compartments; most body fluid (63%) is in the intracellular compartment, and the remaining 37% is in the extracellular compartment. The extracellular compartment contains interstitial fluid, plasma, lymph, and transcellular fluid. The electrolyte composition of the body fluids is important. The chief extracellular cation is sodium; the chief intracellular cation is potassium. Excesses and deficiencies of water and electrolytes cause serious clinical problems.

? Re-Think

Explain the following statement. Aggressive diuresis with a loop diuretic, such as furosemide (Lasix), may cause a person to become hypokalemic, dehydrated, and hypotensive.

ACID–BASE BALANCE

A normally functioning body requires a balance between acids and bases. Acid–base balance is described according to its regulation of pH. Why is the regulation of pH so important? All chemical reactions in the body occur at a particular pH; any alteration in pH interferes with these reactions.

QUICK REFERENCE: ACIDS AND BASES

Chapter 2 describes acids, bases, and pH. You will want to review several terms for quick reference:
- *Acid:* A substance that dissociates (splits) into H^+ and an anion such as Cl^- (e.g., $HCl \rightarrow H^+ + Cl^-$). An acid donates a hydrogen ion (H^+) during a chemical reaction.
- *Base:* A substance that combines with H^+ during a chemical reaction and removes H^+ from solution (e.g., $OH^- + H^+ \rightarrow H_2O$). A base is an H^+ acceptor. The hydroxyl ion (OH^-), for example, combines with H^+ to form water (H_2O).
- *pH:* A unit of measurement that indicates the number of H^+ in solution. Remember that as the number of H^+ increases, the pH decreases. As the number of H^+ decreases, the pH increases. The normal plasma pH ranges from 7.35 to 7.45. A plasma pH of less than 7.35 is called acidosis, and a plasma pH greater than 7.45 is called alkalosis (Figure 25-3, *A*).

WHERE THE ACID (H^+) COMES FROM

Remember that H^+ is acid. Most H^+ comes from the body's chemical reactions during metabolism. For example, when glucose is metabolized in the presence of oxygen, it produces carbon dioxide (CO_2), water, and energy. The CO_2 combines with water and forms an acid (carbonic acid). When glucose is metabolized in the absence of oxygen, it forms lactic acid (H^+). When fatty acids are metabolized very quickly, they yield ketoacids (H^+). Finally, when proteins are metabolized, some of them yield sulfuric acid (H^+). All these acids are produced by metabolizing cells. To maintain acid–base balance, the body must neutralize and excrete the excess acids.

HOW THE BODY REGULATES pH

Three mechanisms work together to regulate pH: buffers, respirations, and kidney function (see Figure 25-3, *B*).

BUFFERS

The buffer system is the first line of defense in the regulation of pH. A buffer is a chemical substance that prevents large changes in pH. There are two parts to a buffer, called a *buffer pair,* which consists of a "taker" and a "giver." A buffer pair works like this: If [H^+] in the blood increases, the taker part of the buffer removes H^+ from the blood. If the [H^+] decreases, the giver part of the buffer donates H^+ to the blood. By removing or adding H^+, the buffer pair can maintain a normal blood pH. The body has numerous buffer pairs; the most important are the bicarbonate buffers, phosphate buffers, hemoglobin, and plasma proteins.

LUNGS

The respiratory system is the second line of defense in the regulation of pH. What does breathing have to do with pH? CO_2 can combine with water to form an acid (H^+). Because breathing controls CO_2 levels, it also affects [H^+] or blood pH (Figure 25-4, *A*).

How Decreasing the Respiratory Rate Decreases pH

By decreasing the respiratory rate, the body retains or accumulates CO_2. The CO_2 combines with H_2O to form H^+. The increase in [H^+] causes the pH to decrease. This is the basis for the development of respiratory acidosis (see Figure 25-4, *B*).

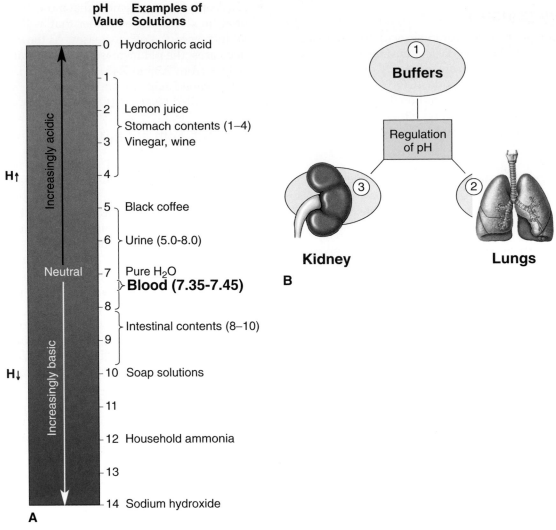

FIGURE 25-3 A, pH scale. **B,** Regulation of pH by buffers, lungs, and kidneys.

How Increasing the Respiratory Rate Increases pH

By increasing respiratory rate, the body exhales, or blows off, CO_2. The decrease in CO_2 causes a decrease in $[H^+]$ and an increase in pH; this is the basis of respiratory alkalosis (see Figure 25-4, C).

How the Respiratory System Knows

How does the respiratory system know that it should increase or decrease the respiratory rate? The medulla oblongata, the respiratory center in the brain, senses changes in $[H^+]$. As plasma pCO_2 increases, the $[H^+]$ in both the plasma and cerebrospinal fluid also increases, thereby stimulating respiratory activity. The respiratory center then increases the rate and depth of breathing, thereby increasing the excretion of CO_2 by the lungs. As plasma $[H^+]$ decreases, the medullary respiratory center sends a slow-down signal, thereby decreasing the rate of breathing and the excretion of CO_2 by the lungs. The ability of the respiratory rate to respond to changing pCO_2 forms the basis for the respiratory compensatory mechanisms in metabolic acidosis and alkalosis.

KIDNEYS

The kidneys are the third line of defense in the regulation of pH. The kidneys help regulate pH by reabsorbing or excreting H^+ as needed. The kidneys also help regulate pH by reabsorbing and excreting bicarbonate (HCO_3^-), a major buffer. Because the kidneys are major H^+ eliminators, patients in kidney failure are generally acidotic.

ACID–BASE IMBALANCES

When the body is unable to regulate pH, acid–base imbalances develop. The acid–base imbalances in the blood are called *acidosis* and *alkalosis*. These imbalances are common, exert generalized effects, and are often life threatening. The acid–base imbalances, their causes, and compensatory mechanisms are summarized in Table 25-2.

A

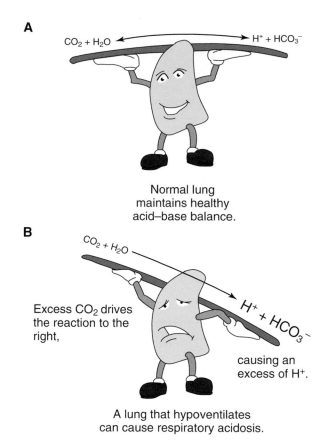

$CO_2 + H_2O$ ⟷ $H^+ + HCO_3^-$

Normal lung
maintains healthy
acid–base balance.

B

$CO_2 + H_2O$

$H^+ + HCO_3^-$

Excess CO_2 drives
the reaction to the
right,

causing an
excess of H^+.

A lung that hypoventilates
can cause respiratory acidosis.

C

$H^+ + HCO_3^-$

$CO_2 + H_2O$

causing a
decrease in H^+.

CO_2 levels decrease,
driving the reaction
to the left, and

A lung that hyperventilates
can cause respiratory alkalosis.

FIGURE 25-4 Respiratory control of acid–base balance. **A,** Normal respiratory rate. **B,** Hypoventilation causes respiratory acidosis. **C,** Hyperventilation causes respiratory alkalosis.

ACIDOSIS

A decrease in plasma pH below 7.35 is acidosis. (Remember that an increase in the plasma [H^+] results in a decrease in pH.) The two types of acidosis are respiratory acidosis and metabolic acidosis. **Respiratory acidosis** is caused by any condition that decreases the effectiveness of the respiratory system or causes prolonged **hypoventilation**. For example, chronic lung disease (emphysema), high doses of narcotics, splinting of the chest, and injury to the medulla oblongata may all cause a decrease in respiratory activity. The

hypoventilation, in turn, increases the plasma levels of CO_2. The excess CO_2 forms H^+, decreases pH, and causes acidosis (see Figure 25-4, *B*). Because the acidosis is caused by a respiratory dysfunction (hypoventilation), it is classified as a respiratory acidosis.

How does the body try to correct respiratory acidosis? First, the buffer systems remove some of the excess H^+. Then the kidneys excrete the excess H^+ and increase plasma bicarbonate (HCO_3^-). The ability of the kidneys to correct respiratory acidosis is called the *renal compensation for respiratory acidosis*. The respiratory system, however, cannot correct this pH imbalance because it is the dysfunctional respiratory system that is causing the acidosis.

Metabolic acidosis is a decrease in pH caused by nonrespiratory conditions. For example, kidney disease, uncontrolled diabetes mellitus, prolonged vomiting of intestinal contents (with loss of bicarbonate), and severe diarrhea (with loss of bicarbonate) are common causes of metabolic acidosis. A patient with poor kidney function is unable to excrete H^+ and becomes acidotic. A patient with uncontrolled diabetes mellitus produces excess ketoacids that overwhelm the buffer systems, accumulate in the plasma, and cause ketoacidosis.

How does the body try to correct metabolic acidosis? First, the buffer system removes some of the excess H^+. Second, the respiratory system helps remove excess H^+ through **hyperventilation** or **Kussmaul** (KOOS-mall) **respirations.** Hyperventilation decreases plasma CO_2 and therefore decreases [H^+] and increases pH. The increased respiratory activity is called the *respiratory compensation for metabolic acidosis*.

🧠 Do You Know...

Why You Can Hyperventilate Yourself into a Hypocalcemic Tetany?

An anxious person often hyperventilates, causing a respiratory alkalosis. Calcium is less soluble in alkalotic blood. Consequently, the plasma levels of calcium decrease. Because calcium is necessary for normal nerve conduction, nerve function is impaired, and the person experiences numbness and tingling. If the person continues to hyperventilate, the plasma levels of calcium may decline so much that an episode of hypocalcemic tetany could occur.

ALKALOSIS

An increase in plasma pH above 7.45 is alkalosis. The two types of alkalosis are respiratory alkalosis and metabolic alkalosis. Respiratory alkalosis develops from hyperventilation and the resulting decrease in plasma CO_2 and [H^+]. Common causes of respiratory alkalosis include anxiety and aspirin (salicylate) poisoning. Any condition that causes hyperventilation causes **respiratory alkalosis** (see Figure 25-4, *C*).

The body tries to correct respiratory alkalosis by the buffers and the kidneys. The buffers donate H^+ to the

Table 25-2	pH Imbalances	
IMBALANCE	**CAUSES**	**COMPENSATIONS**
Acidosis (pH <7.35)		
Respiratory acidosis	Any condition that causes hypoventilation (chronic lung disease such as emphysema, asthma, splinting of the chest, high doses of narcotic drugs, myasthenia gravis)	Kidneys excrete H^+ and reabsorb HCO_3^- (renal compensation for respiratory acidosis)
Metabolic acidosis	Kidney disease, diarrhea, diabetic ketoacidosis, lactic acidosis, vomiting of intestinal contents	Increased respiratory rate to blow off CO_2; Kussmaul respirations (respiratory compensation for metabolic acidosis)
Alkalosis (pH >7.45)		
Respiratory alkalosis	Any condition that causes hyperventilation (anxiety)	Kidneys retain H^+ and excrete HCO_3^- (renal compensation for respiratory alkalosis)
Metabolic alkalosis	Persistent vomiting of stomach contents (loss of HCl), gastric suctioning, overingestion of antacids and bicarbonate-containing drugs	Decreased respiratory activity to retain CO_2 (respiratory compensation for metabolic alkalosis)

plasma, thereby decreasing pH. The kidneys decrease the excretion of H^+; H^+ retention decreases pH. The kidneys also increase the excretion of bicarbonate. The ability of the kidneys to correct respiratory alkalosis is called the *renal compensation for respiratory alkalosis*. The respiratory system cannot correct this pH disturbance because it is the overactivity, or hyperventilation, of the respiratory system that is causing the alkalosis.

Metabolic alkalosis is an increase in pH caused by nonrespiratory disorders. Metabolic alkalosis can be caused by overuse of antacid and bicarbonate–containing drugs; persistent vomiting of stomach contents (loss of HCl); and frequent nasogastric suctioning (loss of HCl). The body tries to correct metabolic alkalosis through buffers, the kidneys, and the respiratory system. The buffers donate H^+, thereby decreasing pH. The kidneys decrease their excretion of H^+. Finally, the respiratory system corrects the pH by hypoventilation. Hypoventilation increases plasma CO_2 and H^+ and decreases pH.

Note that the respiratory system can both cause a pH imbalance and help correct a nonrespiratory pH imbalance. Similarly, the kidneys can both cause and correct pH imbalances. The ability of the lungs and the kidneys to correct a pH imbalance is called a *compensatory function*.

? Re-Think

1. Define acidosis and alkalosis.
2. Explain how the lungs can both cause acidosis (respiratory acidosis) and help correct metabolic acidosis.
3. Explain how the kidneys correct respiratory acidosis as in ketoacidosis.

2+2 Sum It Up!

Plasma $[H^+]$ is expressed as pH. The normal plasma pH range is 7.35 to 7.45. It is regulated by three mechanisms: buffers, respirations, and kidney function. Acid–base balance is essential for the proper functioning of millions of chemical reactions in the body. Thus, acid–base imbalances pose a serious threat to health. The imbalances are classified as acidosis, a plasma pH less than 7.35 (respiratory and metabolic), or alkalosis, a plasma pH higher than 7.45 (respiratory and metabolic). There are respiratory and renal compensatory mechanisms.

As You Age

1. As the kidneys age, the tubules become less responsive to antidiuretic hormone (ADH) and tend to lose too much water. The excess water loss is accompanied by a decrease in the thirst mechanism. As a result, the older person is prone to dehydration.
2. The ability to reabsorb glucose and sodium is also diminished. The presence of excess solute (sodium and glucose) in the urine contributes to excess urination and water loss. In addition, impaired reabsorption of glucose interferes with blood glucose monitoring in diabetes.
3. The kidney tubules are less efficient in the secretion of ions, including the hydrogen ion (H^+). As a result, the older person experiences difficulty in correcting acid–base imbalances.
4. With immobility and diminished exercise, calcium moves from the bones into the renal tubules. There the calcium precipitates, causing kidney stones.

MEDICAL TERMINOLOGY AND DISORDERS Water, Electrolyte, and Acid–Base Imbalances

Medical Term	Word Parts	Word Part Meaning or Derivation	Description
Words			
dehydration	de-	from or down	**Dehydration** is *the loss of water that is necessary for normal body function; it occurs when the body loses more water than it takes in.*
	-hydr/o-	water	
	-ation	process	
edema		From a Greek word meaning "a swelling tumor"	**Edema** is *the accumulation of excess fluid causing swelling.*
Disorders			
pH Imbalances			
acidosis	acid-	From a Latin word meaning "sour" or "sharp," as in vinegar	*A condition in which there is excess H+ (acid) in body fluids. The blood pH is <7.35. Acidosis is classified as either respiratory or metabolic acidosis (described in text).*
	-osis	condition of or increase	
alkalosis	alkali-	From a Greek word meaning "soda ash," a basic or alkaline substance that is slippery and caustic	*A condition in which there is insufficient H+ in body fluids. The blood pH is >7.45. Alkalosis is classified as either respiratory or metabolic (described in text).*
	-osis	condition of or increase	
Electrolyte Imbalances			
hypernatremia	hyper-	above or excessive	**Hypernatremia** is *an elevation in plasma sodium (>145 mmol/L) and can occur in response to a loss of water (most common) or a gain of sodium.* **Hyponatremia** is *a decrease in plasma sodium (<135 mmol/L); it occurs in response to a loss of sodium-containing fluids or excess intake of water (called dilutional hyponatremia).*
	-natr-	From the Latin word *natrium,* meaning "sodium"	
	-emia	in the blood	
hyperkalemia	hyper-	above or excessive	*An elevation of potassium (>5.5 mEq/L) in the blood.* Three causes include: (1) failure to eliminate K+, as in impaired kidney function and the use of drugs such as ACE inhibitors, (2) shift of K+ out of the cells, as occurs in tissue injury or catabolism, and (3) excess intake of K+, as in K+-rich drugs or salt substitutes. Because hyperkalemia affects the depolarization of excitable cells (nerve and muscle), hyperkalemia causes muscle weakness and cramping, nerve paresthesias, and cardiac conduction irregularities.
	-kal/i-	From the Latin word *kalium,* meaning "potassium"	
	-emia	blood condition	
hypokalemia	hypo-	below or deficient	*A decrease of potassium (<3.5 mEq/L) in the blood.* Three causes include: (1) excess K+ loss as occurs in kidney and GI losses (especially diarrhea, vomiting, and GI suctioning), (2) shift of K+ into the cells, and (3) decreased intake of K+.
	-kal/i-	From the Latin word *kalium,* meaning "potassium"	
	-emia	blood condition	
extracellular water imbalances			*Refers to an extracellular volume excess (hypervolemia) or deficit (hypovolemia).* Hypervolemia is also called **volume overload.** It refers to excess extracellular volume and is caused by heart failure, excess steroids, liver failure, impaired kidney function, and excess intravenous fluid infusion. The excess fluid causes weight gain and can accumulate in the extremities (peripheral edema), in the abdominal cavity (ascites), and in the lungs, thereby reducing oxygenation and causing dyspnea and orthopnea. **Hypovolemia** refers to *a diminished volume of blood and is commonly caused by excessive loss of water or reduced intake. If untreated, the condition progresses to hypovolemic shock and death.*

Get Ready for Exams!

Summary Outline

Water, electrolytes, acids, and bases are tightly regulated. Fluids and electrolytes must be distributed in the body compartments in the correct volumes and concentrations.

I. Body Fluids: Distribution and Composition
 A. Major fluid compartments
  1. Two major fluid compartments: intracellular and extracellular compartments
  2. Extracellular compartment: interstitial fluid, intravascular fluid (plasma), lymph, and transcellular fluid
 B. Composition of body fluids
  1. Intracellular fluid: potassium (K^+), phosphate (PO_4^{3-}), and magnesium (Mg^{2+})
  2. Extracellular fluid: sodium (Na^+), chloride (Cl^-), and bicarbonate (HCO_3^-)

II. Water Balance: Intake Equals Output
 A. Intake
  1. The average intake of water is 2500 mL/24 hr.
  2. The primary regulator of fluid intake is thirst.
 B. Output
  1. The average output of water is 2500 mL/24 hr.
  2. Water is excreted by the kidneys, skin, lungs, digestive tract, and sweat.
 C. Water, deficiency, and excess
  1. Deficiency of body water: dehydration
  2. Excess of body water: expanded blood volume and edema

III. Electrolyte Balance
 A. Sodium (Na^+)
  1. Chief extracellular cation
  2. Necessary for water balance and nerve–muscle conduction
  3. Primarily regulated by aldosterone
 B. Potassium (K^+)
  1. Chief intracellular cation
  2. Necessary for nerve–muscle conduction
  3. Primarily regulated by aldosterone
 C. Calcium (Ca^{2+})
  1. Strengthens bones and teeth; necessary for muscle contraction, nerve–muscle conduction, and blood clotting
  2. Primarily regulated by parathyroid hormone
 D. Magnesium (Mg^{2+}) and Chloride (Cl^-)
  1. Magnesium performs important functions in heart, muscles, and nerves.
  2. Chloride: chief extracellular anion; follows Na^+
 E. Bicarbonate (HCO_3^-)
  1. A major extracellular anion
  2. Transports CO_2
  3. Regulates acid–base balance

IV. Acid–Base Balance
 A. pH
  1. The pH refers to the concentration of H^+.
  2. The normal blood pH is 7.35 to 7.45. Acidosis occurs if blood pH is less than 7.35; alkalosis occurs if blood pH is more than 7.45.

 B. Regulation of blood pH
  1. Blood pH is regulated by buffers, the respiratory system, and the kidneys.
  2. Buffers (the buffer pair) can donate or remove H^+.
  3. The respiratory system affects pH by regulating CO_2.
  4. The kidneys can vary their excretion of H^+ and reabsorption of bicarbonate.

V. Acid–Base Imbalances
 A. Acidosis (blood pH <7.35)
  1. Respiratory acidosis is caused by hypoventilation.
  2. Metabolic acidosis has nonrespiratory causes, including kidney disease, uncontrolled diabetes mellitus, diarrhea, and lactic acid production.
 B. Alkalosis (blood pH >7.45)
  1. Respiratory alkalosis is caused by hyperventilation.
  2. Metabolic alkalosis is caused by nonrespiratory conditions, including overingestion of antacids and loss of gastric contents.

Review Your Knowledge

Matching: Water Compartments
Directions: Match the following words with their description below. Some words may be used more than once.

a. interstitial
b. intracellular
c. plasma
d. transcellular

1. ___ Most body water is located within this compartment.
2. ___ Water located within the vascular compartment (blood vessels)
3. ___ Water located between the cells
4. ___ Includes water within the eye, glandular secretions, and cerebrospinal fluid
5. ___ Also called *tissue fluid*

Matching: Ions
Directions: Match the following words with their description below. Some terms may be used more than once.

a. Na^+
b. K^+
c. H^+
d. Ca^{2+}

1. ___ Plasma concentration of this ion determines pH.
2. ___ The chief extracellular cation
3. ___ The chief intracellular cation
4. ___ The ion that is elevated in hyperkalemia
5. ___ Aldosterone stimulates the distal tubule and upper collecting duct to reabsorb this cation.
6. ___ Hypoventilation causes the accumulation of CO_2 and this cation.
7. ___ Many diuretics are kaliuretic and therefore cause a loss of this cation.
8. ___ Most diuretics work by blocking the renal reabsorption of this cation.
9. ___ An increase in this ion causes acidosis.
10. ___ This ion is regulated primarily by parathyroid hormone.

Multiple Choice

1. Hyperkalemia
   a. refers to an elevated serum potassium level.
   b. is never serious.
   c. develops in response to kaliuresis.
   d. refers to dangerously high levels of plasma sodium.
2. Which of the following best indicates the role of albumin in water balance?
   a. Blocks the renal reabsorption of Na^+
   b. Enhances the renal excretion of K^+
   c. Maintains plasma oncotic pressure
   d. "Plugs up" capillary pores, keeping water within the plasma
3. A patient with a history of heart failure is admitted to the hospital in pulmonary edema. Over a 4-day period, his breathing improved and he experienced a loss of 8 lb. Which of the following best explains his clinical improvement?
   a. Increased hematocrit and oxygen-carrying capacity of the blood
   b. Increased secretion of aldosterone and Na^+ reabsorption
   c. Diuresis
   d. Volume expansion
4. Which of the following is not true of Na^+?
   a. Na^+ is the chief extracellular cation.
   b. Na^+ helps regulate extracellular volume.
   c. Na^+ is affected by aldosterone.
   d. Na^+ retention causes diuresis.
5. Impaired respiratory gas exchange and hypoventilation are most apt to cause
   a. volume expansion and heart failure.
   b. diuresis and dehydration.
   c. an increase in blood pH.
   d. respiratory acidosis.
6. Kussmaul respirations are the compensatory mechanism for
   a. pulmonary edema.
   b. respiratory acidosis.
   c. metabolic acidosis.
   d. anxiety-induced hyperventilation.
7. Which of the following is most apt to happen when fatty acids are broken down rapidly and incompletely?
   a. Plasma pH increases.
   b. The patient hypoventilates in an attempt to correct the pH disturbance.
   c. Ketoacids are produced causing metabolic acidosis.
   d. Plasma $[H^+]$ decreases.
8. Hypocalcemia is most apt to
   a. cause blood volume expansion (hypervolemia).
   b. be treated with IV potassium.
   c. cause tetany.
   d. be caused by excess parathyroid hormone activity.

9. An anxiety-induced hyperventilation
   a. decreases blood pH.
   b. causes alkalosis.
   c. increases $[H^+]$.
   d. decreases pO_2.
10. "Tenting" is
    a. a consequence of hypervolemia.
    b. best treated with a diuretic.
    c. due to volume depletion in the interstitial space.
    d. indicative of hyperkalemia.
11. Which of the following is least true of alkalosis?
    a. Can be caused by an anxiety-induced hyperventilation
    b. The blood pH >7.45
    c. Blood $[H^+]$ is decreased
    d. Usually caused by CO_2 retention

Go Figure

1. **According to Figure 25-1**
   a. Most fluid is located in the extracellular space.
   b. Interstitial fluid is the same as intravascular fluid.
   c. Plasma and interstitial fluid are extracellular fluids.
   d. Lymph is located intracellularly.

2. **According to Figure 25-2**
   a. Thirst is a major regulator of water intake.
   b. Most water is lost in the urine.
   c. Water can be lost by organs other than the kidneys.
   d. All of the above are true.

3. **According to Figure 25-3**
   a. As $[H^+]$ increases, pH increases.
   b. The pink end of the pH scale represents a more acidic pH.
   c. The blue end of the pH scale represents an increase in $[H^+]$.
   d. All of the above are true.

4. **According to Figure 25-4 and Table 25-2**
   a. Hypoventilation causes alkalosis.
   b. Hyperventilation causes alkalosis.
   c. Ventilation has no effect on blood pH.
   d. Hypoventilation decreases $[H^+]$ in the blood.

5. **According to Figure 25-4 and Table 25-2**
   a. Kussmaul respirations are compensatory for metabolic acidosis.
   b. Hypoventilation is compensatory for a drug-induced respiratory depression.
   c. An anxious person may hyperventilate, causing a respiratory acidosis.
   d. Persistent vomiting of stomach contents is most apt to induce a metabolic acidosis.

Reproductive Systems

Key Terms

cervix (p. 499)
endometrium (p. 499)
epididymis (p. 492)
estrogen (p. 498)
fallopian tubes (p. 498)
gonadotropins (p. 501)
gonads (p. 490)
graafian follicle (p. 496)

menopause (p. 504)
menses (p. 501)
myometrium (p. 499)
ovarian follicles (p. 496)
ovulation (p. 496)
progesterone (p. 498)
prostate gland (p. 494)
scrotum (p. 490)

semen (p. 494)
spermatogenesis (p. 491)
testes (p. 490)
testosterone (p. 490)
uterus (p. 499)
vas deferens (p. 492)

Objectives

1. List and describe the structures and functions of the male reproductive system.
2. Describe the hormonal control of male reproduction, including the effects of testosterone.
3. List and describe the structures and functions of the female reproductive system.

4. Explain the hormonal control of the female reproductive cycle and the two reproductive cycles.
5. Describe the various methods of birth control.

Few biological drives are as strong as the urge to reproduce. As everyone knows and appreciates, human reproduction is sexual, meaning that both a female and male partner are required. In contrast, reproduction in single-cell organisms is asexual, meaning that no partner is required. They simply divide by themselves. Think of how different your life would be in an asexual environment!

To carry out its role, the reproductive system performs two functions: it produces, nurtures, and transports ova and sperm, and it secretes hormones. The reproductive organs include the primary reproductive organs and the secondary reproductive organs. The primary reproductive organs are the gonads. The female gonads are the ovaries; the male gonads are the testes.

The gonads perform two functions: They secrete hormones, and they produce the gametes. The gametes (GAM-eets) are the ova (eggs) and the sperm. All other organs, ducts, and glands in the reproductive system are secondary, or accessory, reproductive organs. The secondary reproductive structures nourish and transport the eggs and sperm. They also provide a safe and nourishing environment for the fertilized eggs.

MALE REPRODUCTIVE SYSTEM

The male reproductive system performs three roles: it produces, nourishes, and transports sperm; it deposits the sperm within the female reproductive tract; and it secretes hormones. Figure 26-1, *A*, shows the organs of the male reproductive tract.

TESTES

The **testes**, or testicles, are the male gonads. They perform two functions: the production of sperm and the secretion of the male hormone, **testosterone** (see Figure 26-1, *A*). The two oval testes are located outside the abdominal cavity and are suspended in a sac between the thighs called the **scrotum**.

The testes begin their development within the abdominal cavity but normally descend into the scrotum during the last 2 months of fetal development. Failure of the testes to descend into the scrotum is called *cryptorchidism,* a condition that can result in sterility if left untreated.

Why Aristotle Called the Testicle the *Orchis?*

The root of the orchid plant is olive shaped; in Greek the shape is called an *orchis*. Noticing the similarity between the shape of the orchid root and the testicles, Aristotle dubbed the testicle *orchis*. The word *orchis* is still used in medical terms; for example, *orchitis* refers to inflammation of the testicles, and *orchiectomy* refers to the surgical removal of the testicles. The word *testis* comes from the Latin and means "to bear witness to." The word *testes* shares the same Latin root with the word *testify.* In ancient Rome, only men could bear witness, or testify, in a public forum. To show the importance of their testimony, they held their testicles as they spoke.

LOCATION, LOCATION, LOCATION

Why are undescended testicles associated with infertility? It's a temperature thing. Sperm cannot live at body temperature; instead, they prefer the cooler temperature of the scrotum. To avoid infertility, a surgeon pulls the undescended testicles into the scrotum. Wearing tight underwear and jeans can also elevate the temperature in the testes, thereby lowering sperm count. What happens when the outside environmental temperature becomes excessively cold during the winter months? The scrotum, with the assistance of the cremaster muscle, pulls the testes close to the body, thereby keeping the sperm toasty, happy, and motile.

LOBULES

The testis is divided into about 250 smaller units called *lobules* (Figure 26-2, *A*). Each lobule contains seminiferous tubules and interstitial cells. The tightly coiled seminiferous (seh-mih-NIF-er-us) tubules form sperm. The interstitial cells lie between the seminiferous tubules and produce the male hormones called *androgens*. The most important androgen is testosterone. Thus, the testes produce both sperm and testosterone.

SPERM CELLS

Every day, a man makes millions of sperm. Sperm are formed by the epithelium of the seminiferous tubules. The seminiferous tubules contain two types of cells: spermatogenic cells (cells that produce sperm) and supporting cells (cells that support, nourish, and regulate the spermatogenic cells). The supporting cells are also called *sustentacular cells* or *Sertoli cells*.

Spermatogenesis

Spermatogenesis (sper-mah-toh-JEN-eh-sis) is the formation of sperm. The undifferentiated spermatogenic cells are called *spermatogonia*. Each spermatogonium

contains 46 chromosomes—the normal number of chromosomes for human body cells. Under the influence of testosterone, the spermatogonia enlarge to become primary spermatocytes. The primary spermatocytes divide by a special type of cell division called *meiosis*. The important point about meiosis is that it reduces the number of chromosomes by half, from 46 to 23. Thus, a sperm has only 23 chromosomes. When the sperm unites with an egg, which also has only 23 chromosomes (by meiosis), the fertilized egg then contains 46 chromosomes, the normal number for human body cells. Newly formed sperm are not functional and must undergo several maturational changes.

A sperm looks like a tadpole (see Figure 26-2, *B*). The mature sperm has three parts: a head, body, and tail. The head is primarily a nucleus. The nucleus is important because it contains the genetic information. The front part of the head has a specialized structure called the *acrosome,* which contains enzymes that help the sperm penetrate the egg at the time of fertilization. The body, or midpiece, of the sperm is a spiral-shaped structure that contains many mitochondria and supplies the sperm with the energy needed for the "big swim." The tail of the sperm is a flagellum. Its whiplike movements enable the sperm to swim. Most sperm live only hours after being deposited in the female reproductive tract, but the hardier ones may survive for up to 3 days.

 Re-Think

1. What are the names of the male and female gonads? Gametes?
2. Differentiate between the functions of the seminiferous tubules and the interstitial cells.

 Sum It Up!

The purpose of the reproductive system is to produce offspring. Human reproduction is achieved sexually through the union of an egg and a sperm. The primary reproductive organs are the gonads: the ovaries in the female and the testes in the male. The gonads produce the gametes; the ovaries produce the female gametes (eggs), and the testes produce the male gametes (sperm). The mature egg and sperm each contain 23 chromosomes. On union, the fertilized egg contains 46 chromosomes, the number of chromosomes that human cells contain.

GENITAL DUCTS

As the sperm form, they gather in the seminiferous tubules and move into a series of genital ducts, where they mature. They are then transported from the testes to outside the body. The ducts include two epididymides, two vas (ductus) deferens, two ejaculatory ducts, and one urethra.

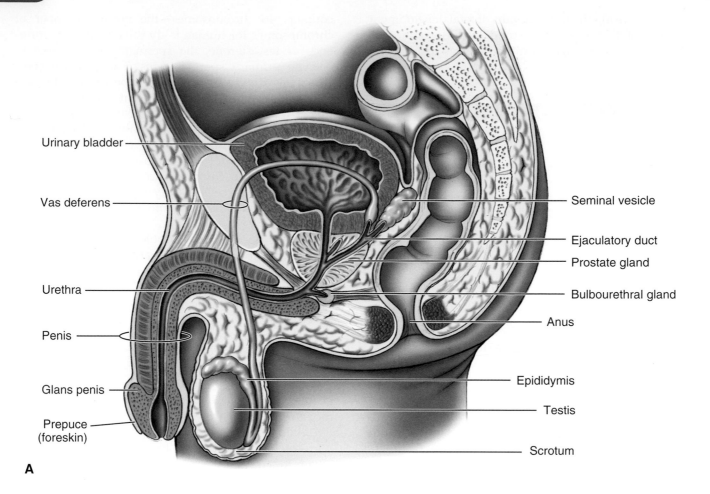

Urinary bladder

Vas deferens

Urethra

Penis

Glans penis

Prepuce
(foreskin)

A

Seminal vesicle

Ejaculatory duct

Prostate gland

Bulbourethral gland

Anus

Epididymis

Testis

Scrotum

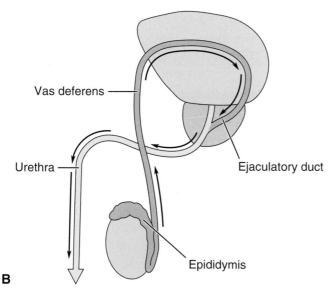

Vas deferens

Urethra

Ejaculatory duct

Epididymis

B

FIGURE 26-1 **A,** Male reproductive organs. **B,** The pathway for semen.

EPIDIDYMIS

The **epididymis** (ep-i-DID-i-miss) is the first part of the duct system. It is about 20 feet (6 m) in length, is tightly coiled, and sits along the top and posterior side of the testis (see Figure 26-1). While in the epididymis, the sperm mature, becoming motile and fertile. The walls of the epididymis contract and push the sperm into the next structure, the vas deferens.

VAS DEFERENS AND EJACULATORY DUCTS

The **vas deferens** (DEF-er-enz) is continuous with the epididymis. It ascends as part of the spermatic cord

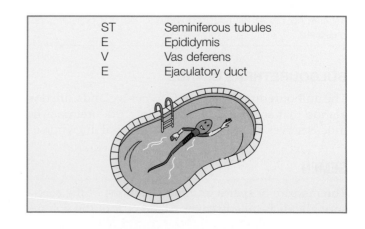

FIGURE 26-2 **A,** Male gonad. The testis consists of lobules containing seminiferous tubules surrounded by interstitial cells. **B,** Sperm.

through the inguinal canal in the groin region into the pelvic cavity. There are two spermatic cords: one coming from the right and one from the left groin region. In addition to the vas deferens, the spermatic cord includes blood vessels, lymphatic vessels, nerves, muscles, and connective tissue.

As the vas deferens courses through the pelvic cavity, it curves over the urinary bladder and joins with the duct of the seminal vesicle to form the ejaculatory duct (see Figure 26-1). The two ejaculatory ducts, from the right and left sides, pass through the prostate gland and join with the single urethra. Trouble remembering the directions? Let swimmer STEVE help!

ST	Seminiferous tubules
E	Epididymis
V	Vas deferens
E	Ejaculatory duct

URETHRA

The urethra extends from the base of the urinary bladder to the tip of the penis. The male urethra serves two organ systems: the reproductive and urinary systems. The urethra carries urine from the urinary bladder to the outside. It also carries semen from the ejaculatory ducts to the outside. However, the urethra can only do one thing at a time. It passes either urine or semen, but never both simultaneously.

ACCESSORY GLANDS

Various secretions are added to the sperm as they travel through the genital ducts. The secretions come from three glands: the seminal vesicles, the prostate gland, and the bulbourethral glands (see Figure 26-1, *A*).

SEMINAL VESICLES

The seminal vesicles are located at the base of the bladder and secrete a thick yellowish material rich in substances such as fructose (sugar), vitamin C, and prostaglandins. These substances nourish and activate the sperm as they pass through the ducts.

PROSTATE GLAND

The single doughnut-like **prostate gland** encircles the upper urethra just below the bladder. The prostate gland secretes a milky alkaline substance that plays a role in increasing sperm motility. It also counteracts the acidic environment of the vagina and so helps protect the sperm as they enter the woman's body. During ejaculation, the smooth muscle of the prostate gland contracts and forces the secretions into the urethra.

 Do You Know...

If It Is a Prostrate or a Prostate Gland?

The doughnut-shaped gland of the male surrounds the urethra as it leaves the bladder. The word *prostate* means "one who stands before"; the prostate gland stands before the exit from the bladder. It sort of has a noble ring to it! However, sometimes the gland is mistakenly called the "prostrate" gland. A prostrate position is flat and helpless—definitely not a flattering name for such equipment. So, it's *prostate*, not prostrate.

BULBOURETHRAL GLANDS

The bulbourethral glands, or Cowper's glands, are tiny glands that secrete thick mucus into the urethra. The mucus serves as a lubricant during sexual intercourse.

SEMEN

The mixture of sperm and the secretions of the accessory glands is called **semen**. About 60% of the volume of semen comes from the seminal vesicles. The rest of it comes from the prostate gland. Semen is a milky white liquid with an alkaline pH.

The secretions of the accessory glands perform several other functions; they nourish the sperm, aid in the transport of sperm, and lubricate the reproductive tract. The amount of semen per ejaculation is small, about 2 to 6 mL, or 1 teaspoon. The number of sperm per ejaculation, however, is impressive—50 to 100 million!

EXTERNAL GENITALS

The external genitals (genitalia) of the male consist of the scrotum and the penis (see Figure 26-1). The scrotum is a sac, or pouch of skin, that hangs loosely between the legs and contains the testes.

The penis has two functions; it carries urine through the urethra to the outside of the body, and it acts as the organ of sexual intercourse (copulation). The penis deposits sperm in the female reproductive tract. The shaft, or body, of the penis contains three columns of erectile tissue and an enlarged tip called the *glans penis*. The opening of the urethra penetrates the glans penis.

The loose skin covering the penis extends downward and forms a cuff of skin around the glans called the *foreskin,* or *prepuce* (PREH-poos). Around puberty, small glands located in the foreskin and the glans secrete an oily substance. This secretion and the surrounding dead skin cells form a cheesy substance called *smegma*. As part of daily hygiene, a man should pull back the foreskin to remove the smegma. Occasionally, the foreskin is too tight and cannot be retracted (phimosis). The foreskin is often surgically removed after birth in a process called *circumcision*. Although parents often have their sons circumcised to promote cleanliness, circumcision is also a common religious ritual.

 Re-Think

Trace the movement of a sperm from the seminiferous tubules to the urinary meatus.

MALE SEXUAL RESPONSE: ERECTION, EMISSION, EJACULATION, AND ORGASM

The urethra extends the length of the penis and is surrounded by three columns of spongy erectile tissue. When a man is sexually stimulated, the parasympathetic nerves fire, the penile arteries dilate, and the erectile tissue fills with blood. The accumulation of blood in the erectile tissue causes the penis to enlarge and become rigid. This process is an erection. It enables the penis to penetrate the reproductive tract of the female. For various reasons, a man may be unable to achieve an erection and is said to have erectile dysfunction (ED). (The older term is *impotence*.)

Orgasm refers to the pleasurable sensations that occur at the height of sexual stimulation. Orgasm in the male is accompanied by emission and ejaculation. Emission is the movement of sperm and glandular secretions from the testes and genital ducts into the proximal urethra, where they mix to form semen. Emission is caused by the influence of the sympathetic nervous system on the ducts, causing rhythmic, peristalsis-type contractions.

An Autonomic Summary—Up and Out!

Up: Erection	Parasympathetic
Out: Emission	Sympathetic

Ejaculation is the expulsion of semen from the urethra to the outside. Ejaculation begins when the urethra fills with semen. Motor nerve impulses from the spinal cord stimulate the skeletal muscles at the base of the erectile columns in the penis to contract rhythmically. The rhythmic contraction provides the force necessary to expel the semen. (The flow of semen during ejaculation is illustrated in Figure 26-1, *B*.) Immediately after ejaculation, sympathetic nerve impulses cause the penile arteries to constrict, thereby reducing blood flow into the penis. This process is accompanied by increased venous drainage of blood from the penis. As a consequence, the penis becomes flaccid and returns to its unstimulated tiny size.

Up and Down!

Up: Erect	Parasympathetic
Down: Flaccid	Sympathetic

MALE SEX HORMONES

EFFECTS OF TESTOSTERONE

The male sex hormones are called *androgens*, the most important being testosterone. Most of the testosterone is secreted by the interstitial cells of the testes. A small amount is secreted by the adrenal cortex.

Secretion of testosterone begins during fetal development and continues at a very low level throughout childhood. When a boy reaches the age of 10 to 13, testosterone secretion increases rapidly, transforming the boy into a man. This phase in reproductive development is called *puberty*. After puberty, testosterone is secreted continuously throughout the life of the male.

Testosterone is necessary for the production of sperm and is responsible for the development of the male sex characteristics. The primary sex characteristics include the enlargement and development of the testes and the various accessory organs such as the penis. Secondary sex characteristics refer to special features of the male body and include the following:

- Increased growth of hair, particularly on the face, chest, axillary region, and pubic region
- Deepening of the voice, caused by enlargement of the vocal cords
- Thickening of the skin and increased activity of the oil and sweat glands; at puberty, the adolescent is faced with new challenges, such as acne and body odor
- Increased musculoskeletal growth and development of the male physique (broad shoulders and narrow waist)

HORMONAL CONTROL OF MALE REPRODUCTION

The male reproductive system is controlled primarily by the hormones secreted by the hypothalamus, anterior pituitary gland, and testes. The hypothalamus secretes a releasing hormone, which then stimulates the anterior pituitary gland to secrete two gonadotropins: follicle-stimulating hormone (FSH) and luteinizing hormone (LH) (Figure 26-3). FSH promotes spermatogenesis by stimulating the spermatogenic cells to respond to testosterone. Note that spermatogenesis comes about through the combined action of FSH and testosterone. LH, also known as *interstitial cell–stimulating hormone* (ICSH) in the male, promotes the development of the interstitial cells of the testes and the secretion of testosterone.

After puberty, a negative feedback loop regulates testosterone production. When the level of testosterone in the blood increases, it causes the hypothalamus and the anterior pituitary gland to decrease their hormonal secretions, thereby decreasing the production of testosterone. As blood levels of testosterone decrease, the anterior pituitary gland increases its secretion of LH (ICSH), thereby stimulating the interstitial cells to secrete testosterone once again. The negative feedback

FIGURE 26-3 Hormonal control of sperm production and testosterone secretion.

mechanism maintains constant blood levels of testosterone.

? Re-Think

1. Differentiate between the following: erection, emission, and ejaculation.
2. Regarding male contraception, why is it medically more acceptable to ligate the vas deferens than to remove the testes?

FEMALE REPRODUCTIVE SYSTEM

The female reproductive system produces eggs, secretes hormones, and nurtures and protects a developing baby during the 9 months of pregnancy. Figure 26-4, *A*, shows the organs of the female reproductive system.

OVARIES

The female gonads are two almond-shaped ovaries, located on either side of the uterus in the pelvic cavity. The ovaries are anchored in place by several ligaments, including the ovarian and the broad ligaments. The ovaries, although not attached directly to the fallopian tubes, are close to them.

EGG DEVELOPMENT: THE OVARIAN FOLLICLE

Within the ovary are many tiny, saclike structures called ovarian follicles. A female is born with 2 million follicles—enough to start a small family. This number steadily declines with age, however, so that at puberty only about 400,000 follicles remain. Of these, only about 400 follicles ever fully mature, because a female usually produces only one egg per month throughout her reproductive years. The production of eggs begins at puberty and continues until menopause, at about 45 to 55 years of age. As with sperm, the supply of eggs far exceeds the actual need. This is Mother Nature's way of ensuring future generations.

Each ovarian follicle consists of an immature egg, called an *oocyte,* and the surrounding cells called *follicular cells* (see Figure 26-4, *B*). Beginning at puberty, several follicles mature every month, although usually only one fully matures. As the egg matures, it begins to undergo meiotic cell division, which reduces the number of chromosomes by half, from 46 to 23.

At the same time, the follicle enlarges, a fluid-filled center is formed, and the follicular cells begin to secrete estrogen. The mature ovarian follicle is known as the graafian (GRAH-fee-en) follicle. The graafian follicle looks like a blister on the surface of the ovary.

OVULATION

Once a month the ovarian follicle bursts—an "eggsplosion"! The ovary ejects a mature egg (ovum) with a surrounding layer of cells. This ejection phase is called ovulation. The egg travels from the surface of the ovary into the peritoneal cavity, where it is immediately swept into the fallopian tubes by the swishing motion of the fimbriae (finger-like projections at the end of the fallopian tubes). The egg travels through the fallopian tubes to the uterus. If the egg is fertilized, it implants itself in the uterine lining and grows into a baby. If the egg is not fertilized, the egg dies and is eliminated in the menstrual blood. Some women feel twinges of pain at the time of ovulation; the pain is called *mittelschmerz* (MIT-el-schmertz) (from the German, meaning "middle pain").

Once ovulation has occurred, the follicular cells that remain in the ovary develop into a glandular structure called the *corpus luteum* ("yellow body"). The corpus luteum secretes two hormones: large amounts of progesterone (proh-JES-ter-ohn) and smaller amounts of estrogen. If fertilization does not occur, the corpus luteum deteriorates in about 10 days and becomes

FIGURE 26-4 **A,** Female reproductive organs. **B,** Maturation of the ovarian follicle, ovulation, and formation of the corpus luteum.

known as the *corpus albicans* ("white body"). The dead corpus albicans is not capable of secreting hormones. If fertilization occurs, however, the corpus luteum does not deteriorate. It stays alive and continues to secrete its hormones until this role can be taken over by the placenta—a structure you will read about in Chapter 27.

Sometimes, the corpus luteum fills with fluid and forms an ovarian cyst. A blood-filled cyst is called a *chocolate cyst*. These cysts can resolve on their own but may require surgery.

OVARIAN HORMONES

At puberty, the ovaries begin to secrete the sex hormones estrogen and progesterone. The follicular cells of the maturing follicles secrete estrogen, and the corpus luteum secretes large amounts of progesterone and smaller amounts of estrogen. These hormones transform a girl into a woman.

Estrogen

Estrogen exerts two important effects: it promotes the maturation of the egg, and it helps develop the female secondary sex characteristics. Just as the male looks male because of testosterone, the female looks female because of estrogen. The feminizing effects of estrogen include the following:

- Enlargement and development of the organs of the female reproductive system
- Enlargement and development of the breasts
- Deposition of fat beneath the skin, especially in the thighs, buttocks, and breasts
- Widening of the pelvis
- Onset of the menstrual cycle
- Closure of the epiphyseal discs in long bones, thereby stopping further growth in height

Progesterone

The corpus luteum secretes **progesterone**. Progesterone has three important effects: it (1) works with estrogen in establishing the menstrual cycle, (2) helps maintain pregnancy, and (3) prepares the breasts for milk production after pregnancy, increasing their secretory capacity. Although the corpus luteum secretes enough progesterone to maintain pregnancy in the early months, the woman's body needs larger amounts of both estrogen and progesterone during the later stages of pregnancy. This role is performed by the placenta.

? Re-Think

1. Name the steps in the progression from the oocyte to the corpus albicans.
2. Explain the function of the corpus luteum.
3. List two ovarian hormones.

2+2 Sum It Up!

The female gonad is the ovary. Once a month, an ovarian follicle matures, forming a graafian follicle. The follicle contains an egg and estrogen-secreting follicular cells. Under the influence of LH, the egg is expelled from the mature follicle; this event is ovulation. Following ovulation, the corpus luteum begins to secrete large amounts of progesterone. Estrogen helps the egg mature and is primarily responsible for the secondary sex characteristics of the female. Progesterone plays an important role in preparing the reproductive system for pregnancy.

GENITAL TRACT

The female genital tract includes the fallopian tubes, uterus, and vagina (see Figure 26-4, *A*).

FALLOPIAN TUBES

The **fallopian** (fal-LOH-pee-an) **tubes** are also called the *uterine tubes* or the *oviducts*. Each of the two fallopian tubes is about 4 inches (10 cm) long and extends from either side of the uterus to the ovaries. The funnel-shaped end of the fallopian tube nearest the ovary is called the *infundibulum* and has fingerlike projections called *fimbriae* (FIM-bree-ay). The fallopian tube does not attach directly to the ovary; the fimbriae hang over the ovary.

At ovulation, the fimbriae sweep the egg from the surface of the ovary into the fallopian tube. Once in the fallopian tube, the egg moves slowly toward the uterus. Because the egg cannot swim like sperm, the peristaltic activity of the fallopian tubes moves it forward.

The fallopian tubes have two functions. First, the tube transports the egg from the ovary to the uterus. Second, the tube is the usual site of fertilization of the egg by the sperm. The fertilized egg moves through the fallopian tube into the uterus, where it implants and grows into a baby. The journey through the fallopian tubes takes about 4 to 5 days.

Tube Troubles

- Occasionally, the fertilized egg implants in the fallopian tube rather than in the uterus. This condition is known as an *ectopic pregnancy*. The word *ectopic* means "in an abnormal site"; a tubal pregnancy is therefore an ectopic pregnancy. An ectopic pregnancy usually results in a miscarriage. It causes maternal bleeding, possible hemorrhage, and even death.
- What happens if the tubes scar and close? Scarring and closing, as occurs with repeated gonorrheal infections, blocks the movement of the egg through the tubes. This can cause sterility.
- Pelvic inflammatory disease (PID). The fallopian tubes open directly into the pelvic cavity. An infection of the female reproductive tract can spread through the tubes into the pelvic cavity, causing PID. PID is most frequently associated with sexually transmitted diseases.

UTERUS

The **uterus**, or *womb*, is shaped like an upside-down pear and is located between the urinary bladder and the rectum. The broad ligament holds the uterus in place. The primary function of the uterus is to provide a safe and nurturing environment for the growing baby. It is the baby's cradle for 9 comfortable months. During pregnancy, the size of the uterus increases considerably to hold the growing baby and the placenta.

The uterus has three parts. The fundus is the upper dome-shaped region above the entrance of the fallopian tubes. The body is the central region. The **cervix** is the lower narrow region that opens into the vagina.

The uterus has three layers: an outer serosal layer called the *epimetrium,* or *perimetrium;* a middle, smooth muscular layer called the **myometrium**; and an inner layer called the **endometrium**. The endometrial uterine lining has two layers: the basilar layer and the functional layer. The basilar layer is thin and vascular and lies next to the myometrium. The functional layer responds to the ovarian hormones and thickens in preparation for the fertilized egg. It is also the layer that sloughs off during menstruation, when fertilization has not occurred.

The cervix is often associated with the Pap smear. The Pap smear is a diagnostic procedure used for detecting cancer of the cervix. The technique involves scraping cells from around the cervix and examining them for evidence of cancer. This simple and painless procedure has been used successfully to diagnose cancer in its early stages, when cure rates are high. The technique is named for its developer, Dr. George Papanicolaou.

 Do You Know...

What Plato, Hysteria, and the Concept of the Wandering Womb Have in Common?

Plato believed that the womb (uterus), if unused for a long period, became "indignant." This indignant womb then wandered around the body, inhibiting the body's spirit and causing disease. According to the male thinkers of the day, a woman was so thoroughly controlled by her wandering womb that she was considered irrational and prone to emotional outbursts and fits of hysteria. This belief was the reason that the womb was named the *hystera.* The term has persisted in medical terminology; a hysterectomy refers to the surgical removal of the uterus.

VAGINA

The vagina is a 4-inch muscular tube that extends from the cervix to the vaginal opening in the perineum. The vaginal opening is usually covered by a thin membrane called the *hymen.* The definition of hymen comes from the image of the vagina as a sanctuary of the virgin love goddess, Aphrodite. The hymen may be torn in a number of ways, such as during first intercourse, use of tampons, or strenuous exercise. Much

has been written about the hymen and whether or not it is intact. The upper portion of the vagina receives the cervix of the uterus. The cervix dips into the vagina so that pockets, or spaces, form around the cervix. The pockets are called *fornices.* The deepest is the posterior fornix, located behind the cervix.

 Do You Know...

What the Spots Are on the Outer Surfaces of These Organs?

These spots represent endometrial tissue adhering to the outer surface of the ovary, fallopian tube, rectum, and urinary bladder. How did the endometrial tissue get there? In some women, a portion of the menstrual discharge flows backward, into the fallopian tubes, and then into the pelvic cavity. The endometrial tissue adheres to the outer surface of the organs in the pelvic cavity. This condition is called *endometriosis*. The endometrial tissue acts as though it were still in the uterus. It responds to the ovarian hormones by thickening, becoming secretory, and then sloughing off. A woman feels the discomfort of menstruation throughout the pelvic cavity. In addition to causing severe pain, endometriosis causes scarring and the formation of adhesions.

 Do You Know...

About Xtreme Sex "Down-Under"?

A little Aussie mouse, *Antechinus*, engages in sex for up to 12 hours, ignoring eating, drinking, and sleeping. He's definitely in a loop! Alas, the happy little fellow dies of exhaustion. What about Ms. Mouse? Going at a more leisurely pace, she calmly stores the sperm throughout the breeding season and in due time gives birth to an adorable litter. What's in this sex frenzy for Mother Nature? Preservation of the species, and more food for mama mouse and babies.

The mucosal lining of the vagina lies in folds (rugae) that are capable of expanding. The folding is important for childbearing because it permits the vagina to stretch and accommodate the baby during birth. In addition to forming a part of the birth canal, the vagina is also the organ that receives the penis during intercourse and serves as an exit for menstrual blood. The bacterial population (normal flora) in the vagina creates an acidic environment that discourages the growth of pathogens.

FIGURE 26-5 External genitals of the female.

The female genital tract consists of the fallopian tubes, uterus, and vagina. The fallopian tube, the usual site of fertilization, transports the egg from the ovary to the uterus. The uterus is where the fetus lives and grows for 9 months. The vagina receives the penis during intercourse and serves as part of the birth canal. A baby makes its entrance into the world through the vagina.

EXTERNAL GENITALS

The female external genitals (genitalia) are together called the *vulva* (Figure 26-5). The vulva includes the labia majora and labia minora, clitoris, and vestibular glands. (The external genitalia of the female are also called the *pudendum,* from a word meaning "shameful." Go figure!)

The two labia majora are folds of hair-covered skin that lie external to the two smaller labia minora. The labia (the word means "lips") are separated by a cleft containing the urethral and vaginal openings. The labia prevent drying of the mucous membranes. The labia majora merge anteriorly (in front) to form the rounded hair-covered region over the symphysis called the *mons pubis.*

The clitoris is the structure that resembles the penis. Although small, the clitoris contains erectile tissue and is capped by a thin membrane called the *glans.* The labia minora extend forward and partially surround the clitoris to form a foreskin. Like the penis, the clitoris contains sensory receptors that allow the female to experience pleasurable sexual sensations.

The vestibule is a cleft between the labia minora. It contains the openings of the urethra and the vagina. A pair of vestibular glands (Bartholin's glands) lies on either side of the vaginal opening and secrete a mucus-containing substance that moistens and lubricates the vestibule. Note that the female urinary system and the reproductive system are entirely separate, unlike in the male. The female urethra carries only urine, whereas the male urethra carries urine and semen.

The perineum refers to the entire pelvic floor. The common use of the word, however, is more limited. Most clinicians use the word *perineum* to mean the area between the vaginal opening and anus (called the "obstetric perineum").

FEMALE SEXUAL RESPONSE

The female responds to sexual stimulation with erection and orgasm. Erectile tissue in the clitoris and the tissue surrounding the vaginal opening swell with blood in response to parasympathetically induced dilation of the arteries. Erectile tissue in the vaginal mucosa, breasts, and nipples also swell. Other responses include an engorgement of the vagina and secretion by the vestibular glands. At the height of sexual stimulation, a woman experiences orgasm.

The orgasm also stimulates a number of reflexes. These reflexes cause muscle contractions in the perineum, uterine walls, and uterine tubes; the muscular activity is thought to aid in directing and transporting the sperm through the genital tract.

? Re-Think

1. What is the function of the fallopian tubes?
2. List the layers of the uterus.
3. Trace the movement of the egg from ovulation to implantation.

HORMONAL CONTROL OF THE REPRODUCTIVE CYCLES

Let us review the female reproductive cycle. Each month, an egg is produced by the ovary in anticipation of producing a baby. As the egg develops in the ovary, the uterus prepares to receive the fertilized egg. Its preparation consists of the building up of a thick, lush endometrial lining. If the egg is not fertilized, the endometrial lining is no longer needed to nourish the fetus, so it is shed in the menstrual flow. Then the monthly process begins again. A second egg ripens in the ovary, and the uterine lining starts the rebuilding process. This process repeats itself throughout the female reproductive years, all for the purpose of reproducing.

A number of hormones control the female reproductive cycle. Unlike male hormones, female hormonal secretion occurs in a monthly cycle, with a regular pattern of increases and decreases in hormone levels. In fact, the word menses (MEN-seez) comes from the Greek word for "month" or "moon." The hypothalamus, anterior pituitary gland, and ovaries secrete most of the hormones involved in the menstrual cycle. The hypothalamus secretes a releasing hormone that stimulates the anterior pituitary gland to secrete the two gonadotropins, FSH and LH. FSH and LH then stimulate the ovaries, causing them to secrete estrogen and progesterone. The hormones that regulate the female reproductive cycle are summarized in Table 26-1.

TWO REPRODUCTIVE CYCLES

There are two components of the female reproductive cycle: the ovarian cycle and the uterine cycle. These cycles begin at puberty and last about 40 years. (Refer to Figure 26-6 as you read about the cyclic changes.) Figure 26-6, *A*, illustrates the secretions of the anterior pituitary gland, FSH and LH, over a 28-day monthly cycle. (The 28-day cycle is an average length; a normal cycle may be shorter or longer than 28 days.) The hypothalamic-releasing hormones are responsible for stimulating the anterior pituitary secretion of the gonadotropins.

For each day of the cycle, you should be able to identify the secretions of the anterior pituitary gland, maturation of the ovarian follicle, changes in the blood levels of ovarian hormones, and growth of the endometrial lining of the uterus. Figure 26-6, *B*, illustrates the growth and maturation of the ovarian follicle, which results in ovulation and the development of the corpus luteum. Figure 26-6, *C*, shows the blood levels of the ovarian hormones estrogen and progesterone. Figure 26-6, *D*, illustrates the monthly changes in the uterine lining. Together, the parts of Figure 26-6 describe events that occur over a 28-day period.

OVARIAN CYCLE

The ovarian cycle consists of two phases: the follicular phase and the luteal phase.

Follicular Phase

The follicular phase (see Figure 26-6, *B*) begins with the hypothalamic secretion of releasing hormones. These hormones, in turn, stimulate the release of gonadotropins by the anterior pituitary gland. The FSH and small amounts of LH stimulate the growth and maturation of the ovarian follicle. The maturing ovarian follicle secretes large amounts of estrogen,

Table 26-1	Female Hormones		
HORMONE	**GLAND**	**TARGET ORGAN**	**EFFECTS**
Releasing hormone	Hypothalamus	Anterior pituitary	Stimulates the secretion of the gonadotropins (FSH and LH)
Follicle-stimulating hormone (FSH)	Anterior pituitary	Ovary	Initiates development of the ovarian follicle Stimulates the secretion of estrogen by the follicular cells
Luteinizing hormone (LH)	Anterior pituitary	Ovary	Causes ovulation Stimulates the corpus luteum to secrete progesterone
Estrogen	Ovary (follicle)	Locally (ovary) Uterus (endometrium) Other tissues and organs	Stimulates maturation of the ovarian follicle Stimulates the proliferative phase of endometrial development Causes the development of the secondary sex characteristics
Progesterone	Ovary (corpus luteum)	Uterus (endometrium)	Stimulates the secretory phase of endometrial development
Human chorionic gonadotropin (hCG)	Trophoblastic cells of the embryo	Corpus luteum	Maintains the corpus luteum during early pregnancy

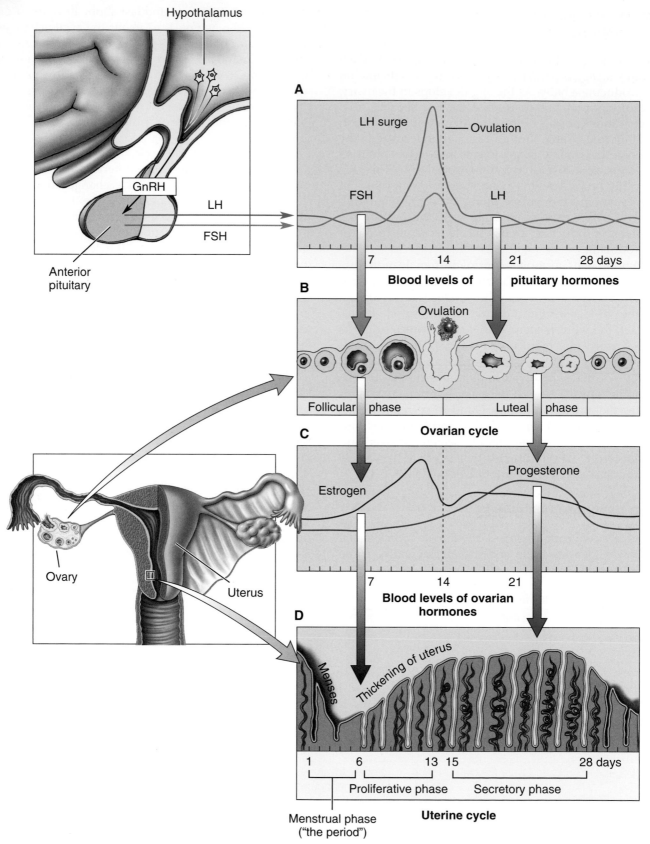

FIGURE 26-6 Hormonal control of the female reproductive cycle (28-day cycle). **A,** The anterior pituitary gland secretes the gonadotropins FSH and LH in response to hypothalamic-releasing hormones. **B,** Ovarian events. **C,** Blood levels of the ovarian hormones estrogen and progesterone. **D,** The uterine cycle.

causing the blood levels of estrogen to increase (see Figure 26-6, *C*).

Estrogen dominates the follicular phase. Estrogen affects both the ovary and uterus. Estrogen stimulates the maturation of the ovarian follicle and helps build up the uterine lining in the first half of the uterine cycle, days 1 to 14 (see Figure 26-6, *D*).

The follicular phase ends when a sharp rise (midcycle surge) of LH on day 14 causes ovulation. See Figure 26-6, *A*, for the midcycle surge of LH and Figure 26-6, *B*, for ovulation.

Luteal Phase

The luteal phase immediately follows ovulation. Follicular cells of the ruptured follicle on the surface of the ovary form the corpus luteum. LH then stimulates the corpus luteum to secrete progesterone and small amounts of estrogen. The progesterone and estrogen exert a negative feedback effect on the anterior pituitary gland, thereby inhibiting further secretion of FSH and LH. Progesterone also supports the endometrial lining of the uterus during the second half of the cycle (days 14 to 28). Progesterone dominates the luteal phase.

When the corpus luteum dies, secretion of progesterone and estrogen declines. As a result of the decrease in estrogen and progesterone, FSH and small amounts of LH are once again secreted, and the cycle is repeated.

UTERINE CYCLE

The uterine cycle, also called the *menstrual cycle,* consists of the changes that occur in the endometrium over a 28-day period (see Figure 26-6, *D*). Estrogen and progesterone secreted by the ovaries cause the endometrial changes; thus, the ovarian cycle controls the uterine cycle. The uterine cycle has three phases: the menstrual phase, the proliferative phase, and the secretory phase.

Menstrual Phase

Bleeding characterizes the menstrual phase. It begins on the first day and continues for 3 to 5 days, varying from person to person. During the menstrual phase, the functional layer of the endometrial lining and blood leave the uterus through the vagina as menstrual flow. This process is also called "having your period."

Proliferative Phase

The proliferative phase begins with the end of the menstrual phase. Repair and growth of the inner endometrial lining characterize the proliferative phase. The lining grows primarily because of estrogen secreted by the ovaries (see Figure 26-6, *B* and *C*). The proliferative phase is so named because the cells proliferate and thus repair the endometrial lining. Note in Figure 26-6, *D,* that the endometrial lining becomes thicker and acquires additional blood vessels during the proliferative phase.

Secretory Phase

The secretory phase is caused by the secretion of progesterone by the corpus luteum of the ovary (see Figure 26-6, *C* and *D*). Progesterone causes the endometrial lining to thicken, thereby forming a nutritious environment awaiting the arrival of a fertilized ovum.

2+2 Sum It Up!

Let's highlight the events of the ovarian and uterine cycles. Refer again to Figure 26-6.

- The development of the ovarian follicle, during the follicular phase of the ovarian cycle, is caused primarily by FSH. FSH stimulates the follicle to secrete estrogen. The estrogen performs two functions: it stimulates the growth of the follicle, and it is responsible for the proliferative phase of the uterine cycle.
- Ovulation is the expulsion of the egg at midcycle (day 14) and is caused by a surge of LH from the anterior pituitary gland.
- The follicular cells that remain on the surface of the ovary form the corpus luteum. The corpus luteum secretes progesterone and some estrogen. Blood carries the hormones to the uterus.
- Progesterone stimulates the uterine lining to become thick and lush, thereby forming a rich lining for the fertilized egg.
- When blood levels of estrogen and progesterone decline, the endometrial lining sloughs off and causes bleeding (menstruation).
- The ovarian hormones (estrogen and progesterone) exert a negative feedback effect on the anterior pituitary gland.

When blood levels of the ovarian hormones rise, secretions of FSH and LH are low. When the corpus luteum degenerates into the corpus albicans, however, the blood levels of estrogen and progesterone decrease. The decrease in the ovarian hormones in turn allows the anterior pituitary gland to secrete FSH and LH. The stimulated ovary then develops another follicle.

? Re-Think

1. List the two phases of the ovarian cycle.
2. List the three phases of the uterine cycle.
3. Explain how the ovarian cycle controls the uterine cycle.

IMPLANTATION: KEEPING THE CORPUS LUTEUM ALIVE

NOTE: The endometrial lining does not slough off if blood levels of estrogen and progesterone are adequate. These levels are adequate if the corpus luteum does not deteriorate. How does the body prevent the deterioration of the corpus luteum?

If fertilization occurs, preserving the uterine lining is crucial, for this is where Baby will live and grow. Menstruation must be prevented. How? Soon after fertilization, the egg implants in the uterine lining. Some of the cells at the site of implantation in the uterus secrete a hormone called *human chorionic gonadotropin* (hCG). Blood carries hCG from the uterus to the ovary, where it stimulates the corpus luteum. Deterioration of the corpus luteum is prevented by hCG, thereby ensuring the continued secretion of estrogen and progesterone. The life of the corpus luteum is prolonged for 11 to 12 weeks by hCG, until the placenta can take over as the major estrogen- and progesterone-secreting gland. (See Chapter 27 for the rest of this story.)

 Do You Know...

What the Missing Words in This "Scientific" Observation Are?

According to the ancient scientist Pliny, "When a _____ approaches, fermenting wine will be soured, seeds she touches become infertile, grass withers, garden plants shrivel, and fruit falls from the trees."

The missing words are "menstruating woman." Menstruating women were often feared, and a great lore grew up around menstrual blood. Casual observation might have suggested that the above charges were false. Pliny pondering periods! Not too observant for a scientist.

? Re-Think

1. Explain why the corpus luteum deteriorates to the corpus albicans in the nonpregnant state.
2. Explain why the corpus luteum does not deteriorate in the pregnant state.

MENARCHE, MENSES, AND MENOPAUSE

In the female, puberty is marked by the first period of menstrual bleeding, or menarche (meh-NAR-kee). Thereafter, the menstrual periods (menses) occur regularly until the woman reaches her late 40s or early 50s. At this time, the periods gradually become more irregular until they cease completely. This phase is called menopause. Menopause is also called the change of life, or the climacteric. Female reproductive function lasts from menarche to menopause.

The effects of menopause are caused by a decrease in the ovarian secretion of estrogen and progesterone. Without ovarian hormones, the uterine cycle ceases and the woman stops menstruating. Other symptoms associated with menopause include hot flashes, sweating, depression, irritability, and insomnia. The symptoms are highly variable. Some women experience severe disturbances; others hardly notice any systemic effects.

METHODS OF BIRTH CONTROL

Birth control is the voluntary regulation of reproduction. Birth control can limit the number of offspring produced and help determine the timing of conception. Methods of contraception are forms of birth control that prevent the union of egg and sperm.

BARRIER METHODS OF BIRTH CONTROL

Barriers prevent the sperm from entering the female—no union means no baby. Barrier methods are mechanical or chemical. The female and male condoms and the diaphragm are mechanical barriers; spermicidal creams, foams, and jellies are chemical barriers. The effectiveness of the chemical barriers is improved considerably when they are used with a mechanical barrier.

HORMONAL CONTRACEPTIVES

The birth control pill is a pharmacological agent that contains estrogen and progesterone. As the blood levels of estrogen and progesterone increase, negative feedback inhibits the secretion of FSH by the anterior pituitary gland. This process, in turn, prevents ovulation; no egg means no baby.

Implants containing progesterone act in much the same way. Progesterone-containing capsules, or rods, can be surgically implanted under the skin of a woman's upper arm or scapular region. The progesterone is slowly but continuously released from the implant. As with the birth control pill, the elevated blood levels of progesterone prevent ovulation. The same effect can be achieved by the injection of synthetic progesterone two to four times per year.

A contraceptive patch can also be used as a form of birth control. A contraceptive patch is a transdermal patch applied to the skin, which releases synthetic estrogen and progestin hormones to prevent pregnancy.

SURGICAL METHODS OF BIRTH CONTROL

Surgical methods of contraception include a vasectomy in the male and a tubal ligation in the female (Figure 26-7). A vasectomy involves removing a small section of each vas deferens and tying the cut ends. A vasectomy is contraceptive because the sperm cannot leave the epididymis; no sperm means no baby.

In the female, a tubal ligation involves removing a small section of each fallopian tube and tying the cut ends. After a tubal ligation, the egg cannot be transported from the ovary through the fallopian tubes, where fertilization normally takes place. No egg means no baby.

INTRAUTERINE DEVICES

An intrauterine device (IUD) is a small solid object placed in the uterine cavity. The IUD prevents pregnancy because it stimulates the uterus to prevent implantation of the fertilized egg. Note that the IUD is not technically contraceptive. In other words, it does not prevent conception; instead, it prevents implantation.

BEHAVIORAL METHODS OF BIRTH CONTROL

Sexual partners can behave in ways to prevent pregnancy. Behavioral methods include abstinence, the

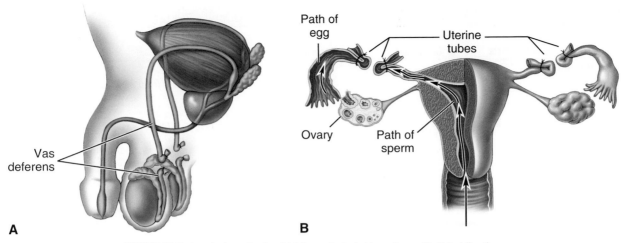

FIGURE 26-7 Surgical methods of birth control. **A,** Vasectomy. **B,** Tubal ligation.

rhythm method, and coitus interruptus. Abstinence, or the avoidance of sexual intercourse, is the most effective method of birth control.

The rhythm method, also called *natural family planning* or *timed coitus,* requires avoiding sexual intercourse at a time when the female is ovulating, generally at midcycle. Because the menstrual cycle (and ovulation) are not always regular, the rhythm method is associated with a high pregnancy rate. Coitus interruptus involves the withdrawal of the penis from the vagina before ejaculation. It too is associated with a high pregnancy rate.

EMERGENCY CONTRACEPTION

Emergency contraception refers to contraception that is implemented after intercourse. It is accomplished by two types of drugs. One group of drugs contains both estrogen and progesterone and works like "the pill" by preventing ovulation and inhibiting implantation in the event that fertilization occurs. A second drug group causes the loss of the implanted embryo by blocking progesterone receptors in the endometrium. The loss of progesterone receptors causes the endometrium to slough, carrying the implanted embryo with it.

2+2 Sum It Up!

In the female, puberty is marked by the first period of menstrual bleeding. This event is called *menarche*. Thereafter, monthly menstrual periods (menses) occur regularly until menopause. Menopause, also called the *climacteric* or *change of life,* generally occurs when a woman is in her late 40s or early 50s. Menopause is caused by the decreased ovarian secretion of estrogen and progesterone. Birth control is the voluntary regulation of reproduction. There are numerous methods of contraception.

🍂 As You Age

1. As a woman ages, her ovaries begin to atrophy, or shrink. Between the ages of 40 and 50, estrogen secretion decreases and symptoms of menopause appear; menstrual periods cease, signaling the end of her reproductive years.
2. The decrease in estrogen secretion causes a change in the accessory organs of reproduction. Tissues become thinner, with a decrease in secretions. The changes in these structures make the woman more prone to vaginal infections. Also, a decrease in vaginal secretions can make intercourse uncomfortable. The decrease in estrogen is also thought to cause weakening of bone, causing osteoporosis, and an increase in the incidence of cardiovascular diseases.
3. By the age of 50, the size of the uterus has decreased by 50%. The ligaments that anchor the uterus, urinary bladder, and rectum weaken, allowing these organs to drop down. Surgical correction is sometimes needed.
4. Breast tissue changes; the supporting ligaments weaken; fibrous cells replace glandular cells; and the amount of fat tissue decreases. These changes cause breast tissue to sag.
5. Around the age of 40, testicular function declines. This decline is accompanied by a decrease in the secretion of testosterone and a decreased sperm count (up to 50%). Despite these changes, a man continues to produce sperm and is capable of fathering children throughout most of his life span.

MEDICAL TERMINOLOGY AND DISORDERS — Disorders of the Reproductive Systems

Medical Term	Word Parts	Word Part Meaning or Derivation	Description
General Terminology			
congenital	con-	together or with	*Refers to a condition that is present from birth,* as in a congenital heart defect.
	-gen/o-	origin or production	
	-al	pertaining to	
gonad		From the Greek word *gonos,* meaning "seed or act of generation"	**Gonads** are *organs that produce the seeds of generation or reproduction.* The female gonad is the ovary and the male gonad is the testis.
heredity	here(s)	From the Latin word *heres,* meaning "heir or heiress"	*Refers to the passing on of characteristics genetically from generation to generation.*
lactation	lact/o-	milk	*The formation or secretion of milk by the mammary (mammo- = breast) glands.* Lactation is stimulated by the hormone called *prolactin* (pro- = in favor of) or *lactogenic hormone.*
	-tion	process	
myometrium and the other "metriums"	my/o-	muscle	The **myometrium** is *the smooth muscle layer of the uterus.* The **endometrium** (endo- = within) is *the inner lining of the uterus.* The **perimetrium** (peri- = around) or **epimetrium** (epi- = upon) is *the outer serosal layer of the uterus.*
	-metr/o-	uterus or womb	
natal	nat/i-	birth	*Refers to the place or time of one's birth.* A **neonate** (neo- = new) is *a newborn infant.* The **prenatal period** is *the time before the birth;* the **perinatal period** is *the time around the birth;* and the **postnatal period** is *the time immediately after the birth.*
	-al	pertaining to	
placenta		From a Latin word meaning "a flat cake"	Called a "uterine cake" by the Italians, the **placenta** is *the vascular organ that develops within the uterus of a pregnant female in order to nourish the developing fetus.*
ovum	ov/i	egg	*Refers to the ovum or egg.* **Ovulation** is *the expulsion of the egg at midcycle from the* **ovary.** The **oviduct** is *the egg-carrying vessel also known as the fallopian tube.* The prefix oophor/o- derives from the Greek and also refers to the ovary, as in **oophorectomy** (removal of the ovary).
Disorders: General			
infertility	in-	not, opposite	**Infertility** can be caused by the male (accounts for one third of the cases), female (one third), or both partners (one third). **Male infertility** may be due to abnormal production of sperm (number or motility), problems with the delivery of sperm, and general health. **Female infertility** may be caused by blockage of the fallopian tubes, endometriosis, ovulation disorders, and hormonal imbalances. Cancer treatment and advancing age can adversely affect both male and female fertility.
	-fertile	From the Latin word *fertilis,* meaning "bearing in abundance"	
sexually transmitted diseases			Abbreviated as STDs; also known as *sexually transmitted infections* (STIs). STDs are a major health concern and are easily spread through sexual contact. Some STDs affect primarily the reproductive structures, whereas others extend their effects to major organ systems throughout the body. The common bacterial STDs include chlamydia (most common), gonorrhea (*Neisseria gonorrhoeae*), and syphilis (*Treponema pallidum*). The most common virally induced STDs are hepatitis B virus (HBV), herpes simplex virus type 2 (HSV-2), human immunodeficiency virus (HIV, progression to AIDS), and human papillomavirus (HPV, also called *genital* or *venereal warts*). Trichomoniasis (*Trichomonas vaginalis*) is the most common STD and is caused by a protozoan or parasitic organism.

MEDICAL TERMINOLOGY AND DISORDERS Disorders of the Reproductive Systems—cont'd

Medical Term	Word Parts	Word Part Meaning or Derivation	Description
Disorders: Male			
benign prostatic hypertrophy	benign	From the Latin word *bene*, meaning "well"	Also called **benign prostatic hyperplasia (BPH).** Hyperplasia of the prostate gland (not cancerous) is age related and commonly occurs in elderly men. Early symptoms include urinary dribbling, urinary incontinence, and incomplete emptying of the bladder.
	prostat/o-	prostate	
	-ic	pertaining to	
	hyper-	above or excessive	
	-troph/o-	nourishment, development	
	-y	condition of	
cancer		From a Latin word meaning *crab;* a reference to its tendency to extend outward and penetrate like claws	**Cancer,** or **malignant neoplasms,** can develop in any part of the male reproductive system. Cancer of the prostate is the second most frequently diagnosed cancer in the United States, whereas testicular cancer is the most common cancer in U.S. males from late teens to mid-30s.
erectile dysfunction			Also called **EDF** or **impotence;** refers to the inability to have or maintain an erection.
gynecomastia	gynec/o-	woman	**Gynecomastia** is *the development of mammary glands in the male; it occurs in response to altered hormonal secretion or as a side effect of drug therapy.*
	-mast/o-	breasts	
	-ia	condition of	
hydrocele	hydro-	water	A **hydrocele** is *a fluid-filled sac surrounding a testicle; it presents as a swollen scrotum.*
	-cele	pouching or hernia	
hypospadias	hypo-	deficient	A **hypospadias** is *a congenital opening of the urethra on the undersurface of the penis.*
	-spadias	to draw away	
prostatitis	prostat/o-	prostate	**Prostatitis** is *the inflammation of the prostate gland; usually caused by an infection.*
	-itis	inflammation	
varicocele	varic/o-	twisted vein	A **varicocele** is *an enlargement and distortion (varicosity) of the veins that drain the testis. It appears bluish through the scrotum, feels like a sac of worms, and often causes discomfort.*
	-cele	pouching or hernia	
vasectomy	vas/o-	vessel	A **vasectomy** is *the removal of a segment of the vas deferens in order to produce sterility in the male.* A **vasovasostomy** is *a surgical procedure performed to restore the vas deferens and fertility in the male; it reverses the effects of vasectomy.*
	-ectomy	removal	
Disorders: Female			
cervicitis	cervic/o-	cervix	*Inflammation of the cervix, the lower necklike part of the uterus that extends into the vagina.*
	-itis	inflammation of	
colporrhaphy	colp/o-	vagina (sheath)	A **colporrhaphy** is *the surgical repair of a tear in the vaginal wall. The defect may be a cystocele, a protrusion of the bladder into the vagina. The defect may also be a rectocele, the bulging of part of the rectum into the vagina.*
	-orrhaphy	repair	
displacement of the uterus			**Anteflexion** (ante = before; flexus = bend) is *the forward bending of the uterus.* **Retroflexion** (retro = back) is *an abnormal bending backward of the uterus.* **Retroversion** (retere = to turn) is *an abnormal backward turn of the whole uterus.*
dyspareunia	dys-	difficult or painful	**Dyspareunia** means *painful intercourse,* usually in women.
	-pareunia	From the Greek word *pareunos,* meaning "lying beside"	
endometriosis	endo-	within	**Endometriosis** is *a condition in which endometrial tissue grows in other parts of the body, particularly within the pelvic cavity.* Structures most commonly affected are the intestines, fallopian tubes, and ovaries (described in text).
	-metr/o-	uterus	
	-osis	condition of	

Continued

MEDICAL TERMINOLOGY AND DISORDERS Disorders of the Reproductive Systems—cont'd

Medical Term	Word Parts	Word Part Meaning or Derivation	Description
episiotomy	episi/o-	vulva (covering)	An **episiotomy** is *an incision into the perineum, the area between the vagina and anus; it is done during the delivery of a baby in order to prevent the tearing of the perineum during delivery.*
	-otomy	a cutting into	
leukorrhea	leuk/o-	white	**Leukorrhea** is *an abnormal white to yellow vaginal discharge.*
	-rrhea	discharge	
mammogram	mamm/o-	breast	**Mammogram** is *a screening procedure for the early diagnosis of breast cancer.*
	-gram	record	
mastitis	mast/o-	breast	**Mastitis** is *inflammation of the breasts.* A **mastectomy,** commonly performed for breast cancer, is *the surgical removal of a breast;* **amastia** refers to *the absence of a breast.* **Hypermastia** and **macromastia** refer to *abnormally large breasts,* whereas **hypomastia** and **micromastia** refer to *abnormally small breasts.*
	-itis	inflammation	
menarche	men/o-	menstruation; monthly	**Menarche** refers to *the beginning of menstruation.* **Amenorrhea** is *the absence of menstruation.* **Dysmenorrhea** is *painful or difficult menstruation.* **Menorrhagia** is *excessive bleeding at menstruation.* **Metrorrhagia** is *bleeding from the uterus at any time other than normal menstruation.* **Menopause** means *the cessation of menstruation.*
	-arche	beginning	
neoplasms	neo-	new	There are benign and malignant tumors that can develop in all reproductive structures. There is a benign **fibroid tumor** of the uterine muscle, or **leiomyoma** (leios- = smooth; -my/o- = muscle; -oma = tumor). **Fibrocystic breast disease** is characterized by multiple benign cysts in the breasts. **Breast cancer** is a common malignancy of the breast tissue. There are many types of benign **ovarian cysts,** some of which are permanently and successfully eliminated; others (e.g., **polycystic ovary syndrome [PCOS]**) may persist chronically and interfere with fertility and create other serious health issues. **Carcinoma in situ** (in situ = in place) refers to an early form of cancer in which there has been no spread of the malignant cells into surrounding tissue.
	-plasia	growth	
salpingitis	salping/o-	uterine or fallopian tube; comes from the Greek word meaning "trumpet" (because of its appearance)	**Salpingitis** is *the inflammation of the uterine or fallopian tubes.*
	-itis	inflammation of	

Get Ready for Exams!

Summary Outline

The reproductive system produces the cells and hormones necessary for reproduction.

I. Male Reproductive System
A. Testes
  1. The testes, or testicles, are the male gonads.
  2. Lobules with two types of cells: the seminiferous tubules and the interstitial cells
B. Genital ducts and glands
  1. The sperm move through a series of genital ducts: epididymis, vas deferens, ejaculatory ducts, and urethra.
  2. Three glands—the seminal vesicles, the prostate gland, and the bulbourethral glands—secrete into the genital ducts. The mixture of sperm and glandular secretions is called *semen.*
C. External genitals
  1. The male genitals consist of the scrotum and the penis.
  2. The penis performs two functions: It is the organ of copulation (sexual intercourse), and it carries urine.
D. Male sexual responses: erection, emission, ejaculation, and orgasm
E. Male sex hormones
  1. The most important is testosterone, determining the primary and secondary sex characteristics.
  2. Controlled by hormones from the hypothalamus and from the anterior pituitary gland

II. Female Reproductive System

A. Ovaries
  1. The ovaries are the female gonads.
  2. Each ovarian follicle consists of an oocyte and follicular cells.
  3. On day 14 (of a 28-day cycle), ovulation occurs.
  4. The ovarian follicular cells become the corpus luteum.
  5. The ovaries secrete two hormones: estrogen and progesterone.

B. Genital tract
  1. The genital tract includes the fallopian tubes, uterus, and vagina.
  2. The fallopian tubes transport the egg from the ovaries to the uterus, and are where fertilization takes place.
  3. The uterus is the baby's cradle during pregnancy.
  4. The uterus has three layers: epimetrium, myometrium, and endometrium.

C. External genitals are called the *vulva* (labia majora, labia minora, clitoris, and the vestibular glands).

D. Female sexual response: erection and orgasm

E. Hormonal control of the female reproductive cycles
  1. The two cycles are the ovarian cycle and the uterine cycle.
  2. The ovarian cycle is divided into the follicular phase and the luteal phase.
  3. During the follicular phase, the ovarian follicle matures and secretes estrogen.
  4. The luteal phase of the ovarian cycle begins immediately after ovulation and is dominated by the secretion of progesterone by the corpus luteum.
  5. In the nonpregnant state, the corpus luteum deteriorates. In the pregnant state, the corpus luteum stays alive because of human chorionic gonadotropin (hCG).
  6. The uterine cycle is divided into the menstrual phase, proliferative phase, and secretory phase.
     a. The menstrual phase refers to the loss of a part of the endometrial lining and blood ("having your period").
     b. During the proliferative phase, the inner endometrial lining thickens and becomes vascular, primarily in response to estrogen.
     c. During the secretory phase, the endometrial lining becomes lush and moist from increased secretory activity; the secretory phase is dominated by progesterone.
  7. See Figure 26-6 for a summary of the daily hormonal relationships among the anterior pituitary gland, ovaries, and uterus.

III. Methods of Birth Control

A. The regulation of childbearing can be achieved with the use of barrier methods, hormonal contraceptives, surgical methods, intrauterine devices, behavioral methods, and drugs used for emergency contraception.

Review Your Knowledge

Matching: Female Structures

Directions: Match the following words with their description below. Some words may be used more than once.

a. fallopian tubes
b. uterus
c. ovaries
d. vagina

1. ___ Fertilization occurs here.
2. ___ Female gonads
3. ___ Contains the fundus, body, and cervix
4. ___ Contains the endometrium, myometrium, and epimetrium
5. ___ Home of the corpus luteum
6. ___ Where implantation occurs
7. ___ Home of the graafian follicle
8. ___ Menstrual phase, proliferative phase, and secretory phase
9. ___ Follicular phase and luteal phase
10. ___ Birth canal; distal to the cervix

Matching: Male Structures

Directions: Match the following words with their description below. Some words may be used more than once.

a. interstitial cells
b. seminiferous tubules
c. urethra
d. epididymis
e. scrotum

1. ___ Structure that forms sperm
2. ___ Testosterone-secreting cells
3. ___ Tightly coiled ducts that sit on top of the testes
4. ___ Structure that is shared by both the reproductive and urinary tracts
5. ___ Pouch that contains the testes

Matching: Hormones

Directions: Match the following words with their descriptions below. Some words may be used more than once.

a. estrogen
b. progesterone
c. hCG
d. gonadotropins
e. testosterone

1. ___ Primary androgen secreted by the testes
2. ___ What FSH and LH are called
3. ___ The proliferative phase (uterus) is dominated by this ovarian hormone.
4. ___ The secretory phase (uterus) is dominated by this ovarian hormone.
5. ___ Secreted by trophoblastic cells; preserves the secretion of the corpus luteum
6. ___ The ovaries are the targets of this anterior pituitary secretion.
7. ___ Its secretion is a response to interstitial cell–stimulating hormone (ICSH).
8. ___ This hormone makes a female look like a woman.
9. ___ This hormone makes a male look like a man.
10. ___ The corpus luteum secretes large amounts of this hormone; it makes the endometrium juicy, or lush

Multiple Choice

1. In the male, the gonadotropins
   a. are aimed at the testes.
   b. include FSH and LH (ICSH).
   c. stimulate sperm development and the secretion of androgen.
   d. All of the above are true.
2. In the male, luteinizing hormone
   a. is also called ICSH and stimulates the interstitial cells to secrete testosterone.
   b. stimulates sperm production.
   c. causes emission.
   d. causes orgasm.
3. Estrogen and progesterone
   a. are gonadotropins.
   b. are secreted by the trophoblastic cells as they implant in the uterine wall.
   c. are secreted by the ovaries.
   d. exert their effects only on reproductive structures.
4. In the nonpregnant state
   a. the corpus albicans becomes hormonally active, secreting estrogen and progesterone.
   b. the endometrium secretes hCG.
   c. hormonal secretion of the corpus luteum gradually declines.
   d. the zygote becomes hormonally active.
5. Human chorionic gonadotropin (hCG)
   a. promotes the maturation of the egg.
   b. is responsible for female characteristics.
   c. maintains the corpus luteum.
   d. transforms the corpus luteum into the corpus albicans.
6. The luteal phase of the ovarian cycle
   a. is responsible for menstruation.
   b. is responsible for the uterine secretory phase.
   c. elevates plasma levels of estrogen, progesterone, and hCG.
   d. precedes the LH surge.
7. Menstruation occurs in response to
   a. an LH surge.
   b. diminished plasma levels of estrogen and progesterone.
   c. elevated plasma levels of hCG.
   d. elevated plasma levels of FSH and LH.
8. Which of the following is not true of testosterone?
   a. Classified as androgen
   b. Secreted by the anterior pituitary gland
   c. Is necessary for the maturation of sperm
   d. Is responsible for most of the male secondary sex characteristics
9. Which structure ejects both semen and urine?
   a. Epididymis
   b. Oviducts
   c. Urethra
   d. Vas deferens
10. The graafian follicle
    a. matures under the influence of hCG.
    b. is an ovarian structure.
    c. implants in the endometrial lining.
    d. secretes FSH and LH in an attempt to ripen an oocyte.

Go Figure

1. **According to Figure 26-1**
   a. The epididymis is located within the pelvic cavity.
   b. The testes are located within the pelvic cavity.
   c. The vas deferens is shared by both the urinary and reproductive tracts.
   d. The urethra extends the length of the penis.

2. **According to Figures 26-1 and 26-2**
   a. The seminiferous tubules are located within the testes.
   b. Testosterone is secreted by the prostate and seminal vesicles.
   c. Sperm are kept warm by migrating to the prostate gland until released.
   d. The acrosome is another name for the foreskin.

3. **According to Figure 26-4**
   a. Ovulation involves the expulsion of the ovum from the corpus albicans.
   b. The corpus luteum forms before the graafian follicle.
   c. The graafian follicle and corpus luteum develop within the uterus.
   d. The corpus luteum forms after ovulation.

4. **According to Figure 26-4**
   a. The reproductive tract opens into the pelvic cavity.
   b. The myometrium is the muscle layer of the ovary.
   c. The fallopian tubes attach to the cervix of the uterus.
   d. The endometrium refers to the hormonally sensitive ovarian tissue.

5. **According to Figure 26-6**
   a. The ovarian cycle includes the proliferative and secretory phases.
   b. The LH surge precedes the development of the graafian follicle.
   c. LH and FSH are gonadotropins secreted by the adenohypophysis and aimed at the endometrium.
   d. FSH stimulates the development of the graafian follicle in the ovary.

6. **According to Figure 26-6**
   a. Elevated blood levels of estrogen and progesterone prevent the secretion of gonadotropins through negative feedback control.
   b. The uterine lining is built up in direct response to FSH and LH.
   c. A surge of ovarian progesterone is responsible for ovulation.
   d. The source of estrogen and progesterone is the anterior pituitary gland.

Human Development and Heredity

Key Terms

amnion (p. 514)
blastocyst (p. 513)
chorion (p. 514)
chromosomes (p. 525)
embryo (p. 514)
fertilization (p. 511)

fetus (p. 518)
genes (p. 525)
human chorionic gonadotropin (hCG) (p. 513)
karyotype (p. 525)
mammary glands (p. 522)

placenta (p. 514)
sex-linked trait (p. 527)
teratogens (p. 518)
umbilical cord (p. 517)
zygote (p. 512)

Objectives

1. Describe the process of fertilization: when, where, and how it occurs.
2. Do the following regarding prenatal development:
   - Describe the process of development: cleavage, growth, morphogenesis, and differentiation.
   - Explain the three periods of prenatal development: early embryonic, embryonic, and fetal.
   - State two functions of the placenta.
3. Explain hormonal changes during pregnancy.
4. Describe the hormonal changes and stages of labor.
5. Describe the structure of the breast and lactation.
6. Describe immediate postnatal changes and lifelong developmental stages.
7. Discuss heredity and how genetic structures are related, including:
   - Describe the relationships among deoxyribonucleic acid (DNA), chromosomes, and genes.
   - Define *karyotype*.
8. Explain how the gender of the child is determined.
9. State the difference between congenital and hereditary diseases.

Nine months after conception, the reproductive process produces a baby. The "bundle of joy" has arrived on the scene. Note that this term of endearment does not suggest "up, awake, and playing at 2 AM," and diapers, diapers, and more diapers. Nonetheless, Baby is cute, and the urge to reproduce is very strong. Let us follow Baby's start from fertilization through development and birth. Finally, we'll see what is meant by statements like "He's got his father's nose and his mother's smile." This is the genetic story.

FERTILIZATION

Fertilization, also called *conception*, refers to the union of the nuclei of the egg and the sperm. When, where, and how does this union take place?

WHEN FERTILIZATION OCCURS

Timing is everything. In the female, ovulation occurs at midcycle, around day 14 (see Chapter 26). The egg lives for about 24 hours after ovulation. Sperm usually live between 12 and 48 hours, with some surviving up to 72 hours. Generally speaking, for fertilization to occur, sexual intercourse must take place around the time of ovulation, generally no earlier than 72 hours (3 days) before ovulation and no later than 24 hours (1 day) after ovulation.

ALERT: Evidence suggests that some women are reflex ovulators. These women ovulate in response to having intercourse. Think about it; the chance of pregnancy goes *waaay* up. Remember that rabbits are reflex ovulators, and we all know about the rabbit population.

WHERE FERTILIZATION OCCURS

After ovulation, the egg enters the fallopian tube. Fertilization normally occurs in the first third of the fallopian tube.

HOW FERTILIZATION OCCURS

During intercourse, about 200 to 600 million sperm are deposited in the vagina, near the cervix of the uterus. Although many of the sperm are killed by the acidic environment of the vagina, about 100,000 survive and swim through the uterus and into the fallopian tube toward the egg. Within 1 to 2 hours after intercourse, thousands of sperm are gathered around the egg in the fallopian tube. Life comes at you fast!

The acrosome on the head of the sperm ruptures and releases enzymes. The enzymes digest the linings of cells that surround the egg. Then, one (and only one) sperm penetrates the membrane of the egg. Upon penetration of the egg, the nuclei of the egg and sperm unite, thereby completing fertilization. The fertilized egg is called a **zygote** (ZYE-goht). "Zygote" was your first name!

The single-cell zygote has 46 chromosomes: 23 from the egg and 23 from the sperm. The zygote begins to divide, forming a cluster of cells that slowly makes its way through the fallopian tube toward the uterus. When this cluster of cells reaches the uterus, it implants itself into the plush endometrial lining, where it grows and develops into a human being with billions of cells.

? Re-Think

1. Where does fertilization occur?
2. Why is it possible for a fertilized ovum to take up residence within the abdominal cavity rather than the uterus?

HUMAN DEVELOPMENT

Development is a process that begins with fertilization and ends with death. Human development is divided into two phases: prenatal development and postnatal development. Prenatal development begins with fertilization and ends at birth. The time of prenatal development is called *pregnancy,* or *gestation.* The normal gestation period lasts 38 weeks, or about 9 months. Pregnancy is divided into trimesters (3-month periods): the first trimester is the first 3 months of pregnancy; the second trimester is months 4, 5, and 6; and the third, or last, trimester is months 7, 8, and 9. Postnatal development begins with birth and ends with death; it is what we are all doing now—living *life.*

PRENATAL DEVELOPMENT

What does prenatal development include? Prenatal development includes cleavage, growth, morphogenesis, and differentiation. Cleavage is cell division by mitosis. Mitosis produces two identical cells from a single cell. Thus, one cell splits into two cells, the two cells split into four cells, four cells split into eight cells, and so on. Each new cell is identical to the parent cell. Mitotic cell division increases the numbers of cells but not their actual size. The size of the cell increases through growth. As development progresses, therefore, both the number and size of the cells increase.

Morphogenesis (mohr-foh-JEN-eh-sis) is the shaping of the cell cluster. Certain cells migrate to specific areas in the cell cluster. This process changes the shape of the cell mass. For example, cells migrate to the side of the cell mass and take the appearance of tiny buds. These buds eventually become legs. Through morphogenesis, the round cluster of cells develops into an intricately and wondrously formed infant. Baby is shaping up!

Differentiation is the process whereby a cell becomes specialized. A cell differentiates to become a nerve cell, muscle cell, blood cell, or some other cell.

What are the periods of prenatal development? There are three periods: early embryonic, embryonic, and fetal periods.

EARLY EMBRYONIC PERIOD

FROM ZYGOTE TO BLASTOCYST ... OR FROM ZYGOTE TO EGGPLANT

The early embryonic period lasts for 2 weeks after fertilization. During this period, the zygote undergoes mitosis and travels from the fallopian tube into the uterus. After fertilization (Figure 27-1, *A*) the zygote undergoes cleavage. Cleavage is accomplished by mitosis, or cell division that increases the numbers of cells. The cells formed by mitotic cell division are blastomeres (see Figure 27-1, *B*). Note the two-cell, four-cell, and eight-cell cluster.

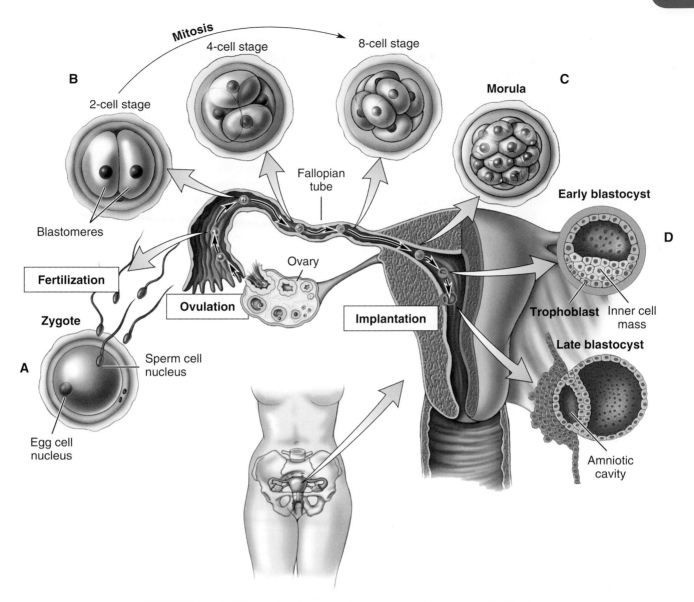

FIGURE 27-1 **A-D,** Stages of early embryonic development, from zygote to blastocyst.

When the number of cells increases to 16, the collection of cells is called a *morula* (see Figure 27-1, *C*). The morula looks like a raspberry, so tiny that it is visible only through a microscope. Transformation from the zygote to a morula takes about 3 days. The morula enters the uterine cavity, where it floats around for 3 to 4 days and continues to undergo mitosis. By the end of the fifth day, the morula has developed into a blastocyst.

Note the structure of the early blastocyst (see Figure 27-1, *D*). The early blastocyst contains a hollow cavity surrounded by a single layer of flattened cells and a cluster of cells at one side. The single layer of flattened cells surrounding the cavity is called the *trophoblast*. These cells will help form the placenta and also secrete an important hormone. The cluster of cells within the blastocyst is called the *inner cell mass*. These cells will eventually form Baby.

The late blastocyst develops by day 7. This stage shows the beginnings of the amniotic cavity. The late blastocyst burrows into the endometrial lining of the uterus, where it is gradually covered over by cells of the endometrial lining. The burrowing process is called *implantation*. We now have an "eggplant"!

During implantation, the blastocyst also functions as a gland. The trophoblast, the flattened layer of cells that surrounds the cavity, secretes a hormone called human chorionic gonadotropin (hCG), which travels through the blood to the ovary, where it prevents the deterioration of the corpus luteum. In response to hCG, the corpus luteum continues to secrete estrogen and progesterone. The estrogen and progesterone stimulate the growth of the uterine wall and prevent menstruation.

The secretion of hCG continues at a high level for about 2 months and then steadily declines as the placenta develops. The placenta eventually takes over the role of the corpus luteum by secreting large amounts of estrogen and progesterone. The blastocyst thus helps preserve its own survival through its secretion of hCG. Think about it: Baby helps Baby survive. With the implantation of the blastocyst and the organization of the inner cell mass, the early embryonic period comes to a close.

hCG forms the basis of pregnancy tests. hCG is secreted in early pregnancy and can be detected in the mother's urine or blood. A pregnancy test may indicate positive results within about 8 to 10 days after fertilization.

> **? Re-Think**
>
> 1. List the stages of development from fertilization to implantation.
> 2. Explain the significance of the trophoblastic secretion of hCG.

SEEING DOUBLE: TWINS

Each cell within the morula or blastocyst can become a complete individual. Sometimes, these cells split and two embryos begin developing at the same time, thereby producing two offspring (twins) rather than one. These are identical, or monozygotic (mon-oh-zye-GOH-tik), twins because they develop from the same zygote and have identical genetic information. For monozygotic twins to develop, one sperm fertilizes one egg, and the zygote then splits.

Sometimes a woman ovulates two eggs, which are then fertilized by two different sperm. Because two babies are produced, they are called *twins*. These twins, however, are not identical. They do not develop from the same egg and do not have the same genetic information. They are called *fraternal,* or *dizygotic* (dye-zye-GOH-tik), *twins* (meaning that they come from two different zygotes). Triplets, quadruplets, and other multiple births can develop in the same two ways.

> **? Re-Think**
>
> 1. What is the difference between monozygotic and dizygotic twins?
> 2. Identical twins are always the same gender. Why is that not true for fraternal twins?

EMBRYONIC PERIOD

Embryonic development lasts for 6 weeks, from week 3 through week 8. During this period, the baby-to-be is called an **embryo**. The embryonic period involves the formation of extraembryonic membranes, the placenta, and all of the organ systems in the body.

EXTRAEMBRYONIC MEMBRANES

The extraembryonic membranes form outside the embryo; hence, the term *extra*embryonic. The membranes help protect and nourish the embryo; they are also involved in the embryonic excretion of waste. At birth, the membranes are expelled along with the placenta as the afterbirth. The four extraembryonic membranes are the amnion, chorion, yolk sac, and allantois.

The **amnion** (AM-nee-on) enlarges and forms a sac around the embryo (Figure 27-2). The sac is called the *amniotic sac* and is filled with a fluid called the *amniotic fluid*. The amniotic fluid forms a protective cushion around the embryo and helps protect it from bumps and changes in temperature. The amniotic fluid also nourishes embryos as they drink and digest it. About 1 L of amniotic fluid occupies the amniotic sac at full term. Interestingly, much of the amniotic fluid is from the urine produced by the fetal kidneys!

The embryo secretes waste and sheds cells into the amniotic fluid. This process is the basis for a diagnostic test called an *amniocentesis,* in which a sample of amniotic fluid is aspirated from the amniotic cavity and examined for evidence of fetal abnormalities (see Figure 27-2, *B*). The amniotic sac is often called the *bag of water*. It breaks before delivery and generally signals the onset of labor.

A second extraembryonic membrane is the chorion. The **chorion** develops many finger-like projections called *chorionic villi*. The chorionic villi penetrate the uterine wall and interact with the tissues of the mother's uterus to form the placenta. Sampling of the cells of the chorionic villi is another way to detect genetic defects (Figure 27-3 and Figure 27-2, *C*).

A third extraembryonic membrane is the yolk sac. The yolk sac in birds and reptiles helps nourish the offspring, but the yolk sac in humans serves different functions: it produces red blood cells and immature sex cells. After the sixth week, the yolk sac ceases to function. The embryonic liver and spleen then produce red blood cells, and by the seventh month the bone marrow has assumed this function. By then, the yolk sac has become part of the umbilical cord.

The allantois (ah-LAN-toh-is) is the fourth extraembryonic membrane. The allantois contributes to the formation of several structures, including the urinary bladder. The blood vessels of the allantois also help form the umbilical blood vessels, which transport blood to and from the placenta. After the second month, the allantois deteriorates and becomes part of the umbilical cord.

> **? Re-Think**
>
> List four extraembryonic membranes and provide a function of each.

PLACENTA

The **placenta** is a disc-shaped structure about 7 inches (15 to 20 cm) in diameter and 1 inch (2.5 cm) thick. Normally, the placenta develops in the upper portion of the uterus. The placenta is a highly vascular

Chorionic villi

Placenta

Chorion

Yolk sac

Embryo

Amniotic fluid

Allantois

Amnion

Umbilical cord

A

Chorionic villi

Chorionic villi sampling

Amniotic fluid

Amniotic cavity

B   **Amniocentesis**

Sample from chorionic villi

C

FIGURE 27-2 Extraembryonic membranes and the formation of the placenta. **A,** The embryo is surrounded by the amnion and the amniotic fluid. **B,** Amniocentesis. **C,** Chorionic villi sampling.

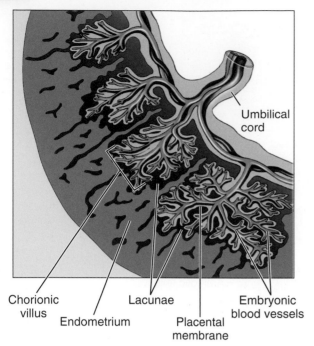

Chorionic villus
Endometrium
Lacunae
Placental membrane
Embryonic blood vessels
Umbilical cord

FIGURE 27-3 Cross-section of the chorionic villi.

uterus (see Figure 27-3). The chorionic villi contain blood vessels that are continuous with the umbilical arteries and umbilical vein of the embryo. The chorionic villi sit in blood-filled spaces (lacunae) in the mother's endometrium.

Pay special attention to the arrangement of the embryonic and maternal blood vessels. The chorionic villi contain blood that comes from the embryo. The endometrial spaces (lacunae) contain blood from the mother. The embryonic and maternal blood supplies, although intimately close, are separated by the placental membrane. The placental membrane thus maintains two separate circulations: the embryonic and maternal circulations. The two circulations do not mix!

Functions of the Placenta

The placenta plays two important roles. First, it is the site across which nutrients and waste are exchanged between mother and baby. Oxygen, food, and other nutrients diffuse from the mother's blood into the blood of the embryo. Carbon dioxide and other waste diffuse from the embryo's blood into the mother's blood and are then excreted. Baby-to-be "breathes," "eats," and excretes at the placenta. If the placenta is injured in any way, the oxygen supply to the embryo may be cut off, causing irreversible brain damage and possibly death.

Secondly, the placenta acts as a gland. It secretes hormones that help maintain the pregnancy, prepare the body for the birthing process, and promote postnatal events such as breast-feeding. The hormones of pregnancy are listed and described in Table 27-1.

structure formed from embryonic and maternal tissue. By the end of the embryonic period (8 weeks), the placenta is functional. After the birth of the baby, the placenta is expelled as part of the afterbirth.

Formation of the Placenta

The placenta develops as the chorionic villi of the embryo burrow into the endometrial lining of the

Table 27-1	Hormones of Pregnancy	
HORMONE	**SECRETED BY**	**EFFECTS**
Human chorionic gonadotropin (hCG)	Embryonic cells (trophoblasts) during implantation	Maintains the function of the corpus luteum; forms the basis of the pregnancy test
Estrogen and progesterone	Corpus luteum during the first 2 months; placenta after 2 months	Both estrogen and progesterone stimulate the development of the uterine lining and mammary glands. Progesterone inhibits uterine contractions during pregnancy. Estrogen causes relaxation of the pelvic joints. At the beginning of labor, estrogen opposes the quieting effects of progesterone on uterine contractions and sensitizes the myometrium to oxytocin.
Prolactin	Anterior pituitary gland	Prolactin stimulates the breast to secrete milk.
Oxytocin	Posterior pituitary gland	Oxytocin causes the release of milk from the breast (part of the milk let-down reflex initiated by suckling). It causes uterine contractions (participates in labor and postpartum uterine contractions to decrease bleeding).
Prostaglandins	Placenta	Prostaglandins stimulate uterine contractions.
Aldosterone	Adrenal cortex	Aldosterone expands blood volume.
Human placental lactogen (HPL)	Placenta	HPL affects the maternal energy metabolism to make more nutrients available to the fetus.

? Re-Think

What are two functions of the placenta?

HOOK UP: THE UMBILICAL CORD

How does the embryo connect with the mother? The **umbilical cord** is the structure that connects embryo and mother at the placenta (see Figure 27-2). The umbilical cord contains two umbilical arteries and one umbilical vein (see Figure 18-8). Because the umbilical cord carries oxygen-rich blood to the developing infant, it is literally the baby's lifeline. Compression or injury to the umbilical cord can cause severe distress and possibly the death of the baby.

When the baby is delivered, the umbilical cord is cut, severing the placenta. The stump of the cord shrivels up, drops off, and leaves the navel (belly button). The baby's organs, such as the lungs, kidneys, and digestive system, must then take over the functions previously performed by the placenta.

? Re-Think

Why can umbilical cord compression or premature separation of the placenta cause fetal death?

ORGANOGENESIS

The embryonic period is a time of organogenesis (or-gah-no-JEN-eh-sis), or the formation of body organs and organ systems. The inner cell mass of the blastocyst forms a flattened structure called the *embryonic disc*. The embryonic disc, in turn, gives rise to three primary germ layers: the ectoderm, mesoderm, and endoderm.

All the tissues and organs of the body develop from these germ layers. For example, the ectoderm gives rise to the nervous system, portions of the special senses, and the skin. The skin is one of the earliest organs to develop and forms during the third week. The mesoderm gives rise to muscle, bone, blood, and many of the structures of the cardiovascular system. The endoderm gives rise to the epithelial lining of the digestive tract, respiratory tract, and parts of the urinary tract. By the end of the embryonic period (week 8), the main internal organs are established. The embryo weighs about 1 g, is about 1 inch (2.5 cm) in length, and has a human appearance (Figure 27-4).

BE CAREFUL: TERATOGENS

Because the organs of the body are being formed at this time, the embryonic period is most critical for

8 weeks

Umbilical cord **3 months**

6 weeks

Umbilical stalk

28 days

5 months

9 months

FIGURE 27-4 From embryo to fetus to baby.

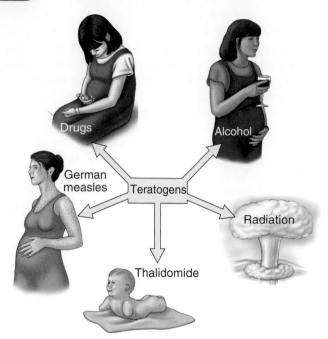

FIGURE 27-5 Teratogens: "monster-producing" agents.

development. Toxic substances such as alcohol, drugs, and certain pathogens can cross the placental membrane and interfere with embryonic development, causing severe birth defects. These toxic substances are called **teratogens** (TER-ah-toh-jens), a word that means "monster-producing" and attests to the severity of teratogenic birth defects. Hazardous conditions such as exposure to radiation can also act as teratogens (Figure 27-5).

 Do You Know...

How You Get That Extra Inch, or "Slackus the Urachus"?

Following delivery of a baby, the umbilical cord is tied off or clamped. Traditionally, the cord of a girl baby was tied close to the abdominal wall. The cord of a male baby, however, was tied farther away from the abdominal wall. Why the difference in cord length?

In the baby, a cordlike structure called the *urachus* extends from the top of the urinary bladder to the navel. It was thought that the urachus would be pulled up tight if the cord were tied too close to the abdominal wall. The tight urachus in turn would pull up on the penis, thereby stunting its growth. Conversely, by leaving the umbilical cord long, the urachus would relax, and the penis would grow longer. This obsession with penile length gave rise to the motto "slackus the urachus." Today, the umbilical cord in both male and female babies is clamped about 1 to 2 cm from the abdominal wall. No penile shortening has been recorded.

Alcohol is a potent teratogen. It can cause a cluster of birth defects known as *fetal alcohol syndrome*. In addition to causing facial deformities, alcohol interferes with neurological and mental development. The tranquilizer thalidomide is another drug that produces teratogenic effects. The development of finlike appendages instead of arms and legs has been correlated with the ingestion of thalidomide during pregnancy. Because of the sensitivity of the embryo to teratogenic agents, the mother must be extremely careful to protect her unborn child from toxic substances and hazardous conditions. Many drugs are teratogenic and most pharmacological clinical trials do not involve pregnant women!

 Do You Know...

What a Sonogram Is?

A sonogram is an image produced by sound waves as they encounter different tissues and organs. During the procedure, sound waves are directed through the mother's abdomen. As the sound waves "hit" the fetus, an image appears on the scope, showing an outline of the fetus. The size, position, and gender of the fetus can be determined by sonography, as can certain fetal abnormalities.

FETAL PERIOD

The fetal period extends from week 9 to birth. At this time, the developing offspring is called a **fetus**. The fetal period is primarily a time of growth and maturation; only a few new parts appear. Body proportions, however, continue to change. For example, at 8 weeks, the head is almost as large as the body. At birth, the head is proportionately much smaller than the body. Note the changes in body size and proportion in Figure 27-4.

Table 27-2 summarizes prenatal development. Note that a primitive nervous system begins to form in the third week. The heart and blood vessels originate during the second week. The heart is pumping blood to all the organs of the embryo by the second month, and a heartbeat can be detected during the third month, when the gender of the fetus can also be determined. Once the testes differentiate, they produce the male sex hormone testosterone. Testosterone stimulates the growth of the male external genitals. In the absence of testosterone, female genitals form.

The mother first feels the fetus move during the fifth month; this experience is called *quickening*. As the fetus grows, its skin becomes covered by a fine downy hair called *lanugo* (lah-NOO-go) (during the fifth month). The skin is covered by a white, cheeselike substance called the *vernix caseosa*. The vernix is thought to protect the delicate fetal skin from the amniotic fluid. By the fifth month, the fetus is in crowded quarters and is flexed in the fetal position. During the last 2 months, the baby is gaining weight rapidly as fat is deposited in the subcutaneous tissue. As the time for birth approaches, the fetus rotates so that the head is pointed toward the cervix. At the end of 38 weeks, the fetus is full term. During this period, the fetal weight has increased from less than 0.5 oz (14 g) to 7.5 lb (3.4 kg; average weight of a full-term infant). The fetus has grown in length from about 1 to 21 inches (2.5 to 53 cm). Baby is ready to face the world!

Table 27-2   **Human Development**

TIME	DEVELOPMENTAL EVENT
Embryonic	
Second week	Implantation occurs. The inner cell mass is giving rise to the primary germ layers; beginning of placental development.
Third week	Beginning of the nervous system
Fourth week	Appearance of limb buds. Heart is beating. Embryo has tail. Other organ systems begin.
Fifth week	Enlarged head; nose, eyes, and ears are noticeable.
Sixth week	Fingers and toes are present; appearance of cartilage skeleton
Second month	All organ systems are developing. Cartilaginous skeleton is being replaced by bone (ossification). Embryo is about 1.5 inches (3.8 cm) long.
Fetal	
Third month	Facial features present in crude form. Can determine gender (the external reproductive organs are distinguishable as male or female).
Fourth month	Sensory organs are present; eyes and ears attain shape and position. Eyes blink and the baby begins sucking movements. Skeleton is visible.
Fifth month	Vernix caseosa and a fine downy hair (lanugo) cover the skin. Heartbeat can be heard during a prenatal visit. Quickening occurs.
Sixth month	Continues to grow. Myelination of the spinal cord begins.
Seventh month	Eyes are open. Testes descend into scrotum. Weighs about 3 lb (135 g). Bone marrow becomes the only site of blood cell formation.
Eighth month	Body is lean and well proportioned. Subcutaneous fat begins to be deposited.
Ninth month	Full term and ready to be delivered. Average weight is 7.5 lb (338 g), average length is 21 inches (53.3 cm).

Sometimes, the embryo or fetus is born too early, before the 9-month gestation period is completed. A number of terms are used to describe early birth. An *abortion* is the loss of an embryo or fetus any time during the gestational period; most commonly, abortion refers to the termination of the pregnancy before the twentieth week of development. A *spontaneous abortion* occurs naturally, with no artificial interference. Usually, a spontaneous abortion is caused by some fetal abnormality. A *miscarriage* is the layperson's term for a spontaneous abortion. An *induced abortion* is an abortion deliberately caused by some artificial or mechanical means. An unwanted pregnancy is a common cause of an induced abortion. A *therapeutic abortion* is performed by a physician as a form of treatment for the mother. For example, a pregnancy that threatens the life of the mother may be terminated to save her life or improve her medical condition.

A baby born before 38 weeks but capable of living outside the womb is a premature or preterm infant. A 20-week-old fetus is considered viable—that is, able to live outside the womb. A premature baby is small but, more importantly, it is immature and may require medical support. In particular, the hypothalamus is too immature to regulate body temperature well, and the surfactant produced by the fetal lungs is inadequate to maintain breathing. Generally, the more premature the birth, the greater the need for medical support.

2+2 Sum It Up!

Fertilization takes place in the fallopian tube, when the nuclei of a sperm and egg unite, producing a zygote. The zygote gradually moves through the fallopian tube into the uterus, where it develops into an infant over a 9-month period. Prenatal development includes the processes of cleavage (mitosis), growth, morphogenesis, and differentiation. Prenatal development is divided into three periods: the early embryonic period (2 weeks), the embryonic period (6 weeks), and the fetal period (7 weeks to birth at 38 weeks). The zygote undergoes mitosis and develops into a blastocyst; trophoblastic cells help the blastocyst to implant. Other major accomplishments of the embryonic period include the formation of extraembryonic membranes and the development of the placenta and umbilical cord. The embryonic period is also the period of organogenesis. The fetal period is primarily a period of rapid growth and maturation. Baby shapes up, fattens up, and moves about.

? Re-Think

Why is the embryo more susceptible to teratogens than a seventh-month fetus?

CHANGES IN THE MOTHER'S BODY DURING PREGNANCY

Throughout pregnancy, the mother supplies all the food and oxygen for the fetus and eliminates all the waste. This added burden requires many changes in the mother's physiology:

- The rate of metabolism increases. For example, the mother secretes greater amounts of the thyroid hormones triiodothyronine (T_3) and thyroxine (T_4). Human placental lactogen circulates within the maternal circulation; among other growth-promoting actions, this hormone makes additional amounts of glucose available to the growing fetus.
- The mother's blood volume expands by as much as 40% to 50%. The increase in blood volume is caused by an increase in the secretion of aldosterone by the adrenal cortex. To pump the additional blood and meet the demands of an increased metabolism, the activity of the cardiovascular system increases. For example, heart rate, stroke volume, and cardiac output increase.
- Respiratory activity increases to provide additional oxygen and eliminate excess carbon dioxide.
- The kidneys work harder and produce more urine because they must eliminate waste for both the mother and fetus.
- Under the influence of estrogen and progesterone, the size and weight of the uterus increase dramatically as the fetus grows to full term. To accommodate the growth of the uterus, the pelvic cavity expands as the sacroiliac joints and symphysis pubis become more flexible. With growth, the uterus pushes the abdominal organs upward. In the later months of pregnancy especially, the upward displacement of abdominal organs exerts pressure on the diaphragm and hampers the mother's breathing.
- The mother's nutritional needs increase as the maternal organs (uterus and breasts) grow and she provides for the growing fetus. In particular, the need for calcium increases, because an increase in parathyroid hormone (PTH) extracts calcium from the mother's bone, making it available to the growing fetus.

Pregnancy brings some discomforts for some women. Nausea and vomiting, generally referred to as *morning sickness,* commonly occur in the first 3 months. Morning sickness may be caused by hormonal changes, especially to the elevated levels of hCG. During the later months of pregnancy, the woman gains approximately 2 to 3 lb/month. The added weight causes a shift in the mother's center of gravity, thereby affecting her balance and forcing her to adjust her walking style. Eventually, many women appear to be waddling.

The added weight may also cause discomfort in the lower back and many other aches as the uterine ligaments and other supporting structures stretch. The expanding uterus stretches the abdominal skin, causing stretch marks, or striae (STRYE-ay). It also displaces the stomach upward, causing heartburn. Frequent urination results from increased urine formation and compression of the urinary bladder by the uterus. Finally, the expanded uterus hampers the return of blood through the veins of the lower body region. This inhibited blood flow, in turn, may cause varicose veins and hemorrhoids. No wonder the mother-to-be looks forward to giving birth!

Although these discomforts of pregnancy are normal, several pregnancy-related conditions are not normal but are dangerous to both the mother and child. For example, the mother may develop a toxemia of pregnancy. This condition is characterized by an elevated blood pressure and progresses in severe cases to generalized seizures. The early stage is called *pre-eclampsia,* and the later seizure stage is called *eclampsia.*

2+2 Sum It Up!

Pregnancy causes many changes in the mother. Hormonal changes are numerous and complex. Secretion of hCG, estrogen, and progesterone help maintain the pregnancy and prepare the organs of reproduction for 9 months of pregnancy. Other hormones, such as aldosterone, thyroid hormones, and parathyroid hormone, prepare the mother's body to nourish and sustain the growing unborn child. Almost every maternal organ responds to the presence of the fetus; the heart pumps more blood, the kidneys excrete more waste, and the increased metabolic rate indicates that every cell is working harder.

BIRTH OF BABY

Finally, Baby is ready to face the world. The birth process is called *parturition* (pahr-too-RIH-shun). Labor is the process whereby forceful contractions expel the fetus from the uterus. Once labor starts, forceful and rhythmic contractions begin at the top of the uterus and travel down its length, forcing the fetus through the birth canal.

LABOR

HORMONAL BASIS OF LABOR

The precise mechanism that starts labor is unknown. A number of hormonal stimuli do, however, play a role. For example, progesterone, which normally quiets uterine contractions during pregnancy, is secreted in decreasing amounts after the seventh month. This decrease coincides with an increase in the secretion of estrogen. Estrogen has two effects on the uterus: it opposes the quieting effect of progesterone on uterine contractions, and it sensitizes the myometrium (uterine muscle) to the stimulatory effects of oxytocin.

The secretion of prostaglandins by the placenta also plays a role in initiating labor. Prostaglandins stimulate uterine contractions. Finally, the stretching of the uterine and vaginal tissue in the late stage of pregnancy stimulates nerves that send signals to the hypothalamus. The hypothalamus, in turn, stimulates the release of oxytocin from the posterior pituitary gland. Oxytocin exerts a powerful stimulating effect on the myometrium and is thought to play an important role in labor.

 Do You Know...

Why Aspirin and Ibuprofen Can Inhibit the Onset of Labor?

Aspirin and ibuprofen are antiprostaglandin drugs. Because prostaglandins stimulate uterine contractions, suppression of prostaglandin secretion by these drugs may inhibit uterine contractions, thereby inhibiting labor.

Labor can, however, have a false start. Sometimes, a very pregnant and embarrassed mother is admitted to the hospital in false labor. What has happened? She has indeed felt uterine contractions. However, these contractions—called *Braxton Hicks contractions*—are weak, irregular, and ineffectual, and they normally occur during late pregnancy. These contractions are caused by the increased responsiveness of the uterus to various hormones, particularly changing concentrations of estrogen and progesterone. The mother returns home to await the onset of true labor.

STAGES OF LABOR

The three stages of true labor are the dilation stage, expulsion stage, and placental stage (Figure 27-6). The dilation stage begins with the onset of labor and ends with full dilation of the cervix (10 cm). This stage is characterized by rhythmic and forceful contractions, rupture of the amniotic sac (the bag of water), and cervical dilation. It is the longest stage of labor and generally lasts between 6 and 12 hours. The expulsion stage extends from complete cervical dilation to the expulsion of the fetus through the vagina (birth canal). This stage generally lasts less than 1 hour. During this stage, the mother has the urge to push with her abdominal muscles.

In a normal delivery, the head is delivered first. A head-first delivery allows the baby to be suctioned free of mucus and to breathe even before the body has fully exited from the birth canal. Because the vaginal orifice may not expand enough to deliver the baby, however, an episiotomy may be performed. An episiotomy (eh-piz-ee-OT-oh-mee) is a surgical incision into the perineum, the tissue between the vaginal opening and the anus. The incision enlarges the vaginal opening and facilitates the delivery of the baby.

The third stage is the placental stage and occurs 10 to 15 minutes after the birth. It involves the separation of the placenta from the uterine wall and expulsion of the placenta and attached membranes by forceful uterine contractions. The placenta and the attached membranes are collectively called the *afterbirth*. In addition to expelling the fetus and the placenta, the uterine contractions also cause vasoconstriction of the uterine blood vessels, thereby minimizing blood loss. Uterine contractions also help the uterus return to its nonpregnant size and shape. About 500 mL of blood is lost during delivery.

FIGURE 27-6 Stages of labor. **A,** Before labor begins. **B,** Dilation stage. **C,** Expulsion stage. **D,** Placental stage.

Sometimes, the fetus does not come out head first. Instead, another part of the body, such as the buttocks, is delivered first. This presentation is called a *breech birth*. A breech presentation makes delivery more difficult for both the mother and the infant.

There are a number of conditions that prevent a safe vaginal delivery, thereby requiring surgery. A cesarean section (C-section) refers to the delivery of the infant through a surgical incision in the abdominal and uterine walls.

Do You Know...

What Placenta Previa and Abruptio Placentae Are?

Sometimes, the placenta forms too low in the uterus, near the cervix. When the cervix dilates during the later stages of pregnancy, the placenta detaches from the uterine wall, causing bleeding in the mother and depriving the fetus of an adequate supply of oxygen and nutrients. This condition is called *placenta previa*. *Abruptio placentae* refers to the premature separation of an implanted placenta at about 20 or more weeks of pregnancy. Without immediate treatment, abruptio placentae results in severe hemorrhage in the mother and death for the fetus.

FEMALE BREAST AND LACTATION

STRUCTURE OF A BREAST: THE MAMMARY GLANDS

The anterior chest contains two elevations called *breasts* (Figure 27-7, *A*). The breasts are located anterior to the pectoralis major muscles and contain adipose tissue and mammary glands. **Mammary glands** are accessory organs of the female reproductive system. They secrete milk following the delivery of the baby. At the tip of each breast is a nipple surrounded by a circular area of pigmented skin called the *areola*. Each mammary gland contains 15 to 20 lobes. Each lobe contains many alveolar glands and a lactiferous duct. The alveolar glands secrete milk, which is carried toward the nipple by the lactiferous duct. Connective tissue, including the suspensory ligaments, helps support the breast.

Until a child reaches puberty, the mammary glands of male and female children are similar. At puberty, however, the female mammary glands are stimulated by estrogen and progesterone. The alveolar glands and ducts enlarge, and adipose tissue is deposited around these structures. The male breast does not develop because there is no hormonal stimulus to do so. If a male is given female hormones, however, he too develops breasts.

GOT MILK?

HORMONES OF LACTATION

During pregnancy, the increased secretion of estrogen and progesterone has a profound effect on the breasts. The breasts may double in size in preparation for lactation (milk production) following birth. Usually, there is no milk production during pregnancy because lactation requires prolactin, a hormone secreted by the anterior pituitary gland (see Figure 27-7, *B*). High plasma levels of estrogen and progesterone inhibit prolactin secretion during pregnancy. After delivery, however, plasma levels of estrogen and progesterone decrease, allowing the anterior pituitary gland to secrete prolactin. Milk production takes 2 to 3 days to begin. In the meantime, the mammary glands produce colostrum (koh-LOH-strohm), a yellowish watery fluid rich in protein and antibodies.

Prolactin is necessary for milk production, but a second hormone, oxytocin, is necessary for the release of milk from the breast. How does the release of milk happen? When the baby suckles, or nurses, at the breast, nerve impulses in the areola are stimulated. Nerve impulses then travel from the breast to the hypothalamus; the hypothalamus, in turn, stimulates the posterior pituitary gland to release oxytocin. The oxytocin travels through the blood to the breast, causing contraction of the smooth muscle of the lobules. This process squeezes milk into the ducts, where it can be sucked out of the nipple by the nursing infant (see Figure 27-7, *B*).

The effect of suckling and oxytocin release is called the *milk let-down reflex*. Note that the stimulus for the milk let-down reflex is suckling at the breast. Thus, nursing mothers are encouraged to suckle their infants often. Breast-feeding encourages a good flow of milk. Also note the distinction between the effects of prolactin and oxytocin. Prolactin stimulates milk production, or lactation. Oxytocin stimulates the milk let-down reflex and stimulates the flow of milk.

In addition to its effect on the flow of milk, oxytocin causes the uterus to contract. Uterine contraction helps minimize blood loss and more quickly returns the uterus to its nonpregnant state. (The return of the uterus to its nonpregnant size is called *involution*.) A class of drugs called *oxytocic agents* are sometimes administered to the mother after childbirth. Like oxytocin, these drugs (ergot preparations) cause uterine contractions and minimize postpartum bleeding.

 Re-Think

1. List three pregnancy-induced physiological adjustments.
2. Differentiate between the effects of prolactin and oxytocin with regard to lactation.
3. What is colostrum?

POSTNATAL CHANGES AND DEVELOPMENTAL STAGES

IMMEDIATE ADJUSTMENTS

Immediately after birth, the baby must make many important adjustments to survive. Most importantly,

FIGURE 27-7 **A,** Breast and mammary glands. **B,** Hormones involved in breast-feeding; the milk let-down reflex.

the baby must begin breathing. The first deep breaths, drawn as the baby cries, expand the lungs and provide the infant with life-giving oxygen. The cardiovascular system also makes major adjustments, the most important being the establishment of blood flow to the lungs. Pulmonary blood flow occurs when the fetal heart structures, such as the foramen ovale and ductus arteriosus, close. (Review fetal circulation in Chapter 18.)

Other organ systems continue functioning as they did before birth. For example, the kidneys, having once secreted their urine into the amniotic fluid, become diaper-seeking organs, and the digestive system continues its lifelong career of eating, digesting, and excreting. The first stool produced by the newborn—meconium (meh-COH-nee-um)—is soft and dark green. (During a long difficult labor the baby may become stressed and excrete meconium into the amniotic fluid—not good.)

DEVELOPMENT AS A LIFELONG PROCESS

After the newborn makes the immediate adjustments, the infant continues to grow and develop. Throughout life, the person will pass through the following developmental stages:

- *Neonatal period.* The neonatal period begins at birth and lasts for 4 weeks. During this time, Baby is called a *neonate,* or *newborn.*
- *Infancy.* The period of infancy lasts from the end of the first month to the end of the first year. Baby's first birthday marks the end of this stage.
- *Childhood.* The period of childhood lasts from the beginning of the second year to puberty.
- *Adolescence.* The period of adolescence lasts from puberty to adulthood. One word characterizes this stage: hormones. The period of adolescence is a period of tremendous growth and upheaval. Adolescents are physically capable of reproduction. The teen moves toward adulthood, leaving behind childish ways and coming to grips with becoming an adult.
- *Adulthood.* Adulthood is the period from adolescence to old age. During this period, the person is usually concerned with family matters and career goals. (Most of us are still trying to give up childish ways!)
- *Senescence.* Senescence is the period of old age, ending in death. It is not only a time to reflect on a life well lived, but also a time to pursue other goals and to pass on the collected wisdom of a lifetime.

2+2 Sum It Up!

After the birth of the baby, both baby and mother make many physiological adjustments. The mother's body returns to its nonpregnant state. For example, cardiac output and blood volume decrease. She is physiologically prepared to breastfeed. Through the actions of prolactin and oxytocin, her mammary glands are producing milk and making it readily available to the suckling infant. The baby has made an initial adjustment to life on the outside and is breathing, urinating, and eating. The newborn continues postnatal development as a neonate. From there, it is on to infancy, childhood, adolescence, adulthood, and senescence.

HEREDITY

"He has his father's nose and his mother's smile." How often have we made that type of statement when we recognize the traits of a parent in a child? The transmission of characteristics from parent to child is called *heredity,* and the science that studies heredity is called *genetics.* The work of an Austrian monk, Gregor

Mendel, in the early nineteenth century paved the way for the modern science of genetics. Using garden peas, Mendel demonstrated a pattern of specific traits passed on from parent to child.

DNA, GENES, AND CHROMOSOMES

How are genetic structures related? Genetic information is located in the deoxyribonucleic acid (DNA) molecule and, more specifically, in the DNA base

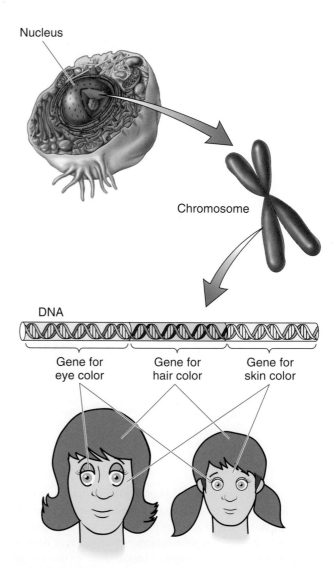

FIGURE 27-8 Chromosomes and genes.

Table **27-3** Examples of Genetic Traits		
TRAIT	**DOMINANT**	**RECESSIVE**
Hairline	Widow's peak	Continuous hairline
Hair color	Dark	Light
Hair texture	Curly	Straight
Hair on back of hand	Present	Absent
Freckles	Present	Absent to few
Dimples	Present	Absent
Eye color	Dark	Light
Color vision	Normal	Color-blind
Ear lobes	Unattached	Attached
Cleft chin	Present	Absent
Rh factor	Present	Absent

sequencing (Figure 27-8; see Chapter 4). DNA is tightly wound into threadlike structures called **chromosomes** found in the nucleus of most cells in the body. **Genes** are segments of the DNA strand and carry information for a specific trait such as skin color, freckles, and blood type. See Table 27-3 for other genetically determined characteristics. Some traits are determined by a single pair of genes, whereas other traits, such as height, require input from several genes. Each chromosome may carry thousands of genes, and each gene occupies a specific position on a chromosome.

Chromosomes exist in pairs. With the exception of the sex cells (egg and sperm), there are 23 pairs, or 46 chromosomes, in almost all human cells (red blood cells are the other exception). During fertilization, the egg and sperm each contribute 23 chromosomes to the zygote for a total of 23 pairs, or 46 chromosomes. One member of each pair comes from the egg; the other comes from the sperm. Thus, for each trait, genetic instructions come from both the mother and the father. Forty-four chromosomes (22 pairs) are called *autosomes* (AW-toh-sohms). The autosomal gene pairs are numbered from 1 to 22. Two (one pair) of the 46 chromosomes are sex chromosomes; each is either an X or Y chromosome.

Re-Think

What happens to the chromosomal number during meiotic cell division? Why is this important?

GENETIC ART: THE KARYOTYPE

It is possible to photograph the chromosomes in the cell. The photograph of the chromosomes is then cut apart, and the chromosomes are arranged in pairs by size and shape. The resulting display of the paired chromosomes is called a **karyotype** (KAIR-ee-oh-type)

(Figure 27-9). This genetic artwork displays 22 pairs of autosomes and one pair of sex chromosomes. The karyotype is a diagnostic tool. It can reveal structural abnormalities and errors in the numbers of chromosomes.

DOMINANT, RECESSIVE, AND CODOMINANT GENES

Remember that each cell inherits two genes for each trait—tall or short, straight nose or curved nose, stubby fingers or long fingers, dark eyes or light eyes. Hence, the choice. Will it be long or short, or curved or straight? Genes can be dominant, recessive, or codominant. A dominant gene expresses itself; it gets noticed. The dominant gene overshadows the recessive gene and keeps it unnoticed, or unexpressed. Thus, a recessive gene is not expressed if it is paired with a dominant gene. For example, the genes for dark eyes are dominant, whereas the genes for light eyes are recessive. If the dominant genes (dark) and the recessive (light) genes are paired, the genes for dark eyes will be expressed (Figure 27-10). The genes for light eyes will not be expressed. Codominant genes express a trait equally. AB blood type is an example of codominance.

If recessive genes carry light eye coloring, how can an offspring develop blue eyes? Although blue eye coloring is recessive, a baby develops blue eyes because both the mother and father are carrying the genes for blue eyes, a recessive trait (see Figure 27-10). If either the mother or father had passed on a dominant gene for dark eyes, the child would have brown eyes.

The question can be put another way. If I have brown eyes, can any of my children have blue eyes? Yes! If I am carrying both a dominant (brown) and recessive (blue) gene for eye color, my child has a chance of having blue eyes. My recessive gene might pair with a recessive gene from my mate. If so, the pairing of two recessive genes produces a blue-eyed offspring. Brown-eyed me is a carrier, one who shows no evidence of a trait (like blue eyes) but carries a recessive gene for that trait.

TOO MANY OR TOO FEW CHROMOSOMES

A person normally inherits 22 pairs of autosomal chromosomes. Sometimes, however, a person inherits too many or too few autosomal chromosomes. The most common autosomal abnormality is called *trisomy 21*, or *Down syndrome*. A child with trisomy 21 has three copies of chromosome 21 instead of two copies. Other types of trisomy occur very infrequently in live births. Trisomy 18, called *Edwards syndrome*, is caused by three copies of chromosome 18, whereas trisomy 13, called *Patau syndrome*, is caused by three copies of chromosome 13. Autosomal abnormalities are usually caused by nondisjunction.

Nondisjunction is the failure of the chromosomes to separate during meiosis, thereby causing the

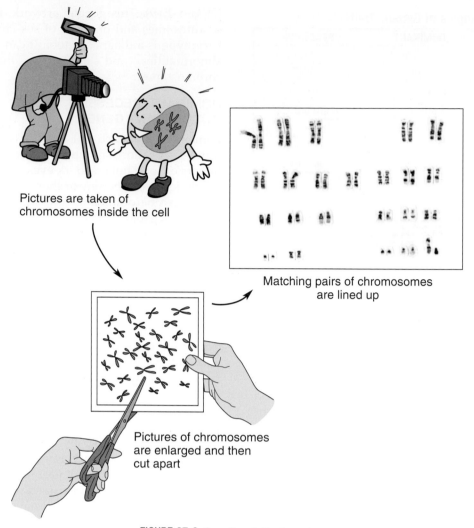

Pictures are taken of
chromosomes inside the cell

Matching pairs of chromosomes
are lined up

Pictures of chromosomes
are enlarged and then
cut apart

FIGURE 27-9 Genetic art: the karyotype.

formation of eggs or sperm with too many or too few chromosomes. If these eggs and sperm lead to pregnancy, the embryo may have one too many or too few chromosomes. Most pregnancies with an unbalanced number of chromosomes miscarry in the first trimester. Down syndrome is the most common chromosomal abnormality because the condition is least likely to cause the pregnancy to miscarry. Even so, an estimated 70% of pregnancies with Down syndrome spontaneously miscarry, usually in the first trimester.

GENETIC EXPRESSION

Genetic expression determines what the offspring looks like. A person's genetic expression can be influenced by a number of factors, including the person's gender, the influence of other genes, and environmental conditions. For example, certain types of baldness and color blindness may be inherited by males and females, but these traits are more apt to appear in the male. A child may also have the genetic capability of growing very tall. If the child is deprived of adequate nutrition and exercise, however, that child may not grow as tall as the genetic makeup has predicted.

GENETIC MUTATIONS

Normally, DNA replicates all information with few mistakes. Because of this precision, information is passed along reliably and efficiently to the next generation. Sometimes, however, a change occurs in a gene, or a chromosome breaks in some unexpected way. The result may be a unique feature or a birth defect. This change in the genetic code is called a *mutation*. Some mutations occur spontaneously; others are caused by mutagenic agents, such as chemicals, drugs, and radiation. Mutations can be beneficial or harmful and may even cause the death of the offspring. For example, a mutation in the cells of the immune system may render a child resistant to a particular disease, thereby enhancing health. Another mutation, however, may weaken the immune system, making it more susceptible to pathogens.

A

B

FIGURE 27-10 Eye color, with dominant and recessive genes. **A,** The dominant brown-eye gene is expressed over the recessive blue-eye gene. **B,** Two recessive blue-eye genes produce a blue-eyed offspring.

 Re-Think

Define *nondisjunction, trisomy,* and *genetic mutation.*

IT'S A BOY, IT'S A GIRL: HOW THE SEX OF THE CHILD IS DETERMINED

Xs AND Ys

Each human cell has 22 pairs of autosomal chromosomes and one pair of sex chromosomes (X and Y chromosomes). The female has two X chromosomes in her cells, a pair designated XX. A male has both an X and Y chromosome in his cells, a pair designated XY (Figure 27-11).

SEX DETERMINATION: A MALE THING

The sex cells, the egg and the sperm, divide by a special type of cell division called *meiosis*. The important step in meiosis is the reduction (by half) of the chromosomes. In other words, meiosis reduces the numbers of chromosomes from 46 to 23. The meiotic cell reduction also reduces the numbers of sex chromosomes by half. Consequently, each egg contains one X chromosome, and the sperm contains either an X chromosome or a Y chromosome. If a sperm containing an X chromosome fertilizes an egg, the child has an XX sex chromosome pair and is therefore female. If a sperm containing a Y chromosome fertilizes an egg, the child has an XY chromosome pair and is therefore male. Thus, the sperm (male) determines the sex of the child.

Sometimes, a person inherits an abnormal number of sex chromosomes. For example, a female with Turner syndrome inherits only one sex chromosome, an X chromosome. Turner syndrome is designated as XO. The X signifies the female chromosome; the O signifies the absence of the second sex chromosome. A child with Turner syndrome does not develop secondary sex characteristics, is shorter than average, and has a webbed neck. People with Turner syndrome have normal intelligence.

 Re-Think

Explain why the father determines the gender of the child.

SEX-LINKED TRAITS

The X and Y chromosomes differ structurally. The female X chromosome is larger than the Y chromosome and carries many genes for traits in addition to determining sex. The male Y chromosome is much smaller than the X chromosome and does not carry as much genetic information as the X chromosome. Any trait that is carried on a sex chromosome is called a **sex-linked trait**. Because the X chromosome has more genetic information than the Y chromosome, most sex-linked traits are carried on the female X chromosome. Sex-linked traits carried on the X chromosomes are also called *X-linked traits*.

Although most sex-linked traits are carried on the X chromosome, they are expressed, or appear, in the male. Sex-linked diseases include hemophilia, Duchenne muscular dystrophy, and fragile X syndrome. Less serious sex-linked traits include baldness and red–green color blindness.

CONGENITAL AND HEREDITARY DISEASE

You need to distinguish between hereditary diseases and congenital diseases and defects. Hereditary diseases are genetically transmitted; congenital conditions are present at the time of birth. Congenital disorders include those that are inherited and those that are not. For example, hemophilia is genetically transmitted and is therefore inherited. Because hemophilia is present at birth, it is also congenital.

A disease can, however, be congenital but not inherited. For example, a mother may give birth to an infant who was exposed to the rubella virus (German measles) during her first trimester of pregnancy. This child may be born with cardiovascular, ocular, and neural tube defects. These defects were not transmitted genetically from the parents to the child and are therefore not hereditary. The defects are congenital, however, because they were present at birth. Only 15% of congenital defects have a known genetic cause. For 70% of congenital birth defects, the cause is unknown.

Gene therapy offers hope for the treatment and eventual cure of genetic disorders. *Gene therapy* refers to the insertion of normal genes into cells that have abnormal genes. For example, a person with congenitally high cholesterol levels might be successfully treated with genes that code for normal cholesterol production. Although still in its early experimental stages, gene therapy provides hope for those with such genetic conditions as sickle cell disease, cystic fibrosis, and muscular dystrophy.

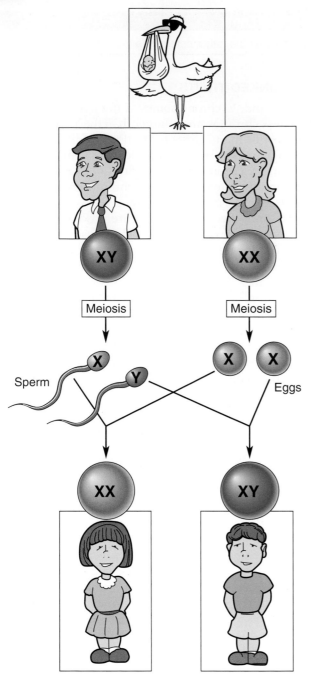

FIGURE 27-11 Determination of sex; Xs and Ys.

? Re-Think

1. What is a sex-linked trait?
2. Explain how a disorder can be congenital but not hereditary.

2+2 Sum It Up!

A child resembles the parents because he or she inherits genetic information from each parent. Genetic information is stored in the DNA molecules, which are arranged in strands called *chromosomes*. Almost every human cell contains 22 pairs of autosomal chromosomes and one pair of sex chromosomes. Genes are segments of DNA that contain codes for specific traits such as eye color or blood type. The child receives two genes for each inherited trait—one from the mother and one from the father.

Genes are dominant, recessive, or codominant. The sex chromosomes are designated X and Y. At fertilization, an XX combination produces a female child, whereas an XY combination produces a male. The father, with his Y chromosome, determines the sex of the child. Genetic information is passed along efficiently and reliably. Occasionally, incorrect or unhealthy information is passed along, thereby producing genetic diseases.

Note: The Medical Terminology and Disorders table related to this chapter appears in Chapter 26.

Get Ready for Exams!

Summary Outline

The purpose of the reproductive system is to produce off-spring whose genetic information is faithfully transmitted from generation to generation.

I. Fertilization to Birth
  A. Fertilization
    1. *Fertilization* (conception) refers to the union of an egg and a sperm, called a *zygote*.
    2. Fertilization takes place around the time of ovulation.
    3. Fertilization normally occurs within the fallopian tube.
  B. Human development: begins with fertilization and ends with death
  C. Prenatal development
    1. Prenatal development processes: cleavage, growth, morphogenesis, and differentiation
    2. Prenatal period: early embryonic, embryonic, and fetal periods
      a. The early embryonic period lasts for 2 weeks after fertilization. The zygote develops and

implants into the uterine endometrial lining; its trophoblastic cells secrete hCG (maintains the corpus luteum).

b. There are two types of twins: monozygotic (identical) twins and dizygotic or fraternal (nonidentical) twins.

c. The embryonic period lasts for 6 weeks and involves the formation of the extraembryonic membranes, the placenta, and all the organ systems.

d. The four extraembryonic membranes are the amnion, chorion, yolk sac, and allantois.

e. The placenta develops as the chorionic villi of the embryo burrow into the endometrial lining of the uterus.

f. The placenta has two functions: the site of "exchange" and glandular function.

g. The embryo is hooked up to the placenta by the umbilical cord.

h. The embryonic period is a period of organogenesis.

i. The fetal period extends from week 9 to birth; it is a time of growth and maturation.

j. Hormonal changes during pregnancy are summarized in Table 27-1.

D. Birth (parturition)

1. Labor is the forceful contractions that expel the fetus from the uterus.

2. Labor is caused by hormones.

E. Breasts and lactation

1. The breasts contain mammary (milk-secreting) glands and adipose tissue.

2. Hormonal control of breast function: prolactin and oxytocin (milk let-down reflex)

II. Postnatal Development

A. Immediate postnatal changes

1. The baby takes a first breath and the cardiovascular system makes some major adjustments.

2. Baby is no longer eating, drinking, and breathing at the placenta.

B. Developmental periods: neonatal period, infancy, childhood, adolescence, adulthood, and senescence

III. Heredity

A. DNA, genes, and chromosomes

1. Genetic information is stored in the DNA of genes, which are arranged into chromosomes.

2. Chromosomes exist in pairs. With the exception of sex cells, most human cells have 23 pairs of chromosomes, or 46 chromosomes.

3. Genes are dominant, recessive, or codominant.

4. The sex chromosomes are designated X and Y. A female has two X chromosomes and a male has one X chromosome and one Y chromosome. Because only the male has the Y chromosome, the father determines the sex of the child.

5. Sex-linked traits are carried on the sex chromosomes. Most are carried on the X chromosome and are therefore also called *X-linked traits*.

B. Congenital and hereditary diseases

1. A congenital disorder is a condition present at birth.

2. Congenital disorders include inherited and noninherited birth defects and diseases. A hereditary disease is transmitted genetically from parent to child.

Review Your Knowledge

Matching: Fertilization and Development

Directions: Match the following words with their descriptions below.

a. primary germ layers
b. fetus
c. zygote
d. fertilization
e. embryo
f. parturition
g. trophoblasts
h. placenta
i. implantation
j. umbilical cord

1. ___ The fertilized ovum
2. ___ Cells that secrete hCG
3. ___ A zygote-making event
4. ___ The site where Baby breathes, eats, and excretes
5. ___ Baby's lifeline; contains the umbilical blood vessels
6. ___ Baby's name at age 3 to 8 weeks
7. ___ Process whereby the blastocyst baby-to-be burrows into the endometrium
8. ___ The birth process
9. ___ Endoderm, mesoderm, and ectoderm
10. ___ Baby's name from 9 weeks to birth

Matching: Hormones

Directions: Match the following words with their descriptions below. Some words may be used more than once.

a. hCG
b. prolactin
c. oxytocin
d. aldosterone

1. ___ Hormone that stimulates the mammary glands to make milk
2. ___ Posterior pituitary hormone involved in the milk let-down reflex
3. ___ Hormone that sustains the corpus luteum
4. ___ Hormone that stimulates the contraction of the myometrium
5. ___ Secretion of this hormone continues at a high level for about 2 months and then steadily declines as the placenta takes over.
6. ___ Hormone that stimulates Na^+ reabsorption and expands blood volume during pregnancy

Matching: Heredity

Directions: Match the following words with their descriptions on the next page.

a. sex-linked trait
b. mutation
c. autosomes
d. sex chromosomes
e. genes

1. ___ Segments of a DNA strand that carry the code for a specific trait, such as eye color
2. ___ Twenty-two pairs (numbered 1 to 22) of chromosomes
3. ___ X and Y chromosomes
4. ___ Any trait that is carried on an X or Y chromosome
5. ___ A change in the genetic code that may express itself as a change in a particular trait

Multiple Choice

1. Implantation
   a. normally occurs within the fallopian tubes.
   b. is achieved by the morula.
   c. is a uterine event achieved by the blastocyst.
   d. occurs within the ovaries.
2. Human chorionic gonadotropin (hCG)
   a. promotes the maturation of the egg.
   b. is responsible for female characteristics.
   c. maintains the corpus luteum.
   d. promotes the transformation of the corpus luteum into the corpus albicans.
3. Trophoblastic cells
   a. secrete oxytocin.
   b. are responsible for the milk let-down reflex.
   c. assist with implantation.
   d. are incorporated within the graafian follicle.
4. The morula
   a. only is formed if there is an ectopic pregnancy.
   b. is the unfertilized ovum that gets discharged with the menstrual blood.
   c. refers to the pre-embryonic cluster of cells.
   d. spends its life embedded within the endometrium.
5. Which of the following is least true of the placenta?
   a. Is the site at which the baby-to-be breathes
   b. Is very vascular
   c. Replaces the glandular secretion of the corpus luteum
   d. Nourishes the zygote as it matures into the morula
6. The chorion is an extraembryonic membrane that
   a. develops finger-like projections that penetrate the uterine wall forming the placenta.
   b. forms the inner cell mass.
   c. secretes the hormones that initiate labor.
   d. secretes vernix caseosa that covers the fetus.
7. The myometrium
   a. sloughs during menstruation.
   b. is responsive to oxytocin and oxytocic drugs.
   c. is the uterine lining that is most responsive to estrogen and progesterone.
   d. forms finger-like projections that penetrate the uterine lining forming the placenta.
8. Which of the following happens first?
   a. Zygote formation
   b. Fertilization
   c. Ovulation
   d. Early blastocyst
9. Prolactin and oxytocin
   a. are secreted by the adenohypophysis.
   b. stimulate the milk let-down reflex.
   c. stimulate the mammary glands to make milk.
   d. target the mammary glands.
10. Colostrum is
    a. secreted by the mammary glands.
    b. located within the amniotic sac.
    c. the vernix caseosa that covers the fetus.
    d. a hormone that initiates labor and terminates pregnancy.

Go Figure

1. **According to Figure 27-1**
   a. The morula splits to form a zygote.
   b. A zygote forms within the fallopian tube.
   c. The late blastocyst is a fallopian tube dweller.
   d. Implantation is an ovarian event.

2. **According to Figure 27-1**
   a. Repeated mitosis of the zygote forms a morula.
   b. Trophoblastic cells, located in the ovary, assist in the implantation of the embryo.
   c. Fertilization usually occurs within the corpus luteum.
   d. Trophoblastic cells secrete LH, which is responsible for ovulation.

3. **According to Figures 27-2 and 27-3**
   a. The chorionic villi are located within the umbilical cord.
   b. Figure 27-2, C, illustrates the procedure for amniocentesis.
   c. None of the extraembryonic membranes are illustrated in Figure 27-2, A.
   d. The chorionic villi interact with the maternal uterine lining to form the placenta.

4. **According to Figure 27-7**
   a. Alveolar glands secrete milk into the lactiferous ducts.
   b. Oxytocin is secreted reflexively in response to suckling.
   c. Prolactin stimulates the breast to make milk.
   d. All of the above are true.

5. **According to Figure 27-7**
   a. The stimulus for the milk let-down reflex is the level of prolactin in the mother's blood.
   b. Oxytocin is a posterior pituitary hormone that causes milk to flow in response to suckling.
   c. Prolactin is a neurohypophyseal hormone that mediates the milk let-down reflex.
   d. All of the above are true.

6. **According to Figure 27-11**
   a. The father determines the gender of the offspring.
   b. The father provides sperm that only carry the Y chromosome.
   c. The mother provides ova that only carry the Y chromosome.
   d. An infant with an X and Y chromosome is female.

Answers to Review Your Knowledge and Go Figure Questions

Chapter 1: Introduction to the Human Body

Matching: Directions of the Body
1. c
2. e
3. b
4. f
5. d

Matching: Regional Terms
1. d
2. f
3. i
4. h
5. g
6. b
7. c
8. e
9. a
10. j

Multiple Choice
1. c
2. d
3. c
4. d
5. b
6. b
7. c
8. c

Go Figure
1. d
2. d
3. a
4. d
5. c

Chapter 2: Basic Chemistry

Matching: Atoms and Elements
1. a
2. b
3. d
4. c
5. e

Matching: Structure of the Atom
1. f
2. a
3. b
4. d
5. d

Matching: Ions and Electrolytes
1. c
2. b
3. a
4. d
5. e

Matching: Acids and Bases
1. e
2. c
3. b
4. f
5. f

Multiple Choice
1. c
2. a
3. d
4. d
5. b
6. c
7. c
8. c

Go Figure
1. b
2. b
3. a
4. c
5. c
6. b

Chapter 3: Cells

Matching: Cell Structure
1. f
2. d
3. a
4. b
5. c
6. e
7. g

Matching: Transport and Tonicity
1. g
2. h
3. i
4. c
5. f
6. e
7. a
8. d
9. b
10. d

Multiple Choice
1. b
2. d
3. c
4. a
5. c
6. d
7. b

Go Figure
1. b
2. d
3. d
4. c
5. d
6. c

Chapter 4: Cell Metabolism

Matching: Carbohydrates, Proteins, and Fats
1. d
2. b
3. c
4. g
5. f
6. b
7. h
8. a
9. e
10. a

Matching: Biochemistry Terms
1. b
2. a
3. c
4. d
5. a
6. e

Matching: Genetic Code and Protein Synthesis
1. d
2. e
3. c
4. a
5. b

Multiple Choice
1. a
2. d
3. c
4. c
5. a
6. a

Go Figure
1. c
2. b
3. a
4. a
5. c
6. b
7. b
8. a
9. d

Chapter 5: Microbiology Basics

Matching: Microorganisms and Other Pathogens
1. b
2. a
3. e
4. d
5. d
6. c
7. e
8. b
9. c
10. b
11. f

Multiple Choice
1. a
2. b
3. c
4. c
5. d

Go Figure
1. c
2. d

Chapter 6: Tissues and Membranes

Matching: Tissues
1. a
2. b
3. a
4. a
5. b
6. c
7. b
8. b
9. b
10. d

Matching: Membranes
1. d
2. e
3. b
4. a
5. c

Multiple Choice
1. c
2. a
3. d
4. a
5. a
6. b
7. d

Chapter 7: Integumentary System and Body Temperature

Matching: Skin
1. d
2. b
3. a
4. c
5. d
6. b

Matching: Glands
1. b
2. b
3. a
4. c
5. d
6. a
7. b
8. a

Matching: Colors
1. c
2. b
3. a
4. d
5. e

Multiple Choice
1. b
2. b
3. c
4. c
5. b
6. c
7. a
8. d
9. b

Go Figure
1. c
2. b
3. c
4. c
5. d

Chapter 8: Skeletal System

Matching: Long Bone
1. d
2. c
3. g
4. i
5. j
6. a
7. b
8. f
9. h
10. e

Matching: Names of Bones
1. e
2. f
3. b
4. d
5. g
6. h
7. j
8. a
9. c
10. i

Matching: Joints and Joint Movement
1. c
2. j
3. i
4. h
5. c
6. a
7. f
8. b
9. d
10. g

Multiple Choice
1. b
2. c
3. c
4. d
5. b
6. a
7. d
8. c
9. a
10. b

Go Figure
1. a
2. c
3. c
4. c
5. d
6. d
7. d
8. a
9. b

Chapter 9: Muscular System

Matching: Muscle Terms

1. l	5. k	9. h
2. j	6. b	10. i
3. j	7. f	
4. d	8. g	

Matching: Names of Muscles

1. c	5. j	9. b
2. k	6. a	10. b
3. g	7. d	
4. f	8. i	

Multiple Choice

1. a	5. a	9. c
2. c	6. b	10. b
3. b	7. d	
4. d	8. b	

Go Figure

1. c	4. d	7. b
2. a	5. c	8. c
3. b	6. d	9. c

Chapter 10: Nervous System: Nervous Tissue and Brain

Matching: Nerve Cells

1. e	5. c	9. h
2. d	6. b	10. i
3. f	7. j	
4. a	8. g	

Matching: Brain

1. b	3. d	5. e
2. a	4. c	

Multiple Choice

1. b	5. a	9. b
2. d	6. b	10. d
3. c	7. c	11. d
4. d	8. b	

Go Figure

1. b	4. c	7. d
2. a	5. c	
3. d	6. c	

Chapter 11: Nervous System: Spinal Cord and Peripheral Nerves

Matching: Reflexes

1. f	3. e	5. a
2. b	4. c	6. d

Matching: Nerves

1. a	5. e	9. h
2. b	6. c	10. a
3. h	7. f	
4. g	8. d	

Multiple Choice

1. c	5. d	9. d
2. d	6. a	10. d
3. a	7. a	
4. a	8. b	

Go Figure

1. c	3. b	5. d
2. d	4. d	

Chapter 12: Autonomic Nervous System

Matching: Sympathetic or Parasympathetic

1. S	5. S	9. P
2. P	6. S	10. S
3. S	7. P	
4. S	8. P	

Matching: Norepinephrine or Acetylcholine

1. NE	5. ACh	9. NE
2. NE	6. NE	10. ACh
3. ACh	7. NE	
4. ACh	8. ACh	

Multiple Choice

1. c	5. b	9. b
2. b	6. b	10. c
3. a	7. c	
4. c	8. d	

Go Figure

1. c	3. a	5. a
2. a	4. d	

Chapter 13: Sensory System

Matching: Senses

1. a	4. e	7. d
2. d	5. b	
3. c	6. a	

Matching: Structures of the Eye

1. h	5. f	9. h
2. e	6. b	10. g
3. c	7. e	
4. a	8. d	

Matching: Structures of the Ear

1. b	5. c	9. b
2. b	6. c	10. c
3. a	7. a	
4. c	8. b	

Multiple Choice

1. b	5. a	9. d
2. c	6. b	10. d
3. b	7. c	
4. c	8. b	

Go Figure

1. b	5. a	9. d
2. b	6. a	10. d
3. d	7. b	11. d
4. c	8. b	

Chapter 14: Endocrine System

Matching: Glands

1. a	5. h	9. d
2. b	6. c	10. g
3. b	7. f	
4. e	8. a	

Matching: Hormones

1. e	5. c	9. d
2. g	6. f	10. a
3. b	7. j	
4. i	8. i	

Multiple Choice

1. b	5. d	9. b
2. a	6. a	10. d
3. c	7. c	
4. d	8. b	

Go Figure

1. d	3. d	5. a
2. c	4. d	6. b

Chapter 15: Blood

Matching: Blood Cells

1. c	5. a	9. b
2. c	6. a	10. c
3. c	7. b	
4. b	8. c	

Matching: Blood Clots

1. e	3. a	5. c
2. d	4. b	

Matching: Blood Types

1. d	3. c	5. d
2. d	4. a	

Multiple Choice

1. b	5. d	9. d
2. b	6. d	10. b
3. a	7. b	
4. c	8. a	

Go Figure

1. d	3. d	5. d
2. b	4. d	

Chapter 16: Anatomy of the Heart

Matching: Structures of the Heart

1. g	5. d	9. d
2. b	6. a	10. h
3. f	7. a	
4. c	8. e	

Matching: Valves

1. d	5. a	9. d
2. d	6. c	10. c
3. b	7. c	
4. c	8. d	

Multiple Choice

1. d	5. c	9. d
2. d	6. b	10. d
3. a	7. a	
4. b	8. b	

Go Figure

1. b	3. a	5. c
2. c	4. c	

Chapter 17: Function of the Heart

Matching: Cardiac Function Terms

1. b	5. d	9. c
2. c	6. d	10. b
3. b	7. f	
4. e	8. a	

Matching: Loads and Effects

1. b	4. b	7. b
2. c	5. e	8. c
3. a	6. d	

Multiple Choice

1. d	4. d	7. d
2. d	5. c	8. d
3. b	6. a	

Go Figure

1. b	4. a	7. c
2. c	5. a	
3. c	6. a	

Chapter 18: Anatomy of the Blood Vessels

Matching: Blood Vessels: Structure and Function

1. c	5. d	9. a
2. b	6. d	10. c
3. c	7. d	
4. c	8. a	

Matching: Names of Blood Vessels

1. f	6. a	11. k
2. i	7. j	12. b
3. e	8. g	13. h
4. a	9. d	14. l
5. e	10. c	15. m

Matching: Fetal Circulation

1. a	3. c	5. b
2. e	4. d	

Multiple Choice

1. d	5. a	9. c
2. a	6. d	10. a
3. b	7. c	
4. b	8. d	

Go Figure

1. b	3. b	5. b
2. c	4. c	

Chapter 19: Functions of the Blood Vessels

Matching: Blood Pressure Terms

1. d	5. g	9. b
2. f	6. a	10. e
3. a	7. b	
4. h	8. c	

Matching: Blood Pressure Readings

1. a	5. b	9. a
2. a	6. a	10. b
3. b	7. b	
4. c	8. c	

Matching: Changes in Blood Pressure

1. a	5. a	9. a
2. b	6. b	10. a
3. a	7. a	
4. a	8. b	

Multiple Choice

1. c	4. a	7. c
2. d	5. c	8. c
3. b	6. b	9. b

Go Figure

1. c	4. b	7. b
2. b	5. c	
3. c	6. c	

Chapter 20: Lymphatic System

Matching: Lymph Terms

1. e	3. b	5. a
2. c	4. d	

Multiple Choice

1. c	4. c	7. a
2. c	5. b	8. b
3. c	6. c	

Go Figure

1. a
2. b
3. d

Chapter 21: Immune System

Matching: Nonspecific Immunity

1. d	3. c	5. a
2. b	4. b	

Matching: Specific Immunity

1. e	3. d	5. b
2. a	4. c	

Matching: Active and Passive Immunity

1. a	3. b	5. b
2. b	4. a	6. a

Multiple Choice

1. b	5. b	9. d
2. d	6. c	10. b
3. c	7. c	
4. c	8. a	

Go Figure

1. d	3. b	5. b
2. d	4. c	6. c

Chapter 22: Respiratory System

Matching: Structures of the Respiratory Tract

1. d	5. b	9. d
2. c	6. h	10. g
3. e	7. h	
4. a	8. f	

Matching: Thoracic Cavity and Ventilation

1. d	4. e	7. c
2. b	5. f	
3. c	6. a	

Multiple Choice

1. c	4. c	7. c
2. c	5. b	
3. c	6. d	

Go Figure

1. b	5. d	9. c
2. b	6. d	10. a
3. d	7. d	
4. c	8. d	

Chapter 23: Digestive System

Matching: Structures: Making the Connections

1. c	4. e	7. f
2. d	5. h	8. a
3. b	6. g	

Matching: Enzymes, Hormones, and Digestive Aids

1. f	6. g	11. e
2. b	7. a	12. h
3. c	8. d	13. c
4. e	9. g	
5. i	10. f	

Multiple Choice

1. c	5. c	9. b
2. d	6. c	10. d
3. c	7. a	
4. c	8. b	

Go Figure

1. b	4. c	7. d
2. b	5. a	8. a
3. b	6. b	9. d

Chapter 24: Urinary System

Matching: Plumbing...More or Less

1. c	5. d	9. b
2. b	6. c	10. d
3. a	7. d	
4. d	8. d	

Matching: Nephron Unit

1. d	5. b	9. f
2. b	6. e	10. d
3. a	7. c	
4. g	8. h	

Matching: Hormones and Enzymes

1. b	5. f	9. d
2. a	6. a	10. g
3. e	7. e	
4. a	8. c	

Multiple Choice

1. d	5. c	9. c
2. d	6. b	10. b
3. d	7. b	
4. c	8. b	

Go Figure

1. d	4. a	7. d
2. b	5. b	
3. b	6. b	

Chapter 25: Water, Electrolyte, and Acid–Base Balance

Matching: Water Compartments

1. b	3. a	5. a
2. c	4. d	

Matching: Ions

1. c	5. a	9. c
2. a	6. c	10. d
3. b	7. b	
4. b	8. a	

Multiple Choice

1. a	5. d	9. b
2. c	6. c	10. c
3. c	7. c	11. d
4. d	8. c	

Go Figure

1. c	3. b	5. a
2. d	4. b	

Chapter 26: Reproductive Systems

Matching: Female Structures

1. a	5. c	9. c
2. c	6. b	10. d
3. b	7. c	
4. b	8. b	

Matching: Male Structures

1. b	3. d	5. e
2. a	4. c	

Matching: Hormones

1. e	5. c	9. e
2. d	6. d	10. b
3. a	7. e	
4. b	8. a	

Multiple Choice

1. d	5. c	9. c
2. a	6. b	10. b
3. c	7. b	
4. c	8. b	

Go Figure

1. d	3. d	5. d
2. a	4. a	6. a

Chapter 27: Human Development and Heredity

Matching: Fertilization and Development

1. c	5. j	9. a
2. g	6. e	10. b
3. d	7. i	
4. h	8. f	

Matching: Hormones

1. b	3. a	5. a
2. c	4. c	6. d

Matching: Heredity

1. e	3. d	5. b
2. c	4. a	

Multiple Choice

1. c	5. d	9. d
2. c	6. a	10. a
3. c	7. b	
4. c	8. c	

Go Figure

1. b	3. d	5. b
2. a	4. d	6. a

Glossary

A

abdominopelvic cavity (ab-DOM-i-no-PEL-vik) Part of the ventral cavity that lies inferior to the diaphragm; includes the upper abdominal cavity and lower pelvic cavity.

abduction (ab-DUK-shun) Movement of a body part away from the midline.

absorption Taking in of substances across cells or membranes; more specifically, referring to the movement of digested food from the digestive tract into the blood and lymph.

accommodation Adjustment of the curvature of the lens to focus an image on the retina.

acetylcholine (ass-ee-til-KOH-leen) Neurotransmitter that is secreted from the nerve terminals of cholinergic fibers; found in the CNS, neuromuscular junction, and synapses of the parasympathetic nerves.

acid (ASS-id) Substance that donates or releases hydrogen ions when it ionizes in water.

acidosis (ass-i-DOH-sis) Imbalance caused by excess H^+ concentration in the blood, causing the blood pH to decrease below 7.35; respiratory acidosis and metabolic acidosis.

actin (AK-tin) One of the contractile proteins in muscle; forms the thin filaments.

action potential Sequence of changes in the membrane potential that occurs when an excitable cell (neuron or muscle) is stimulated. It has two phases—depolarization and repolarization; also called the *nerve impulse* and the *cardiac impulse*.

active immunity Immunity achieved when the body makes antibodies against an antigen.

active transport Transport process that requires an input of energy (ATP) to move a substance from an area of low concentration to an area of high concentration.

adaptation Adjustment to a stimulus, such as the adaptation to odor.

adduction (ad-DUK-shun) Movement of a body part toward the midline of the body.

adenohypophysis (ad-eh-no-hye-POF-i-sis) Anterior pituitary gland.

adenosine triphosphate (ATP) Energy-storing and energy-transferring molecule found in all cells.

adipose (AD-i-pohs) tissue Type of connective tissue that stores fat.

adrenal gland Endocrine gland that consists of an outer cortex and inner medulla. The cortex secretes steroids and the medulla secretes catecholamines.

adrenergic fiber A neuron that secretes norepinephrine (noradrenaline) as its neurotransmitter.

aerobic catabolism (air-OH-bik kah-TAB-oh-liz-em) Chemical reactions that break down complex substances into simpler substances in the presence of oxygen.

aerobic metabolism Chemical reactions that require oxygen; includes aerobic anabolism and catabolism.

afferent (AF-fer-ent) neuron Carrying toward a center, such as afferent nerves carrying information toward the central nervous system.

afterload The force against which the heart contracts, such as the blood pressure.

agglutination (ah-GLOO-tin-ay-tion) Clumping of cells in response to an antigen-antibody reaction.

albumin (al-BYOO-min) Plasma protein that helps regulate plasma osmotic pressure, thereby "holding" water within the blood vessels; responsible for the oncotic pressure.

aldosterone (al-DOS-ter-own) Mineralocorticoid (steroid) secreted by the adrenal cortex; stimulates the kidney to reabsorb sodium and water and to excrete potassium.

alkalosis (al-kah-LOH-sis) Imbalance associated with a decrease in H^+ concentration and an increase in blood pH higher than 7.45; respiratory alkalosis and metabolic alkalosis.

allergen (AL-er-jen) Foreign substance or antigen that stimulates an allergic reaction.

alpha-adrenergic receptor A type of receptor that is activated by norepinephrine.

alveolus (al-VEE-oh-lus) (*pl.,* alveoli) Tiny grapelike sac in the lungs; the site of gas exchange (oxygen and carbon dioxide) between the air and the blood.

amino acids Small nitrogen-containing organic compounds; the building blocks of protein.

amnion (AM-nee-on) One of the four extraembryonic membranes that surrounds the fetus.

amylase (AM-eh-lays) Enzyme that digests carbohydrates.

anabolism (ah-NAB-oh-liz-em) Metabolic reactions that build complex substances from simpler substances.

anaerobic catabolism (an-air-OH-bik kah-TAB-oh-liz-em) Chemical reactions that break down complex substances into simpler substances without the presence of oxygen.

anaerobic (an-air-OH-bik) metabolism Chemical reactions that do not require oxygen.

anastomosis (ah-nas-toh-MOH-sis) A connection between two tubular structures.

anatomical position Position of the body; the body is standing erect with the face forward and the arms at the sides (palms and toes face in a forward direction).

anatomy (ah-NAT-o-mee) Study of the structure of the body.

anemia Condition characterized by abnormally low amounts of hemoglobin or low numbers of red blood cells.

angiotensin (an-jee-oh-TEN-sin) Hormone produced by the action of renin on angiotensinogen; angiotensin II elevates blood pressure and stimulates the secretion of aldosterone by the adrenal cortex.

anion (AN-eye-on) Negatively charged ion.

antagonist A muscle that exerts an opposing effect.

antibodies Substances that react with a specific antigen.

antibody-mediated immunity A type of immunity engaged in by the B lymphocyte. The B cell secretes antibodies that attack the antigen; also called *humoral immunity*.

antidiuretic hormone (ADH) Posterior pituitary hormone that stimulates the collecting duct in the kidney to reabsorb water, thereby decreasing urinary output; also called *vasopressin*.

antigen (AN-ti-jen) Foreign substance that stimulates the production of antibodies.

aorta (ay-OR-tah) Large artery that conducts blood from the left ventricle of the heart.

aortic valve Semilunar valve located between the left ventricle and aorta.

apocrine (AP-oh-krin) gland One of the sudoriferous (sweat) glands.

aponeurosis (ap-oh-nyoo-ROH-sis) Broad, flat sheet of fibrous connective tissue that connects muscle to another structure.

appendicular skeleton Part of the skeleton that includes the bones of the upper extremities, lower extremities, pelvic girdle, and pectoral girdle.

appendix Worm-shaped outpouching of the wall of the cecum.

areolar (ah-REE-oh-lar) tissue Loose connective tissue.

arteriole (ar-TEER-ee-ohl) Small artery that is composed largely of smooth muscle, found between the larger artery and the capillaries; also called *resistance vessel*.

artery Blood vessel that carries blood away from the heart.

articulation Joining of structures at a joint.

artificially acquired immunity Immunity acquired through the use of agents such as vaccines, toxoids, and immunoglobulins.

atom Fundamental unit of an element; the smallest part of the element that has the characteristics of that element.

ATP See *adenosine triphosphate*.

atrioventricular valves Cuspid valves located between the atria and ventricles; include the tricuspid and bicuspid (mitral) valves.

atrium (*pl.*, atria) Upper chamber of the heart that receives blood from veins.

atrophy (AT-ro-fee) A wasting or a decrease in the size of an organ or tissue, usually referring to a muscle.

autoimmunity (aw-toh-i-MYOO-ni-tee) Immunity against one's own tissue.

autonomic nervous system Involuntary or automatic nervous system that controls the organs, glands, cardiac muscle, and smooth muscle; two divisions: the sympathetic and parasympathetic nervous systems.

axial skeleton The part of the skeleton that includes the skull, vertebral column, ribs, and sternum.

axon (AK-son) Elongated part of the neuron that conducts nerve impulses away from the cell body.

B

bacteria Single-cell organisms classified as cocci, bacilli, and curved rods.

baroreceptor (bar-oh-ree-SEP-tor) Receptor that detects or senses changes in blood pressure; located in the carotid sinus and aortic arch.

baroreceptor (bar-oh-ree-SEP-tor) reflex An autonomic reflex that restores blood pressure to normal; the reflex is initiated by a sudden change in blood pressure.

basal metabolic rate (BMR) The rate at which cells metabolize (use oxygen) in a resting state.

base Substance such as the hydroxyl ion (OH⁻) that combines with hydrogen ion (H⁺).

base pairing Pairing of the bases of the nucleotides; adenine and thymine (DNA), guanine and cytosine (DNA and RNA), and adenine and uracil (RNA).

base sequencing Sequence or arrangement of the bases in a strand of DNA or RNA; carrier of the genetic code.

basophil (BAY-so-fil) Type of granular leukocyte; stains blue.

belly The thick part of a skeletal muscle between its origin and insertion.

beta-adrenergic receptor A type of receptor that is activated by norepinephrine.

bicuspid (bye-KUSS-pid) valve The atrioventricular valve between the left atrium and left ventricle; also called the *mitral valve*.

bile A digestive aid secreted by the liver and stored in the gallbladder; emulsifies fats.

biliary (BILL-ee-air-ee) tree Arrangement of ducts that transports bile from the liver to the gallbladder and duodenum; includes hepatic ducts, cystic duct, and common bile duct.

bilirubin (bill-ee-ROO-bin) Pigment produced from the breakdown of hemoglobin and secreted into the bile; an accumulation of bilirubin in the skin causes jaundice.

blastocyst Early pre-embryonic cluster of cells with a hollow interior; the late blastocyst implants into the inner uterine lining.

blood pressure The force that the blood exerts against the vessel wall.

B lymphocytes (B cells) Lymphocytes that engage in antibody-mediated immunity.

Bowman's capsule C-shaped tubular structure that partially surrounds the glomerulus. Water and dissolved substances are filtered from the glomerulus into the Bowman's capsule.

brain stem Lower part of the brain that connects the brain with the spinal cord; consists of the midbrain, pons, and medulla oblongata.

breast Milk-secreting glandular (mammary) organ on the chest.

bronchioles (BRONK-ee-ohls) Small airway tubes in the respiratory tract that are composed largely of smooth muscle; connect the bronchi and alveoli.

bronchus (*pl.*, bronchi) Large airway in the lungs that connects the trachea and bronchioles; there is a right and left bronchus.

buffer Substance that resists changes in pH. A buffer can remove or add H⁺, thereby adjusting pH.

C

calyces (KAY-liss-ees) Cuplike structures that collect urine from the collecting ducts of the nephron units.

capacitance (cah-PAS-it-ance) vessels Refers to the veins and specifically to their ability to store blood.

capillary Smallest and most numerous of the blood vessels; site of exchange of nutrients and waste between the blood and tissue fluid. The capillaries are called the *exchange vessels*.

capillary exchange The movement of nutrients, oxygen, and waste across the capillary membranes; the exchange is between the blood and interstitium.

carbaminohemoglobin (karb-a-MEE-no-HEE-moh-GLOH-bin) Hemoglobin that has combined with carbon dioxide.

carbohydrates Organic compounds that include simple sugars, starch, and glycogen; primary source of energy.

carbon dioxide (CO₂) The waste product of cellular metabolism.

cardiac conduction system Specialized cardiac cells that create and conduct the electrical cardiac impulse (action potential); includes the SA node, AV node, and His-Purkinje system.

cardiac cycle Events that occur in the heart during one heartbeat.

cardiac muscle Type of striated muscle found in the heart; the myocardium.

cardiac output Amount of blood pumped by the heart in 1 minute (about 5000 mL/min); determined by heart rate and stroke volume.

cardiac reserve The potential increase in cardiac output above resting cardiac output.

cardiology The study of the heart.

carrier A living organism that harbors a pathogen and acts as a source of infection.

catabolism (kah-TAB-oh-liz-em) Metabolic breakdown of complex molecules into simpler molecules; the breakdown is accompanied by the release of energy.

catalyst (KAT-ah-list) Any substance that speeds up the rate of a chemical reaction; see *enzyme*.

catecholamine (kat-eh-KOHL-ah-meen) Classification of hormones secreted by the adrenal medulla; includes epinephrine (adrenaline) and norepinephrine (noradrenaline).

cation (KAT-eye-on) Positively charged ion.

cecum (SEE-come) Part of the large intestine that connects the ileum of the small intestine and ascending colon of the large intestine.

cell Basic unit of life; the structural and functional unit of a living organism.

cell cycle The phases that a cell goes through as it divides.

cell-mediated immunity Type of immunity engaged in by the T cell; cell-to-cell combat.

cell membrane Membrane that surrounds the cell and regulates what enters and leaves the cell; also called the *plasma membrane*.

cerebellum (sair-eh-BELL-um) Part of the brain located under the cerebrum; it coordinates skeletal muscle activity.

cerebrospinal fluid Cushioning fluid that circulates within the subarachnoid space around the brain and spinal cord.

cerebrum (seh-REE-brum) Largest and uppermost part of the brain, divided into two cerebral hemispheres. There are four lobes: frontal, parietal, temporal, and occipital.

ceruminous (seh-ROO-mi-nus) glands Modified sweat glands found in the external ear canal; they secrete cerumen, or ear wax.

cervix Constricted portion (neck) of an organ, usually referring to the lower portion of the uterus.

chemoreceptor (KEE-moh-ree-SEP-tor) Receptor that detects changes in the chemical composition of a substance.

cholinergic (koh-lin-ER-jik) fiber A neuron that secretes acetylcholine (ACh) as its neurotransmitter.

chondrocytes (KON-droh-sytes) Cartilage-forming cells.

chordae tendineae (KORD-ay ten-din-EE-ay) Tough fibrous bands of connective tissue that attach the cusps of the AV valves to the walls of the ventricles of the heart.

chorion (KOH-ree-on) The outermost extraembryonic membrane surrounding the fetus; helps form the placenta.

chromosome Coiled, threadlike structures that contain segments of DNA called *genes*.

chronotropic (KRON-oh-TROH-pik) effect A change in heart rate (HR). A positive chronotropic effect is an increase in HR, whereas a negative chronotropic effect is a decrease in HR.

chyle (kile) Milky fluid found in the lacteals of the villi; consists of emulsified fats and lymph.

chyme (kime) Pastelike mixture of partially digested food, water, and digestive enzymes that is formed in the stomach.

cilia (SIL-ee-ah) (*sing.*, cilium) Hairlike processes on the surface of many cells.

clone A group of cells that come from a single cell and are therefore genetically identical.

coagulation Clotting of blood.

cochlea (KOHK-lee-ah) Part of the inner ear that contains the organ of Corti, the receptors for hearing.

collecting duct The nephron structure that receives urine from the distal tubule and delivers it to the renal pelvis.

colon (KOH-lon) Major portion of the large intestine that extends from the cecum to the rectum.

columnar epithelium Type of epithelium that has column-shaped cells.

common bile duct The biliary duct that connects the liver, gallbladder, and duodenum; allows bile to enter the duodenum.

communicable disease A disease that can be spread from one host to another.

complement (KOM-pleh-ment) proteins Group of proteins in the blood that are concerned with phagocytosis.

compliance The degree of stretch of a hollow organ; the change in volume in response to a change in pressure.

compound Substance composed of two or more chemical elements, such as water (H_2O).

conductance (con-DUC-tans) vessels Blood vessels that are primarily concerned with carrying blood to smaller blood vessels; functional name for arteries.

conduction Loss of heat energy as it is transferred from the warm body to a cooler object, such as a cooling blanket.

congenital (kon-JEN-i-tall) Present at birth.

connective tissue One of the four basic types of tissue that generally binds and supports body structures.

contracture (con-TRAK-ture) An abnormal formation of fibrous tissue within a muscle, causing it to freeze in a flexed position.

convection Loss of heat energy to the surrounding cooler air. The layer of heated air next to the body is constantly being removed by a fan (or breeze) and replaced by cooler air.

cornea (KOR-nee-ah) Transparent portion of the sclera that covers the anterior portion of the eye.

coronary arteries Right and left coronary arteries deliver oxygenated blood to the heart muscle.

corpus luteum (KOHR-pus LOO-tee-um) Yellow body formed from the ovarian follicle after ovulation; secretes large amounts of progesterone and smaller amounts of estrogen.

covalent (ko-VAYL-ent) bond Bond or attraction formed by the sharing of electrons between atoms.

cranial cavity Part of the dorsal cavity that contains the brain.

cranial nerves The 12 pairs of nerves that emerge from the brain; with the exception of the vagus nerve (CN X), the cranial nerves innervate the head and shoulders.

craniosacral (kray-nee-oh-SAY-kral) outflow Parasympathetic nerve activity.

creatinine (cree-AH-tuh-neen) A nitrogenous waste product that is excreted by the kidney.

cuboidal epithelium (KYOO-boyd-al ep-i-THEE-lee-um) Type of epithelium that has cells shaped like cubes.

cutaneous (kyoo-TAYN-ee-us) membrane Skin.

cytoplasm (SYE-toh-plaz-em) Gel-like substance surrounded by the cell membrane but outside of the nucleus.

D

dehydration State in which there is a deficiency in body water.

dendrite (DEN-dryte) Treelike process of the neuron that receives the stimulus and carries it toward the cell body.

deoxyribonucleic (dee-OK-see-rye-boh-nook-LAY-ik) acid (DNA) Nucleotide that stores the genetic information of the organism.

depolarize (dee-POH-lar-ize) Change in the membrane potential across the cell membrane, with the inside of the cell becoming less negative or less polarized than the resting membrane potential.

dermatome (DER-mah-tohm) Area of the body supplied by a spinal nerve.

dermis The thicker layer of the skin; dense connective tissue under the epidermis of the skin.

detrusor (dee-TROO-sor) muscle Smooth muscle located in the urinary bladder.

dialysis (dye-AL-i-sis) A passive transport process that allows small particles to diffuse through a semipermeable membrane.

diaphragm (DYE-ah-fram) Dome-shaped skeletal muscle that separates the thoracic and abdominal cavities; chief muscle of inspiration (inhalation).

diaphysis (dye-AF-i-sis) Shaft of a long bone.

diastole (dye-ASS-toh-lee) Relaxation phase of the cardiac cycle.

diastolic (dye-ah-STOL-ik) pressure Blood pressure in the large arteries when the heart is resting (diastole); the bottom number of a blood pressure reading.

differentiation (dif-er-EN-shee-AY-shun) Process whereby a cell becomes specialized.

diffusion Passive transport process that causes movement of a substance from an area of higher concentration to an area of lower concentration.

digestion Process of breaking down food into absorbable particles; mechanical and chemical.

disease Failure of the body to function normally.

diuresis (dye-yoo-REE-sis) Increased excretion of urine.

dominant gene Gene whose trait is expressed.

dorsal cavity Body cavity located toward the back part of the body; divided into the cranial cavity and spinal cavity.

dorsal root Sensory nerve of a spinal nerve as it attaches to the spinal cord.

dromotropic effect A change in the speed of the action potential (electrical signal) as it moves from the SA node through the His-Purkinje system.

duodenum (doo-oh-DEE-num) First part of the small intestine.

E

eccrine (EK-rin) gland Type of sweat gland that secretes a watery substance; plays an important role in the regulation of body temperature.

edema (eh-DEE-mah) Abnormal collection of fluid, usually causing swelling.

efferent (EF-fer-ent) Movement away from a central point, such as a motor neuron that carries information away from the central nervous system.

efferent neuron (EF-fer-ent NOO-ron) A motor neuron; brings information from the CNS to the periphery.

ejection fraction The percent of the ventricular volume that is pumped or ejected during ventricular systole (contraction).

electrocardiogram (ECG) (eh-lek-troh-KAR-dee-oh-gram) Graphic recording of the electrical events that occur during the cardiac cycle.

electrolyte (eh-LEK-troh-lyte) Compound that dissociates into ions when dissolved in water.

electrolyte (eh-LEK-troh-lyte) balance Having normal amounts of electrolytes in each fluid compartment.

element Substance composed of only one type of atom.

embryo (EM-bree-oh) The developing human between the gestational ages of 2 and 8 weeks.

emulsification (ee-MULL-seh-feh-KAY-shun) The physical breakdown of a large fat globule into many smaller fat globules.

endocardium (en-doh-KAR-dee-um) Inner lining of the heart wall.

endocrine (EN-doh-krin) glands Ductless glands that secrete hormones, usually into the blood for transport throughout the body.

endocytosis (en-doh-sye-TOH-sis) Uptake of material through the cell membrane by forming a vesicle; includes pinocytosis and phagocytosis.

endometrium (en-doh-MEE-tree-um) Inner lining of the uterus.

endoplasmic reticulum (ER) (en-doh-PLAZ-mik reh-TIK-yoo-lum) Intracellular membrane system concerned with the synthesis and transportation of protein and steroids; called the *rough ER* if ribosomes are attached, called the *smooth ER* if there are no ribosomes.

energy Ability to perform work.

enzyme (EN-zyme) Organic catalyst; speeds up the rate of a chemical reaction.

eosinophil (ee-oh-SIN-oh-fil) Type of granular leukocyte; stains a rose color.

epicardium (ep-i-KAR-dee-um) Outer layer of the heart; forms part of the pericardium.

epidermis (ep-i-DER-mis) Outer epithelial layer of the skin.

epididymis (ep-i-DID-i-miss) Coiled tube that carries sperm from the testis to the vas deferens.

epiglottis (ep-i-GLOT-iss) Cartilage that guards the opening into the larynx; directs food and water into the esophagus.

epiphysis (eh-PIF-i-sis) End of a long bone.

epithelial (ep-i-THEE-lee-al) tissue One of the four types of tissues; found on the surface of the body (skin) and lining the body cavities; it also forms glands.

equilibrium Balance.

erythrocyte (eh-RITH-roh-syte) Red blood cell.

erythropoietin (eh-RITH-roh-POY-eh-tin) Hormone secreted by the kidneys that stimulates the bone marrow to produce red blood cells.

esophagus (eh-SOF-ah-gus) The tubelike structure that connects the pharynx to the stomach; the food tube.

estrogen (ES-troh-jen) Female sex hormone secreted by the developing ovarian follicle.

eustachian (yoo-STAY-shun) tube Tube that connects the pharynx with the middle ear; also called the *auditory tube*.

evaporation Loss of heat as water changes from the liquid to the vapor or gas state.

exchange vessels Refer to the *capillaries*, which allow for the movement of nutrients, oxygen, and waste across their membranes.

exhalation Process of moving air out of the lungs; the breathing-out phase of ventilation, also called *expiration*.

exocrine (EKS-oh-krin) glands Type of glands that secrete their products into ducts that open onto a surface.

exocytosis (eks-o-sye-TOH-sis) Elimination of material from a cell through the formation of vesicles.

extension Increase in the angle of a joint.

extracellular fluid Fluid located outside the cell, such as the plasma and interstitial fluid.

F

facilitated diffusion Passive process whereby a substance moves with the assistance of a carrier molecule from an area of higher concentration to an area of lower concentration.

fallopian (fal-LOH-pee-an) tube Passageway through which the egg or zygote moves from the ovary to the uterus; also called the *oviduct* or *uterine tube*.

fascia (FASH-uh) Fibrous connective tissue membrane that covers individual skeletal muscles or certain organs.

fertilization Union of an ovum and a sperm to form a zygote; also called *conception*.

fetus Name given to the developing human at the end of the embryonic period, from the end of the eighth week of pregnancy to birth.

fibrin (FYE-brin) Protein strands formed by the action of thrombin on fibrinogen; the clot.

filtration Process whereby water and dissolved substances move through a membrane in response to pressure.

flexion Decrease in the angle of a joint; a bending movement.

fontanel (FON-tah-nel) Membranous gap between the cranial bones of an infant's skull.

frontal lobe Anterior portion of the cerebrum that controls voluntary skeletal activity, motor speech, and plays an important role in emotions, critical thinking, and ethical decision making.

frontal plane Vertical plane that divides the body into front (anterior) and back (posterior parts); the coronal plane.

fungus Plantlike organisms such as mushrooms; cause mycotic infections.

G

gallbladder Small pear-shaped organ concerned with the concentration and storage of bile.

gene Part of the chromosome that codes for a specific trait; the biological unit of heredity.

glomerular (gloh-MAIR-yoo-lar) filtration The filtration (pushing) of water and dissolved solute through the pores of the glomerular membrane. The rate of glomerular filtration is called the *glomerular filtration rate* (GFR).

glomerulus (gloh-MAIR-yoo-lus) Tuft of capillaries located in the Bowman's capsule of the nephron unit of the kidney.

glottis (GLOT-iss) Opening between the vocal cords; an air passage for the respiratory tract.

gluconeogenesis (gloo-koh-nee-oh-JEN-eh-sis) Biochemical process that makes glucose from nonglucose substances, especially protein.

glucose A monosaccharide, or simple sugar, that serves as the principal fuel for the cells of the body.

glycogen (GLY-koh-jen) Polysaccharide that is the storage form of glucose; also called *animal starch*.

glycolysis (gly-KOHL-i-sis) Anaerobic catabolism of glucose into lactic acid.

Golgi (GOAL-jee) apparatus Membranous organelle concerned with the final trimming and packaging of protein for exocytosis.

gonadotropin (go-NAD-oh-TROH-pin) Hormone "aimed at" the gonads; includes follicle-stimulating hormone (FSH), luteinizing hormone (LH), and human chorionic gonadotropin (hCG).

gonads (GO-nads) Organs that produce gametes (ova or sperm); term for ovaries and testes.

graafian (GRAH-fee-en) follicle Mature ovarian follicle.

gray matter Part of the central nervous system that is composed of cell bodies and unmyelinated fibers.

H

haversian (hah-VER-shun) system Structural unit of compact bone; bone is layered in concentric circles around an osteonic canal; an osteon.

heart failure The inability of the heart to pump blood in sufficient quantities to meet the requirements of the body; characterized by a low ejection fraction and signs of organ congestion, such as pulmonary edema.

helminths (HEL-minths) Parasitic worms.

hematocrit (hee-MAT-oh-krit) Laboratory test that expresses the percentage of red blood cells present in a volume of blood.

hemoglobin (hee-moh-GLOH-bin) Iron-containing protein in the red blood cell can form a weak bond with oxygen; also transports carbon dioxide.

hemolysis (hee-MAWL-ih-sis) Breakdown of erythrocytes.

hemopoiesis (hee-muh-poy-EE-sis) Production of blood cells.

hemostasis (hee-moh-STAY-sis) The stopping of blood loss.

homeostasis (ho-me-o-STAY-sis) Ability of the body to maintain a constant internal environment.

hormone Substance secreted by an endocrine gland into the blood.

human chorionic gonadotropin (KOH-ri-on-ik go-nad-oh-TROH-pin) Hormone secreted by the trophoblastic cells of the embryonic blastocyst; maintains the corpus luteum until the placenta can take over its glandular function.

hydrogen bond Weak intermolecular bond formed between hydrogen and a negatively charged atom such as oxygen or nitrogen.

hyperkalemia (hye-per-kah-LEE-mee-ah) Abnormally high blood potassium level.

hypertension Blood pressure that is higher than normal.

hypertonic (hye-per-TON-ik) Having a solute concentration greater than that of a reference solution.

hypertrophy (hye-PER-tro-fee) Increase in the size of a body part, usually referring to a muscle.

hyperventilation (hye-per-ven-ti-LAY-shun) Abnormally rapid, deep breathing.

hypokalemia (hye-poh-kah-LEE-mee-ah) A lower-than-normal amount of potassium in the blood.

hypophysis (hye-POF-is-sis) Pituitary gland; adenohypophysis (anterior) and neurohypophysis (posterior).

hypotension Blood pressure that is lower than normal.

hypothalamus (hye-poh-THAHL-ah-mahs) Part of the diencephalon that regulates the pituitary gland, autonomic nervous system, water balance, appetite, temperature, and emotions.

hypotonic (hye-poh-TON-ik) Having a solute concentration less than that of a reference solution.

hypoventilation (hye-poh-ven-ti-LAY-shun) Abnormally slow and/or shallow respiratory rate.

I

ileum (IL-ee-um) Distal end of the small intestine.

immunity Ability to resist and overcome injury by pathogens or antigenic substances.

immunoglobulin (i-myoo-noh-GLOB-yoo-lin) Antibodies produced by plasma cells in response to antigenic stimulation.

infection Disease caused by a pathogen.

inflammation Body's response to infection or injury; characterized by redness, heat, swelling, and pain.

inhalation Process of moving air into the lungs; the breathing-in phase of ventilation, also called *inspiration*.

inotropic (in-o-TROH-pik) effect A change in the strength or force of myocardial contraction that does not involve stretching the myocardial fibers.

insertion The more movable attachment point of a muscle to a bone.

intake Amount of fluid taken into the body.

integument A natural covering, such as the skin.

integumentary (in-teg-yoo-MEN-tar-ee) system Organ system that consists of the skin and its accessory organs.

intercellular Between the cells.

interferons (in-ter-FEER-ons) Substances produced by a virus-infected cell; protect other cells from viral infection.

interneuron Neuron that links the sensory and motor neurons in the central nervous system.

interstitial (in-ter-STISH-al) fluid Fluid located between the cells; tissue fluid.

intracellular fluid Fluid located within cells.

intrapleural (in-trah-PLOR-al) pressure The pressure within the intrapleural space (between the visceral and parietal pleurae); must be negative for the lungs to be expanded.

ion (EYE-on) An electrically charged atom or group of atoms; cation (positive) or anion (negative).

ionic (eye-ON-ik) bond Bond formed by the exchange of electrons between atoms.

ischemia (is-KEE-mee-ah) Insufficient blood flow to a tissue, sometimes resulting in tissue damage and death (gangrene).

isotonic (eye-soh-TON-ik) Having the same concentration as the reference solution.

isotope (EYE-so-tohp) Atom that has the same number of protons and electrons but a different number of neutrons; the same atomic number, but a different atomic mass.

J

jaundice (JAWN-dis) Yellow coloring of the skin and whites of the eyes caused by an increase of bilirubin in the blood.

jejunum (jeh-JOO-num) Second or middle part of the small intestine.

joint Union of two or more bones; an articulation.

juxtaglomerular apparatus A specialized structure in the kidney formed by the distal convoluted tubule and the afferent arterioles; the renin-secreting cells.

K

kaliuretic Refers to the effect of a hormone or drug that causes the elimination of potassium in the urine.

karyotype (KAIR-ee-oh-type) Arrangement of the chromosomes by pairs in a fixed order.

keratin (KER-ah-tin) A protein found in the skin, hair, and nails; it hardens the cells and makes them water resistant.

ketone bodies Products of rapid and incomplete fatty acid catabolism; includes acetone, acetoacetic acid, and beta-hydroxybutyric acid.

kidney Organ of the urinary system that produces urine; contains the nephron units.

Korotkoff sounds The sounds (tap tap tap) heard when blood pressure is being recorded; the sounds are due to the flow of blood through the constricted artery.

Kussmaul (KOOS-mall) respirations Increase in the rate and depth of respirations to correct a metabolic acidosis.

L

lacrimal (LAK-ri-mal) gland Gland that secretes tears.

lacteal (LAK-teal) Lymph vessel in a villus of the small intestine.

larynx (LAIR-inks) Structure that contains the vocal cords; voice box.

leukocyte (LOO-koh-syte) White blood cell; functions primarily to defend the body against infection.

ligaments Strong bands of connective tissue that join bone to bone.

limbic (LIM-bik) system The emotional brain.

lipase Enzyme that digests fats into fatty acids and glycerol.

lipids Organic molecules that include fats, oils, and steroids.

liver lobule A unit of the liver made up of liver cells (hepatocytes) surrounding a central vein. Hepatocytes process sinusoidal blood, secreting bile into surrounding canaliculi.

loop of Henle (HEN-lee) A hairpin-looped tubular structure of the nephron unit that receives urine from the proximal tubule and delivers it to the distal tubule.

lymph (limf) Fluid that has the same composition as tissue fluid and is carried by the lymph vessels.

lymph node Mass of lymphoid tissue located along the course of a lymphatic vessel.

lymphatic duct Large tube or vessel that carries lymph, such as the thoracic duct; same as lymphatic vessel.

lymphatic vessels Vessels that transport lymph from lymphatic capillaries and larger lymphatic ducts to the subclavian veins.

lymphocyte (LIM-foh-syte) Agranular leukocyte; T and B lymphocytes engage in specific immunity.

lysosome (LYE-so-sohm) Organelle that contains powerful enzymes; engages in phagocytosis and does the "intracellular housecleaning."

M

macrophage (MAK-roh-fayj) Enlarged monocyte that eats foreign material; a "big eater." Macrophages may be wandering or fixed.

mammary (MAM-mah-ree) gland Gland of the female breast that secretes milk.

matter Anything that occupies space; may occur as solid, liquid, or gas.

mechanoreceptor (meh-KAN-o-ree-SEP-tor) Receptor that is stimulated by bending, pressing, or pushing.

mediastinum (MEE-dee-ass-TI-num) Space between the lungs that contains the heart and pericardial cavity, trachea, thymus gland, esophagus, and large blood vessels.

medulla oblongata (meh-DOOL-ah oh-blohn-GAHT-ah) Most inferior part of the brain stem that controls vital functions, such as respiratory and cardiovascular function.

meiosis (my-OH-sis) Type of cell division used by the sex cells to reduce the number of chromosomes in each from 46 to 23.

melanin (MEL-ah-nin) Pigment responsible for the color of the skin and hair.

melanocyte (mel-AN-o-syte) Melanin-producing cell.

meninges (meh-NIN-jeez) Membranes that cover the brain and spinal cord; include the dura mater, arachnoid mater, and pia mater.

menopause Normal developmental stage in women that marks the end of the ovarian and uterine cycles.

menses (MEN-seez) Menstruation; the monthly discharge of blood from the uterus.

metabolic acidosis A condition in which blood pH decreases below 7.35; the cause is nonrespiratory.

metabolic alkalosis A condition in which blood pH increases above 7.45; the cause is nonrespiratory.

metabolism All the chemical reactions that occur within the cells; consists of anabolism and catabolism.

micturition (mik-tor-RISH-un) Urination.

milk let-down reflex An oxytocin-mediated reflex that results in the release of milk from the breast in response to suckling.

mineral Inorganic substance such as sodium or potassium.

mitochondria (my-toh-KON-dree-ah) Organelles that produce most of the ATP; the "power plants" of the cell.

mitosis (my-TOH-sis) Type of cell division that produces two identical daughter cells, each containing 46 chromosomes.

mitral (MY-tral) valve See *bicuspid valve*.

mixed nerve Nerve that contains both sensory and motor fibers.

mixture Combination of two or more substances that can be separated by ordinary physical means.

molecule Chemical combination of two or more atoms.

monocyte (MON-oh-syte) Agranular phagocytic leukocyte that can become a macrophage.

monosaccharide (mon-oh-SAK-ah-ride) A simple sugar consisting of hexoses (e.g., glucose, fructose, galactose) or pentoses (e.g., ribose, deoxyribose).

motor nerve Collection of motor neurons that carries information away from the central nervous system.

motor unit Refers to the somatic motor neuron and the muscle fibers innervated by the motor neuron.

mucous membranes Type of membranes that line the cavities and tubes that open to the exterior of the body.

muscarinic (mus-kar-IN-ik) receptor Cholinergic receptor activated by acetylcholine; located primarily on the target organs of the parasympathetic nerves.

muscle tissue Type of tissue composed primarily of contractile protein; includes skeletal, smooth, and cardiac muscle.

myelin (MY-eh-lin) White fatty material that covers some nerve fibers.

myocardium (my-oh-KAR-dee-um) Heart muscle.

myometrium (my-oh-MEET-ri-um) Muscle layer of the uterus that contracts and causes the delivery of the infant.

myosin (MY-oh-sin) Muscle protein that interacts with actin to cause muscle contraction; also called the *thick filament*.

N

natriuresis The excretion of sodium into the urine.

natriuretic peptides Protein hormones that promote the excretion of sodium into the urine; include atrial natriuretic peptide and brain natriuretic peptide.

naturally acquired immunity Immunity acquired through natural means, such as getting a disease or receiving antibodies from your mother.

negative feedback A mechanism activated by an imbalance; activation of the mechanism then corrects the imbalance.

nephron unit Structural and functional unit of the kidney that makes urine.

nerve Bundle of nerve fibers and blood vessels.

nerve impulse Action potential that occurs in neurons.

nerve tract Group of neurons that share a common function within the central nervous system; may be ascending (sensory) or descending (motor).

nervous tissue A type of tissue that includes neurons and neuroglia.

neuroglia (noo-ROG-lee-ah) Nerve cells that support, protect, and nourish the neurons.

neurohypophysis (noo-roh-hye-POF-i-sis) The posterior pituitary gland; secretes oxytocin and antidiuretic hormone.

neuromuscular junction Junction or space that occurs between a motor neuron and a muscle fiber.

neuron Nerve cell that conducts the action potential (nerve impulse).

neurotransmitters (noo-roh-TRANS-mit-ters) Chemical made within the axon terminal responsible for transmission of the signal across the synapse or junction.

neutrophil (NOO-troh-fil) Granular, motile, and highly phagocytic leukocyte.

nicotinic receptor A type of cholinergic receptor that is activated by acetylcholine; located in the autonomic ganglia and within the neuromuscular junction.

nociceptor (noh-see-SEP-tor) Pain receptor.

norepinephrine (nor-ep-i-NEF-rin) A neurotransmitter secreted by the adrenergic fibers of the sympathetic nervous system; activates adrenergic receptors.

normal flora A population of microorganisms that normally inhabit an area such as the skin, intestines, or vagina.

nosocomial (noh-soh-CO-mee-al) infection Hospital-acquired infection.

nucleus (pl., nuclei) Large organelle separated from the cytoplasm by a nuclear membrane; stores the DNA in chromosomes and acts as the control center of the cell.

O

occipital (ok-SIP-it-al) lobe Cerebral lobe located in the back of the head; concerned primarily with vision.

olfactory (ol-FAK-tor-ee) receptor Chemoreceptor associated with the sense of smell.

oliguria (ohl-i-GOO-ree-ah) Scanty urine formation, usually defined as less than 400 mL/24 hr.

oncotic pressure The part of the osmotic pressure of the blood caused by the plasma proteins.

optic chiasm (OP-tik kye-AS-m) Site for the crossing of the medial fibers of the optic nerve to the opposite side of the brain; located in front of the pituitary gland.

organ Group of tissues that performs a specialized function, such as the lungs.

organelle (or-gah-NELL) Structure within the cytoplasm, such as the mitochondria, that performs a specific function.

organic compound Carbon-containing substance.

organ of Corti (KOR-tee) Hearing receptors (mechanoreceptors) located in the inner ear.

organ system Group of organs that perform a particular function, such as the organs of digestion.

origin The part of the muscle attached to the more immovable structure.

osmosis (os-MO-sis) Movement of water across a membrane from an area where there is more water to an area where there is less water.

osseous (OS-ee-us) tissue Bone tissue.

ossicles (OSS-eh-kuls) Tiny bones found in the middle ear: malleus, incus, stapes.

osteoblast Bone-building cell; immature osteocyte.

osteoclast Cell that causes the breakdown of bone.

output Refers to a quantity that is ejected, such as urinary output and cardiac output.

ovarian follicle Ovarian structure that releases an egg at maturation; graafian follicle.

ovulation Discharge of the mature ovum from the graafian follicle.

oxyhemoglobin (ahk-see-HEE-moh-gloh-bin) Hemoglobin that contains oxygen.

P

pain receptor Nociceptor; free nerve endings that sense pain.

pancreas (PAN-kree-ass) Organ that has both endocrine and exocrine functions. The islets of Langerhans secrete the hormones insulin and glucagon. The exocrine glands secrete the most important of the digestive enzymes.

parasites Organisms that require another living organism for their growth and survival.

parasympathetic (pair-ah-sim-pah-THET-ik) nervous system Division of the autonomic nervous system concerned with "feeding and breeding."

parathyroid (pair-ah-THYE-royd) gland Gland that secretes parathyroid hormone (PTH) and helps regulate calcium and phosphate.

parietal (pah-RYE-i-tal) Pertaining to the wall of a cavity, as in the parietal pleura that lines the wall of the thoracic cavity.

parietal layer The layer of the pleural or peritoneal membranes that lines the walls of their cavities.

parietal (pah-RYE-i-tal) lobe Lobe of the cerebrum concerned primarily with somatosensory function.

partial pressure Pressure exerted by one gas in a gas mixture.

passive immunity Short-acting immunity achieved when the person is given antibodies made by another animal.

passive transport Transport process that requires no additional energy in the form of ATP.

pathogens Disease-causing organisms.

pectoral girdle Portion of the skeleton that supports and attaches to the upper extremities; scapula and clavicle.

pelvic girdle Portion of the skeleton to which the lower extremities are attached; formed by two coxal bones.

peptide bond Bond formed between two amino acids.

pericardial cavity The thoracic cavity that contains the heart and great vessels.

pericardium (pair-ee-CARD-ee-um) Slinglike serous membrane that partially encloses the heart; supports the weight of the heart.

perineum (pair-i-NEE-um) Pelvic floor; extends from the anus to the vulva in the female and from the anus to the scrotum in the male.

periosteum (pair-ee-OS-tee-um) Fibrous connective tissue that covers the surface of a long bone.

peripheral nervous system Nerves and ganglia that lie outside the central nervous system.

peristalsis (pair-i-STAL-sis) Rhythmic contraction of smooth muscle that propels a substance forward; peristalsis in the digestive tract moves food from the esophagus toward the anus.

peritoneum (pair-i-toh-NEE-um) Serous membrane located in the abdominal cavity; there is a parietal peritoneum and a visceral peritoneum.

peritubular capillaries The capillaries that surround the tubular structures of the nephron unit; primarily concerned with reabsorption and secretion in the formation of urine.

pH A measure of the hydrogen ion concentration.

phagocytosis (fag-oh-sye-TOH-sis) Eating of pathogens or cellular debris.

pharynx (fair-inks) The throat; three parts—nasopharynx, oropharynx, and laryngopharynx.

photoreceptors Receptors stimulated by light; include the rods and cones of the retina.

physiology (fiz-ee-OL-o-jee) Study of the functioning of the body.

pineal (PIN-ee-al) gland Small gland located in the brain; secretes melatonin and is involved in regulating biorhythms.

placenta (plah-SEN-tah) A gland and site of exchange of nutrients, oxygen, and waste between the mother and baby-to-be.

plasma The yellow liquid portion of blood.

platelet (PLAYT-let) A fragment of a megakaryocyte that functions in hemostasis; also called a *thrombocyte*.

pleura (PLOO-rah) Serous membrane located in the thoracic cavity. There is a visceral pleura and a parietal pleura.

pleural cavities Thoracic cavities that contain the lungs.

plexus Network of nerves such as the cervical plexus.

polysaccharide (pahl-ee-SAK-ah-ride) Carbohydrate made of more than two simple sugars, such as glycogen.

precordium (pree-KOR-dee-um) Area of the anterior chest that overlies the heart.

preganglionic fiber A neuron that transmits action potentials from the central nervous system to a ganglion.

preload The degree of ventricular myocardial stretch; end-diastolic volume.

postganglionic fiber A neuron that transmits action potentials from a ganglion to a distal target organ.

prime mover The muscle that is most responsible for a particular movement.

progesterone (proh-JES-ter-ohn) Hormone secreted by the corpus luteum of the ovary; stimulates the growth of the endometrium and helps maintain the pregnancy.

projection Process whereby the brain causes a sensation to be felt at the point of stimulation.

proprioception (proh-pree-oh-SEP-shun) Sensation of movement and position of the body.

prostaglandins (pross-tah-GLAN-dins) Group of compounds made from fatty acids in cell membranes; exert powerful and local hormone-like effects.

prostate gland Gland that surrounds the proximal portion of the urethra in the male and contributes to the formation of semen.

protease (PROH-tee-ayz) Enzyme that digests protein.

proteins Large nitrogen-containing molecules composed of many amino acids.

protozoa (pro-toe-ZO-ah) Single-cell animal-like microbe; classified as amebas, ciliates, flagellates, and sporozoa.

pulmonary circulation Path of blood through vessels that takes unoxygenated blood from the right ventricle to the lungs and oxygenated blood from the lungs to the left atrium.

pulmonary edema Abnormal collection of fluid in the lungs causing difficulty in the oxygenation of hemoglobin.

pulse Vibration of the arteries caused by rhythmic expansion and recoil of the large arteries following contraction of the ventricles.

pulse pressure Calculated as the difference between the systolic and diastolic blood pressures.

Purkinje (pur-KIN-jee) fibers Fast-conducting fibers located in the ventricular walls; conduct the electrical impulses from the bundle of His to the ventricular myocardium.

pyramidal (pi-RAM-i-dal) tract Major motor tract that descends from the precentral gyrus of the frontal lobe to the spinal cord; also called the *corticospinal tract*.

R

radiation Loss of heat as it leaves a warm object, such as the body, to the surrounding cooler air.

receptor Sensory structure that responds to a specific stimulus, such as light, chemicals, or touch.

recessive gene Gene whose trait is not expressed.

recruitment Enlistment of additional motor units to increase the force of muscle contraction.

red blood cell Blood cell that contains mostly hemoglobin; an erythrocyte.

referred pain Pain that feels like it originates in an area other than the part being stimulated.

reflex Automatic response (nervous or chemical) to a stimulus.

reflex arc A nerve pathway that includes a receptor, sensory neuron, motor neuron, and effector organ.

refraction Bending of light waves so as to focus them on the retina.

refractory period Period during which nervous tissue cannot respond to a second stimulus.

renal artery The artery that delivers oxygenated blood to the kidney.

renal tubule Tubular part of the nephron unit that helps make and transport urine; consists of Bowman's capsule, proximal convoluted tubule, loop of Henle, distal convoluted tubule, and collecting duct.

renal vein The vein that carries unoxygenated blood from the kidney to the inferior vena cava.

renin (REE-nin) Enzyme secreted by the kidneys that activates angiotensinogen.

repolarize (ree-POH-lahr-ize) Return of the membrane potential to its resting state after the nerve impulse.

resistance vessel Blood vessel that can change its diameter and therefore determine resistance to the flow of blood; functional name for the arterioles.

respiratory acidosis Increased H^+ concentration (decreased pH) caused by hypoventilation.

respiratory alkalosis Decreased H^+ concentration (increased pH) caused by hyperventilation.

reticular formation Complex network of nerve fibers that arises within the brain stem and projects into the lower cerebrum; causes arousal of the cerebrum so that the person does not slip into a coma.

reticulocyte (reh-TIK-yoo-loh-syte) Immature red blood cell.

retina (RET-i-nah) Nervous inner layer of the eye; contains the photoreceptors, rods, and cones.

Rh factor Type of antigen on the surface of the red blood cell.

ribonucleic (rye-boh-noo-KLAY-ik) acid (RNA) Nucleotide that copies or transcribes the genetic code from DNA; also involved in translation.

ribosomes (RYE-bo-sohms) Organelles concerned with the synthesis of protein; ribosomes are bound to the endoplasmic reticulum or are free in the cytoplasm.

rickettsia (rik-ETS-see-ah) Type of small bacteria that must reproduce in a living organism.

S

sagittal (SAJ-i-tal) plane Vertical plane that divides the organ or body into right and left parts. A midsagittal plane divides the body into right and left halves.

sarcomere (SAR-koh-meer) Contractile unit of a muscle extending from Z line to Z line; contains the contractile proteins and the thick and thin filaments.

sarcoplasmic reticulum (sar-koh-PLAZ-mik reh-TIK-yoo-lum) Calcium-storing endoplasmic reticulum located in muscle.

sclera (SKLEH-rah) Outer layer of the posterior eyeball.

scrotum Pouch of skin that encloses the testes.

sebaceous (seh-BAY-shus) glands Exocrine glands located in the skin that secrete sebum.

sebum (SEE-bum) Oily secretion of a sebaceous gland.

second messenger Chemical activated in response to hormone stimulation, such as cAMP.

semen Sperm-containing secretion of the male.

semilunar valve Valve shaped like a half-moon located between the ventricles and their attached vessels: pulmonic valve and aortic valve.

sensory nerves Collection of sensory neurons that carry information toward the central nervous system.

serous membrane Epithelial membrane that lines the abdominopelvic and thoracic cavities and the organs within the cavities.

serum Blood plasma minus the clotting factors.

sex-linked trait Any trait that is carried on a sex chromosome (X or Y chromosome).

sinus Cavity such as the paranasal sinuses in the head.

sinusoid (SINE-u-soid) Large, highly permeable capillary that permits free movement of proteins between the tissue fluid and the blood.

skeletal muscle Striated voluntary muscle that lies over parts of the skeleton; causes movement of the skeleton.

skin turgor (TUR-ger) Turgor is a condition of normal tension within a cell. Skin turgor refers to the degree of elasticity of the skin.

smooth muscle Nonstriated, involuntary muscle found in tubes and organs.

solute A substance that is dissolved in another substance (solvent).

solution Mixture in which the particles that are mixed together remain evenly distributed.

solvent Substance in which the solute is dissolved or mixed.

somatic nervous system Part of the peripheral nervous system that stimulates the skeletal muscles.

specific gravity When referring to urine, density of urine compared with the density of an equal volume of water.

spermatogenesis (sper-mah-toh-JEN-eh-sis) Formation of sperm.

sphincter (SFINGK-ter) Circular muscle that opens and closes a tube, such as the anal sphincter.

spinal (vertebral) cavity Elongated cavity that contains the spinal cord.

spinal cord Part of the central nervous system located in the vertebral canal.

spinal nerves Nerves that arise from the spinal cord.

splanchnic (SPLANK-nik) circulation Blood supply of the abdominal organs of digestion.

spleen Lymphoid organ located in the left upper quadrant of the abdominal cavity.

spores An encasement that allows the organism to withstand harsh environmental conditions.

sporozoa Parasitic protozoans that increase by sporulation and that cause many serious diseases such as malaria.

squamous (SKWAY-muss) epithelium Flattened, scalelike epithelial cells; simple or stratified.

Starling's law of the heart Refers to the relationship between myocardial stretch and strength of myocardial contraction.

steroid Lipid-soluble hormone such as estrogen, testosterone, and cortisol.

stomach A digestive organ located between the esophagus and duodenum.

stratum corneum (STRAH-tum KOR-nee-um) Outermost layer of the epidermis.

stratum germinativum (STRAH-tum jer-mi-nah-TIV-um) Innermost layer of the epidermis where cell division takes place.

stroke volume Amount of blood that the ventricle pumps in one heartbeat.

subcutaneous (sub-kyoo-TAY-nee-us) layer Tissue beneath the dermis that contains fat cells.

sudoriferous (soo-doh-RIF-er-us) glands Sweat glands.

surfactant (sur-FAK-tant) Chemical substance that reduces surface tension, thereby preventing the collapse of alveoli.

suspension Mixture in which the large particles gradually settle to the bottom unless continuously shaken or agitated.

suture (SOO-chur) Type of immovable joint found between the bones of the skull.

sympathetic nervous system A division of the autonomic nervous system that causes the fight-or-flight response; also called *thoracolumbar outflow.*

synapse (SIN-aps) The interaction between two nerves where chemical transmission of the electrical signal occurs.

synergist (SIN-er-jist) A muscle that assists or works with another muscle.

synovial (si-NO-vee-all) joint Freely movable joint.

systemic circulation Part of the circulatory system that serves all parts of the body except the lungs.

systole (SIS-toh-lee) Contraction of the myocardium.

systolic pressure The blood pressure in the large arteries during cardiac contraction (systole); the upper number of a blood pressure reading.

T

target tissue Tissue at which a hormone is aimed.

temporal (TEM-poh-ral) lobe Lobe of the cerebrum responsible for hearing, smelling, speech, and memory.

tendons Strong bands of connective tissue that anchor muscle to bone.

teratogen (TER-ah-toh-jen) Means "monster-producing"; anything that causes developmental abnormalities in the embryo or fetus, such as the rubella virus, alcohol, or radiation.

testes (TES-tees) (*sing.,* testis) Male gonads that produce sperm and testosterone.

testosterone (tes-TOS-teh-rohn) Most important androgen (male hormone); makes a male look male.

tetanus Sustained muscle contraction; also a disease caused by the *Clostridium tetani* pathogen.

thermoreceptor (THER-moh-ree-SEP-tor) Receptor that detects changes in temperature.

thermoregulation Homeostatic regulation of body temperature by adjustments in the heat-producing and heat-losing mechanisms.

thoracic (thoh-RASS-ik) cavity Upper part of the ventral cavity superior to the diaphragm; filled largely by the lungs and heart.

thoracic (thoh-RASS-ik) duct Large lymphatic vessel that receives lymph from most of the body and empties it into the left subclavian vein.

thoracolumbar outflow Sympathetic nerve activity; fight-or-flight response.

thrombocyte (THROM-boh-syte) See *platelet.*

thymus gland Lymphoid organ located in the mediastinum; plays an important role in immunity.

thyroid gland Gland that secretes T_3 (triiodothyronine), T_4 (tetraiodothyronine, thyroxine), and calcitonin.

tidal volume Amount of air inhaled and exhaled during one ventilatory cycle.

tissue Group of cells that perform a similar function.

T lymphocytes (T cells) Type of lymphocyte that engages in cell-mediated immunity; thymus-derived lymphocyte.

tonsil Patches of lymphoid tissue embedded in the throat region; pharyngeal (adenoids), lingual, and palatine tonsils.

tonus (TOE-nus) The continuous contraction of a muscle.

toxoid Inactivated toxin that retains its antigenic properties.

trachea (TRAY-kee-ah) Large airway located between the larynx and bronchus; windpipe.

transcellular fluid Extracellular fluid that includes cerebrospinal fluid, aqueous and vitreous humor, synovial fluid of the joints, serous fluid within body cavities, and exocrine gland secretions (e.g., gastric juice).

transverse plane Plane that divides the body into a top (superior) and bottom (inferior) part.

tricuspid (try-KUS-pid) valve Atrioventricular valve found between the right atrium and right ventricle.

tubular reabsorption Movement of water and dissolved substances from the tubules into the peritubular capillaries.

tubular secretion Movement of substances from the peritubular capillaries into the tubules.

turgor See *skin turgor.*

twitch A muscle response to a single electrical stimulus.

U

umbilical (um-BIL-i-kul) cord Long structure that connects the fetus to the placenta; contains the umbilical arteries and umbilical vein.

urea (yoo-REE-ah) Nitrogenous waste product formed by the liver and excreted by the kidneys.

ureter (YOOR-eh-ter) Tube that conducts urine from the kidney to the urinary bladder.

urethra (yoo-REE-thrah) Tube that conducts urine from the bladder to the exterior of the body.

urinary bladder The hollow pelvic organ that receives urine from the kidneys and stores it until it can be expelled.

urinary specific gravity The density of urine as compared to water; the greater the solute in urine, the higher is its specific gravity.

urine The product of nephron unit function of the kidneys; composed mostly of water, waste, and ions.

uterus Hollow reproductive organ in which the fetus grows; the womb.

V

vaccine Antigens that have been altered in order to produce active immunity without causing the disease.

vascular resistance The amount of opposition that the blood vessels offer to the flow of blood; most resistance is caused by the arterioles (resistance vessels).

vas deferens (DEF-er-enz) Tube that carries sperm from the epididymis to ejaculatory duct; the ductus deferens.

vasoconstriction (vay-soh-kon-STRIK-shun) Narrowing of blood vessels; usually refers to arterioles.

vasodilation (vay-soh-DYE-lay-shun) Widening of blood vessels; usually refers to arterioles.

vasopressin See *antidiuretic hormone (ADH)*.

vasopressors Hormones or drugs that cause an elevation in blood pressure.

vector A carrier of pathogens from host to host; mechanical or animal.

vein Blood vessel that takes blood toward the heart.

venae cavae (VEE-nee KAY-vee) Large veins that take unoxygenated blood to the right atrium; superior and inferior venae cavae.

ventilation Moving air into and/or out of the lungs; two phases: inhalation (breathing in) and exhalation (breathing out).

ventral cavity Cavity located toward the front part of the body; divided by the diaphragm into the upper thoracic cavity and lower abdominopelvic cavity.

ventral root Attachment of a motor branch of a spinal nerve to the spinal cord.

ventricle (VEN-tri-kul) Cavity in an organ, such as the ventricles in the heart and brain.

venule (VEN-yool) Tiny vein that connects capillaries to a larger vein.

vernix caseosa (vern-IKS kah-see-OH-sah) Cheeselike substance covering the skin of the fetus; secreted by the sebaceous glands.

vestibule (VES-ti-byool) Part of the inner ear concerned with equilibrium.

villus (*pl.*, villi) Finger-like projections such as the villi that line the intestine; function in absorption of digestive end products.

viruses Pieces of DNA or RNA surrounded by a protein shell; viruses are parasitic in that they require other living cells for reproduction.

viscera (VISS-er-ah) Internal organs of the body.

visceral layer The layer of the pleural and peritoneal serous membranes that adheres to the outer surface of an organ, such as the lungs.

vital capacity The greatest amount of air that can be exhaled following maximal inhalation.

vitamin Organic substance necessary for normal metabolism.

W

white blood cell See *leukocyte*.

white matter Myelinated fibers, mostly axons, located in the central nervous system.

Z

zoonosis (zo-ON-o-sis) A disease that occurs primarily in the wild but can be transmitted from animals to humans.

zygote (ZYE-goht) Fertilized ovum.

Index

Note: Page numbers followed by f indicate figures; t, tables; and b, boxes.